Dietary Proteins *and* Atherosclerosis

Dietary Proteins *and* Atherosclerosis

G. Debry

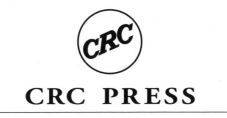

CRC PRESS

Boca Raton   London   New York   Washington, D.C.

Library of Congress Cataloging-in-Publication Data

Debry, Gérard.
    Dietary proteins and atherosclerosis / G. Debry.
        p. ; cm.
    Includes bibliographical references and index.
    ISBN 0-8493-2102-6
      1. Atherosclerosis—Etiology. 2. Coronary heart disease—Etiology. 3. Proteins in human nutrition. 4. Proteins in animal nutrition. 5. Proteins—Pathophysiology. I. Title.
      [DNLM: 1. Dietary Proteins—adverse effects. 2. Arteriosclerosis—etiology. QU 55 D288d 2003]
    RC692.D43 2003
    616.1'36071—dc22

                                                2003055434

Visit the CRC Press Web site at www.crcpress.com

© 2004 by CRC Press LLC

No claim to original U.S. Government works
International Standard Book Number 0-8493-2102-6
Library of Congress Card Number 2003055434
Printed in the United States of America 1 2 3 4 5 6 7 8 9 0
Printed on acid-free paper

To Annick

Acknowledgment

I wish to extend very sincere thanks to Moyra Barbier for her help in reviewing the translation of this work.

Foreword

To most scientists and to all of the general public, heart disease begins and ends with fat and cholesterol. Only those scientists who have done research in the field know that the earliest purely nutritional studies of experimental atherosclerosis were predicated on finding an atherogenic principle in animal protein. The early experiments did point to a connection between food of animal origin and atherosclerosis, but the observation that dietary cholesterol induced arterial lesions overwhelmed the earlier studies. It was assumed that the cholesterol content of the animal protein was responsible for the observed effects.

The obsession with dietary cholesterol exists to this day and the role(s) of animal and vegetable proteins have been investigated for brief periods and are rarely cited. There was a period of interest in the 1920s when Newburgh and Clarkson demonstrated the atherogenicity of animal protein even in the absence of cholesterol. The first comparison of the effects of animal and vegetable proteins was carried out by Meeker and Kesten in 1940, but this observation was not exploited for another two decades. There has been a steady output of papers in this field since the early 1970s but it has remained a trickle in comparison to the cholesterol and fat literature. This situation may change, now that we recognize risk factors such as homocysteine, C-reactive protein and the role of infection, and we realize that the disease goes beyond dietary fat.

In this book, Professor Debry has succinctly summarized and discussed the role that dietary protein may play in the etiology of atherosclerosis and atherosclerotic heart disease. The book is encyclopedic in scope and, remarkably for its size, summarizes virtually all aspects of the protein–atherosclerosis connection.

Data are presented on every animal species available for experimental work. The effects of proteins from different sources and of proteins within each source category are discussed, as are the additional effects of other dietary components (fat, fiber, minerals).

The possibility that levels or ratios of specific amino acids may exert special influences is addressed as well. The possible mechanisms of protein effects (which have still not been clarified) are also summarized. The effects of the nonprotein components of plant protein are also mentioned. Finally, there is a discussion of dietary protein effects in humans. Two of the conditions that play a role in atherosclerosis — hypertension and thrombosis — can also be affected by dietary protein and these, too, are discussed.

In the 1950s when the relationship between dietary fat and atherosclerosis was becoming established epidemiologically, Yerushalmy and Hilleboe used the same epidemiologic data to show that there was a protein effect that was as strong as that of fat. This book provides data that support and expand their observation.

Professor Debry has provided an invaluable source of data concerning dietary protein and atherosclerosis. It is not meant to displace the interest in fat and cholesterol in this disease, but rather to offer another area of interest and investigation that has been generally neglected. This book should become part of the library of every person working in atherosclerosis research or in public health. It will expand the horizons of research workers in the fields of biology and medicine related to atherosclerosis and heart disease. Combining the many new research tools now available with the long-neglected data presented in this volume should yield greater comprehension of the etiology of atherosclerosis and may lead to an earlier solution of this major health problem.

David Kritchevsky
Philadelphia, PA

Preface

Although food lipids are now recognized as the major nutritional factors in atherosclerosis, it is interesting to remember that the first experimental research projects investigating the possible relationships among nutrition, blood lipids, and atherosclerosis studied the effects of animal proteins and meat in particular. Indeed, dietary meat induces various forms of pathologic damage to hepatic tissues in rabbits (Garnier and Simon 1907) and dogs, and also liver necrosis and arterial lesions (D'Amato 1908). The results of these studies on rabbits were confirmed by Ignatowski (1908a, 1908b) and Fahr (1912). Later, investigators assessed the effects of different animal proteins: meat (Lubarsch 1909, 1910) or various associations such as meat, egg yolk, egg white, and milk (Starokadomsky and Ssobolew 1909; Stuckey 1911, 1912). Anitschkow and Chalatow established the cholesterol-fed rabbit as a model for atherosclerosis research (Anitschkow and Chalatow 1913; Finking and Hanke 1997). On the basis of their results, the investigators came to the conclusion that proteins were not the only factors responsible for arterial injuries and that the initially suspected effects of cholesterol should be accepted (Chalatow 1912; Wesselkin 1913; Anitschkow and Chalatow 1913; Wacker and Hueck 1913).

The respective roles of animal proteins and cholesterol already studied (Kon 1913, 1914; Steinbiss 1913; Knack 1915; Newburgh 1919; Newburgh and Squier 1920; Newburgh and Clarkson 1922, 1923a, 1923b; Diecke 1926; Clarkson and Newburgh 1926) are discussed later. A positive correlation has been established between animal protein consumption and serum cholesterol concentrations and the extent of atherosclerosis, despite the absence of cholesterol in the diet (Newburgh and Clarkson 1923a, 1923b). However, according to Diecke, no correlation can be established between atherosclerosis and hypercholesterolemia (Diecke 1926). The arterial hypertension observed in rabbits on a diet including meat could also be the cause of atherosclerotic lesions (Schmidtmann 1926). The prevalence of cardiovascular diseases, as assessed by epidemiologic studies over the same period, is positively and equally correlated with animal protein or fat consumption (Yerushalmy and Hilleboe 1957; Yudkin 1957).

Meeker and Kestens (1940, 1941) demonstrated that in contrast to animal proteins, vegetable proteins do not induce an increase in serum cholesterol concentrations. Atherosclerosis is not observed in rabbits fed maize oil and casein or wheat gluten. Nevertheless, plasma cholesterol concentrations were higher when the rabbits were fed casein rather than wheat gluten (Enselme et al. 1963).

The experiments by Kritchevsky et al. (1959) and Howard et al. (1965) confirmed the results obtained by Meeker and Kestens. When cholesterol was added to the diet of rabbits, the nonpurified soybean protein provided decreased serum cholesterol concentrations, and not only was harmless but prevented atherosclerosis. Two general reviews have summarized the effects of dietary proteins on plasma cholesterol concentrations and atherosclerosis in animals (Yudkin 1957; Enselme et al. 1962).

In young women, the capacity of vegetable proteins compared to animal proteins to lower plasma cholesterol levels was first observed by Walker et al. (1960). In men, Hodges et al. (1967) showed that vegetable proteins decrease the serum cholesterol concentrations induced by diets containing various proportions of fats and simple or complex carbohydrates. In spite of these results, investigations on the relationship between proteins and atherosclerosis have been replaced by others focusing on the rapid development of the lipidic theory of atherosclerosis.

Nevertheless over the past 30 years, there has been renewed interest in the protein theory (Connor and Connor 1972; Carroll and Hamilton 1975; Hermus 1975; Kritchevsky 1976; Hamilton and Carroll 1976; Debry 1976; Carroll 1978a, 1978b; Kritchevsky 1980a, 1980b; Carroll 1981b; Kritchevsky and Czarnecki 1982, 1983; Laurent 1983, Terpstra et al. 1983a, 1983b; Kritchevsky 1983a, 1983b; Kritchevsky et al. 1983, 1984; Debry et al. 1984; Goldberg and Schonfeld 1985; West and Beynen 1986; Forsythe et al. 1986; Kritchevsky et al. 1987; Kritchevsky and Klurfeld 1987; Debry 1987a, 1987b; Guzman and Strong 1987; Kritchevsky 1987; Foley et al. 1988; West and Beynen 1988; Barth and Pfeuffer 1988; Kritchevsky 1990; Debry 2001a, 2001b). The history of these relationships was reviewed by Kritchevsky and Czarnecki (1983) and Terpstra et al. (1983a, 1983b), and more recently by Kritchevsky (1993, 1995). However, in one general review on diet, plasma cholesterol, and coronary heart disease by Smith and Pickney (1989), none of the 1700 references quoted dietary proteins as a possible factor involved in atherosclerosis, and in a recent review on coronary heart disease risk factors (Ferns and Lamb 2001), the eventual role of proteins is not mentioned.

The results of experiments with varying diet components have shown that serum cholesterol concentrations are positively correlated with animal protein content, and casein in particular. However, according to the authors, these effects could also be due to other diet components (Carroll and Hamilton 1975; Hamilton and Carroll 1974, 1976; Carroll 1978a), and cannot be generalized since the serum cholesterol levels induced by certain animal and vegetable proteins are not significantly different. This is the case, for example, with pork protein or raw egg white, wheat gluten, and peanut protein (Carroll and Hamilton 1975) or with beef and vegetable proteins (Kritchevsky et al. 1981). Moreover, since animal growth depends on the biological value of proteins, this value should be taken into account (Hermus 1975).

Although the results of epidemiologic studies and clinical trials support the notion of a positive correlation between the consumption of dietary proteins and the prevalence of atherosclerosis or coronary thrombosis, this theory cannot be attested with certainty since the collection of data on animal and vegetable protein consumption remains relatively inaccurate in humans. In contrast, the numerous experimental studies carried out in animals of various species as well as in humans have partly identified, although only in a limited number of studies, the pathophysiologic mechanisms of the effects of proteins on atherosclerosis.

The damage caused by some animal proteins and the protective effects of certain vegetable proteins have been clearly demonstrated. Although dietary proteins are considered to be of minor importance in the etiology of hypercholesterolemia and atherosclerosis in humans (Carroll 1978a; Kris-Etherton et al. 1988), their effects on plasma lipids, various factors of blood coagulation, endocrinologic balance, arterial hypertension, and arterial wall properties have been demonstrated. The effects of nonprotein substances associated with vegetable proteins in plants have been the subjects of numerous studies over recent years. Results have shown that the direct influence of these proteins on plasma lipid levels and the development of atherosclerosis remains unclear and further studies are still required to establish the real effects (Smith 1998).

The Author

Professor G. Debry is currently Professor Emeritus at the Department of Nutrition at the University Henri Poincaré in Nancy, France. He achieved the degree of M.D. in 1956 and has been a professor of human nutrition and metabolic diseases at University Henri Poincaré since 1967. He founded the Training for Dietitians at French Technological Universität Institutes in 1968 and was the Director of the INSERM Unit of Human Nutrition from 1963 to 1983. In 1984 he founded the Human Nutrition Center of the University Henri Poincaré, which he also managed until 1996. From 1970 to 1994, Professor Debry held a joint appointment at the University Hospital as the head of the Diabetes, Nutrition and Metabolic Diseases and of the Enteral Nutrition Departments.

Professor Debry has served and headed several French ministerial committees, notably, the Ministries of Health, of Research, and of Agriculture. He was an expert in nutrition for the World Health Organization from 1970 to 2000, and has been a corresponding member of the French Academy since 1986 and a member of the European Academy of Nutritional Science since 1988. He has won several research awards from the French Academy of Medicine and the French Academy of Sciences, as well as the Research Prize in Nutrition from the French Nutrition Foundation in 1980 and the André Mayer Award in 1983. He has also received several medals including Officer of the Legion of Honour in 1991.

Professor Debry has written numerous publications, including 37 contributed chapters to edited volumes and nine monographs. He has also served as editor for five International Congresses.

Contents

Introduction: Epidemiologic and Clinical Data

EPIDEMIOLOGIC DATA

In some epidemiologic surveys, a strong positive correlation has been observed between the consumption of animal proteins and the incidence of coronary morbidity and mortality (Yudkin 1957; Yerushalmy and Hilleboe 1957; Connor and Connor 1972; Armstrong et al. 1975; Kritchevsky 1976; Stamler 1979; Kritchevsky and Czarnecki 1982; Debry et al. 1984, 1987a, 1987b). Data from epidemiologic studies regarding the relationships between protein consumption, plasma lipids, and atherosclerosis in vegetarians and vegetalians cannot be considered significant since these diets contain few saturated fats and a high quantity of dietary fibers (Hardinge and Stare 1954; Sacks et al. 1975; Burslem et al. 1978). In the same way, the results of several epidemiologic surveys in Western countries cannot be considered significant even though the consumption of animal proteins is high because, in these foods, the proteins are associated with animal fats. In addition, these foods are cooked with animal fats. The nature of the fats associated with the proteins must also be taken into account. As an example, the plasma cholesterol concentrations in the Masaï population who drink considerable quantities of milk (Mann et al 1964) and in Eskimos who consume large quantities of fish fats (Bang et al. 1971) are significantly lower than those of Western populations. Nevertheless, more accurate surveys are still necessary to provide a correct interpretation of these results.

In conclusion, epidemiologic data relating to a possible effect of certain food proteins on the development of atherosclerosis in humans are still inadequate for any conclusive association to be confirmed. This explains the absence of consensus statements in the international literature (Dawber 1980; Bulpitt 1985; Lee et al. 1990).

CLINICAL DATA

The influence of malnutrition and the incidence of cardiovascular diseases with atheroma remain unclear. The consumption of proteins, animal fats, minerals, vitamins, and antioxidant substances are indeed reduced. During starvation the incidence of coronary heart disease and of myocardial infarction is reduced, whereas that of hypertension and congestive heart failure remains unchanged. Plasma cholesterol concentrations do increase during the progression of kwashiorkor but the disease duration is too short, invariably interrupted by death or nutritional rehabilitation, to allow any progression of the atherosclerosis.

Kwashiorkor may be induced by an unbalanced diet containing adequate energy supplies or by a diet of poor protein quality whereas marasmus is induced by either a balanced or an unbalanced diet with inadequate energy supplies (Sidransky 1990). In both of these diseases, plasma lipid concentrations are very likely reduced via a mechanism of reduced protein synthesis that diminishes lipoprotein formation (Truswell and Hansen 1969). Total heparin lipolytic activity is reduced, particularly as a result of reduced hepatic lipase activity in children with kwashiorkor (Agbedana et al. 1979a, 1979b). In infants with kwashiorkor, plasma cholesterol concentrations are restored to normal levels by a low-fat diet enriched with amino acids or various proteins (Schendel and Hansen 1958). These diets have the same effects in under-nourished adults (Tripathy et al. 1970). In patients with chronic renal insufficiency, the Kempner diet, which is low in proteins and fats, reduces plasma lipid concentrations (Kempner 1948; Loschiavo et al. 1988; Coggins et al. 1994). However, Olson et al. (1958b) suggested that this reduction may not be due to reduced protein intake alone.

With the exception of the anatomopathologic study by Moore et al. (1981), we have not found any other anatomopathologic work relating to the association between protein consumption and atherosclerosis. In this study, however, the correlations that were established between protein consumption and the extent of atherosclerotic lesions cannot be interpreted since the confounding influence of the consumption of fats is too great.

1 Protocol Design for Experimental Data on the Effects of Food Proteins on Plasma Lipids and Lipid Metabolism

1.1 GENERAL CONDITIONS FOR PROTOCOL DESIGN

Although a large number of experiments have been conducted in humans, the majority are based on animal models. Results, and how they should be interpreted, depend on the choice of several parameters made by the investigators regarding study designs and protocols. These include species, strains, sex, and age of animals, but also diet composition and study duration (Sidransky 1990; van Raaij et al. 1983; Westerterp 1999). These experimental data are discussed along with analysis of their results.

1.2 ANIMAL SPECIES

The effects of proteins on cholesterol and lipid metabolism can vary according to animal species (Pfeuffer and Barth 1990; Sidransky 1990). In addition, the extrapolation of experimental results is discussed with relation to the metabolic specificity of each species (see section on similarities and contrasts between animals and humans). The response to animal and vegetable proteins is not the same in rabbits and rats as it is in primates and humans. As described later, the hypercholesterolemic effect of casein is species dependent, apparently influenced by the lower intestinal phosphatase activity (van der Meer 1983; van der Meer et al. 1985a, 1985b; van der Meer and Beynen 1987; van der Meer 1988; van der Meer et al. 1988) and by the high ratio of glycine-conjugated to taurine-conjugated bile acids that are specific metabolic characteristics of rabbits but not of rats or humans (van der Meer and de Vries 1985). Although an increase in serum cholesterol levels is easily obtained in rabbits by feeding a cholesterol-free casein diet (Carroll and Hamilton 1975), cholesterol has to be added to the diet in rats (Yadav and Liener 1977), chickens (Kritchevsky et al. 1959), and pigs (Kim et al. 1978). Rats have a very efficient reduction of hepatic cholesterol synthesis and enhancement of bile acid formation and excretion, which counteract the effect of increased loading of cholesterol in the diet (Dietschy and Wilson 1970a, 1970b, 1970c).

The cholesterol lipoprotein distribution varies according to the animal species. For example, in guinea pigs, most cholesterol is carried by the low-density lipoprotein (LDL) fraction (Fernandez and McNamara 1991), and in hamsters by the high-density lipoprotein fraction (HDL) (Fernandez et al. 1999a, 1999b). However, lipoprotein distribution in *Cynomolgus* monkeys is similar to that of humans and sensitive to dietary modifications (Wilson et al. 1998a). It is therefore particularly important that studies are conducted to assess the specific influence of diets for each species.

1.3 GENETIC FACTORS

Certain genes are of considerable significance both in animals and humans: genes and nutritional adaptations (Roberts 1985), gene–diet interaction in lipoprotein metabolism (Després et al. 1990; Dreon and Krauss 1992; Simopoulos and Nestel 1997; Ordovas 1999; Rainwater et al. 1999; Simopoulos 1999; Friedlander et al. 2000), genes contributing to atherosclerosis (Lusis and Sparkes 1989; Warden et al. 1992; Berg 1992), and to arterial hypertension (Cowley 1997; Kurokawa and Okuda 1998; Luft 1998; Dominiczak et al. 1998; Gavras et al. 1999; Gerber and Halberstein 1999). These should be the focal point of studies since their presence or absence modifies the response of lipid metabolism and blood pressure to the diet, and also the results of experiments and the significance of data obtained during epidemiologic surveys on atherosclerosis and hypertension (Roberts et al. 1974; Lovenberg and Yamori 1990; Dreon and Krauss 1992; Warden et al. 1992; Clifton and Abbey 1997; Tikkanen 1997; Krauss 1997; Luft 1998; Simopoulos 1999; Westerterp 1999; Friedlander et al. 2000; Guillaume et al. 2000).

In rats, it as been shown that the cholesterolemic response to dietary cholesterol is strain dependent. After cholesterol intake, serum cholesterol concentrations increase strongly in certain strains, whereas in others this increase is less marked (Dietschi and Wilson 1970a, 1970b, 1970c; van Zuphten and den Bieman 1981).

The accumulation of cholesterol differs in hyper-responding and hypo-responding rabbits (van Zuphten et al. 1981; Beynen et al. 1984; Beynen et al. 1986a). Rabbits of the *WWHHL* strain, which have a defect in the LDL receptor, show a similar susceptibility to hyperlipidemia and atherosclerosis as that seen in humans with familial hypercholesterolemia and having the same defect (Watanabe 1980; Kita et al. 1981). Likewise, a new strain of genetically spontaneously hypertensive rats (*SHR*-rats) with similar pathologic conditions to those observed in humans exhibits a very high incidence of stroke (Okamoto and Aoki 1963; Okamoto et al. 1974) and a similar pathology to humans (Okamoto 1969).

Transgenic mice express high plasma concentration of human apolipoprotein B-100 and lipoprotein(a) (Linton et al. 1993). Serum cholesterol response to dietary cholesterol is dependent on apoprotein E phenotype (Miettinen et al. 1988). A deficiency in important genes, such as the apolipoprotein E (apo E), apo C-I, and hepatic lipase genes, increases the response of plasma lipids to the intake of fats and cholesterol. On the other hand, this response is decreased when the apo B gene is deficient and when the LDL receptor is overexpressed. According to the species and strain, the genetic factors and mechanisms that influence plasma lipid responses to the intake of fats and cholesterol can vary (Doucet et al. 1987). Indeed, some strains of mice, such as the *C3H* strain, are resistant to atherosclerotic factors, whereas the *C57BL/6J* strain is particularly vulnerable (Shih et al. 1995; Paigen 1995; Rader and Puré 2000). In rats fed with a high-protein cafeteria diet, serum and lipoprotein cholesterol concentrations are greater in the corpulent phenotype of the *LA/N-cp* strain than in lean specimens (Tulp et al. 1984). In genetically obese and lean growing pigs, the interactions of a high-fat/high-cholesterol diet with a low or high dietary protein diet over a 9-week period are different. Indeed, in pigs, plasma cholesterol concentrations are increased by a low-protein diet and by a high-fat/high-cholesterol diet and these concentrations are highest with a high-protein, high-fat/high-cholesterol diet. Plasma cholesterol concentrations are higher in genetically lean than in genetically obese growing pigs (Pond et al. 1986). In baboons the baseline concentrations and diet response of lipoprotein(a) are influenced by multiple genes (Rainwater et al. 1999).

In humans, the various genetic markers involved in different responses of post-prandial lipemia have not yet been adequately identified (Kushawaha and McGill 1997; Clifton and Abbey 1997; Tikkanen 1997), although progress in this field is advancing relatively rapidly. In the Swedish Twins Study, the risk of cardiovascular atherosclerotic disease is three times greater in monozygotic twins than in dizygotic twins (Marenberg et al. 1994). The phenotype with a prevalence of small, dense LDL is associated with increased concentrations of intermediate-density lipoproteins (IDL) that are rich in triacylglycerols, reduced levels of HDL, insulin resistance, and an increased risk of atherosclerotic cardiovascular disease (Krauss 1997). The apo E-4 phenotype is associated with higher plasma cholesterol values than the apo E-3 phenotype (Utermann et al. 1984; Assmann et al. 1984; Miettinen et al. 1988; Tikkanen et al. 1990; Mänttäri et al. 1991; Gylling and Miettinen 1992; Lehtimäki et al. 1992; Miettinen et al. 1992; Lopez-Miranda et al. 1994), and this may well be the major reason for the enhanced coronary artery disease risk (Davignon et al. 1988). However, these different cholesterol values in apo E-3 and E-4 phenotypes are not confirmed by other studies (Xu et al. 1990; Boerwinkle et al. 1991; Glatz et al. 1991; Cobb et al. 1992; Cobb and Risch 1993; Martin et al. 1993; Jones et al. 1993; Sarkkinen et al. 1994; Zambón et al. 1995; Rantala et al. 2000). The magnitude of dietary effects on plasma lipid and lipoproteins level varies among individuals (Katan et al. 1986; Beynen and Katan 1986; Beynen et al. 1987a). The contribution of candidate genes to the response of plasma lipids and lipoproteins to dietary challenge has been reviewed by Friedlander et al. (2000). In hyperlipidemic humans, as in animals, genetic variations contribute to the basal plasma levels of lipids and lipoprotein and to the diet response (Sarkinen et al. 1994). In hyperlipidemic humans, as in animals, genetic variations contribute to the basal plasma levels of lipids and lipoprotein and to the diet response (Sarkinen et al. 1994).

In 44 healthy, middle-aged subjects receiving four different diets successively for 1 month each (baseline diet, fat-controlled low-cholesterol diet, high-fat high-cholesterol diet, baseline diet), serum lipid levels varied during the high-fat, high-cholesterol diet according to the genetic factors relating to the role of apo B

DNA polymorphisms. In particular, the apo B*Eco*RI and *Msp*I polymorphisms were associated with responsiveness to diet, such as an increase in LDL cholesterol (Rantala et al. 2000). A meta-analysis including 15 eligible reports confirms these results (Rantala et al. 2000). In 214 Israeli individuals, the response of lipid and lipoprotein levels to the diet is similar among apo E and CETP genotypes, but different for serum cholesterol and LDL-cholesterol concentrations among apo B genotypes, and also for serum triacylglycerol and HDL-cholesterol concentrations in lipoprotein lipase genotypes (Friedlander et al. 2000).

1.4 AGE

The age-related variations in lipoprotein metabolism must be taken into consideration when interpreting results (Yamamoto and Yamamura 1971; Sullivan et al. 1971; Story et al. 1976; Malhotra and Kritchevsky 1978; Murawski and Egge 1978; Uchida et al. 1978; Cryer and Jones 1978; Kritchevsky 1980a; Carlile and Lacko 1981; Beynen et al. 1983a; Fukuda and Iritani 1984; Herzberg and Rogerson 1984; Stange and Dietschy 1984; Vahouny et al. 1985; Carlile et al. 1986; Pfeuffer and Barth 1986a; Park et al. 1987; Choi et al. 1989a, 1989b, 1990; Pfeuffer and Barth 1990; de Schriver 1990).

Digestive absorption of cholesterol (Story et al. 1976) and its synthesis by the liver decline with increasing age (Story et al. 1976; Malhotra and Kritchevsky 1978; Kritchevsky 1980a; Stange and Dietschy 1984; Pfeuffer and Barth 1986a). In older rats, serum cholesterol and triacylglycerol concentrations as well as those of free fatty acids in lipoproteins are increased, whereas the polyunsaturated fatty acids/saturated fatty acids ratio (P/S) is reduced (Story et al. 1976; Kritchevsky 1980a). The turnover of cholesterol esters, which is faster in older rats, is not modified by the nature of proteins in the diet (Pfeuffer and Barth 1986a; Carlile et al. 1986; Park et al. 1987; de Schriver 1990). In contrast, with young rats, the activity of lecithin-cholesterol acyltransferase (LCAT), the secretion of cholesterol, and the extent of its esterification and turnover are all reduced in older rats (de Schriver 1990). Excretion of bile acids and fecal steroids is also reduced with increasing age (Uchida et al. 1978; Park et al. 1987; de Schriver 1990).

The interactions among dietary proteins, cholesterol, and age on the regulation of lipid metabolism in rats are complex (Choi et al. 1989a). In young and adult rats and pigs, the interactions between age and diet have been clearly demonstrated by the differences in the responses of serum and liver cholesterol to casein, soybean protein, and whey protein, depending on whether the diet is free of or enriched with cholesterol (Nagata et al. 1980, 1981b; Bosisio et al. 1981; Sautier et al. 1983; Eklund and Sjöblom 1986; Pfeuffer and Barth 1986a; Norton et al. 1987; Park et al. 1987; Choi et al. 1989a). In young but not in older rats, the activity of hepatic hydroxymethylglutaryl-CoA reductase (HMG-CoA reductase) is reduced by a soybean protein diet without cholesterol (Choi et al. 1989a). Lipoprotein lipase (LPL) activity is also affected by age (Cryer and Jones 1978). The level of cholesterol secretion, which is greater with casein than with soybean protein, is lower in adult than in young rats (Pfeuffer and Barth 1986a). Nevertheless, results may well be influenced by the duration of experiments, which is twice as long for adults than for young rats. These data concord with those of previous studies (Fillios and Mann 1954; Yamamoto and Yamamura 1971; Story et al. 1976; Murawski and Egge 1978; Uchida et al. 1978; Malhotra and Kritchevsky 1978; Kritchevsky 1980a; Raheja and Linscheer 1982; Stange and Diestchy 1984; Carlile et al. 1986; Park et al. 1987), with the exception of one study on cholesterolemia where no modification was observed (Story et al. 1976). In fasting animals fed with soybean protein or casein, cholesterol levels and triacylglycerol secretion were both reduced in older subjects but serum concentrations of cholesterol can increase at any age in nonfasting animals. The age-related increase in serum cholesterol concentrations is not prevented by the consumption of various proteins such as casein, wheat gluten, soybean protein, and potato (de Schriver 1990).

The lipotropic effect of protein on the liver and that of methionine or cystine supplementation on liver cholesterol may vary markedly with the age and sex of rats (Okey and Lyman 1954, 1957). Liver synthesis and triacylglycerol secretion are both reduced in older rats (Sullivan and Miller 1971; Herzberg and Rogerson 1984; Fukuda and Iritani 1984; Pfeuffer and Barth 1986a). When 4-week-old male *Wistar* rats are put on a diet containing either casein or soybean protein for 6 weeks (rats then aged 10 weeks), or for 21 weeks (until aged 25 weeks), the level of triacylglycerol secretion in the serum is lower in subjects fed on soybean protein than in those fed on casein, but this difference is not significant in adult rats (Pfeuffer and Barth 1986a).

1.5 SEX

The influence of sex has been discussed in some experiments (Pfeuffer and Barth 1990). Female rats show greater response levels than male rats, and growing animals respond more than adult subjects (review in Barth et al. 1990a, 1990c). Female rats were more susceptible than male rats to protein-induced hypercholesterolemia in some studies (Fillios et al. 1958; West et al. 1982; Terpstra et al. 1982a, 1983a), but not in another experiment (Beynen et al. 1983b). In humans, the sensitivity to differential effects of casein and soybean protein diets is greater in men than in women (Meinertz et al. 1990).

1.6 DIET

If the results of experiments are to be considered valid, energy intake and protein levels must cover energy and protein requirements. One example in rabbits showed that undernutrition enhances atherosclerosis and hypercholesterolemia (Goldner et al. 1954).

Diet components differ from one experiment to another. Dietary protein contents can be balanced, high, or low, and cholesterol and/or fats may be added or not to these protein diets. In rabbits, the most sensitive species, hypercholesterolemia may be obtained with a cholesterol-free or a sucrose-containing diet, whereas in rats or pigs, a cholesterol supplement is necessary to induce an increase in serum cholesterol concentrations.

The food proteins used are of animal or vegetable origin, with the occasional addition of an amino acid such as lysine or arginine, but in other experiments only a mixture of amino acids similar to those of these proteins is utilized. The technological processes used in the development of these proteins (textured proteins, protein isolates, soybean protein alcohol extracts of high or low molecular weight, undigested fractions of soybean protein, germinated or fermented soybean protein, soybean protein hydrolysates, formaldehyde or thermal treatment of casein and soybean protein) can also modify the results.

The protein quality has to be taken into account (Young 1991). In male *Sprague-Dawley* weanling rats fed on balanced diets containing 11% or 12% protein (casein, heat-treated casein, egg albumin, wheat gluten, soybean protein isolates, or a wheat–gluten–soybean protein mixture), plasma cholesterol and HDL-cholesterol concentrations were inversely correlated with protein quality evaluated by the protein-energy ratio (Lefevre and Schneeman 1983). These effects of protein quality are consistent with those of low-protein diets. The lipotropic effect of protein in quantities greater than those required for a normal rate of growth might vary markedly with the age and sex of animals (Okey and Lyman 1956).

As will be highlighted later, the food environment may modify the effects of proteins (Pfeuffer and Barth 1990). The nature and quantity of fats, carbohydrates, minerals and vitamins, and the possible influence of nonproteic substances that may be components of the food proteins should be taken into account.

1.7 SIMILARITIES AND CONTRASTS BETWEEN ANIMALS AND HUMANS

Experimental studies based on various designs have identified various factors such as lipoprotein distribution that, to varying degrees, modify plasma lipid concentrations and influence the development of atherosclerosis. In 1953, Mann et al. clearly pointed out that numerous experiments with a variety of species had shown that common laboratory animals, other than rabbits and chickens, do not develop hypercholesterolemia or atherosclerosis when fed large amounts of cholesterol. In dogs the development of atherosclerosis is inconsistent, even in the presence of marked hypercholesterolemia (Mann et al. 1953).

Experiments in rabbits, rats (the most numerous), mice, dogs, and *Squirrel* monkeys cannot be, except rarely, extrapolated to humans since the distribution of plasma lipids, liver cholesterol flow, and/or lipemic response to dietary cholesterol overload are different in these species compared to those of humans (Nicolosi 1997; Harris 1997). The serum lipid levels of rats, in comparison to humans, are relatively low and lipoprotein distribution is very different. The LDL levels are much lower, and although the HDL concentrations are comparable, the flotation rate in the rat is slightly faster (Boyd 1942; Lewis et al. 1952).

Data from experiments in various species such as hamsters, guinea pigs, pigs or *Cynomolgus, Cebus, African green, Macaca fascicularis*, and *Rhesus* monkeys and baboons can generally be extrapolated to humans since their levels of hepatic cholesterol synthesis are weak compared to that of total body synthesis

(Kris-Etherton and Dietschy 1997). On the other hand, these species have a limited capacity to stimulate the synthesis of bile acids when the cholesterol content of the diet is enhanced. The increased concentration of hepatic cholesterol induces a decrease in LDL-receptor activity (Kris-Etherton and Dietschy 1997). The lipid metabolism of the *Macaca fascicularis* monkey is very similar to that of humans (Rudel and Pitts 1978; Tall et al. 1978; Vesselinovitch and Wissler 1980). Since the particular mechanisms involved in the effects of diet on plasma lipid levels are likely to be very similar to those in humans, hamsters and guinea pigs have been extensively used (review in Fernandez et al. 1999a). Nevertheless, the plasma lipoprotein cholesterol distribution in hamsters and guinea pigs is different from that of humans. In guinea pigs and hamsters, most cholesterol is transported in LDL and in HDL particles, respectively (Fernandez and McNamara 1991; Fernandez et al. 1999a). However, these two animal species show similar responses to dietary cholesterol and, in comparison with a casein-based diet, a soybean protein diet decreases their plasma cholesterol concentrations (Fernandez et al. 1999b). The plasma lipid distribution in humans, monkeys, and pigs is relatively similar (Chapman 1980; Jacobsson and Lindholm 1982; Richard et al. 1983; Barth et al. 1990a; Wilson et al. 1998a). The majority of serum cholesterol is transported by the LDL fraction in humans but by the HDL fraction in rabbits and rats (Brattsand 1976; Day et al. 1979; Myant 1981; Terpstra et al. 1982c).

The effects of cholesterol-containing diets are greater in certain animals such as hamsters because their liver cholesterol synthesis is weaker than that of other animals such as rats (Schaeffer 1997). There is less likelihood of occurrence of diet-related atherosclerotic lesions in rats and pigs than in chickens, rabbits, monkeys, and humans (Barth et al. 1990a). Atherosclerotic lesions and their diffusion throughout the wall of the aorta are similar in humans and monkeys and occur to a lesser degree in pigs, but are varied in rats, chickens, and rabbits (Barth et al. 1990a). The high cost of experimental studies in monkeys would appear to make minipigs the best model (Barth et al. 1990a; Kris-Etherton and Diestchy 1997) and, to a lesser degree, hamsters and guinea pigs (Kris-Etherton and Diestchy 1997; Smith 1998).

Vegetable proteins have been reported to have a greater hypocholesterolemic effect than animal proteins in certain studies in humans (Olson et al. 1958b; Walker et al. 1960; Hodges et al. 1967; Keys and Hodges 1967). Nevertheless, these effects were not observed by other researchers (Keys and Anderson 1957; Anderson et al. 1971). In several experimental trials with amino acid mixtures, the results were not conclusive except when they contained glutamic acid (Olson et al. 1970a, 1970b; Garlich et al. 1970).

1.8 CONCLUSION

In the early 20th century, the importance of the relation between food protein consumption and atherosclerosis was first suggested and then studied in epidemiologic, clinical, anatomopathologic, and experimental studies in both humans and several animal species. In contrast to vegetable proteins, the increasing effect of animal proteins on serum lipid concentrations and the positive correlation between serum lipid levels and atherosclerosis gave rise to these research projects. Likewise, the increase in serum cholesterol levels induced by a diet that is either too low or too high in proteins highlights the importance of respecting protein requirements. However, the effects of proteins on cholesterol and lipid metabolism vary according to a great number of factors including animal species, genetic factors, age, sex, composition and energy level of diet, and duration of experiment. Moreover, it is only in pigs and monkeys that these effects show considerable similarity to those of humans. Extrapolating animal observations to human data must therefore only be made with the greatest caution (Finot 1992).

2 Experimental Data on Animals

2.1 EFFECTS OF DIETARY PROTEIN LEVEL

The effects of proteins on plasma lipids depend on diet balance and the nature and amount of proteins in the diet but also on its fat and cholesterol content. Both the diet balance and study duration must be taken into account. Numerous investigations have been conducted with different methods, such as progressive decrease or increase of protein level in the diet. Because results differ according to the species, results for each species must be examined. Terpstra et al. (1983a, 1983b) and Sidranski (1990) have reviewed this subject.

The amount of dietary protein is negatively correlated to serum cholesterol concentrations as has been demonstrated with casein or soybean protein, often with a high-fat, high-cholesterol diet in several animal models such as chickens (Léveillé and Sauberlich 1961), cockerels (Pick et al. 1965), rats (Moyer et al. 1956; Bydlowski et al. 1986), mice (Mayer and Jones 1953; Léveillé and Sauberlich 1964), and *Cebus* monkeys (Mann et al. 1953). However, in male *Sprague-Dawley* rats fed on a low-protein (2.6%), cholesterol-free diet, total plasma cholesterol, triacylglycerol, and phospholipid concentrations were decreased (Bydlowski et al. 1984), whereas if cholesterol (2%) was added to the low-protein (2.6%) diet, the results were opposite. Indeed, plasma cholesterol and triacylglycerol levels were higher than with a standard (27.6%) protein diet (Bydlowski et al. 1986).

Data on the effects of soybean protein and casein are discussed in Section 2.2.1 and Section 2.2.2. The evidence that an amino acid imbalance causes significant changes in the amino acid profile has been reviewed by Harper (1964), and the effects of a protein-deficient diet or the various amino acids on liver protein synthesis have been extensively studied by Sidransky (1976). Discrepancies in the results are probably due to the varying experimental conditions.

2.1.1 BIRDS

2.1.1.1 Chickens and Cockerels

In chickens, there is a negative correlation between the level of protein in a cholesterol-free or cholesterol-rich diet and serum cholesterol concentrations (Pick et al. 1965; Mol et al. 1982; Terpstra et al. 1983a), and also with the cholesterol concentrations in several tissues except the liver (de Schriver et al. 1990). The turnover rate of plasma cholesterol is higher when chickens are fed a high-protein diet (30%) compared with those fed a low-protein diet (15%). In addition, fecal cholesterol excretions are increased (Yeh and Léveillé 1969, 1972, 1973).

In chickens, laying hens, and cockerels, plasma cholesterol concentrations generally increase when the dietary protein content, with or without cholesterol, is restricted, and regardless of the nature of the protein, as in

1. Soybean protein or sesame diets (Léveillé and Fisher 1958; Johnson et al. 1958; Nishida et al. 1958; Stamler et al. 1958a, 1958b, 1958c; Kokatnur et al. 1958b; Pick et al. 1959; Fisher et al. 1959; March et al. 1959; Léveillé et al. 1960, 1961; Léveillé and Sauberlich 1961; Kokatnur and Kummerow 1961; Léveillé et al. 1962a; Pick et al. 1965; Kenney and Fisher 1973; Mol et al. 1982);
2. Casein diets (Johnson et al. 1958; Kokatnur et al. 1958a; Stamler et al. 1958a; Fisher et al. 1959; Kenney and Fisher 1973; Mol et al. 1982); and
3. Mixtures of casein and soybean protein (Kokatnur et al. 1956).

However, in other experiments, serum cholesterol concentrations are only reduced if cholesterol is added to the diet (Nikkilä and Ollilla 1957; Marion et al. 1961) and they are not significantly modified in cockerels when the level of soybean protein is reduced. Serum and liver lipid concentrations are increased (Rose and Baloun 1969). The incorporation of [1-^{14}C]acetate into liver cholesterol in chickens fed a low-protein diet is greater than in those fed a high-protein diet. Dietary cholesterol causes a significant decrease. The rate of fatty acid biosynthesis is increased more by a low-protein diet than by cholesterol (Nishida et al. 1960). Chickens react differently from other species of animals. Indeed, when fed on cholesterol-enriched, semipurified diets containing two levels (20% and 50%) of casein or soybean protein for 29 days, serum cholesterol concentrations are higher with casein than with soybean protein at the 20% level. However, if chickens are fed the 50% protein diets, serum triacylglycerol and phospholipid levels and liver cholesterol concentrations are lower than those of chickens fed on 20%-protein diets (Terpstra et al. 1983d).

When the protein level of a diet increases, lipogenesis, liver malic enzyme and fatty acid concentrations decrease in the liver (Yeh and Léveillé 1969; Peret et al. 1975), whereas that of cholesterol is enhanced. However, plasma cholesterol concentrations decrease (Nishida et al. 1958, 1960) because of the increase in cholesterol turnover and in cholesterol and bile acid excretions (Yeh and Léveillé 1969, 1972, 1973). When the dietary protein content is increased from 10%, to 30% and 45%, digestive absorption of peptide amino acids in the duodenum and low jejunum is more rapid (Hevia and Visek 1979a; Sklan 1980).

To summarize, in chickens, unless the intake level is particularly high, the source of dietary protein in a cholesterol-free or cholesterol-rich diet has no significantly different effect on serum cholesterol levels. There is a negative correlation between dietary protein levels and serum cholesterol concentrations (Mol et al. 1982; Terpstra et al. 1983d); the same applies to cholesterol concentrations in other tissues except the liver (de Schriver et al. 1990). However, these effects of the dietary protein level are more distinct with casein than with vegetable proteins.

2.1.1.2 Pigeons

The effects of casein at the 5%, 15%, and 30% levels have been investigated in *White Carneau* pigeons that are particularly susceptible to atherosclerosis, with or without a cholesterol-rich diet. Plasma cholesterol concentrations increase when cholesterol is added to a high-casein diet (Lofland et al. 1961; Clarkson et al. 1962; Lofland et al. 1966). Similar results are obtained in pigeons fed on 20% or 40% casein diets with 0.25% cholesterol (Little and Angell 1977), and in pigeons fed 7.5% or 15% casein in a cholesterol-free diet (Subbiah 1977).

2.1.1.3 Quails

In *Coturnix coturnix japonica* quails plasma and aortic cholesterol concentrations are lower when the soybean protein levels in an atherogenic diet are high (40% or 60%) than when they are low (10% or 20%). Excretion of neutral steroids, cholesterol, and bile acids is enhanced (McClelland and Shih 1988).

2.1.2 RABBITS

The data from several experiments performed in rabbits are conflicting because of varying diet composition: nature and amount of proteins in relation to protein requirements, amino acid composition of proteins, and diet balance (review in Nath et al. 1959). Increasing the level of dietary beef protein (from 27% to 36%) enhances serum cholesterol concentrations (Newburgh and Clarkson 1922).

Serum cholesterol concentrations are unchanged with the following modifications of protein levels in the diet: vegetable proteins derived from gluten flour, ground soybean, and alfalfa meal (38%, 22%, 13%; Freyberg 1937); soybean protein (54%, 27%; Huff et al. 1977); and casein (30%, 8%; Munro et al. 1965). In contrast, an increase in serum cholesterol levels is observed with other changes of casein levels in the diet (36%, 27%, Huff et al. 1977; 54%, 27%, Terpstra et al. 1981; Terpstra and Sanchez-Muniz 1981).

Reducing vegetable protein content (6.5%) in the diet of *Fauve de Bourgogne Oryctolagus cuniculus Dom. L.* rabbits induces a moderate increase in plasma cholesterol levels, particularly the esterified fraction, and LDL-cholesterol and triacylglycerol concentrations, but only after 2 months. A similar evolution is observed, but after a slightly shorter time (12 weeks), when the diet is rich in cholesterol (2% w/w) (Laurent 1983).

Morphologic observations have shown an earlier onset of atherosclerosis with 36% of lean beef muscle in the diet than with 27% (Newburgh and Clarkson 1923a). Serum cholesterol concentrations are lower when meat (5%) is added to an atherogenic diet containing 10% casein and 1% cholesterol (Polcak et al. 1965).

To summarize, in rabbits, although the experimental data are sometimes conflicting, enhancing the animal protein content in the diet raises serum cholesterol concentrations, whereas a higher vegetable protein content has no effect. However, a low-vegetable protein diet moderately increases serum cholesterol concentrations. It is therefore particularly important to adapt protein intake to the level required.

2.1.3 RODENTS

2.1.3.1 Rats

The data from several experiments on rats are conflicting because of varying diet composition (nature of proteins, amount of proteins in relation to protein requirements, amino acid composition, cholesterol content, and balance of the diet) (review in Nath et al. 1959).

The relationship between diet protein level and serum cholesterol concentrations is complex. In rats, during the period of rapid growth, a diet containing proteins of poor nutritional quality increases plasma cholesterol concentrations. It is necessary to use a diet with proteins of good nutritional quality or supplemented with DL-methionine (Jones and Huffman 1956a, 1956b; de Groot 1958; Olson 1958a; Chen et al. 1972; Torre et al. 1980; Lefevre and Schneeman 1983; Moundras et al. 1997). When 72-day-old male *Sprague-Dawley* rats were starved for 3 days, and then fed for the following 3 days on a high-protein diet (88.5% casein), the lipid components of the liver returned to the control level (or approximately). However, in 490-day-old rats, the total lipid, phospholipid, and cholesterol concentrations remained at the starvation level (Weigand et al. 1980).

In male and female *Sprague-Dawley* albino rats fed on a casein, cholesterol-free diet for 17 weeks, serum cholesterol concentrations increased when the casein level in the diet was very low (5% or 10%). They decreased to 20% and increased again to 40% and then 60%. Whatever the casein levels in the diet, serum cholesterol concentrations were always higher in female than in male rats (Fillios et al. 1958). A progressive increase of the protein (casein or soybean protein) level (10%, 20%, 40%, 60%), in a cholesterol-rich (2%) and cholic-acid (1%) diet of male *Charles River* strain rats induced different changes in serum cholesterol concentrations, which increased with the low-protein level and then decreased (Moyer et al. 1956). In female *Wistar* rats, increasing dietary protein levels in soybean protein or casein diets from 8% to 20% (Leclerc et al. 1989), or from 10% to 20% to 30%, for 30 days in male *Wistar* rats (Okita and Sugano 1990), decreased the serum cholesterol level in particular when diets contained cholesterol. The plasma levels of cholesterol esters, triacylglycerols, and phospholipids were positively correlated with the level (8% or 20%) of casein in the diet of female *Wistar* rats (Leclerc et al. 1989). In male weanling *Sprague-Dawley* rats fed on a cholesterol-rich casein diet (1.2%) for a 25-week period, serum cholesterol concentrations were significantly lower with a 12.5% casein content compared to 7.5%, 9%, or 25% content. However, the long duration of the experiment was an essential parameter since after an 8-week period, serum cholesterol concentrations were only mildly higher with 12.5% casein than with the other casein levels in the diet (Jones and Huffman 1956a, 1956b). The plasma levels of cholesterol esters, triacylglycerols, and phospholipids were positively correlated with the level (8% or 20%) of casein in the diet of female *Wistar* rats (Leclerc et al. 1989). A casein-rich, cholesterol-free diet increases serum cholesterol and triacylglycerol concentrations according to the proportion of casein, and to an even greater extent with a cholesterol-rich diet (Bagchi et al. 1963; Léveillé and Sauberlich 1964; Chen et al. 1972; Rao and Rao 1977; Leelamma et al. 1978;

Hevia et al. 1980a, 1980b; Okita and Sugano 1989, 1990) or one containing casein and corn oil (Takeuchi et al. 2000). However, the effect of this increase is only observed with casein. In *Sprague-Dawley* rats, the reduction of casein level from 25% to 10% in a cholesterol-free diet increased serum cholesterol concentrations (Chen et al. 1972), and the reduction of casein (from 60% to 40% to 10%) in a diet containing 2% cholesterol increased serum cholesterol concentrations. Stepwise increases (from 6% to 40%) in the casein level of a diet enriched in cholesterol (1%) and cholic acid (0.5%) fed to male weanling *Sprague-Dawley* rats caused a progressive reduction of serum cholesterol concentrations. The liver total lipid and total cholesterol contents were slightly lower with 40% casein than with the other levels. The cholesterolemic effect of fibrin and pork protein are similar to those obtained with casein at the same concentrations, whereas zein has a higher hypercholesterolemic effect. At high or low levels, a soybean protein diet induces lower or higher serum cholesterol concentrations, respectively. The substitution of wheat gluten for casein increases serum cholesterol levels (Nath et al. 1959).

Soybean protein is less hypercholesterolemic than casein (Moyer et al. 1956; Terpstra et al. 1982b; Vahouny et al. 1984), and other studies on cholesterol-rich diets have only demonstrated a hypercholesterolemic effect in females (Terpstra et al. 1982a). The successive addition of 5% of various proteins (dried whole egg, wheat gluten, fish and meat meal) to a basal diet containing 15% casein decreased the serum cholesterol level. However, the addition of casein results in the highest serum cholesterol concentration (de Groot 1959).

Although serum cholesterol concentrations remained unchanged in male *Wistar* rats fed on a cholesterol-free diet, with 27% or 12% casein intake levels (Chang and Johnson 1980) they did vary in male weanling *Sprague-Dawley* rats consuming at three other levels of casein: weak change at 12% to 18%, moderately elevated at 7.5%, and highest at 40% (Jones and Huffman 1956a, 1956b).

The effects of the amount of casein on serum cholesterol concentrations can be biphasic: an increase at levels of 7.5% or 40%, and a decrease at 12% to 18% in male weanling *Sprague-Dawley* rats (Jones and Huffman 1956a, 1956b). This biphasic response was confirmed by Nath et al. (1959) in the same strain of rats. However, whereas an absence of change is observed with casein intake levels of 12% or 27% (Chang and Johnson 1980), serum cholesterol levels increase with a high level of casein in the diet (18%>10%>4%, Bagchi et al. 1963; 30%>15%>7.5%, Hevia et al. 1980a; 8%, 20%, Leclerc et al. 1989), and decrease with a high level of wheat gluten (Moyer et al. 1956; Kato et al. 1980; Takeuchi et al. 2000).

Variation in serum cholesterol concentrations may also be multiphasic according to the level of protein in the diet, showing an increase with 10% casein, a decrease with 30%, a further increase with a 69% casein diet, or a decrease with 40% pork or soybean protein or wheat gluten and an increase with 10%. These data were obtained in male *Charles River* rats (Moyer et al. 1956) and in male weanling *Sprague-Dawley* rats (Nath et al. 1959); similar results were observed in other experiments with casein (de Groot 1958; Seidel et al. 1960; Chen et al. 1972).

Plasma and liver cholesterol concentrations of male weanling *Sprague-Dawley* rats are higher when they are fed for 21 weeks on a diet containing 45% instead of 15% of lactalbumin, with both diets being adjusted to contain similar levels of calcium and phosphorus. Plasma triacylglycerol, HDL-cholesterol, and phospholipid concentrations were unchanged. A diet including a high level of lactalbumin (45%) increases plasma and liver LDL-cholesterol concentrations but has no effect on plasma triacylglycerol levels (Kassim et al. 1984). The serum cholesterol concentrations induced by the addition of 0.1% polychlorinated biphenyl (PCB) increased as the protein level of the diet was enhanced up to around 35% in male *Wistar* rats (Kato et al. 1980).

In male weanling *Wistar* rats with nephritis due to a nephrotoxic agent, the reduction of hyperlipidemia by a diet low (8.5%) in soybean protein isolates is partially due to decreased liver cholesterol synthesis. Growth retardation can be alleviated by the addition of methionine (0.3%) (Fujisawa et al. 1995). The same result was obtained in male *Wistar* rats with a low casein diet supplemented with a low meat-protein diet (8.5%) or if this diet was supplemented by 0.5% L-valine (Yagasaki et al. 1994).

The exact nature of plasma lipid modifications has been defined by more recent studies performed in rats (Meghelli-Bouchenak et al. 1987, 1989a, 1989b, 1991a, 1991b; Gouache et al. 1991; Narce et al. 1992; Bouziane et al. 1992, 1994a, 1994b; Sato et al. 1996). When the protein level of the diet of male *Wistar* rats was reduced over a period of 28 days (casein, 18% to 6%), the triacylglycerol level of VLDL, decreased, whereas plasma free-cholesterol and phospholipid concentrations were elevated. Plasma and liver cholesterol levels decrease with an increasing dietary protein content, in particular with cholesterol-enriched diets. The fecal excretion of acidic but not neutral steroids and the arachidonate/linoleate ratio in plasma and liver phosphatidylcholine levels increase more with soybean protein than with casein (Okita and Sugano 1989).

2.1.3.2 Mice and Hamsters

In *white Swiss* mice, a low-protein diet induces hypercholesterolemia (Fillios and Mann 1954). Increasing the level of casein (9%, 18%, 27%, 36%) in a cholesterol-free diet of *Swiss Webster* mice decreased plasma and liver cholesterol levels. When these diets were enriched in cholesterol (1%) and cholic acid (0.2%), serum cholesterol concentrations were higher than with the cholesterol-free diet at all casein levels. However, at the 36% casein level, serum cholesterol concentrations were similar with the cholesterol-free or cholesterol-rich diets. The addition of 0.6% L-cystine or 0.6% cystine plus 1.19% DL-methionine to the cholesterol-rich diet depressed plasma and liver cholesterol levels but had no effect with the cholesterol-free diet (Léveillé and Sauberlich 1964).

To summarize, in rodents, a diet with an excessively elevated or deficient protein level produces an increase in serum cholesterol concentrations. Of all the proteins investigated, casein exerts the greatest effect on serum cholesterol concentrations. The protein level of a diet is therefore of particular importance and must be balanced with the protein requirements.

2.1.4 DOGS

Serum lipid and cholesterol concentrations were enhanced by a low-protein diet (4.4 g/kg/day of casein). When cholesterol was added to the diet, serum cholesterol concentrations were similar to those of control animals (Li and Freeman 1946).

2.1.5 CALVES

Serum cholesterol concentrations are negatively correlated with the soybean protein level of the diet. Serum cholesterol levels of calves are higher when the diet contains 9% protein derived mainly from soybean meal compared to 25% (Coccodrilli et al. 1970). Similar results were obtained when diets containing different levels of soybean protein in the range of 0% to 28% were used (Chandler et al. 1968) or with a diet supplemented with alfalfa pellets containing 15% protein (Bohman et al. 1962). However, these changes could be due to the fiber content of alfalfa (36%) since a lower cholesterol level has been obtained in rabbits with a high alfalfa-fiber dietary content (Kritchevsky et al. 1977). In growing *Holstein* calves, the increase in dietary protein content from 16% to 25% lowered total serum and free cholesterol levels. In the same example, serum HDL-cholesterol concentrations were increased and LCAT was enhanced (Park 1985).

2.1.6 PIGS

The results are different for pigs. After 18 months on a diet that was rich in fats and cholesterol but very low in protein (5%), serum cholesterol concentrations were the same as those of control animals fed on a normal level of protein (25%) (Gupta et al. 1974).

Variations in dietary soybean protein content induce different effects on serum cholesterol concentrations in young and adult swine (Barnes et al. 1959a, 1959b; Greer et al. 1966, Gupta et al. 1974). However, the serum cholesterol concentrations of adult pigs increased when the protein level of the diet was reduced from 18% to 12% (Greer et al. 1966) but did not vary if it was reduced from 13.7% to 4.9% (Barnes et al. 1959a). When young weaned swine were fed either a high- or low-protein (corn and soybean protein) diet varying from 4.9% to 13.7% or from 9% to 16%, the dietary lipid content being low (3%) or high (13%), and either high- or low-fat (beef tallow) for 36 weeks, the increase in serum cholesterol levels in all groups (maximum level reached after 4 to 8 weeks) was followed by a decline to nearly the minimum level; however, this minimum was reached more quickly by the two high-protein groups. The delayed return to minimal cholesterol levels by the low-protein high-fat group was related to the greater severity of protein malnutrition (Barnes et al. 1959b).

2.1.7 MONKEYS

Rhesus monkeys on a low-protein (3.8% kilocalories) purified diet since birth have higher plasma concentrations of very low density lipoprotein (VLDL) and HDL particles than the control group (Portman et al. 1985). In baboons, serum cholesterol concentrations are higher with a dietary casein level of 25% than with an 8% or 10% level (Strong and McGill 1967). In *Vervet Cercopithecus aethiops* monkeys fed on a semipurified diet containing 12.5%, 25.0%, or 37.5% casein for 36 weeks, serum lipid and lipoprotein concentrations were higher than initial levels but only significantly for the two groups on 25% or 37.5% proteins and more so with 25% proteins than 37.5% (Kritchevsky et al. 1988a). Likewise, in *Squirrel* monkeys, increasing the protein level of the diet from 9% to 25% produced only an insignificant effect on serum cholesterol concentrations (Middleton et al. 1967). In all of these experiments, a cholesterol-rich diet enhanced the effect on serum cholesterol concentrations. When cholesterol was added to the diet, a moderate reduction in protein level (25% versus 8%) reduced cholesterol concentrations, whereas if the protein level was 4%, serum cholesterol concentration and cholesterol level in α-lipoproteins increased, whether or not the diet contained cholesterol (Srinivasan et al. 1977, 1979). However, in other species such as *Spider* monkeys, the casein levels (4% or 8% or 25%) in a diet containing cholesterol had no interacting effects on serum cholesterol concentrations (Srinivasan et al. 1977).

2.1.8 SUMMARY

Although the results are sometimes conflicting, in some species, such as rabbits, calves, pigs, monkeys, and dogs (although the data are insufficient in the latter), variations below or above protein requirements would appear to globally increase serum cholesterol concentrations. These data indicate that the diets used in experiments ought to contain a similar percentage and level of protein to those of individual requirements.

2.1.9 EFFECTS OF LOW-PROTEIN DIET ON PLASMA LIPIDS, LIVER ENZYMES, LIPID METABOLISM, AND BILIARY FLOW

2.1.9.1 Plasma Lipids

The exact nature of plasma lipid modifications have been defined by more recent studies performed in rats (Flores et al. 1970a, 1970b; Meghelli-Bouchenak et al. 1987, 1989a, 1989b, 1991a, 1991b; Gouache et al. 1991; Narce et al. 1992; Bouziane et al. 1992, 1994a, 1994b; Sato et al. 1996; Boualga et al. 2000). When the dietary protein level was reduced over a period of 28 days (18% versus 6% casein) the triacylglycerol level of VLDL decreased, whereas plasma free-cholesterol and phospholipid concentrations were increased.

Overall plasma lipoprotein concentrations, and also those of apo BH, apo A-1, and apo E, were unchanged but those of apo A-1V and particularly apo B-I and apo C were significantly reduced (Gouache et al. 1991). However, Sato et al. (1996) observed elevated apo A-1V and apo E levels. The synthesis of apo B, a major apoprotein of hepatic VLDL, was decreased via a transcriptional mechanism that significantly reduces the hepatic secretion of lipoproteins that are rich in triacylglycerols (Flores et al. 1970a, 1970b; Seakins and Waterlow 1972; Yagasaki and Kamataka 1984; Davis et al. 1985; Sato et al. 1996). Apo B serum concentrations were lowered and positively correlated with an abundance of apo B mRNA (Sato et al. 1996). Apoproteins A-1, A-1I, and A-1V of HDL, 50% of which are synthesized in the intestines, remained unchanged, whereas apo C and B (particularly apo B-100 and B-48) of VLDL, which are synthesized by the liver, were reduced (Meghelli-Bouchenak et al. 1987, 1989b, 1991a, 1991b; Aubert and Flament 1991; Bouziane et al. 1992). However, in *ExHC* rats fed on a low-protein diet, mRNA for apo A-1V, apo B, and apo E, but not apo A-1 mRNA were decreased by 20% to 50% compared with rats fed on a diet containing an adequate level of protein. A period of protein depletion of 3 days resulted in a 30% to 40% decrease in mRNA levels for apo E (de Jong and Schreiber 1987). A low-protein diet decreases apo B synthesis through a post-transcriptional mechanism that reduces secretion of triacylglycerol-rich lipoproteins from the liver (Sato et al. 1996).

2.1.9.2 Liver Enzymes and Lipid Metabolism

In chickens, hypercholesterolemia was associated with increased liver fatty acid synthesis (Nishida et al. 1960). In other experiments, however, this association was only observed if cholesterol was added to the diet (Nikkilä and Ollilla 1957; Marion et al. 1961; Rose and Balloun 1969). Plasma cholesterol turnover and fecal excretion of cholesterol and bile acids were reduced (Yeh and Léveillé 1973). A low-protein soybean diet increases plasma and hepatic lipids but not plasma cholesterol concentrations.

In rats, a low-protein diet, with casein or whey protein, induced hepatic steatosis and increased liver HMG-CoA reductase activity. It also increased serum cholesterol concentrations, decreased fatty acid synthase activity and liver bioavailability of sulfur amino acids. Intracellular glutathione and taurine levels were reduced and liver lipid transport impaired. The same diet also enhanced the susceptibility of VLDL and LDL particles to peroxidation and increased liver triacylglycerol concentrations (Flores et al. 1970a; Seakins and Waterlow 1972; Yagasaki and Kamataka 1984; Meghelli-Bouchenak et al. 1987; Aubert and Flament 1991; Moundras et al. 1997). The accumulation of triacylglycerols in the liver is the result of a decrease in the secretion of triacylglycerol-rich lipoproteins caused by the reduced synthesis of their lipoprotein constituents such as apoproteins, phospholipids, and cholesterol (Davis et al. 1985; review in Sato et al. 1996). In growing (Wiener et al. 1963) and lactating female *Wistar* rats (Leclerc et al. 1985), a low-protein diet increased the liver concentrations of neutral lipids, namely triacylglycerols. The liver lipidosis observed in growing rats fed with a low-protein diet supplemented with methionine would not appear to result from a threonine deficiency since it is not suppressed by threonine supplementation (Leclerc et al. 1989).

Liver and serum cholesterol and apoprotein concentrations, with the exception of apo B, were lower in elderly male *ExHC* rats on whey protein than with a casein-deficient diet (Sato et al. 1996). However, probably as a result of differences between strains, and in particular the degree of cholesterol sensitivity of rats, and also in the composition of diets, no significant difference was observed in two other experiments in male *Wistar* rats (Marquez-Ruiz et al. 1992) or weanling female *Wistar* rats (Zhang and Beynen 1993b).

The quality and the quantity of protein in the diet of rats induce different levels of activity of certain enzymes involved in carbohydrate metabolism. The activities of malic enzyme and pyruvate kinase decrease with increased intake of proteins and with the enhancement of their biological values. In contrast, the activity of glucose-6-phosphate dehydrogenase and phosphoenolpyruvate carboxykinase is enhanced in *Wistar CF* male rats when the protein level of the diet increases, whereas that of glucose-6-phosphatase is unchanged (Peret et al. 1975).

The activity of several enzymes is modified when the level of casein in the diet of young growing rats is reduced. Enzymatic activities of Δ5-, Δ6-, and Δ9-desatu-rases are decreased by the reduction of protein intake, which also impairs the metabolism of arachidonic and eicosapentenoic acid precursors of prostaglandins, thromboxanes, and leukotrienes. Their levels in VLDL phospholipids and the ratio of saturated/unsaturated fatty acids are reduced in growing male *Wistar* rats (Narce et al. 1992; Bouziane et al. 1994b). In male pathogen-free-specific *Sprague-Dawley* rats, the activities of liver and kidney superoxide dismutase, thiobarbituric acid-reactive substance, and glutathione peroxidase were all increased by dietary soybean protein or casein restriction (5%). Lipid peroxidation may be also enhanced (Sambuichi et al. 1991).

The changes in the lipogenic activities of several enzymes in the liver of young growing rats are related to protein quality as is demonstrated by varying the proteins in the diet (casein, lactalbumin, soybean protein, gluten, and gelatin). Total and specific activities of acetyl-CoA carboxylase, fatty acid synthase, ATP-citrate lyase, and glucose-6-phosphate dehydrogenase are all positively correlated to protein qual-ity, as are the total activities but not the specific activities of glucokinase and malic enzymes in male weanling *Sprague-Dawley* rats (Herzberg and Rogerson 1981, 1984). In the same strain of rats fed on a protein-free diet, liver neutral glyceride, total cholesterol, phospholipid, and plasmalogen concentrations were increased, decreased, or unchanged by the addition of one amino acid to the diet (Williams and Hurlebaus 1965a, 1965b), as described in Section 2.7. During prolonged protein depletion, the loss of protein, succinic oxidase, and succinic deshydrogenase activ-ities are protected by the addition of methionine (0.3%) or cystine (0.3%) in male *Sprague-Dawley* rats (Williams 1964).

An increase in plasma cholesterol levels could be due to a deficiency in methio-nine (Mizuno et al. 1988). However, in another experiment in young female *Wistar* rats, with or without methionine supplements, a casein diet (8%) or soybean protein diet (8%) inconsistently induced fatty liver syndrome (Yokogoshi et al. 1985). Regardless of the diet allowed, pregnancy seems to be a contributing factor to an increase in the free carnitine fraction and phospholipid levels in the liver, whereas in nonpregnant *Sprague-Dawley* rats, serum levels of free carnitine decrease and triacylglycerols increase when they are fed on a low-protein, lysine-deficient diet (Fernandez Ortega 1989).

LPL activity is reduced in adipose tissue but not in the heart or liver of young albino rats fed on a low-protein diet (Agbedana 1980). The plasma lipolytic activity due to LPL and hepatic lipase was also low in the experiments of Lamry et al. (1995). LPL activities were measured in a control group of weaning male *Wistar* rats fed on a balanced diet containing 200 g of protein/kg (160 g of wheat gluten and 40 g of casein) and in another group fed on a low-protein diet (50 g of protein/kg: 40 g of wheat gluten, 10 g of casein), with both diets lasting 28 days. At the end of this period, the epididymal fat-tissue LPL activity and that of the heart (in contrast to the results of Agbedana) and of the gastrocnemius in the group with malnutrition were 36% and 44%, respectively, of those of the control group. After a refeeding period of 28 days with the control group diet, the LPL activity of epididymal fat and liver lipolytic activity were similar to control group values. It is therefore likely that a low-protein diet limits storage in adipose tissue due to the reduced serum VLDL-triacylglycerol bioavailability (Boualga et al. 2000).

2.1.9.3 Biliary Flow

Biliary flow is diminished in female *Sprague-Dawley* rats fed on a low-protein diet but plasma concentrations of cholesterol and bile acids are higher than in animals fed with a chow diet (Villalon et al. 1987).

2.1.10 EFFECTS OF HIGH-PROTEIN DIET ON ENZYMES AND LIVER LIPOGENESIS

In chickens, increased dietary protein content decreases hepatic lipogenesis and liver malic enzyme levels (Yeh and Léveillé 1969; Peret et al. 1975). In young male weanling *Sprague-Dawley* rats, the activity of acetyl-CoA carboxylase, fatty acid synthase, and glucose-6-phosphate dehydrogenase increased with higher dietary protein levels, whereas that of malic enzyme decreased. Glucokinase and pyruvate dehydrogenase activity was not related to dietary protein levels. Increasing dietary protein levels up to 100 g of casein/kg resulted in enhanced activity of several enzymes: fatty acid synthase, glucose-6-phosphate dehydrogenase, ATP-citrate lyase, and liver fatty acid synthesis (Herzberg and Rogerson 1981). However, the changes in the lipogenic activities of several enzymes in the liver of young rats of the same strain are related to protein quality as can be demonstrated by varying the proteins in the diet (casein, lactalbumin, soybean protein, gluten, and gelatin). Total and specific activities of acetyl-CoA carboxylase, fatty acid synthase, ATP-citrate lyase, and glucose-6-phosphate dehydrogenase are all related to protein quality, as are the total but not the specific activities of glucokinase and malic enzymes (Herzberg and Rogerson 1984).

2.1.11 CONCLUSION

It is obvious that our knowledge of the effects of low-protein and high-protein diets for each species is dependent on the number of experiments and experimental conditions. It is therefore quite impossible to suggest an accurate general conclusion. Moreover, as the effects of low- and high-protein diets differ according to species, any extrapolation of the data for human use must take into consideration the species investigated. Whether the level of proteins in the diet decreases or increases, serum cholesterol concentrations are enhanced in birds, rabbits, and rodents (rats, mice, hamsters). Chickens, however, react differently from other species. In calves and monkeys, reactions vary according to strain. In pigs, serum cholesterol would appear to be particularly sensitive to the different levels of proteins in the diet. In dogs, since insufficient experiments have been conducted, no conclusion can be proposed. Of all the proteins investigated, casein produces the greatest increase in serum cholesterol concentrations.

Differences in experimental protocols, particularly the nature and quantity of diet components, as described later, may well explain most conflicting results. The lipid and cholesterol contents of a diet modulate the protein and sulfur amino acid effects. The food environment is therefore an important parameter to be taken into account (Greer et al. 1966). On the whole, the evidence on the effects of protein levels on serum cholesterol concentrations clearly show that only adequate coverage of protein requirements will ensure normal levels of serum cholesterol concentrations. In the experiments, the nutritional values of proteins chosen for the diet is another essential factor, as is the use of protein levels that are similar to protein requirements (Léveillé et al. 1962c; Young 1991). The widely varying reactions observed in different animal species underline the importance, before any extrapolation can be made to humans, of conducting experiments in monkeys and pigs since their metabolic reactions are the closest to those of humans.

2.2 EFFECTS OF THE NATURE OF PROTEINS

The nature of proteins, particularly casein and soybean protein, has to be taken into account since their effects can vary according to species and protocol designs (Carroll and Hamilton 1975; Kritchevsky 1980b; Sugano 1983; Terpstra et al. 1983a; van Raaij et al. 1983; West et al. 1983b; Forsythe 1986; Beynen 1990a, 1990c; Carroll 1992). The review by Waggle and Kolar (1979) clearly illustrates that the several nonprotein components of various soybean protein products should also be taken into consideration because of their potential effect on lipid metabolism and the process of atherosclerosis. As was noted earlier, it is clear that the same recommendation should also be made with regard to genetic factors.

2.2.1 CASEIN VERSUS SOYBEAN PROTEIN: EFFECTS ON SERUM CHOLESTEROL CONCENTRATIONS

Assessment of the respective effects of casein and soybean protein on lipid metabolism has been the subject of a great number of studies in several animal species and in humans (Beynen et al. 1983d; Campbell et al. 1995). Substituting animal proteins with soybean protein in the diet reduces serum concentrations of total and LDL cholesterol (Nestel 1985; Carroll 1991a, 1991b; Kritchevsky 1993; Sirtori et al. 1993; Sugano and Koba 1993; Carroll and Kurowska 1995).

2.2.1.1 Birds

In various bird models such as chickens, cockerels, or pigeons fed with a cholesterol-enriched diet, if casein is replaced by soybean protein, serum cholesterol concentrations are reduced (Kokatnur et al. 1956; Stamler et al. 1958c; Kritchevsky et al. 1959; Kenney and Fisher 1973). On the other hand, this substitution has no or only a very weak effect in the context of a cholesterol-free diet (Johnson et al. 1958; Lofland et al. 1966; Hevia and Visek 1979a; Mol et al. 1982). However, in chickens fed on casein *ad libitum*, the plasma and liver concentrations of cholesterol are increased and the hypercholesterolemia is severe if cholesterol is added to the diet (Choi and Chee 1995a, 1995b).

In contrast to rats and mice, in chickens raising the amount of soybean protein in the diet, with or without cholesterol, does not increase serum cholesterol concentrations (Johnson et al. 1958; Nishida et al. 1958; Stamler et al. 1958a, 1958b, 1958c; Kokatnur et al. 1958b; Léveillé and Fisher 1958; Kokatnur and Kummerow 1959; March et al. 1959; Léveillé et al. 1960; Léveillé and Sauberlich 1961; Léveillé et al. 1961; Rose and Balloun 1969; Kenney and Fisher 1973). In the context of a soybean protein diet, serum cholesterol levels are significantly lower for the upper limit of dietary protein levels (50% protein) (Kokatnur et al. 1956).

With casein, the results vary according to species. Although an increase in casein intake and, to an even greater extent, an increased level of cholesterol, enhance serum cholesterol concentrations in pigeons (Lofland et al. 1961; Little and Angell 1977), they do not exert the same effect in chickens (Stamler et al. 1958a; Johnson et al. 1958; Kokatnur et al. 1958b; Fisher et al. 1959; Kenney and Fisher 1973). In chickens receiving six different diets (a commercial diet without or with cholesterol [1%], semipurified diets containing either casein without or with cholesterol [1%], casein plus arginine [0.85%], or soybean protein), no change in serum cholesterol concentrations were observed if the chickens were fed a cholesterol-free diet, whereas serum cholesterol concentrations increased when cholesterol (1%) was added to the diet. The cholesterol-rich diet induced a shift in the lipoprotein pattern from LDL to IDL and VLDL (Mol et al. 1982). There is a negative correlation between the protein levels of a diet and serum cholesterol concentrations (Mol et al. 1982; Terpstra et al. 1983d), and also between protein levels and cholesterol concentrations in various tissues, except the liver (de Schriver et al. 1990).

2.2.1.2 Rabbits

The variations in serum cholesterol concentrations depend on the level and the nature (animal or vegetable) of proteins in the diet (Sidransky 1990). When the level of soybean protein in the diet was raised from 27% to 54%, serum cholesterol concentrations were similar (Huff et al. 1977). Raising vegetable protein levels (gluten flour, soybean, alfalfa) from 13% to 22% to 38% had no influence on serum cholesterol concentrations (Freyberg 1937).

Since the studies of Meeker and Kesten (1940, 1941), and that of Howard et al. (1965), the hypercholesterolemic effect on rabbits of animal proteins, and casein in particular, and the normo- or hypocholesterolemic effects of vegetable proteins, particularly soybean protein, have been confirmed in several studies (Carroll 1967, 1971; Hermus 1975; Carroll and Hamilton 1975; Hamilton and Carroll 1976; Huff et al. 1977; Carroll et al. 1979; Kritchevsky et al. 1981, 1983; Scholz et al. 1983; Carroll 1983; Beynen et al. 1983a; Terpstra et al. 1983b; van Raaij et al. 1983; Lovati et al. 1990; Carroll 1991a). Casein increases serum free and esterified cholesterol and phospholipid levels, but not those of triacylglycerols, and decreases the molar ratio of free to esterified cholesterol in the liver, whereas it is increased in the serum (Beynen et al. 1983a).

The results of experiments vary according to species, strain, sex, and age of animals. The younger the subjects, the greater their sensitivity (Ignatowski 1909; Huff et al. 1982; West et al. 1982; van Raaij et al. 1983; Beynen et al. 1983d; Pfeuffer 1989).

The variations in serum cholesterol concentrations depend on the proportion and nature (animal or vegetable) of proteins in the diet (Sidranski 1990). The extent of the impact of dietary cholesterol also varies from one animal to another depending on the influence of genetic factors (Beynen et al. 1986a; Lovati et al. 1990; Anonymous 1991). Male rabbits of two inbred strains (*IIIVO/Ju* and *AX/Ju*) that are either hyper- or hyporesponsive to dietary cholesterol were also hyper- or hyporesponsive to the protein source (casein versus soybean protein) with a cholesterol-free diet (Beynen et al. 1986a). When the dietary cholesterol content was very low, serum cholesterol concentrations of male pathogen-free-specified rabbits of the *New Zealand white* strain were similar with casein and soybean protein. A balanced diet increased serum cholesterol concentrations only if the diet was very rich in cholesterol (Lovati et al. 1990).

However, for other researchers, diets containing animal proteins, particularly casein, resulted in increased serum cholesterol concentrations even if the diet was cholesterol free (Meeker and Kesten 1941; Lambert et al. 1958; Wigand 1959; Howard et al. 1965; Carroll 1967, 1971; Carroll and Hamilton 1975; Hamilton and Carroll 1976; Chao et al. 1983; Kroon et al. 1985; Bauer 1987), although in some of these experiments the protein level of the diet was higher than normal.

The addition of soybean protein or substitution of casein with soybean protein in a diet reduces serum and liver cholesterol concentrations and modifies lipoprotein and apoprotein distribution (Howard et al. 1965; Kritchevsky 1976; Roberts et al. 1979; Lacombe and Nibbelink 1980; Terpstra and Sanchez-Muniz 1981; Terpstra et al. 1981; 1982a, 1982b, 1983a, 1983b; Scholz et al. 1983; Beynen et al. 1983a; van Raaij et al. 1983; Bauer and Covert 1984; Havel 1986; Kurowska et al. 1989; Hrabek-Smith et al. 1989; Pacini et al. 1989; Bergeron and Jacques 1989; Kritchevsky et al. 1989; Carroll et al. 1989; Samman et al. 1990c).

With a normolipidic diet (30%), the effects of casein and soybean protein depend on the protein and fat content of the diet and also on the type of fats. The diets used in these experiments were often moderately rich in proteins (25%) (Lambert et al. 1958; Brattsand 1976; Lacombe and Nibbelink 1980; Hrabek-Smith and Carroll 1987). The hypercholesterolemic effect of butter was observed with diets containing either casein or soybean protein. However, if butter was replaced by almond oil, serum cholesterol concentrations were moderately high with a casein diet and normal with a soybean protein diet. The fats and proteins in a diet modify the serum cholesterol concentrations of male *New Zealand white* rabbits (Sanchez et al. 1988a), as was clearly demonstrated by the comparison of serum cholesterol concentrations obtained with several types of diets containing various types of proteins (casein, soybean, fish) and various types of fats (maize oil, coconut oil) (Bergeron et al. 1991). A low dose of simvastatin enhanced the hypocholesterolemic effect of soybean protein but had no influence when male *New Zealand white* rabbits were fed with a diet containing casein or cod proteins (20%), fats (11%), and cholesterol (0.06%) (Giroux et al. 1997).

Unlike a casein diet, a soybean protein diet modifies cholesterol metabolism. The rate of serum cholesterol turnover, the fractional catabolism rate of cholesterol and that of serum esterified cholesterol and steroid synthesis, are increased (Huff and Carroll 1980b; Kritchevsky et al. 1983; Cohn et al. 1984). The extracellular pool of cholesterol is decreased (Nagata et al. 1982; Park and Liepa 1982; Park et al. 1987). In rabbit as in human plasma, but not in rat plasma, the transfer protein is present (Norum et al. 1983). These facts again highlight the inter-species differences that could explain the greater effect of casein on serum cholesterol concentrations in rabbits than in rats (West et al. 1990).

2.2.1.3 Rats

As in rabbits, the effects of proteins are influenced by the species, strain, sex, age, and genetic factors, particularly those relating to obesity. With casein, serum cholesterol concentrations are higher in female than in male rats of the *Wistar* and *Zucker* strains than with soybean protein and they are also higher in obese than in normal-weight animals and in weanling and weaned rats, as in guinea pigs (Fillios et al. 1958; McGregor 1971; Terpstra et al. 1982a, 1982b, 1982d; van Raaij et al. 1983; Edgwin 1985; Yashiro et al. 1985; de Schriver 1990). The hypercholesterolemic effects of casein are higher in genetically obese *Zucker* rats than in *Wistar* rats (Beynen et al. 1983b). With the possible exception of wheat gluten, other proteins (casein, soybean, and potato protein) do not prevent the age-related increase in serum cholesterol concentrations in immature and mature male *Wistar* rats. Total plasma and HDL cholesterol are significantly lower with plant proteins than with casein diets. LCAT activity is not significantly different in rats fed different plant proteins, whereas the esterification rate is lower in rats fed casein. Fecal neutral and acidic steroids excretion is higher with plant proteins (de Schriver 1990). The cholesterol in the plasma of casein-fed rabbits is carried mainly in the VLDL and IDL fraction and the turnover of cholesterol is slower (Carroll 1982).

The results of various experiments have demonstrated complex and conflicting relations between the level of casein in the diet of rats and their serum cholesterol concentrations. As described in Section 2.1, variations in serum cholesterol concentrations would appear to be multiphasic in relation to the casein level and to the presence or absence of cholesterol in the diet. A cholesterol-free diet had no or only a very weak effect (Sautier et al. 1979; Neves et al. 1980; Pathirana et al. 1980; Eklund and Sjöblom 1980, 1986).

The plasma cholesterol concentrations of male *Wistar* rats fed the basal (cholesterol-free, cholic acid-free) semisynthetic diet containing either soybean protein or casein were similar to those observed in chow-fed controls. The increase in plasma cholesterol levels after the addition of exogenous cholesterol to the diet was smaller with the soybean protein diet than with that containing casein (Raheja and Lindscheer 1982). In several experiments, casein has been shown to be hypercholesterolemic and soybean protein hypocholesterolemic (Moyer et al. 1956; Nath et al. 1959; de Groot 1958, 1959, 1960; Terpstra et al. 1982b; Sjöblom et al. 1989; Okita and

Sugano 1990; Kimura et al. 1990). Similar results were obtained in diabetic rats (Kudchodkar et al. 1988). Replacing casein with soybean protein in normo- or hyper-cholesterolemic rats decreased the harmful influence of casein on serum cholesterol concentrations in male rats of the *Holtzman* strain (Seidel 1960), and in male and female *Zucker* rats (Terpstra et al. 1982a, 1982b). However, this effect was only significant in male *Sprague-Dawley* rats fed on a diet that was particularly rich in proteins (36%) for 7 weeks (Baba et al. 1992) or in *Fischer 344* rats fed on a cholesterol-free diet (Carlile et al. 1986). Whereas in young male *Sprague-Dawley* rats the hypocholesterolemic effect of soybean protein was observed regardless of dietary cholesterol, in adult male rats, it was obtained only with a cholesterol-rich diet (Choi et al. 1989a).

Unlike casein, plant proteins significantly reduce plasma total cholesterol and HDL-cholesterol concentrations in immature and mature *Wistar* rat but the plasma cholesterol increase associated with aging is not prevented by consumption of casein, soybean protein or potato protein although wheat gluten would appear to be effective (de Schriver 1990). However, although in male *Sprague-Dawley* rats (Neves et al. 1980), total plasma cholesterol levels varied according to the various proteins, plant protein effects, compared with animal proteins, were not found to be hypocholester-olemic in young rats from the same strain (Eklund and Sjöblom 1980) and casein or soybean protein in a cholesterol-free diet had no differential effects in *Wistar* rats (Sautier et al. 1979) and in *Sprague-Dawley* rats (Pathirana et al. 1980).

Some authors have reported an increase in serum cholesterol and triacylglycerol concentrations when the casein level of a cholesterol-free diet is raised (Bagchi et al. 1963; Hevia et al. 1979b, 1980a, 1980b). These effects were also observed in lean female *Zucker* rats (Terpstra et al. 1982b). Although stepwise addition of 5% casein to a diet containing 15% casein caused a progressive increase in serum cholesterol level, the same successive addition of various proteins such as dried whole egg, wheat gluten, fish, and meat meal resulted in a reduction in serum cholesterol levels (de Groot 1959). The serum cholesterol concentrations of male weanling *Sprague-Dawley* rats were moderately high, low, or very high with the following dietary casein content (7.5%, 12% to 18%, or 40%, respectively) (Jones and Huffman 1956a, 1956b). Similar variations were obtained in the same strain of rats by Nath who observed that serum cholesterol concentrations were high when the casein content of the diet was 10% or 69% and normal when it was 30% (Nath et al. 1959). The serum cholesterol levels of rats fed for 2 weeks on a casein diet were higher than when they were fed on a soybean diet, and regardless of whether or not the diet contained cholesterol; however, these results were only observed when the dietary protein content was high (45%) and not with 30% or 15% (Hevia and Visek 1979b). When the level of casein or soybean protein was increased (10%, 20%, 30%) in the diet for 30 days, the plasma cholesterol but not triacylglycerol concentrations of male *Wistar* rats decreased with the increasing dietary protein level. When cholesterol and sodium cholate were added to the diet at 0.5% and 0.125%, respectively, serum cholesterol concentrations decreased to a greater extent with soybean protein than with casein, and serum triacylglycerol levels were also reduced (Okita and Sugano 1989).

As was previously demonstrated, the cholesterol level of a diet influences the effects of proteins. In short-term (2 weeks) experiments with casein and soybean protein, serum cholesterol concentrations of male *Wistar* rats only varied when the diet was supplemented with cholesterol, but this effect was less pronounced than in mice (Raheja and Lindscheer 1982). If cholesterol was added to the diet, serum cholesterol concentrations increased (de Groot 1958; Seidel et al. 1960; Bagchi et al. 1963; Eklund and Sjöblom 1986; Iwami et al. 1987; Saeki and Kiriyama 1989; Sautier et al. 1990). The hypocholesterolemic effect of soybean protein was patent with a cholesterol-enriched diet in male *Wistar* rats but this effect and the decrease in liver lipid concentrations were irrespective of the presence or absence of dietary cholesterol. The fecal excretion of acidic but not neutral steroids increased with increasing protein level, particularly in rats fed soybean protein. The arachidonate/linoleate ratio in plasma and liver phosphatidylcholine are enhanced with the increase in protein levels and were higher with casein than with protein diets (Okita and Sugano 1989).

In several experiments with purified or unpurified soybean protein cholesterol-free diets, serum cholesterol concentrations of *Wistar* (Sautier et al. 1979) and male *Sprague-Dawley* rats (Saeki and Kiriyama 1988) and the liver cholesterol concentrations (Hevia and Visek 1979b) were identical to those obtained with a casein diet or with a dietary cholesterol content of 0.1% in growing male *Wistar* rats (Madani et al. 1998). In male and female *lean Zucker* strain rats fed on a cholesterol-enriched semipurified diet containing two levels (20% and 50%) of either casein or soybean protein for a 14-week period, the serum cholesterol level was higher in females with casein and even higher when the casein level was increased in the diet. In male rats serum cholesterol concentrations were not significantly different with casein or soybean protein diets. With casein diets, the females exhibited a more pronounced shift of HDL cholesterol to LDL cholesterol than the males. The liver cholesterol concentration of the rats was highest in those fed the 50% casein diet and progressively lower in the animals on diets containing 20% casein, 20% soybean protein and 50% soybean protein (Terpstra et al. 1982a). However, in *Wistar* rats fed on a cholesterol-rich diet, in contrast to whey proteins, soybean protein did not exert a hypocholesterolemic effect (Lefevre and Schneeman 1984; Nagaoka et al. 1992).

In order to explain these discrepancies between the data, Pfeuffer and Barth pointed out the significant impact of the duration of experiments and of the level of protein intake (Pfeuffer and Barth 1990). Indeed, the results of several studies have shown that the response of serum cholesterol concentrations is enhanced when the protein content of a diet is too low or too high (Jones and Huffman 1956b; Fillios et al. 1958; Nath et al. 1959). It is also influenced by the food environment, particularly the addition of cholesterol to a diet, the amount of amino acids, and the nature of fats in the diet. With a low-fat and high-sucrose cholesterol-free diet, casein exerts a weakly hypercholesterolemic effect (Nagata et al. 1980, 1982; Sautier et al. 1986; Pfeuffer and Barth 1986a).

2.2.1.4 Mice

In mice, the results are contradictory and it is not possible to deduce that serum cholesterol levels are higher with casein than with soybean protein (Roy and

Schneeman 1981; Nagata et al. 1981b; Raheja and Lindscheer 1982; Weinans and Beynen 1983). Soybean protein does not increase serum cholesterol concentrations of mice. Indeed in this species the fecal steroid excretion is not increased by a soybean protein diet (Hayashi et al. 1994). A hot ethanol extract from soybean protein decreased serum cholesterol concentrations and increased LDL receptor activity in male *Swiss CD-1* mice (Lovati et al. 1991a).

With casein and soybean protein diets serum cholesterol concentrations are higher in *C57 BL/JG* weanling male mice than with a chow diet (Roy and Schneeman 1981). However, in another experiment on 9-week-old, female, genetically obese mice (*C57BL6J obese ob/ob*) a soybean protein diet, for 27 days, caused a reduction in the serum cholesterol level, whereas a casein diet increased it (Schmeisser and Hrisco 1987).

A 56-day α protein (20% soybean protein) cholesterol-rich (5%) diet that was deficient in sulfur amino acids enhanced serum cholesterol concentrations of adult *Swiss white* mice, and if the protein content of the diet was lowered to 10% and the fat content increased to 15%, serum cholesterol concentrations rose significantly. In the same strain of mice the progression of hypercholesterolemia was partially prevented by DL-methionine supplementation (0.6%) in these diets (Fillios and Mann 1954). Serum triacylglycerol and hepatic and biliary cholesterol concentrations were significantly lower with soybean protein than with casein when cholesterol was added to the diet of *Swiss white* mice. The hypercholesterolemic effect of exogenous cholesterol was more pronounced in mice than in rats (Raheja and Lindscheer 1982).

2.2.1.5   Guinea Pigs and Hamsters

Serum cholesterol concentrations were higher with casein than with soybean protein in guinea pigs (McGregor 1971). If the diets contained 0.04 g/100 g of cholesterol and 22.5 g/100 g of proteins with different casein/soybean protein ratios (60/40 or 20/80 or 0/100), serum cholesterol concentrations of male *Hartley* guinea pigs and *Golden Syrian* hamsters were lowest with 100% soybean protein (Fernandez et al. 1999a, 1999b). In *Golden Syrian* hamsters, on a cholesterol-enriched diet (0.2%) containing 20% of soybean protein or casein and 10% of fat (perilla oil, α-linolenic acid or safflower oil, linoleic acid), the serum and liver concentrations of cholesterol were not significantly different but fecal steroid excretion was stimulated, particularly with safflower oil (Gatchalian-Yee et al. 1995).

Male *Golden Syrian* hamsters fed a semipurified diet containing 25% of either casein or soybean protein, with a low-cholesterol (0,01%) level for a period of 28 days, had significantly higher total serum cholesterol and VLDL- and HDL-cholesterol concentrations with casein than with soybean protein. In contrast, when the same diet contained a high cholesterol level (0.25%), serum cholesterol concentrations were not significantly different between casein and soybean protein-fed animals. With the two diets, hepatic free and esterified cholesterol concentrations were similar, although the mean daily excretion of bile acids was considerably higher in the soybean protein-fed animals (Wright and Salter 1993). In another experiment on *Golden Syrian Mesocricetus auratus* hamsters fed on casein and soybean protein (26.3%) for 28 days, the same authors showed that although total serum cholesterol concentrations were not significantly different, the LDL- and HDL-cholesterol levels were higher and VLDL-cholesterol levels lower in hamsters fed on the soybean protein diet than those fed on casein. Plasma insulin and glucagon concentrations were similar in both groups but plasma triiodothyronine concentrations were higher and plasma thyroxine concentrations lower with the soybean protein diet (Wright and Salter 1998). In comparison, in *Golden Syrian* hamsters, fed for a period of 8 weeks on a cholesterol-enriched semipurified diet containing either casein (40%) or soybean protein concentrates, a significant reduction in total cholesterol and VLDL- and LDL-cholesterol plasma concentrations was observed (Nicolosi and Wilson 1997).

2.2.1.6 Pigs

A mixed, cholesterol-rich (0.6 mg/kcal) diet of vegetable proteins (50% soybean meal, 25% each of corn and wheat) had a significant hypocholesterolemic effect in young male boars (*purebred Yorkshire* or *Yorkshire* x *Hampshire*) compared with a casein diet (90% casein and 10% lactalbumin), the polyunsaturated/saturated fatty acids ratio of the two diets being different (P/S 3 versus 0.3). HDL-cholesterol levels were also reduced in pigs fed on plant protein (Forsythe et al. 1980). The hypo-cholesterolemic effect of soybean protein and the hypercholesterolemic effect of casein were both observed in pigs on a diet that was rich in fat and cholesterol (Kim et al. 1978, 1980a, 1980b; Beynen et al. 1985a; Beynen and West 1987; Ho et al. 1989) or fed on casein protein isolates (Julius and Wiggers 1979). Although lymphatic transport of triacylglycerols was similar (3hrs) with casein and soybean protein diets, that of cholesterol was significantly higher with casein. In the casein group, the greater apo B-48 secretion with higher specificity, as measured by [³H]leucine incorporation, may be responsible for the greater cholesterol transport in chylomicrons. The mechanism of the weaker synthesis of apo B-48 in pigs fed on soybean protein compared with those on casein is still unclear (Ho et al. 1989). However, with low-fat and low-cholesterol diets, the effects of casein and soybean protein were similar (Kim et al. 1980a).

2.2.1.7 Monkeys

When female *Rhesus Macaca mulatta* monkeys were fed on a semipurified diet containing 0.1% cholesterol, and alternately casein or soybean protein (first period: soy 13 weeks, then casein 15 weeks; second period: soy 17 weeks, then casein 17 weeks) the serum cholesterol level increased gradually with casein during the first period then decreased with soybean protein and increased again with casein during the second period. Changes in serum cholesterol level were mainly reflected by changes in LDL cholesterol (Terpstra et al. 1984). In one male and seven female *Macaca fascicularis* monkeys fed on a semipurified cholesterol diet containing corn starch (50%) and sucrose (10%), replacing casein with soybean protein isolates, and vice versa, produced no significant change in total serum cholesterol levels. However, HDL cholesterol and VLDL-cholesterol concentrations were, respectively, higher and lower after the soybean protein diet than after the casein diet (Barth et al. 1984).

In a study by Wilson et al. (1998a), female *Cynomolgus Macaca fascicularis* monkeys were fed on the following three diets for a 6-week period: the "average American diet" "(AAD) (36% energy from fats); American Heart Association Step 1 (AHA Step 1) diet (30% energy from fats); and modified AHA Step 1 diet with the addition of soybean protein isolate (10% of total energy) and guar gum (5.8 g/day). The plasma total cholesterol and LDL-cholesterol concentrations were significantly lower (−19% and −24%, respectively) in monkeys fed on AHA Step 1 diet than in those fed on the AAD diet. These results are interesting because lipoprotein distribution in *Cynomolgus* monkeys is similar to that of humans and sensitive to dietary modifications.

Likewise in pre- and postmenopausal *Cynomolgus* monkeys, a moderately atherogenic soybean protein diet induced different results depending on the phytoestrogen level. Plasma cholesterol concentrations were lower and HDL-cholesterol concentrations higher with the high phytoestrogen content in diet (Anthony et al. 1994). Similar results were also obtained in *Cynomolgus* monkeys (Anthony et al. 1997) and in *Cebus* monkeys, and these were more pronounced when cholesterol was added to the diet (von Duvillard et al. 1992). These data show the importance of the nonprotein components of a diet.

2.2.2 CASEIN VERSUS SOYBEAN PROTEIN: EFFECTS ON LIPID AND CHOLESTEROL METABOLISMS

2.2.2.1 Rabbits

Plasma cholesterol turnover is higher in male *New Zealand white* rabbits fed on soybean protein than in those fed on casein (Huff and Carroll 1980b). The hypercholesterolemia observed in male *New Zealand white* rabbits fed on a wheat-starch/casein diet, in comparison with rabbits fed on laboratory chow, is partially due to the decreased number of specific hepatic LDL receptors reducing the catabolism of plasma cholesterol (Chao et al. 1982). The cholesterol content of the diet modifies the liver metabolism of cholesterol but not that of triacylglycerols. The output of cholesteryl esters from perfused livers of male *English shorthair* rabbits is much greater from the livers of cholesterol-fed than from normal chow-fed rabbits (MacKinnon et al. 1985). Dietary casein increased free and esterified cholesterol concentrations in the liver of *New Zealand white* rabbits but not those of phospholipids or triacylglycerols (Beynen et al. 1983a). A soybean protein diet, in comparison with a casein diet, did not increase hepatic cholesterol concentrations in *New Zealand white* rabbits (Lovati et al. 1990). In male *albino* rabbits fed on semipurified diets containing 20% casein or soybean protein for a 50-day period, the plasma cholesterol, triacylglycerol, and phospholipid levels were lower with soybean protein, and associated with higher activities of LCAT and LPL and also post-heparin lipolytic activity (Alladi et al. 1989a). In male *New Zealand white* rabbits, a cholesterol-free semisynthetic wheat-starch/casein diet compared to a chow diet increased hepatic synthesis and secretion of cholesterol-rich lipoproteins and apoproteins

(Chao et al. 1986). As in human plasma but not in rat plasma, the transfer protein is present in rabbits (Norum et al. 1983). This observation once again demonstrates the interspecies differences that could explain the greater effect of casein on serum cholesterol concentrations in rabbits than in rats (West et al. 1990).

2.2.2.2 Rats

A casein-containing cholesterol-free diet reduces the activity of HMG-CoA reductase and hepatic cholesterol synthesis in male *Wistar* rats (Nagata et al. 1982; Kritchevsky et al. 1984). In mature *Sprague-Dawley* or male *Wistar* rats fed on a cholesterol-free soybean protein diet, compared with casein, the specific activities of HMG-CoA reductase, cholesterol 7-α-hydroxylase, serum cholesterol turnover, and hepatic steroidogenesis were increased. The serum cholesterol level was decreased. The size of the rapidly exchangeable cholesterol pool (pool A) was markedly reduced (Reiser et al. 1977; Nagata et al. 1982; Kritchevsky 1990). However, in male *albino Wistar* rats with a cholesterol-free highly purified soybean protein diet, although fecal excretion of neutral and acid steroids and HMG-CoA reductase activity were enhanced, that of 7-α-hydroxylase was low (Vahouny et al. 1985; Madani et al. 1998). LCAT activity was similar with different plant proteins but the esterification rate was lower in immature and mature *Wistar* rats fed on casein (de Schriver 1990).

A soybean protein diet increased the esterified cholesterol fractional metabolism and the synthesis of steroids, whereas the pool of extra-cellular cholesterol was reduced in male *Wistar*, weanling male *Sprague-Dawley,* and mature and immature *Charles River* rats (Nagata et al. 1982; Park and Liepa 1982; Park et al. 1987), and VLDL catabolism was enhanced in female *Sprague-Dawley* rats (Lovati et al. 1985; Sugano et al. 1990b). The turnover of serum cholesterol esters was unchanged in immature male *Fischer* rats (Park et al. 1987). A soybean protein diet, in comparison with a casein diet, did not increase hepatic cholesterol concentrations in male *Wistar* rats (Lapré et al. 1989) but enhanced the level of serum cholesterol turnover and also that of cholesterol fractional metabolism of male weanling *Sprague-Dawley* rats (Cohn et al. 1984).

In female Spr*ague-Dawley* rats fed a casein or soybean protein diet supplemented with 1.2% cholesterol, HMG-CoA reductase activity was reduced by both diets. However, enzyme activity was significantly higher with the soybean protein diet (Sirtori et al. 1984). Serum cholesterol and triacylglycerol levels, liver cholesterol concentrations, and intestinal cholesterolgenesis, but not hepatic cholesterolgenesis, were lower in rats fed on the cholesterol diet (0.2%) with soybean protein than with the casein diet (Tatcher et al. 1984; Vahouny et al. 1985; Eklund and Sjöblom 1986; Iritani et al. 1986, 1988, 1996; Baba et al. 1992; Galibois et al. 1992; Ide et al. 1992; Prost et al. 1996). Unlike casein, soybean protein did not increase hepatic cholesterol concentrations in male *Wistar* rats (Lapré et al. 1989). VLDL catabolism was increased in female *Sprague-Dawley* rats fed on a soybean protein diet rather than a casein diet (Lovati et al. 1985; Sugano et al. 1990b). Net turnover of serum cholesterol was unchanged in male *Fischer* rats (Park et al. 1987). The increase in serum cholesterol concentrations of male weanling *Sprague-Dawley* rats attributable to a casein diet could well be a consequence of the decreased VLDL catabolism (Cohn et al. 1984).

The changes in lipid metabolism were also observed in suckling young *Sprague-Dawley* rats. Serum cholesterol, triacylglycerol, and phospholipid concentrations are weaker when their mothers are fed with soybean protein than with casein. Total and esterified cholesterol and triacylglycerol liver concentrations are enhanced during breast-feeding (Lu and Jian 1997).

The decrease in intestinal absorption of cholesterol and bile acids in rats or rabbits fed on soybean protein cholesterol-free diets (Fumagalli et al. 1978; Nagata et al. 1981a; Huff and Carroll 1980a) increased the specific activity of HMG-CoA reductase and stimulated the hepatic production in male *Sprague-Dawley* rats (Reiser et al. 1977) in response to the decreased influx of cholesterol into the liver (Fumagalli et al. 1978; Nagata et al. 1981a; Huff and Carroll 1980a). The increase in fecal steroid excretion of male *Wistar* rats may not be completely compensated by the stimulation of sterogenesis in the liver (Sugano et al. 1982a). The secretion of cholesterol, triacylglycerols, and apo A-1 was significantly reduced in perfused livers of male *Wistar* rats fed on soybean protein as compared with those fed on casein. However, no such differences were observed when the rats were fed on amino acid mixtures simulating these proteins. The type of dietary protein does not influence the rate of bile flow or the concentration of biliary bile acids and cholesterol. Thus, it can be concluded that the protein-dependent difference in concentrations of serum cholesterol and apo A-1 might not completely explained by the difference in the amino acid profile alone (Sugano et al. 1982a).

2.2.3 CASEIN VERSUS SOYBEAN PROTEIN: EFFECTS ON LIPOPROTEINS

2.2.3.1 Birds

In chickens receiving six different diets (a commercial diet without or with cholesterol [1%], semipurified diets containing either casein with or without cholesterol [1%], casein plus arginine [0.85%] or soybean protein), no changes in serum cholesterol concentrations were observed in chickens fed a cholesterol-free diet, whereas serum cholesterol concentrations increased when cholesterol was added to the diet. The cholesterol-rich diet induces a shift in the lipoprotein pattern from the LDL fraction to IDL and VLDL particles (Mol et al. 1982).

2.2.3.2 Rabbits

In male *New Zealand white* rabbits, a semisynthetic casein diet increased serum cholesterol concentrations, hepatic secretion of cholesterol-rich lipoproteins, and apoprotein synthesis (Kroon et al. 1982, 1985; Chao et al. 1986). Replacing casein with soybean protein in the diet reduced plasma cholesterol concentrations in LDL and VLDL particles and modified the lipoprotein and apoprotein distribution (Howard et al. 1965; Kritchevsky 1976; Brattsand 1976; Roberts et al. 1979; Lacombe and Nibbelink 1980; Terpstra et al. 1981, 1983a, 1983b; van Raaij et al. 1983; Bauer and Covert 1984; Havel 1986; Hrabek-Smith et al. 1989; Pacini et al. 1989; Bergeron and Jacques 1989; Kritchevsky et al. 1989; Carroll et al. 1989). The cholesterol/protein ratio increased two- or three-fold in lipoproteins in male *New Zealand white* rabbits (Hrabek-Smith and Carroll 1987).

With regard to the conventional diet, a semipurified diet without cholesterol did not modify serum cholesterol concentrations but did increase the levels of cholesterol and proteins in VLDL and LDL and those of free cholesterol in LDL and IDL in *New Zealand white* rabbits; however, the VLDL-triacylglycerol content was reduced. The same diet also resulted in reduced HDL cholesterol levels (Bauer 1987). VLDL, IDL, and LDL from casein-fed rabbits of the same strains contained more cholesteryl ester than that of lipoproteins isolated from chow-fed animals (Chao et al. 1986). Both cholesterol and apo E in VLDL and IDL were enhanced in rabbits fed on casein (Roberts et al. 1981, Scholz et al. 1982) or a cholesterol-rich diet (Kushawaha and Hazzard 1978; Scholz et al. 1982; Shore and Shore 1974). However, 6 weeks after casein was replaced by soybean protein or casein supplemented by a mixture of amino acids (expressed in grams per kilogram of feed: glycine 3.9, arginine 6.9, alanine 1.6) in a cholesterol diet (0.08%), the level of serum cholesterol of male *New Zealand white* rabbits was reduced but the apo E contents remained elevated in VLDL and IDL. The same results were observed after the withdrawal of cholesterol from the diet although the apo E level remained in IDL and decreased in LDL. The effects of these diets on the turnover rate of apo E requires further research (Scholz et al. 1983).

The increase in plasma cholesterol and apo E levels occurs first in LDL and then in VLDL when serum cholesterol concentrations are high. Hepatic binding of apo A and E was reduced and the receptor affinity was lowered before serum cholesterol concentrations were increased. VLDL and LDL turnover was reduced with a casein diet as a result of the decrease in LDL apo B receptor affinities. IDL-cholesterol levels are higher with casein than with soybean protein, and IDL apo B catabolism is slower (Carroll 1967, 1971; Hermus 1975; Brattsand 1976; Roberts et al. 1979; Lacombe and Nibbelink 1980; Terpstra and Sanchez-Muniz 1981; Terpstra et al. 1981, 1983a, 1983b; van Raaij et al. 1983; Samman et al. 1989; Khosla et al. 1989, 1991). A cholesterol-free semisynthetic casein diet increases hepatic secretion of cholesterol-rich lipoproteins and apoproteins (Lambert et al. 1958; Kritchevsky et al. 1977; Huff and Carroll 1980b; Chao et al. 1986). The secretions of cholesteryl-ester-rich lipoproteins and apolipoproteins by the perfused livers of male *New Zealand white* rabbits fed a wheat-starch-casein diet are enhanced (Chao et al. 1986).

2.2.3.3　Rats

Replacing casein by soybean protein in the diet reduces plasma cholesterol concentrations and modifies the lipoprotein and apoprotein distributions (Roberts et al. 1979; Terpstra et al. 1982b; van Raaij et al. 1983; Havel 1986). The serum triacylglycerol level was higher with casein than with soybean protein (Tatcher et al. 1984; Vahouny et al. 1985; Eklund and Sjöblom 1986; Iritani et al. 1986, 1988; Baba et al. 1992; Galibois et al. 1992; Guermani et al. 1992; Ide et al. 1992; Iritani et al. 1996). Compared with a cholesterol-free diet containing the same level of casein, the triacylglycerol concentrations of male *Wistar* rats obtained with a highly purified soybean protein diet were significantly lower at the levels of 200 and 300 g/kg and considerably more than at the level of 100 g/kg (Prost et al. 1996).

The effects of casein and soybean protein diets on lipoprotein levels are also different. In male weanling *Sprague-Dawley* rats fed a high-cholesterol, semipurified diet (1.2 g/100 g feed) for 4 weeks, serum cholesterol, VLDL-cholesterol and apo B concentrations were higher with casein. However, HDL cholesterol and serum triacylglycerol concentrations were similar with casein and soybean protein diets. LDL cholesterol was significantly lower in the casein-fed group. Casein-fed rats had a similar rate of plasma cholesterol production, but at significantly lower plasma cholesterol fractional catabolic rates compared with the rats fed on a soybean protein diet. With casein feeding, the fractional catabolic rate of VLDL was also lower. Cohn et al. (1984) suggest that the accumulation of VLDL in the plasma of rats fed dietary casein is not due to the excess VLDL production but to deficient VLDL removal. The diminished VLDL catabolism may well be a consequence of diminished VLDL catabolism. A casein diet with or without cholesterol increased the VLDL, LDL, and HDL particles, but the addition of cholesterol to the diet suppressed this effect. According to some authors, the HDL-cholesterol/total cholesterol ratio is higher with casein than with soybean protein (Nagata et al. 1981a, 1981b; Terpstra et al. 1983b; Park et al. 1987).

With a casein diet or a soybean protein diet, the serum cholesterol of male albino *Wistar* rats was associated, at varying degrees, with chylomicrons (25% and 9%, respectively) and to HDL and LDL fractions (64.6% and 82%) (Vahouny et al. 1985). VLDL-cholesterol levels (Nagata et al. 1980, 1982; Okita and Sugano 1989, 1990) and HDL-cholesterol levels were increased (Nagata et al. 1980; Park and Liepa 1982; Park et al. 1987; Baba et al. 1992; Madani et al. 1998). The plasma cholesterol concentrations of male *Wistar* rats were similar with three different levels of casein or highly purified soybean protein cholesterol-free diets (100, 200, 300 g/kg, and 50 g soybean oil/kg), but soybean protein resulted in a greater enhancement of VLDL uptake by hepatocytes than casein; it also modified the distribution of VLDL and HDL apoproteins. VLDL binding by hepatocytes was lower with the 100 g or 300 g casein or soybean protein diets than with 200 g (Prost and Belleville 1995, 1996; Prost et al. 1995, 1996). The addition of soybean globulins to a culture medium of human hepatoma cells (HepG2) increases the uptake of hepatocytes and activates LDL metabolism (Lovati et al. 1992, 1996).

When the diet of female *Sprague-Dawley* rats was rich in cholesterol, the binding to hepatic membranes of a cholesterol-rich lipoprotein fraction (β-VLDL) was normal with a soybean protein diet and reduced with a casein diet (Sirtori et al. 1984). The production of VLDL apo B was not affected, but its fractional catabolic rate in male weanling *Sprague-Dawley* rats was reduced (Cohn et al. 1984), and the serum triacylglycerol level was higher than with a soybean protein diet (Vahouny et al. 1985; Eklund and Sjöblom 1986; Iritani et al. 1986, 1988; Baba et al. 1992; Galibois et al. 1992; Ide et al. 1992; Iritani et al. 1996; Prost et al. 1996). In male weanling *Sprague-Dawley* rats, the hypercholesterolemic effect of a casein diet could be due to the decrease in VLDL catabolism (Cohn et al. 1984). However, in male *Wistar* rats, hepatic cholesterol secretion was similar with casein or soybean protein diets (Nagata et al. 1982).

The reduction of casein and soybean protein levels in the diet of male *Wistar* rats is associated on one hand with a negative correlation with plasma thiobarbituric acid-reactive substance levels, which are indicators of lipid peroxidation, and on the other hand with a positive reduced resistance of red blood cells against free-radical insult (Madani et al. 2000).

2.2.3.4 Monkeys

When casein was completely replaced by dietary soybean protein (15 g/100 g) in the diet of *Macaca fascicularis* monkeys, each diet containing cholesterol (0.05 g/100 g) for a 3-week period, serum cholesterol and LDL-cholesterol concentrations remained unchanged, but HDL-cholesterol levels increased and those of VLDL cholesterol decreased. Lipoprotein triacylglycerol levels were unchanged by this protein exchange (Barth et al. 1984). The effects of soybean protein in monkeys have therefore been shown to be different from those observed in rodents (Wolfe and Grace 1984).

2.2.4 CASEIN VERSUS SOYBEAN PROTEIN: EFFECTS ON APOPROTEINS

The turnover of apoproteins of IDL and the transfer of VLDL apoproteins to HDL isolated from rabbits fed on a semipurified diet are more rapid when the diet contains soybean protein isolates than with casein (Roberts et al. 1981). Both cholesterol and apo E in VLDL and IDL are enhanced in *New Zealand white* rabbits (Scholz et al. 1982) fed on casein (Roberts et al. 1981) or a cholesterol-rich diet (Kushawaha and Hazzard 1978; Scholz et al. 1983; Shore and Shore 1974; Shore et al. 1974). However, 6 weeks after casein was replaced by soybean protein or casein supplemented by a mixture of amino acids (glycine 3.9, arginine 6.9, alanine 1.6), the level of serum cholesterol of *New Zealand white* rabbits was reduced, but the apo E content remained elevated in VLDL and IDL. The same results were observed after the withdrawal of cholesterol from the diet, although the apo E level remained in IDL and decreased in LDL. However, the effects of these diets on the turnover rate of apo E require future investigation (Scholz et al. 1983).

Casein and soybean protein diets have different effects on VLDL- and HDL-apolipoprotein distribution in male *Wistar* rats (Prost and Belleville 1996). The production of VLDL apo B of male weanling *Sprague-Dawley* rats was not affected, but its fractional catabolic rate was reduced. Thus, lipoprotein clearance by the liver, which in the rat accounts for at least 90% of VLDL remnant removal, is affected by the nature of proteins (Cohn et al. 1984). The apo A-1 level increases LCAT activity. In contrast to a casein diet, a soybean protein diet reduces the levels of apo A-1 in the plasma (Nagata et al. 1981b, 1982; Tanaka et al. 1983a) and the lymph of male *Wistar* rats (Tanaka et al. 1983a). In the perfused rat liver of male *Wistar* rats, apo A-1 secretion was weaker when the rats had been fed with soybean protein (Sugano et al. 1982a). The plasma level of apo B was higher with soybean protein isolates (Nagata et al. 1981a) than with casein diets, whereas in another study, it was higher with a casein diet (Sanno et al. 1983). In male weanling *Sprague-Dawley* rats, the turnover of VLDL apo B was more rapid with soybean protein than with casein diets (Cohn et al. 1984). The number of lipoprotein (apo B/E) receptors on liver membranes was increased (Beynen 1990b). The levels of HDL_2 and apo E in chylomicrons, VLDL, and HDL were also reduced in male *Wistar* and *Brown-Norway* rats (Sautier et al. 1982, 1990, Sugano 1983). The data on apo B and E are therefore inconsistent. Study duration may well influence the effects of both diets (Carroll 1981b; Nagata et al. 1981a, 1981b, 1982). The incidence of plasma lipoproteins enriched in arginine-rich apolipoprotein depends on genetic factors, thyroid function, and the cholesterol content of the diet (Shore and Shore 1974).

2.2.5 CASEIN VERSUS SOYBEAN PROTEIN: EFFECTS ON POLYUNSATURATED FATTY ACIDS

Compared with casein, soybean protein increases the ratio of 20:4n-6/20:3n-6 fatty acids in liver phospholipids of cholesterol-fed male *Sprague-Dawley* rats and *Swiss albino* mice (Huang et al. 1990). Casein protects linoleate against auto-oxidation, and also acts by forming linoleate complexes that reduce oxidizable monomer fatty acid and stabilize polyunsaturated fatty acids such as cyclodextrines (Laakso 1984).

2.2.6 SUMMARY

Data concerning the respective effects of casein and soybean protein on cholesterol, lipoproteins, and lipid metabolism vary according to the animal species, genetic factors, age, and sex of the animals. In most experiments in rodents and rabbits, soybean protein is hypocholesterolemic, and casein, hypercholesterolemic. These effects also depend on the level of proteins, cholesterol, and fats, and also on the fat composition in the diet. In comparison with soybean protein, casein increases VLDL, LDL, and HDL levels, reduces their turnover because of the diminished LDL apo B receptor affinities, and decreases cholesterol turnover and the enzymatic activities of LCAT and LPL. In monkeys these effects are different when they fed on a low-cholesterol diet since the serum cholesterol and LDL-cholesterol levels are not modified by casein in contrast with a soybean protein diet. To date, too few experiments have been conducted in monkeys for any valid conclusion to be put forward.

2.3 EFFECTS OF VARIOUS TYPES OF SOYBEAN PROTEIN AND CASEIN PRODUCTS

A large number of soybean protein and casein products are now commercially available (Lusas and Riaz 1995). Diverse technological processes are used in manufacture of the products listed below.

- White flakes, made by dehulling, flaking, and defatting soybeans by hexane extraction; these are milled into defatted flour or grits, extracted using ethanol or acidic washes, thus producing soybean protein concentrates, or processed by protein alkali extraction, resulting in soybean protein isolates
- Full-fat products in toasted forms
- Dried soybean foods, chiefly soymilk and tofu
- Mixtures of soybean protein

- Textured soybean protein
- Germinated or fermented soybean
- Soybean hydrolysates
- Casein and soybean protein treated with formaldehyde
- Sodium caseinate

Protein content varies; for instance, content in isolated soybean protein is more than 90%, in textured soybean protein approximately 50%, and in soybean concentrate approximately 70% (Erdman 1995).

Ethanol extraction of soybean protein removes the isoflavones and saponins. These products lose most of their hypocholesterolemic effect, as will be described in Section 2.7.4.4 on isoflavones.

The nutritional significance of soybean protein and soybean products, particularly their protein quality, according to the technological process used, their solubility, and their digestibility (Bau et al. 1978a, 1978b), may be modified by the process of cooking (Sanchez et al. 1981; Friedman et al. 1984; Hafez et al. 1985; Woodward and Carroll 1985; Visser and Thomas 1987; Erdman and Fordyce 1989).

2.3.1 SOYBEAN PROTEIN ISOLATES

2.3.1.1 Gerbils

In normocholesterolemic young male *Mongolian* gerbils fed on a semipurified diet containing two levels (16% or 27%) of either casein or soybean protein isolates, plasma cholesterol levels were similar with both diets. When cholesterol (0.1%) was added to the diets, the increase in plasma cholesterol levels was greater with casein than with soybean protein isolates and even more marked with a diet containing 27% casein than only 16%. Serum cholesterol distribution in plasma lipoproteins was similar in young male gerbils fed either 16% or 27% casein or soybean protein isolates (Mercer 1985). However, in another study, serum cholesterol concentrations were lower in male *Mongolian Meriones unguiculatus* gerbils fed with a soybean protein isolates diet than with casein (18%) or cholesterol (0.1%) diets, although serum triacylglycerol concentrations were similar. Serum HDL-cholesterol and LDL-cholesterol concentrations, and the LDL/HDL-cholesterol ratio were lower with the soybean protein diet. Plasma insulin, thyroxine, and thyroid stimulating hormone concentrations were higher (Forsythe 1986). Hepatic reduced glutathione (GSH) concentrations were lower with soybean protein isolates. HMG-CoA reductase activity was higher in male *Meriones unguiculates* gerbils fed on soybean protein isolates. There was no correlation between GSH and HMG-CoA reductase activities. Thus, the effects of different types of dietary proteins are not due to any change in cholesterol biosynthesis mediated by GSH (Tasker and Potter 1993). Plasma lipid concentrations were similar with casein, soybean protein isolates, wheat gluten, or lactalbumin when the dietary content of cholesterol was 0.3% or 0.1%. However, with a diet containing 0.1% cholesterol, the liver cholesterol concentration of adult gerbils was lower with soybean protein isolates or wheat gluten (Lee et al. 1981).

2.3.1.2 Rabbits

In *New Zealand white* rabbits fed on a cholesterol-free, semipurified diet containing soybean protein isolates, the average total serum cholesterol level was similar to that of rabbits fed on a chow diet. VLDL- and LDL-cholesterol levels increased and HDL-cholesterol levels decreased. When soybean protein isolates were replaced by casein, the total serum cholesterol concentrations were between four and five times higher. LDL-cholesterol levels showed a sharp increase, VLDL a moderate rise, and HDL cholesterol a weak increase. With regard to the chow diet, although soybean protein isolates caused apo B, E, and C levels to rise in VLDL and LDL, the increase was more pronounced with casein (Huff and Carroll 1980b; Huff et al. 1982; Hrabeck-Smith and Carroll 1987; Samman et al. 1990b, 1990c). The turnover of apoproteins of IDL and the transfer of VLDL apoproteins to HDL isolated from young male *New Zealand white* rabbits fed on a semipurified diet were more rapid when the diet contained soybean protein isolates instead of casein (Roberts et al. 1981). In the same strain, cholesterol turnover measured by kinetic analysis, combined sterol balance, or analysis of fecal steroids by gas-liquid chromatography was faster with soybean protein isolates diet than with a casein diet, the three methods giving the same results (Huff and Carroll 1980b).

In comparison with casein, soybean protein isolates in a cholesterol-free purified diet significantly reduced total serum cholesterol, LDL-, and HDL-cholesterol levels in *New Zealand white* rabbits (Jacques et al. 1993a, 1993b). In the same species for the same level of protein (25%), soybean protein isolates, in contrast to casein, reduced lipid peroxides and the cholesterol content of atherogenic lipoproteins (β-VLDL and LDL) (Damasceno et al. 2000).

The plasma, liver, and heart cholesterol levels, and the incidence of atherosclerotic lesions of rabbits consuming soybean protein isolates with cellulose or soybean fibers for 36 weeks were lower than those of rabbits fed on casein and cellulose. Fecal bile excretion was increased in male *New Zealand white* rabbits fed on soybean fibers diet (Lo et al. 1987).

2.3.1.3 Rats and Mice

With a soybean protein isolates diet without cholesterol, the serum cholesterol and LDL-cholesterol concentrations in goldthioglucose-treated mice, genetically obese mice (*C57BL.6J ob/ob*), and rats were lower than with a casein diet, but higher than those observed with laboratory chow. Depending on study duration, fecal neutral steroid (coprostanol, cholesterol) and acid (deoxycholate) excretions were two or three times higher with soybean protein isolates than with casein, although weaker than with laboratory chow. The negative correlation between the amount of fecal steroids and plasma cholesterol levels after diets containing these different proteins proves that the former is an important factor that determines the latter (Samman et al. 1990c; Yamashita and Hayaschi 1990; Yamashita et al. 1990). This hypocholesterolemic effect was also observed in *Sprague-Dawley* rats and female mice of the *ICR* strain fed a cholesterol-free semipurified diet (Yamashita et al. 1990) or in male weanling *Sprague-Dawley* rats fed on a cholesterol-enriched diet (Aljawad et al. 1991).

In male *Wistar* rats, casein increased plasma total cholesterol, VLDL- and LDL-cholesterol, and triacylglycerol levels. HDL particles were also enhanced without any changes to HDL-cholesterol levels and only apo C was significantly increased. Liver cholesterol was not affected by different protein sources and was negatively correlated with HDL-cholesterol and HDL protein levels. These effects were removed by the addition of cholesterol to the diet (Lefevre and Schneeman 1984). The total serum cholesterol and LDL-cholesterol levels of rats were also lower with soybean protein isolates or concentrates (18%) than with casein when 0.08% cholesterol was added to the diet (Van Raaij et al. 1983; Forsythe 1986). HDL cholesterol remained unchanged and the LDL-cholesterol/HDL-cholesterol ratio was reduced with soybean protein isolates (Forsythe 1986). The plasma total cholesterol and triacylglycerol concentrations were higher and that of HDL cholesterol was lower with casein than with soybean protein isolates. During this study, which lasted 17 months, no development of atherosclerosis was observed (DiFrancesco et al. 1990).

The plasma level of apo B was higher with soybean protein isolates (Nagata et al. 1981a) than with casein diets. However, in another study it was higher with a casein diet (Sanno et al. 1983). In male *Fischer* rats, the isonitrogenous substitution for 14 days of soybean protein isolates for 50% casein in a diet containing 13-cis retinoic acid reduced the severity of retinoid-induced hypertriglyceridemia and decreased serum cholesterol concentrations (Radcliffe and Czajka-Narins 1998).

2.3.1.4 Hamsters

In hamsters on a cholesterol-enriched diet (0.2%) containing 20% soybean protein or casein, 10% fat (perilla oil, α-linolenic acid or safflower oil, linoleic acid) for 38 days, the serum and liver cholesterol concentrations were not significantly different with either diet. However, the soybean protein diet stimulated fecal steroid excretion in *Golden Syrian* hamsters, particularly with safflower oil (Gatchalian-Yee et al. 1995). When *F1B* hamsters were fed on cholesterol-enriched (0.1%), semipurified diets containing two levels (20% or 40%) of casein or soybean protein isolates and soybean protein concentrates, the plasma cholesterol levels were higher for both proteins with the 40% protein content than with the 20% level and highest with casein (Terpstra et al. 1994). Likewise, another experiment showed that unlike with a casein diet, serum cholesterol concentrations of male weanling *Golden Syrian* hamsters were lowered by soybean protein isolates or soybean protein concentrates, but cholesterol concentrations in lipoprotein fractions did not vary. Serum thyroxine and free thyroxine concentrations were higher in hamsters fed with soybean protein isolates, whereas serum triiodothyronine concentrations were lower than with a casein diet. Since both these diets decrease serum cholesterol concentrations, but only soybean protein isolates increase serum thyroxine concentrations, it is unlikely that a variation in the thyroid hormone status is the mechanism behind the cholesterol-lowering effect (Potter et al. 1996a).

2.3.1.5 Pigs

In young male *Yorkshire* swine (Kim et al. 1978, 1980a, 1983) and in adult *Göttingen* minipigs (Pfeuffer et al. 1988a), soybean protein concentrates and soybean protein isolates have the same effects, but fecal bacterial protein excretion in male adult *Göttingen* minipigs is increased with the soybean protein diet. In adult *Göttingen* miniature pigs fed on a semisynthetic cholesterol-enriched (1%) diet based on either casein or soybean protein isolates for 6 weeks, the quantitative variations in the serum amino acid concentrations were less marked than expected from the amino acid composition of the dietary proteins (Hagemeister et al. 1990).

2.3.1.6 Monkeys

Total serum cholesterol levels did not change significantly in one male and seven female *Macaca fascicularis* monkeys fed on a semipurified cholesterol diet containing corn starch (50%) and sucrose (10%) after the exchange of casein for soybean protein isolates and vice versa. However, the HDL-cholesterol and VLDL-cholesterol concentrations were higher and lower, respectively, after the soybean protein diet than after the casein diet (Barth et al. 1984).

2.3.2 Soybean Protein Extracts of High or Low Molecular Weight and Undigested Fractions of Soybean Protein

The digestion of soybean by pepsin or by microbial exo- or endo-proteases produces extracts of high- or low-molecular weight. In young male *Sprague-Dawley* rats fed on a supplemented cholesterol-rich diet, the former are significantly more hypocholesterolemic than the latter. The high-molecular-weight fraction binds conjugated bile salts *in vitro* (Sugano et al. 1988b, 1990a) and thereby increases the catabolism of LDL and lower plasma LDL cholesterol in animals (Sugano et al. 1990a; Sugano and Koba 1993) as in women (Wang et al. 1995). The reduction of the serum cholesterol level is dose dependent (Terpstra et al. 1982b; Sugano et al. 1983, 1984, 1988b, 1990a). A cholesterol-rich diet containing soybean extracts of high-molecular weight does not enhance liver cholesterol levels because these extracts act as hydrophobic peptides bound to bile acids in the intestine. They cause a strong and significant increase in neutral and acid steroid fecal excretions. This effect is not due to the soybean saponins contained in these extracts, since at the same dietary level they do not lower serum cholesterol concentrations (Sugano et al. 1990a, 1990b; Sugano and Goto 1990).

In *Sprague-Dawley* rats or *Golden Syrian* hamsters, and irrespective of the cholesterol-content, the undigested fraction of soybean protein in a diet had a greater hypocholesterolemic effect than soybean protein itself (Sugano et al. 1988b; Sugano et al. 1990a, 1990b; Ogawa et al. 1992; Gatchalian-Yee et al. 1994, 1997). Likewise, the debittered undigested fraction of soybean protein is more hypocholesterolemic than soybean protein in hamsters on a cholesterol-enriched diet (0.2%) and its effects are similar to those of the undigested fractions of soybean protein. The HDL-cholesterol/total cholesterol ratio is unchanged. Undigested fractions stimulate fecal excretion of neutral and acidic steroids. Soybean protein reduces the desaturation of linoleic acid to arachidonic acid presumably as a result of the reduced activity of Δ6-desaturase. Both undigested fractions interfere more than soybean protein with the desaturation systems with a stronger influence on the fatty acid composition of liver phospholipids (Gatchalian-Yee et al. 1997).

2.3.3 Germinated or Fermented Soybean

Technological processing of soybean, such as germination (Bau and Debry 1979; Chandrasiri et al. 1990) and fermentation using *Rhizopus oligosporus* (Guermani et al. 1993), breaks up one or several factors responsible for the hypocholesterolemic effect since serum cholesterol concentrations are higher when rats are fed with these products than with heated soybean flour.

Soybean germination increased plasma cholesterol concentrations in *Wistar* rats (Chandrasiri et al. 1990). The addition of methionine (1%) to heated soybean flour increases serum triacylglycerol concentrations in *Wistar* rats, but this effect disappears with proteins from germinated soybean (Chandrasiri et al. 1991). The fermentation of soybeans decreases the isoflavone content, but as it also increases isoflavone urinary recovery, it is probable that it enhances the availability of isoflavones in soybean (Hutchins et al. 1995). Tempeh is a fermented soybean product. The addition of tempeh to a high-cholesterol diet does not improve dyslipemia in *Cynomolgus macaques* (Ungerer et al. 1998). In rats fed with tempeh, total serum cholesterol and triacylglycerol levels were lower than with a casein diet. The lower concentration of malondialdehyde in the tempeh group was correlated with a greater activity of the enzyme superoxidedismutase. Thus, tempeh has the capacity to inhibit lipid peroxidation (Astuti 1996).

2.3.4 Soybean Protein Hydrolysates

Total and non–HDL-cholesterol levels were reduced to a greater extent in mice fed for a 3-week period on soybean peptide meal than in those fed on soybean protein isolates (Komatsu et al. 1998). Soybean protein peptic hydrolysate inhibits cholesterol absorption and reduces serum cholesterol in Caco-2 cells (Nagaoka et al. 1997).

2.3.5 Casein and Soybean Protein Treated
with Formaldehyde

Processing casein with formaldehyde modifies its tertiary structure, reduces its digestibility, and induces an increase in serum cholesterol concentrations when cholesterol is added to the diet of *New Zealand white* rabbits (Beynen et al. 1986a; Kuyvenhoven et al. 1989). The same effect is obtained with male *Zucker* rats, whereas in obese female *Zucker* rats, it increases serum cholesterol concentrations. This increase is significantly weaker in rabbits since it is comparable to that obtained with soybean protein (Terpstra et al. 1982c).

The treatment of soybean protein with formaldehyde has no influence on serum cholesterol concentrations (Terpstra et al. 1982c). Bile acid absorption can be decreased by these proteins when incompletely digested, and also by increased excretion of neutral steroids. Thus, serum cholesterol concentrations appear to be lower (Sklan et al. 1979; Terpstra et al. 1982c). The same results are observed in male *New Zealand white* rabbits (West et al. 1984). Nevertheless, it has not been clearly established whether the digestibility of proteins is an important factor in their effects on serum cholesterol levels of male *New Zealand white* rabbits (West et al. 1984), lean female and obese *Zucker* rats (Beynen et al. 1985b), or male *SPF New Zealand white* rabbits (West et al. 1990). Intestinal absorption of sterols is the same in rabbits fed on casein or casein treated by formaldehyde, but it is different in rabbits fed with soybean protein (West et al. 1989).

2.3.6 Sodium Caseinate

The increase in serum cholesterol concentrations is similar with casein or sodium caseinate. However, with sodium caseinate, the serum triacylglycerol level of male *Wistar* rats is lower than with a casein diet (Guermani et al. 1992).

2.3.7 Summary

Several soybean protein and casein products processed by various techniques are available for animals and humans. The most well known are tofu, tempeh, soymilk, soybean protein isolates, and textured vegetable proteins. Experiments in rabbits, rats, and hamsters have shown that soybean protein isolates are not as hypercholesterolemic as casein in a diet with or without cholesterol. In pigs, soybean protein isolates and concentrates are similarly hypocholesterolemic. In monkeys fed on a semipurified cholesterol-rich diet containing corn and sucrose, the effects of casein are comparable to those of soybean protein isolates on total cholesterol, but HDL cholesterol and VLDL cholesterol are, respectively, higher and lower. In gerbils, they are different for cholesterol only with a cholesterol-rich diet, whereas for serum triacylglycerol concentrations they are similar. The serum insulin and thyroxine concentrations were higher with soybean protein isolates in gerbils and hamsters. The undigested fractions of soybean protein are more hypocholesterolemic than soybean protein in rats and hamsters fed on a cholesterol-rich diet; the same applies to hydrolysates in mice. The high-molecular extracts of soybean protein are also more hypocholesterolemic than the low-molecular extracts. Germinated products, like ethanol extracts, are less hypocholesterolemic because of a partial loss of isoflavones. Lastly, sodium caseinate has the same effects as casein.

2.4 INFLUENCE OF DIETARY FOOD ENVIRONMENTS ON EFFECTS OF SOYBEAN PROTEIN AND CASEIN

Food environments can modify the effects of soybean protein and casein on serum lipids and cholesterol concentrations by several factors. The food environment, especially dietary fats and cholesterol, and also other components such as nonstarch polysaccharides, minerals, dietary fibers, saponins, and isoflavones should therefore be given particular consideration in the context of studies on casein and soybean protein, and also those on vegetable proteins (Greer et al. 1966; review in Shutler et al. 1987a, 1987b).

2.4.1 BALANCE

Casein and soybean protein effects are partly dependent on the balance of the diet. As has often been previously described, they are strongly influenced by the addition of cholesterol to the diet. The nonprotein components of a diet have to be carefully balanced (Lapré et al. 1989). When the diet is well balanced, serum cholesterol concentrations are normal, but since animal proteins increase liver cholesterol and decrease bile acid excretion, it is probable that certain mechanisms, such as decreased liver cholesterol synthesis, have a compensating effect (Lapré et al. 1989).

2.4.2 FATTY ACID CONTENT

The nature and amount of fats in the diet interfere with the effects of proteins on serum lipid and cholesterol (Nagata et al. 1980; Sugano et al. 1988a; Fernandez and McNamara 1991). Numerous study results have already been described in Section 2.2.1.

The serum cholesterol concentrations are similar in young *Single Comb White Leghorn* chickens fed for a 4-week period on casein plus fish oil or soybean protein plus fish oil diets (Choi and Chee 1995a), but in chickens fed on a casein diet, serum cholesterol concentrations are higher when maize oil is added to the diet compared to the addition of fish oil (Choi and Chee 1995b).

With a low-fat diet, the effects of proteins on serum cholesterol concentrations are more pronounced than with a high-fat diet in rabbits (Carroll and Hamilton 1975), *Wistar, Sprague-Dawley,* or *Donryu* rats, and female *ICR* strain mice and obese mice (ob/ob) from the *C57BL/6J* strain (Nagata et al. 1980; Yamashita et al. 1990). Inbred rabbits of the *IIIVO/Ju* and *AX/JU* strains that are either hyper- or hypo-responsive to dietary cholesterol are also hyper- or hypo-responsive with a cholesterol-free diet to the fat source (and more so with coconut fat than with corn oil) (Beynen et al. 1986a), but this difference is not observed if the diet of male *New Zealand white* rabbits is rich in cholesterol (Beynen et al. 1986c). Large amounts of polyunsaturated fat in the diet of rabbits erase the induction of hypercholesterolemia by a casein diet (Lambert et al. 1958; Wigand 1959). When the P/S ratio of the diet is low, the effects of proteins on serum cholesterol concentrations are more patent than if this ratio is high (Carroll and Hamilton 1975; Hamilton and Carroll 1976).

In genetically obese mice (*C57BL/-J ob/ob*) and in obese goldthioglucose-treated female mice of the *ICR* strain fed on low- or high-fat diets (0% or 30%), no difference is observed if they are fed on casein or soybean protein isolates (Yamashita and Hayashi 1990).

Most studies have been performed in rats and with a diet containing 20% proteins and approximately 11% fats. In male weanling *Sprague-Dawley* rats fed on high-fat, cholesterol-enriched diets containing casein, soybean protein or whey protein, liver weight, liver total lipids, and cholesterol levels were higher in rats fed on casein and whey than in those fed on soybean protein. However, although VLDL cholesterol levels were lower in rats fed on soybean protein than in those fed on casein, there were no significant differences between the total serum, HDL-, and LDL-cholesterol concentrations observed in the three protein groups (Aljawad et al. 1991). The effects of casein on *Sprague-Dawley* rats were compared with those of soybean protein and depending on their association with different types of fats: menhaden oil (fatty acids: saturated 28.2%, monounsaturated 23%, linoleic 1.8%, arachidonic 2.3%, eicosapentaenoic 16%, docosahexaenoic 10.8%, cholesterol 5.23 mg/g), or coconut oil (fatty acids: saturated 92% with 48.5% lauric acid, monounsaturated 6.5%, polyunsaturated 1.5%). In addition, these diets contained 10 mg/g of cholesterol and maize oil. With regard to coconut oil, when menhaden oil was associated with soybean protein, but not with a casein diet, serum triacylglycerol concentrations were reduced. The cholesterol level in lipoproteins was not modified by either of these two types of oils, and the lipids and proteins did not interact with the liver cholesterol concentrations (Demonty et al. 1998). On the other hand, in young rats more than in old rats, and compared with casein, soybean protein enhanced the hypocholesterolemic effect of maize oil to a greater extent than sardine oil. However, the reduction in liver cholesterol concentrations of male *Sprague-Dawley* rats is greater in old than in young rats (Choi et al. 1989a, 1989b, 1990). In male *Wistar* rats fed with a casein diet (8% to 35%) and corn oil (5% to 20%), the plasma cholesterol concentrations rose with the increase of casein, but this enhancement was reduced by increased corn oil intake. The effects on plasma triacylglycerol concentrations were similar but weaker. Increased corn oil intake raised liver cholesterol and triacylglycerol concentrations to a greater extent than casein (Takeuchi et al. 2000). The difference in fat content between soybean protein isolates (up to 5%) with polyunsaturated fatty acids, or casein (only about 1% of fat) has to be taken into account.

Perilla oil, which is rich in α-linoleic acid, produced a greater decrease in serum cholesterol concentrations of male *Sprague-Dawley* rats than carthame oil, and this effect was enhanced with soybean protein more so than with casein. Similar effects were observed for serum triacylglycerol concentrations, although there was no synergistic interaction. The arachidonic acid/linoleic acid ratio was lower and that of eicosapentaenoic acid/arachidonic acid higher in male *Sprague-Dawley* rats when perilla oil was combined with soybean protein rather than with casein (Sakono et al. 1993).

Casein stimulates linoleic acid and α-linolenic acid metabolism and prostacyclin production to a greater extent than soybean protein; these effects have been observed in *SHR-SP* rats (Ikeda et al. 1994). However, in another study in *ExHC Takatsuki* substrain rats, the addition of α-linolenic acid-rich perilla oil or linoleic-rich safflower oil to casein or soybean protein diets did not change the respective effects of these proteins (Ikeda et al. 1993). When casein or soybean protein diets were supplemented with 0.4% eicosapentaenoic acid, serum triacylglycerol and cholesterol concentrations of *SHRSP* in *normotensive Wistar-Kyoto* strain rats were only reduced with the casein diet. In rats fed with soybean protein, these effects are observed only if the diet was supplemented by 0.3% L-methionine (Kimura et al. 1990). In male *New Zealand white* rabbits, the effects on lipoprotein levels of the addition of various oils (maize oil, hydrogenated sunflower oil, coconut oil) to a diet containing soybean protein and dextrose have been investigated. Although serum cholesterol concentrations were normal with maize oils or sunflower oil, they were high with coconut oil. Serum concentrations of all lipoprotein fractions were increased, chiefly the IDL fraction. In the liver, concentrations of free and esterified cholesterol and phospholipids were also enhanced (Bauer 1990, 1991).

In adult swine fed either on a human-type diet of mixed foods or on a purified diet with changes in the amount and type of fat (butter, olive oil, corn oil) or in the amount of proteins and fat, serum cholesterol concentrations increased, the greatest rise being observed with saturated fats (Barnes et al. 1959a). The effects of two different polyunsaturated/saturated fat ratios (3.0 and 0.3) were investigated in comparison with a soybean protein control diet in young male pigs fed for 12 to 14 weeks with an isocaloric diet containing cholesterol (0.6 mg/kcal) and 16% of energy from protein (either 50% soybean protein plus 25% each from corn and wheat or 90% from casein plus 10% from lactalbumin). As has frequently been demonstrated, the consumption of a plant protein diet reduces serum cholesterol and HDL-cholesterol levels. Serum cholesterol is also lower, without any modification of HDL-cholesterol levels, with a polyunsaturated fat diet than with saturated fats. These results show that the hypocholesterolemic effect of plant proteins is equivalent to that of polyunsaturated fatty acids in growing male *purebred Yorkshire* or *Yorkshire x Hampshire* pigs (Forsythe et al. 1980) as has already been shown in humans (Bronte-Stewart et al. 1956; Jackson et al. 1978).

2.4.3 CHOLINE AND LECITHIN CONTENT

The biochemical, physiologic, and pharmacologic aspects of choline have been reviewed by Zeisel (1981). The effects of the choline and lecithin content of the diet have been studied above all in rats. Hypercholesterolemia is induced in rats on a diet containing cholesterol, cholic acid, and saturated fat. Hypolipemia, hypocholesterolemia, and hypo-β-lipoproteinemia are observed in rats on soybean protein diets low in choline or methionine. The addition of cholesterol to a choline-deficient diet does not lead to hyperlipemia and hypercholesterolemia. In male *Wistar* rats, dietary cholesterol only induces hypercholesterolemia in the presence of dietary choline (Wilgram et al. 1957). A low-choline diet fortified with choline (0.3%) induces a hyperlipemia in young *Sprague-Dawley* of *Holtzman* strain rats (Olson et al. 1958b). The addition of casein to the choline diet of male *Holtzman* strain rats alleviates hypercholesterolemia, and supplementing a choline diet with quantities of methionine equal to those of casein has the same effect. Cysteine or cystine, but not taurine, were as effective as methionine. However, methionine had two opposing effects on serum cholesterol concentrations in rats fed on a hypercholesterolemic choline-free diet: a cholesterol-elevating effect due to its capacity to spare choline by providing a supply of preformed methyl groups, and a cholesterol-lowering effect common to sulfur-containing amino acids and not dependent on the provision of methyl groups (Seidel et al. 1960).

The substitution of casein for soybean protein without the addition of choline in the diet of young *Sprague-Dawley* male rats of the *Holtzman* strain minimized hypolipemia and the hypo-β-lipoproteinemia presumably because of the increased methionine content (Olson et al. 1958a). There is a close metabolic interdependence between choline and cholesterol in rats (Pilgeram and Greenberg 1955), since marked hyperlipemia and hypercholesterolemia were both observed in *Wistar* rats only in the presence of dietary choline (Wilgram et al. 1957). The addition of cholesterol to diets supplemented with adequate choline resulted in atheroma in the coronary arteries and aorta of older rats (Wissler et al. 1954; Bragdon and Mikelsen 1955; Fillios et al. 1956). In contrast to the data of Ridout et al. (1954), and possibly because of the differences in the diets used, a choline-deficient diet reduced the liver cholesterol content in *Holtzman* strain rats (Seidel et al. 1960). The fat content of the liver was enhanced by cholesterol supplementation of a choline-deficient diet of *Wistar* rats (Wilgram et al. 1957).

Methionine supplementation lowered serum cholesterol concentrations in chickens fed on a hypercholesterolemic diet containing choline (Nishida et al. 1958). A high level of choline in a high-cholesterol diet enhanced serum cholesterol concentrations in rats. The addition of glycine, however, prevented this effect in male *Wistar* rats, whereas adding methionine increased it (Sugiyama et al. 1987).

Soybean lecithin is a phospholipid extract that is particularly rich in phosphatidylcholines. After hydrolysis by a phospholipase A1 and the action of triglyceride lipase, phosphatidylcholines reach the liver via endothelial capillaries. Phosphatidylcholines promote rapid transfer of phospholipids and nonesterified cholesterol from lipoproteins to tissue membranes and contribute a small percentage to biliary phosphatidylcholine (review in Chanussot et al. 1996). The active synthesis of phosphatidylcholine is necessary for very low-density lipoprotein secretion from rat hepatocytes (Yao and Vance 1988). In normolipidemic rats, the cholesterol-lowering effect of soybean lecithin on total plasma and HDL cholesterol is associated with an enhancement of biliary lipid secretion and bile formation. Bile phosphatidylcholine, bile salts, and cholesterol levels are significantly higher. Choline contributes to the beneficial effect of a lecithin diet on bile lipid secretion in male *Wistar* (Polichetti et al. 1996) and male *Sprague-Dawley* rats (LeBlanc et al. 1998). The effects of soybean lecithin have also been investigated in male *New Zealand white* rabbits fed on a cholesterol diet (0.2%) enriched with 5% saturated lard triacylglycerols, 5% polyunsaturated soybean triacylglycerols (HS diet), or a 5% polyunsaturated soybean pure lecithin (LE diet). Compared with the HS diet, the LE diet significantly decreased plasma β-VLDL-cholesterol and triacylglycerol levels. HMG-CoA reductase activity was not increased and there was no additional hepatic accumulation of lipid-rich vesicles (Chanussot et al. 1998).

In eleven young male *New Zealand white* rabbits on a diet containing 1% cholesterol repeated intravenous injection of a relatively saturated lecithin (ovolecithin) suspension diminished hepatic steatosis, but did not protect the aorta against atheroma, whereas similar injections of a polyunsaturated lecithin (Lipostabil) protected these rabbits from both fatty liver and aortic atheroma. This lipotrophic action is probably due to the "detergent" and dispersing action of phospholipids on hydrophobic lipids (Adams et al. 1967).

In male *Cynomolgus Macaca fascicularis* monkeys fed for 8 weeks on an American Heart Association (AHA) Step 1 diet supplemented or not by 3.4% soybean lecithin, the cholesterol-lowering efficacy of the AHA diet was enhanced by the addition of soybean lecithin with no reduction in plasma HDL-cholesterol and triacylglycerol levels. In male *F1B* hamsters, a similar experiment showed the same effects on cholesterol and triacylglycerol levels, but also on aortic fatty streaks.

According to some researchers, the hypocholesterolemic and antiatherogenic properties of soybean lecithin cannot be attributed solely to its linoleate content (Wilson et al. 1998b).

2.4.4 CHOLESTEROL CONTENT

As previously mentioned, the addition of cholesterol to the diet usually modifies the effects of proteins on serum cholesterol concentrations. Several other experiments have studied the influence of the cholesterol content of a diet on lipid levels and cholesterol serum concentrations. Depending on the cholesterol content of the diet, the changes in serum cholesterol concentrations are species dependent. Comparison of the results of different experiments shows that the most sensitive species are (in decreasing order) rabbits, guinea pigs, rats, hamsters, pigs, and monkeys, whereas mice, chickens, and calves are not sensitive to changes of cholesterol levels in the diet (Dietschy and Wilson 1970a, 1970b, 1970c; Mol et al. 1982; Beynen and Schoulten 1983; Terpstra et al. 1983c; Weinans and Beynen 1983; Barth et al. 1984; Mahfouz-Cercone et al. 1984; Cho et al. 1985; West and Beynen 1988; Lin et al. 1992; Fernandez et al. 1999a, 1999b).

With a cholesterol-free diet, the various dietary proteins have only a minor or no effect at all in chickens (Johnson et al. 1958) in male cockerels originating from the cross between *New Hampshire* male and *Columbian* females (Hevia and Visek 1979a) and *White Carneau* pigeons (Lofland et al. 1966). However, in one study of male crossbred broiler chickens, the addition of cholesterol to the diet increased serum cholesterol concentrations and caused a shift in the lipoprotein pattern from LDL to IDL and VLDL, regardless of whether the groups were fed on casein or soybean protein (Mol et al. 1982). Semipurified cholesterol-enriched diets (12 g/kg diet) containing two levels (20% w/w) of casein or soybean protein for 29 days, resulted in a greater increase in the levels of serum cholesterol compared with the same cholesterol-free diets in female broiler chickens. The excess of serum cholesterol and phospholipids in the 20%-protein group affected mainly the VLDL and to a lesser degree, the IDL fraction, whereas the cholesterol and phospholipid levels were decreased in the LDL fraction. However, this effect was prevented by the 50% (w/w) casein or soybean protein diets (Terpstra et al. 1983d).

In male *Wistar* rats, the hypocholesterolemic effect of soybean protein compared to casein was more significant when cholesterol was added to the diet (Okita and Sugano 1989, 1990), but this hypocholesterolemic effect was suppressed by the addition of choline to the diet of young male *Sprague-Dawley* of the *Holtzman* strain rats (Olson et al. 1958a). In male *Sprague-Dawley* rats fed on a cholesterol-rich diet containing soybean protein or casein, liver concentrations of cholesterol were very high and hepatic cholesterol synthesis was reduced (Cohn and Nestel 1985). These effects can be explained by the down-regulation of hepatic B/E receptors (Kovanen et al. 1981), the hepatic E receptor being only partially suppressed in rats (Arbeeny and Rifici 1984).

Age modulates the hypocholesterolemic effect of certain proteins since a soybean protein diet, with or without cholesterol, was hypercholesterolemic in young male *Sprague-Dawley* rats, whereas in adult rats, this effect was only observed with a cholesterol-rich diet. In contrast, whey proteins were hypocholesterolemic irrespective of the age of the rats (Choi et al. 1989a).

In some experiments in rats, however, the effects of different proteins on serum cholesterol concentrations were also obtained with a free-cholesterol diet, and were more pronounced in genetically obese *Zucker* rats (Moyer and Kritchevsky 1956; de Groot 1958; Seidel et al. 1960; Nagata et al. 1980, 1981a, 1981b, 1982; Beynen et al. 1983b; LoPresto and Wada 1988; Carroll et al. 1989; Lapré et al. 1989; Yamashita et al. 1990; Baba et al. 1992; Prost and Belleville 1995). The secretion of liver cholesterol by perfused male *English shorthair* rabbit livers in a lipoprotein-free medium was enhanced by a cholesterol diet (MacKinnon et al. 1985). The addition of cholesterol (0.1%) did not modify serum cholesterol concentrations of growing male *Wistar* rats, but did increase the liver cholesterol and triacylglycerol concentrations. HMG-CoA reductase activity was reduced particularly in soybean protein-fed rats, and 7-α-hydroxylase activity was lowered only in casein-fed rats, whereas desaturase activities were reduced in both groups (Madani et al. 1998). In female *Sprague-Dawley* rats fed on a 1.2% cholesterol diet, casein or soybean protein diets had different effects on the activity of receptor-linked enzymes. Casein caused a greater down-regulation of HMG-CoA reductase than soybean. Both 7-α-hydroxylase and acyl-CoA cholesterol acyltransferase (ACATase) activity levels were significantly increased by casein, but remained in a normal range with a soybean protein diet (Sirtori et al. 1984). However, in another experiment, the same authors reported that when soybean protein was substituted for casein in diets enriched in cholesterol (2%), 7-α-hydroxylase and LCAT activities were unaffected. In contrast, cholesterol ester levels and ACATase activity were enhanced in the liver of *Sprague-Dawley* rats on the soybean protein diet (Bosisio et al. 1981).

A cholesterol-supplemented diet (2%) resulted in mild changes in plasma lipid levels, but increased pre-β-lipoprotein and decreased α-lipoprotein levels in male *Wistar* rats. Dietary cholesterol increases bile secretion and biliary excretion of total bile acids, but not those of cholesterol. Biliary cholic and deoxycholic acids are practically unchanged, but the significant increase in chenodeoxycholic acid is responsible for reductions in tissue and serum cholesterol concentrations (Uchida et al. 1977).

The increase in serum cholesterol concentrations is similar in rats and guinea pigs with a cholesterol-rich diet, but their lipoprotein distributions are different. In male *Golden Syrian* hamsters, HDL cholesterol carries 50% of the total cholesterol, whereas in guinea pigs most cholesterol is carried by LDL lipoproteins. Changes in VLDL and LDL composition were observed in male *Hartley* guinea pigs fed with a cholesterol-rich diet (Lin et al. 1994; review in Fernandez et al. 1999a, 1999b). Moreover, in male *Golden Syrian* hamsters fed with a cholesterol-rich diet (0.16 g/100 g), HDL-cholesterol levels increased reaching 50% of the total cholesterol. Serum triacylglycerol concentrations were also very high (Session et al. 1993; Fernandez et al. 1999a, 1999b). Elevations in hepatic cholesterol concentrations with a high intake of dietary cholesterol resulted in the suppression of hepatic apo B/E receptors in guinea pigs (Lin et al. 1994), and in hamsters, in the decrease in mRNA levels for the apo B/E receptors that were associated with a decrease in LDL uptake (Horton et al. 1993).

In guinea pigs, serum cholesterol concentrations remain constant whether the diet contains casein or a soybean protein high-protein (40%). However, when 1% cholesterol was added to the diet, serum cholesterol concentrations of male F_1B hamsters were higher with the casein diet (Terpstra 1982a). The type of fat and quantity of cholesterol interact and also modify the cholesterol metabolism (Lin et al. 1992).

In *Golden Syrian* hamsters, with soybean protein or casein levels of 25% in a cholesterol-free diet, the serum cholesterol, VLDL-cholesterol, LDL-cholesterol, and HDL-cholesterol concentrations (albeit nonsignificantly for the latter) were only increased with the casein diet. When cholesterol was added, the differences were more significant, but with considerable inter-individual variations (Terpstra et al. 1991).

In mature female *Swiss* mice, the increase in serum cholesterol concentrations was similar with high- and low-cholesterol diets (Weinans and Beynen 1983).

In pigs, the addition of 0.5, 1, 2, 4, or 8 g of cholesterol to casein or soybean protein diets induced an increase in serum cholesterol concentrations that was far weaker with the soybean protein diet. The addition of 8 g of cholesterol to a soybean protein diet produced an equivalent effect to that obtained with 1 g of cholesterol in a casein diet (Kim et al. 1982). In pigs (Beynen et al. 1985a) and lean *Zucker* rats (Terpstra et al. 1982a, 1982b, 1983a), or in *Sprague-Dawley* rats (Sirtori et al. 1984; Cohn et al. 1984; Tatcher et al. 1984), the hypercholesterolemic effect of casein was observed when cholesterol was added to the diet (Yadav and Liener 1977). In nonhuman primates (*Cercopithecus aethiops* monkeys), enriching the diet with cholesterol produced an increase in the size and cholesterol ester content of plasma LDL. Since these cholesterol ester-rich LDL fractions are not found in the perfusate livers of cholesterol-fed monkeys, it can be suggested that large molecular weight plasma LDLs are not directly secreted by the liver, but probably result from further intravascular metabolism of cholesteryl ester-enriched hepatic precursor lipoproteins (Johnson et al. 1983). In *Papio hamadryas* baboons, increasing both dietary fat and dietary cholesterol caused significant increase in serum lipoprotein(a) concentrations and the response to dietary cholesterol was mediated by a gene or suite of genes linked to the LPA locus (Rainwater et al. 1999).

2.4.5 CARBOHYDRATE CONTENT

The carbohydrate composition of soybeans is as follows: soluble carbohydrates, about 17% (monosaccharides 1.3%, disaccharides 8.2%, raffinose 2.4%, stachyose 4.8% [difficult to digest]), and insoluble carbohydrates, about 21%, chiefly dietary fibers (hemicellulose 15.8%, cellulose 3.6%, lignine 1.3%) (Bau 1987).

The type and amount of carbohydrates in the diet can modify the effects of proteins on lipid and cholesterol metabolism, particularly the hypercholesterolemic effect of casein in rabbits (Keys and Hodges 1967; Carroll and Hamilton 1975; Hamilton and Carroll 1976; Bauer and Covert 1984; Bauer 1987; Bergeron and Jacques 1989), in rats (Hevia et al. 1979b; Kritchevsky et al. 1982b; Jacques et al. 1986; Pfeuffer and Barth 1986b, 1992; Hurley et al. 1995) and in monkeys (Srinivasan et al. 1979). The addition of sucrose to casein enhanced its hypercholesterolemic effect in *New Zealand white* rabbits. The IDL- and LDL-cholesterol levels increased, whereas those of HDL cholesterol decreased. Sucrose supplementation in a soybean protein diet produced a weak increase in IDL-cholesterol levels (Bauer and Covert 1984). In the same strain of rabbits, a sucrose-rich diet including casein or soybean protein increased the level of protein and phospholipids in HDL and of cholesterol in IDL (Bauer 1987). Compared to cornstarch and dextrose, molasses-enriched dextrose in a high-fat, cholesterol-free, casein-purified diet, did not significantly increase serum cholesterol concentrations of male *New Zealand white* rabbits. However, the LDL-cholesterol level and liver cholesterol and triacylglycerol concentrations were enhanced. Corn starch and dextrose induced a significant increase in HDL cholesterol and a decrease (4.3-fold) in the LDL-cholesterol/HDL-cholesterol ratio (Bergeron and Jacques 1990).

In a diet containing 20% protein (casein, soybean, or cod proteins), 60% carbohydrate (maize starch or sucrose) and 20% lipids, sucrose (in comparison with maize starch) induced a reduction in hepatic cholesterol and triacylglycerol concentrations in rats, regardless of the type of proteins. The interactions between carbohydrates and lipids affected postprandial insulin secretion, which is higher in *Sprague-Dawley* rats with a combination of casein-sucrose and cod protein-maize starch than with soybean protein and these carbohydrates (Hurley et al. 1995). In male *Wistar* rats fed on a casein or a soybean protein isolates diet containing either sucrose or starch (69 g/100 g) for 6 weeks, the plasma cholesterol levels and the rates of secretion of VLDL cholesterol and triacylglycerols were higher, by 27%, 47%, and 34%, respectively, in animals fed on casein plus sucrose than in those fed on soybean protein isolates plus sucrose. When starch was used to replace sucrose, these differences were weak or nonexistent. Thus, in contrast with dietary starch, dietary sucrose increased hepatic cholesterol secretions (Pfeuffer and Barth 1992).

2.4.6 Dietary Fiber Content

The majority of dietary fibers reduce the hypercholesterolemic effect of proteins: alfalfa, bean products, guar gum, lignin, oat bran, pectin, psyllium extract, raw potato starch, soybean fibers, and sugar-beet fibers. Cellulose and wheat bran, however, have no effect (Kritchevsky et al. 1977; Kritchevsky and Story 1978; Kritchevsky 1979; Anderson and Chen 1979; Kim et al. 1981; Chen et al. 1984; Cho 1985; review in Anderson and Tietyen-Clark 1986; Aritsuka et al. 1989, 1992; Moundras et al. 1998; Fernandez et al. 1999a).

It must not be forgotten that the comparison of casein and soybean protein effects is not only a comparison between these two proteins, but also between the environments of the components. It is therefore important to consider the role of the dietary fiber components of soybean protein when the effects of these proteins are compared with those of casein. Their components are cellulosic and noncellulosic, especially neutral arabinogalactan and pectin-related acidic polysaccharides. The detailed composition of soybean fibers has been described by several authors (Lo 1990; Englyst and Cummings 1990; Slavin 1991; Morris 1992; Asp et al. 1992), as have their physiological effects (Schweizer et al. 1983; Schweizer and Edwards 1992).

In *Golden Syrian* hamsters and male *Hartley* guinea pigs fed for a 4-week period on semipurified diets containing 22.5 g/100 g of soybean protein and three different doses of dietary pectin (2.7; 5.4; 10.7/100 g) added instead of cellulose, the plasma cholesterol concentration was only lowered with the dose of 10.7/100 g. Plasma cholesterol differences concern LDL cholesterol in guinea pigs and both non–HDL and HDL cholesterol in hamsters. If cholesterol was added to a diet containing 10.7/100 g of dietary pectin, the plasma LDL-cholesterol levels were highest in guinea pigs and hamsters with 0.16 g/100 g cholesterol in comparison with 0.04 and 0.08/100 g of cholesterol. These supplements are equivalent to 300, 600, and 1,200 mg/day in humans (Fernandez et al. 1999a).

In 8-week-old pigs fed on either a cholesterol-containing or a cholesterol-free diet and casein or soybean protein, the serum concentrations of triacylglycerols and phospholipids were similar. However, the serum cholesterol concentration increased with casein and soybean protein when the diet was supplemented by cholesterol. With the addition of dietary fibers of soybean, the reduction in serum cholesterol concentrations was more pronounced with a soybean protein diet than a casein diet and had a greater effect on LDL cholesterol than on VLDL or HDL cholesterol (Cho et al. 1985).

In a diet containing fat (20%) and cholesterol (1%), the effects of sweet white and sweet yellow lupin diets (lysine/arginine ratios of 0.5 and 0.4, respectively) on cholesterol metabolism were compared to those of casein (lysine/arginine ratio 1.8) in male Wistar rats after 28 days. The total fiber content was casein 5%, sweet white lupin 22%, and sweet yellow lupin 17%. There was a balanced methionine content in the diet. No significant difference in total serum cholesterol levels was observed between the three groups. Both lupin diets increased glucagon levels, and sweet white lupin significantly decreased plasma triacylglycerol and triacylglycerol-LDL levels and the insulin/glucagon ratio, as well as unesterified liver cholesterol levels. Sweet yellow lupin significantly increased plasma glucose and insulin, as well as liver total cholesterol, and decreased the insulin/glucagon ratio compared to the other diets. The different fiber contents between the sweet white and sweet yellow lupin may well modulate the insulin/glucagon ratio and the effect on cholesterol metabolism (Chango et al. 1998).

Various hypotheses have been suggested to explain the mechanisms behind the effects of dietary fibers:

- Differences in the water-holding capacity of dietary fibers may account for the various effects of dietary fibers on minerals, bile acids, digestive enzymes, and the absorption time of different components of intestinal chyme (Kay 1982; Schneeman and Gallaher 1980; Dutta and Hlasko 1985).
- Enhancement of bacterial conversion of cholesterol (Tanaka et al. 1983a, 1983b).
- Damage to bacterial flora (Enle et al. 1982; Tanaka et al. 1983b).
- Reduced intestinal transit time (Vahouny et al. 1978; Anderson and Chen 1979) and intestinal reabsorption due to the binding of bile acids

(Kritchevsky and Story 1978; Vahouny et al. 1978; Story and Kritchevsky 1978).

- Production of short-chain fatty acids, including propionate, by fermentation of dietary fibers. Supplementing diets with propionate decreases the plasma cholesterol concentrations in pigs (Thacker and Bowland 1981; Thacker et al. 1981), and intracaecal infusion of propionic acid in ileally fistulated rats limits the plasma cholesterol increase caused by a casein diet without any alteration of total liver lipids or cholesterol (Ebihara et al. 1993).

Moreover, according to Pfeuffer and Barth (1990), the morphologic changes in intestinal mucosa caused by dietary fibers (Jacobs 1983) or soybean protein (Seegraber and Morril 1982) may be involved in the effects of dietary fibers and soybean protein fibers.

2.4.7 Mineral and Vitamin Content

Variations in mineral intake, particularly calcium, zinc, and copper, influence the serum and liver concentrations of cholesterol in several experiments in rabbits (Allota et al. 1985) and in male weanling *Sprague-Dawley* rats. Adding minerals to the diet of rats, as recommended by the National Research Council, decreased serum cholesterol concentrations and increased the HDL-cholesterol/LDL-cholesterol plus VLDL-cholesterol ratios. It also reduced liver lipid concentrations (Murthy et al. 1982).

In young male *New Zealand white* rabbits if the mineral content of a casein diet was 2.5% instead of the normal level of 4%, the serum cholesterol concentration was higher, and the levels of cholesterol in LDL, HDL, and LDL were increased. The rate of production of the fractional catabolic rate of VLDL apo B was lower. However, the kinetics of LDL apo B were the same in both groups. These modifications are probably due to reduced LDL-receptor affinity and to a reduction in fecal steroid excretion (Samman et al. 1990a).

The mineral content varies in different soybean products. Mineral content and availability have been assessed in soybeans with oil extract, soybean protein concentrates, and soybean protein isolates (Waggle and Kolar 1979; O'Dell 1979; Steinke 1992). The mineral content, particularly iron, copper, manganese, and zinc, is less efficiently used than that of animal proteins (O'Dell 1979).

2.4.7.1 Calcium Content

In soybeans, phytate binds with almost all the calcium and half the phosphorus. It also binds with others bi- or trivalent cations such as iron, copper, zinc, and molybdenum, but the degree of binding varies according to the soybean product technologies (Chervan 1980; Thompson and Erdman 1982; Graf 1983; Forbes et al. 1984; Fordyce et al. 1987; Erdman and Fordyce 1989).

Increasing dietary calcium content (from 0.84% to 1.44%) reduced the enhancing effect of casein on total and free cholesterol serum concentrations in rats and on the free cholesterol/ phospholipids ratio. In contrast, a calcium supplement in a soybean protein diet had no influence in young male *New Zealand white* rabbits (van der Meer et al. 1985b), probably due to the binding of calcium with the phytate content of soybeans (Grynspan and Cheryan 1989). Thus, the calcium-increasing effect of casein is calcium dependent and the degree of casein-phosphorylation influences the casein effect on serum cholesterol in male *New Zealand white* rabbits (van der Meer et al. 1985a, 1988). This effect is, however, species dependent (van der Meer 1988). Lastly, a diet rich in proteins from soybeans, beef, or lactalbumin induced calciuria, sulfaturia, and aciduria in male *Sprague-Dawley* rats (Whiting and McNally 1989).

2.4.7.2 Zinc, Copper, and Magnesium Content

In order to assess the effects produced by mineral level changes in the diet, the casein and soybean protein levels must be taken into account (Klevay 1994). Soybean protein contains more copper and zinc than casein. The ratio of zinc/copper is far higher in casein than in soybean protein (Allotta et al. 1985; Roberts and Samman 1990). The respective concentrations of zinc and copper in soybean protein are 40 ppm and 12 ppm (40 mg/kg and 12 mg/kg), and the zinc/copper ratio is 3.33 (O'Dell 1979). The copper concentration in soybean flour is higher (40-50 mg/g) especially when the lipid content is low (Human Nutrition Information Service 1993). In soybean protein isolates, the respective concentrations of zinc and copper are 34 ppm and 15 ppm (34 mg/kg and 15 mg/kg) and the zinc/copper ratio is 2.27 (Steinke 1992). In casein, the zinc content is considerably higher than the copper content. Indeed, the zinc and copper contents are, respectively, 3800 µg/L and 150 µg/L in cow's milk (Gueguen 2001), and in casein 84% (3,192 µg/L) and 44% (60 µg/L), respectively, of the cow's milk zinc and copper (Renner et al. 1989).

The mineral bioavailability from soybean products has been studied in several experiments and some extensive reviews have been published (O'Dell 1979; Erdman et al. 1980; Erdman et al. 1981; Erdman and Fordyce 1989). The bioavailability of zinc from soybean-based foods is poor (Erdman and Forbes 1981; Erdman et al. 1983; Lynch 1984; Solomon and Cousins 1984) and lowered by phytate content (review in Erdman and Fordyce 1989).

Samman and Roberts (1988) have suggested that casein-induced hypercholesterolemia in young adult rabbits is due to marginal intake of zinc or zinc and copper since supplementing humans with zinc results in a decrease in LDL cholesterol. Zinc supplementation suppresses the hypercholesterolemic effect of a casein diet compared with a soybean protein diet (Samman and Roberts 1987). Nevertheless, in *Sprague-Dawley* weanling male rats fed on an egg protein (20%), cholesterol-rich, zinc-deficient diet (0.37 ppm of zinc and 7.1 ppm copper) for a 4-week period, total serum cholesterol concentrations were significantly decreased compared with those of pair-fed and ad libitum-fed zinc-supplemented controls (41 ppm zinc). A significant positive correlation was observed between the serum concentration of zinc and HDL cholesterol, whereas the serum concentration of zinc and VLDL- or LDL-cholesterol levels were not correlated. Thus, the selective decline of HDL cholesterol is the principal cause of the total serum cholesterol decrease in response to zinc depletion (Koo and Williams 1981). These data concur with the results of previous experiments (Petering et al. 1977; Philip et al. 1978).

Cow's-milk casein decreases the digestive absorption of zinc in rats (review in Lönnerdal 1984). In male *Sprague-Dawley* rats, the bioavailability of zinc from soybean or casein varies according to the protein source and the length of adaptation (Khan and Weaver 1989).

The results obtained in rabbits contrast also with those in chickens. Chickens require greater amounts of zinc when fed on soybean protein rather than on casein (O'Dell 1979). This difference is due to the action of phytate contained in soybean (Cranwell and Liebman 1989).

The effects of zinc and copper have been studied in male weanling rats fed on a casein or defatted dried milk powder (20%), cholesterol-free diet containing zinc (20 ppm) and copper (0.5 or 8 ppm) or zinc (140 ppm) and copper (0.5 or 8 ppm); serum cholesterol concentrations were increased when the copper level was low (Stemmer et al. 1985). In a group of young male rabbits of the *Castle Hill Laboratory White* strain fed on casein for 12 weeks with a range of copper concentrations (2 to 80 µg/g diet), there was a linear relationship between the cholesterolemic response and the copper concentration: the lower the copper level, the greater the response. LDL-apo B production was reduced to a greater extent when the dietary zinc level was high in the diet (Roberts and Samman 1990). When the copper level is adequate in the diet, the liver glutathione concentration and HMG-CoA reductase levels are low (Klevay 1994). A copper deficiency increases HMG-CoA reductase levels (Valsala and Kurup 1987; Yount et al. 1990; Kim et al. 1992), but only if the glutathione level is not enhanced (Kim et al. 1992). It also reduces LCAT activity (Lau and Klevay 1981; Harvey and Allen 1981) and that of lipoprotein lipase (Lau and Klevay 1982). Cardiomyopathy occurs when the diet is deficient in copper and there is an interaction between the type of protein and the dietary content in zinc and copper (review in Stemmer et al. 1985).

Compared with casein, soybean protein reduces the gastrointestinal absorption of magnesium through its phytate component. The addition of sodium phytate to a casein diet, at identical concentrations to those of a soybean diet, produced the same effect in young male *Wistar* rats (Brink et al. 1991). The phytate content, if any, and the particular concentration are therefore important criteria in the assessment of soybean products used in experimental diets. Indeed, phytate concentrations vary according to the technique of soybean processing (Chervan 1980; Erdman et al. 1983; Forbes et al. 1984; Fordyce et al. 1987).

2.4.7.3 Vitamin A and Vitamin E Content

A number of studies have investigated the interaction between dietary vitamin E, vitamin A, or protein levels and serum cholesterol concentrations in certain animal species. Chen et al. reviewed the often-conflicting results (Chen et al. 1972). The level of cholesterol in rats receiving a vitamin E-free casein diet was higher than when vitamin E was added to diet. The cholesterol lowering effect of vitamin E was proportional to the amount added; the higher the level of vitamin E, the lower the serum cholesterol level in *Sprague-Dawley* rats (Chen et al. 1972). Likewise, in other experiments, a vitamin E-free diet resulted in increased serum cholesterol concentrations in rabbits (Campbell et al. 1952), guinea pigs (Shull et al. 1958), ducklings (Dermers and Alary 1966), and hens (Koyanagi et al. 1966). The relationships between vitamin E and vitamin A have been studied in male *Sprague-Dawley* rats. Plasma cholesterol levels in vitamin E-deficient rats fed 1,200 IU of vitamin A for a 12-week period, were significantly higher than those of matched specimens fed tocopherol. Tocopherol significantly decreased liver cholesterol levels in rats fed 400 or 1,200 IU of vitamin A. Whereas total lipid and cholesterol concentrations in the liver were not significantly affected by vitamin A, they were observed to decrease in rats fed vitamin E with 400 or 1,200 IU vitamin A (Harrill et al. 1965).

However, other studies reported inconsistent observations (Weitzel et al. 1956; Verbeva 1965; Cheraskin and Ringsdorf 1970). When alpha-tocopherol was added to a cholesterol-rich diet, the increase in serum cholesterol concentrations was more rapid in rabbits (Campbell et al. 1952).

2.4.8 CONCLUSION

In most cases, a casein diet is hypercholesterolemic, whereas a soybean protein diet is hypocholesterolemic. Their different effects are influenced by the animal species and genetic factors, but also by the age and sex of the animals. For example, the data in chickens differ from those in rabbits. The impact of proteins also varies according to the dietary concentration and the amount of cholesterol. In comparison with soybean protein, casein increases VLDL, LDL and HDL levels and reduces their turnover as a result of the diminished LDL apo B receptor affinities. Casein also decreases cholesterol turnover and the enzymatic activities of LCAT and LPL. Depending on the species, these effects vary. The food environment is of considerable importance. The nature (saturated or polyunsaturated) and the amount of fats modify the effects of proteins, which are greater when their dietary concentration is either too high or too low. The role of carbohydrates and dietary fibers must also be considered. Lastly, the minerals calcium, zinc, and copper enhance the hypocholesterolemic effect of proteins when phytate is absent from the diet. However, the data collected from different animal species are not always coherent.

Several soybean and casein products, processed by various technologies, are used for both animals and humans. Their capacity to confer hypo- or hypercholesterolemic effects depends on the products, the animal species, and the food environment. Germinated products and ethanol extracts are less hypocholesterolemic because of the partial or total loss of isoflavones.

2.5 EFFECTS OF OTHER FOOD PROTEINS

Although less numerous than those using casein and soybean protein, the experiments with other types of proteins have assessed the respective effects on serum cholesterol concentrations. Thus, in rabbits, a classification can be made of the various proteins according to their respective effects on serum cholesterol concentrations. On the basis of their experiments in rabbits, Carroll and Hamilton (1975) and Sidransky (1990) have suggested the following classification in increasing order of induction: fababean protein, soybean protein, pea protein, peanut protein, wheat gluten, rapeseed flour (detoxified), raw egg white, pork protein, beef protein, fish protein, casein, lactalbumin, skimmed milk powder, and whole-egg extract. Animal proteins are therefore hypercholesterolemic, whereas vegetable proteins are hypo-cholesterolemic. However, the changes in plasma total cholesterol levels of *Sprague-Dawley* rats fed on a cholesterol-free diet were not associated with any particular protein source. Plant proteins were not found to have a hypocholesterolemic effect compared with animal proteins in young growing male *Sprague-Dawley* rats (Neves et al. 1980) or female *Sprague-Dawley* rats (Eklund and Sjöblom 1980). Likewise, in *Wistar* rats (Sautier et al. 1979), or rats (Pathirana et al. 1980) fed cholesterol-free diets, casein and soybean protein had no differential effects.

The effects of proteins depend on their nutritional value (Huff and Carroll 1980a). The quality of protein synthesis has to be sufficient to allow physiologically normal digestive absorption and lipid transport (Glickman and Kirsch 1973; Glick-man 1980). In growing male weanling *Sprague-Dawley* rats fed on various diets, each containing different proteins (casein, heat-treated casein, egg albumin, wheat gluten, soybean protein isolates, and a mixture [50/50] of wheat gluten and soybean protein isolates) there was a negative correlation between protein quality, as evaluated by its protein efficiency ratio (PER), and plasma cholesterol and HDL-choles-terol concentrations (Lefevre and Schneeman 1983).

2.5.1 Vegetable Proteins

Purified, cholesterol-free or cholesterol-enriched diets containing 15% proteins of various types (either casein or beef, fish, soybean protein isolates, pea, peanut, rapeseed, oatmeal, wheat gluten) were given alternately to male *Sprague-Dawley* rats for 3-week periods. The effects of the different diets were comparable, but more pronounced when they were enriched with cholesterol (Jacques et al. 1990). However, similar results were not obtained by other authors, as will be described later.

2.5.1.1 Wheat and Corn Gluten

In male weanling *Sprague-Dawley Holtzman* or *Rolfsmeyer* strain rats fed on either a cholesterol-free or a cholesterol-supplemented atherogenic gluten diet (100 g/kg) versus a casein diet, the serum cholesterol level remained low (Nath et al. 1959, 1961; McGregor 1971). In male weanling rats of the *Charles-River* strain supple-mentation of a wheat gluten, cholesterol-free diet with 2.8 or 0.3 g/kg threonine and 9 or 6.5 g/kg lysine (the limiting amino acids of this protein source), did not diminish the hypocholesterolemic effect of wheat gluten in rats, in comparison with a casein diet. Thus, the hypocholesterolemic effect of wheat gluten occurs independently of the low quality of the protein or its specific deficiency in lysine or threonine (Bassat and Mokady 1985). On the other hand, as the results are the same when an athero-genic diet is supplemented by lysine and threonine, the hypocholesterolemic effect of wheat gluten clearly does not depend on its lysine/arginine ratio in male weanling rats of the *Charles River CD* strain (Mokady and Einav 1978) or male weanling *Holtzman* rats (Mokady and Liener 1982). The fact that the serum cholesterol control level is lowest with a cholesterol-free diet can probably be explained by the increased fecal excretion of cholesterol. Hepatic lipogenesis and cholesterol synthesis are enhanced (Mokady and Einav 1978). However, the effect of wheat gluten on serum cholesterol concentrations varies, in lean female random-bred *Zucker* rats, according to the duration of experiments. Indeed, serum cholesterol concentrations reach their lowest level on day 14 of experiments in comparison with casein, fish, and soybean protein diet, but are comparable by the end of the month (Kuyvenhoven et al. 1987).

In young weanling male *Holtzman* rats fed on an atherogenic diet containing 2% cholesterol, 0.5% bile acids, and 10% proteins of various types (casein, soybean protein, wheat gluten, or wheat gluten supplemented with lysine and threonine), the serum cholesterol, LDL-cholesterol, HDL-cholesterol, and triacylglycerol concentrations were lower, and those of HDL cholesterol higher, than those of rats fed with a casein diet. When the diet was supplemented with lysine and threonine, serum cholesterol concentrations were similar to those obtained with soybean protein with no modifications in serum triacylglycerol concentrations (Mokady and Liener 1982).

Serum cholesterol concentrations were similar in young male *Wistar* rats fed with a diet containing 15% proteins such as casein, wheat gluten, or corn gluten, but if 1% cholesterol was added to the diet, serum cholesterol levels rose significantly with casein, but only weakly with the other two diets. Although hypercholesterolemia was induced with polychlorinated biphenyls (PCB), serum cholesterol concentrations of both groups on wheat and corn gluten were lower than those in the soybean protein group (Yoshida et al. 1990b).

2.5.1.2 Rice and Rice-Protein Concentrates

A rice diet is deficient in lysine and threonine. In rats fed a rice diet, the cholesterol content of whole liver and the hepatic Golgi apparatus is lower than is observed with a casein diet. Cholesterol synthesis and turnover are reduced in growing male *Wistar* rats, but these effects can be reversed by lysine and threonine supplements (Ghosh and Misra 1987).

In hamsters fed for 7 weeks on a diet containing 10% fat (coconut oil 69%, corn oil 19%, olive oil 12%), 0.1% cholesterol, and 20% proteins (casein or soybean protein isolates or rice protein concentrates), and 0.1% cholesterol, the plasma cholesterol and non HDL-cholesterol concentrations were reduced on average by 23% for the soybean protein and 42% and 53% for the rice protein concentrates, respectively. The hypocholesterolemic effect of rice is therefore at least as effective as that of soybean protein isolates (Tran and Nicolosi 1997).

Serum cholesterol concentrations and fecal bile acid and neutral steroid excretion were lower and higher, respectively, in male *Sprague-Dawley* rats fed on soybean protein, potato protein, or rice protein than in those fed casein diets. A stronger positive correlation was observed between cholesterol concentrations and dietary methionine concentrations or the methionine/glycine ratio (Morita et al. 1997).

If *Wistar* rats, with hypercholesterolemia induced by the addition of either 1% cholesterol and 25% cholic acid or 200 or 300 ppm of polychlorinated biphenyls (PCB), were fed an identical soybean protein isolates diet to that of hamsters, but with a protein level of 15%, the total serum cholesterol, HDL-cholesterol, liver cholesterol, and triacylglycerol concentrations were lower with soybean protein isolates than with rice protein or casein. The fecal excretion of acidic steroids in rats fed on soybean protein isolates or rice protein was greater than that of rats fed casein. The increased fecal excretion of bile acids observed with soybean protein and rice protein concentrates only partly explains the lower serum cholesterol concentrations due to soybean protein. It is likely that soybean proteins have an inhibiting effect on the absorption of bile acids from the enterohepatic circulation (Yoshida et al. 1990a, 1990b).

2.5.1.3 Other Vegetable Proteins

The total serum cholesterol levels of male *Wistar* rats fed casein or whey or alfalfa are higher than those of rats fed with soybean or fababean or peabean or sunflower proteins (Scarino et al. 1979; Sautier et al. 1983, 1990). The effects of processing on the nutritional value of sunflower or colza proteins have been studied by Bau et al. (Bau et al. 1983; Bau et al. 1987). Low plasma cholesterol levels can be maintained in hypercholesterolemic rabbits by whole haricot bean despite continued cholesterol intake (Finnigan 1983). Since fababean protein concentrates extracted by ethanol have no effect in male *Sprague-Dawley* rats, it is likely that the cholesterol-lowering action of fababean is due to other components than the proteins (Mengheri et al. 1982). In male *Wistar* rats, fecal total and neutral steroid excretion is greater with soybean protein, alfalfa, peabean, or gluten diets than with casein, whey, or sunflower protein (Sautier et al. 1990). In rabbits and rats, but not in hamsters, serum cholesterol concentrations were lower with a cottonseed protein diet than with a casein diet (Beynen and Liepa 1987). However, McGregor (1971) found that wheat gluten induced higher serum cholesterol levels than casein in rats.

The effects of isocaloric semisynthetic rations with varying protein components (casein, wheat gluten, cotton isolates, soybean, and rice proteins) on lipid transport processes in the serum can be caused by several mechanisms including altered lipolysis activity in the serum, modified hepatic production of high-density lipoproteins and free cholesterol, and impaired LDL degradation (Sharmanov et al. 1988).

Albino rats fed with 12% bengal gram (*Cicer arietinum*), black gram (*Phaseolus mungo*), red gram (*Cajanus cajan*), lentils (*Lens culinaris*), or arrowroot have a high cholesterol content and a lower phospholipid content in different tissues. Supplementing pulse protein with a mixture of methionine, lysine, threonine, and tryptophan (0.3% each) decreased the cholesterol content and increased the phospholipid content of the tissues. Supplementing lentil protein with either methionine or threonine, or those of black gram with methionine, prevented the accumulation of cholesterol in the tissues. However, supplementing these proteins with tryptophan, lysine, or threonine was ineffective (Banerjee and Chakrabarti 1973).

The effects of 20% golden pea protein and pea protein were compared, in old male *Sprague-Dawley* rats, with those of casein in a cholesterol-free or a cholesterol-containing diet. With the cholesterol-free diet, plasma cholesterol and triacylglycerol concentrations were reduced by −61% and −47%, respectively, and hepatic cholesterol by −94%. When cholesterol was added to the diet, the plasma cholesterol and triacylglycerol concentrations were reduced by −27% and −40%, respectively, whereas hepatic cholesterol concentrations were twice as high as with casein. Plasma glucose and insulin concentrations were not significantly different, and plasma apo A-1 concentrations were lower than with a casein and cholesterol-free or cholesterol-rich diet (Lasekan et al. 1995).

In young male *Sprague-Dawley* rats fed on a cholesterol-rich diet containing buckwheat protein for 3 weeks, serum cholesterol concentrations decreased considerably (Kayashita et al. 1995) and fecal excretion of neutral sterols, but not acidic sterols, increased. However, if the diet of young male *Wistar* rats was cholesterol-free, these effects were weak (Kayashita et al. 1996). The action of buckwheat protein would appear to be similar to that of dietary fibers and to be due to its low digestibility. Indeed, although buckwheat protein is partially digested by trypsin, the hypocholesterolemic effect is partially decreased. The lysine/arginine ratio is lower in buckwheat protein than in a casein diet, but an arginine-supplemented casein diet does not modify the results in young male *Sprague-Dawley* rats (Kayashita et al. 1997). Total cholesterol and LDL- and HDL-cholesterol serum concentrations were lower in male *New Zealand white* rabbits fed on peanut meal in a purified diet than with a casein diet, but the triacylglycerol serum levels were higher with a peanut-meal diet than with a casein or a soybean protein isolates diet (Jacques et al. 1993a, 1993b).

The protein quality of proso millet is poor since its biological value is 63.8. Indeed, the scores of its first and second limiting amino acids, lysine, and threonine, are 25 and 75, respectively as calculated on the basis of a joint effort by the Food and Agriculture Organization, World Health Organization, and United Nations University (FAO/WHO/UNU 1985; Nishizawa et al. 1989). In male *BALB/c CrSlc* mice (Nishizawa and Fudamoto 1995), and in male *Sprague-Dawley* rats (Nishizawa et al. 1996) fed on proso millet protein the total serum cholesterol and HDL-cholesterol levels increased without any rise in serum LDL-cholesterol concentrations.

The effects of leaf proteins on lipid metabolism have been investigated by several authors (Choi et al. 1988; Cho et al. 1985; Satoh et al. 1993, 1995). With a protein level of 15%, radish or spinach leaf protein isolates, supplemented or not with methionine to balance the methionine-content with that of casein, have been compared to casein for their effects on serum cholesterol levels in *Wistar* rats fed with a cholesterol-enriched diet for a 14-day period. The serum cholesterol level was significantly lower with both leaf protein isolates, and also with spinach leaf protein isolates supplemented with methionine, than with a casein diet, but the effect of radish leaf protein isolates supplemented with methionine was not significantly different from that of casein. The amount of fecal cholesterol and bile acids excreted was greater with both proteins supplemented with methionine and with spinach leaf protein isolates than with a casein diet (Satoh et al. 1993).

Spinach leaf protein concentrates (20%) in a cholesterol-free diet containing between 2% and 10% fats, reduced total serum cholesterol, triacylglycerol, and phospholipid concentrations of weanling *Wistar* rats and increased those of cystine, glutamine, glycine, isoleucine, serine and threonine to a greater extent than casein. These effects are partly due to the inhibition of intestinal absorption of cholesterol and bile acids (Satoh et al. 1995). Italian ryegrass and alfalfa protein concentrates also exert a hypocholesterolemic effect in rats (Cho et al. 1985).

In *Sprague-Dawley* male albino rats on a protein diet (16%), replacing garlic protein with casein significantly decreased the total serum, VLD-, LDL-, and HDL-cholesterol levels, the activity of HMG-CoA reductase, and the atherogenic indices. The cholesterol and triacylglycerol contents of the liver and aorta were also reduced. The effect of garlic protein on HMG-CoA reductase is equivalent to about 85% that of garlic oil (100 mg/kg body weight/day). These results were obtained with either a cholesterol-free or a cholesterol-rich diet. The presence of large amounts of sulfur amino acids in garlic protein and possibly the low lysine/arginine ratio of 0.77 compared to soybean protein (0.84) and casein (2) may well account for the hypolipidemic action of garlic protein (Mathew et al. 1996). Unlike casein, plant protein significantly reduced plasma total cholesterol and HDL-cholesterol concentrations in immature and mature *Wistar* rats. LCAT activity is similar with different plant proteins, but the esterification rate is lower in rats fed casein (de Schriver 1990).

2.5.1.4 Summary

Although a large number of experiments have investigated the effects of various vegetable proteins on cholesterol metabolism, essentially in rats, and sometimes in rabbits and hamsters, it would appear that none have been conducted in animal models applicable to humans, such as pigs and monkeys. Numerous vegetable proteins including casein, soybean, fababean, peabean, haricot bean, rice, pulse, lentil, cottonseed, golden pea, peanut, wheat gluten, buckwheat, sunflower, radish, spinach leaf, garlic, ryegrass, arrowroot, and various grams (bengal black or red) have been studied. All the data available show a negative correlation between the nutritional value of vegetable proteins and serum cholesterol concentrations. The importance of the nutritional value has also been well demonstrated by the effects of protein supplementation with amino acids in which they are deficient. In comparison with animal proteins, vegetable proteins are hypocholesterolemic.

2.5.2 Animal Proteins

The serum cholesterol concentrations of male weanling *Wistar* albino rats are higher with diets containing animal proteins, including poultry and fish, than with proteins from plant sources (Adeyeye et al. 1989). When the diets of *New Zealand white* rabbits were supplemented with a large amounts of cholesterol (1.5 g/kg), serum cholesterol concentrations increased according to the following increasing order of animal protein diets: whey protein, casein, and fish protein. Casein, ovalbumin, and soybean protein produced similar levels of serum cholesterol when they were incorporated into low-cholesterol diets (0.08 g/kg) (Lovati et al. 1990).

2.5.2.1 Fish Protein

The effects of fish protein on serum cholesterol vary according to the animal species, the nature of proteins, and the type and amount of fat content in the diet (Jacques 1990; West et al. 1990). In rabbits, replacing fish protein with casein in a hypolipidic diet without or with only a very small amount of cholesterol leads to a reduction in serum cholesterol, VLDL, and triacylglycerol concentrations, but increases the serum concentrations of LDL and HDL, and also the LDL-cholesterol/HDL-cholesterol ratio (Hermus 1975; Hamilton and Carroll 1976; Hermus et al. 1983; Bergeron and Jacques 1989; Zhang and Beynen 1990; Bergeron et al. 1991; Zhang 1992; Bergeron et al. 1992a; Jacques et al. 1993a, 1993b). In *New Zealand white* rabbits fed on a semipurified diet containing 40% sucrose, 14% coconut oil, 15% cellulose, 5% salt mix, and 1% vitamin mix (a diet known to be hypercholesterolemic) for an 8-month period, the total serum cholesterol, HDL-cholesterol, triacylglycerol levels were lower and aortic atherosclerosis less extensive with 25% fish protein than with 25% casein (Kritchevsky et al. 1982a).

If a casein-containing low-cholesterol diet is well balanced, no hypercholesterolemic effect is detected in *New Zealand white* rabbits (Lovati et al. 1990). On the other hand, replacing fish protein with soybean protein in the diet of *New Zealand white* rabbits did not modify the serum cholesterol and triacylglycerol concentrations, but did reduce the LDL-cholesterol/HDL-cholesterol ratio (Bergeron and Jacques 1989; Jacques 1990; Bergeron et al. 1992b, 1992c). The increase in serum HDL cholesterol with fish protein was greater than that of LDL cholesterol (Bergeron et al. 1989). Nevertheless, in one study, serum cholesterol and triacylglycerol concentrations were higher with fish protein. This discordance is very likely due to the high-fat content of the diet (maize oil and coconut oil) (Goulding et al. 1983). The increased activity of lipoprotein lipase with fish protein suggests an enhanced assembly of circulating HDL via the stimulated lipoprotein lipase activity (Bergeron et al. 1992b). According to West et al. (1990), hypercholesterolemia in rabbits may well be due to changes in lipoprotein patterns such as the accumulation of LDL and HDL with fish, and of VLDL with casein.

Fish protein may have different effects on serum cholesterol concentrations of weaning female *Wistar* rats (Zhang and Beynen 1990; Zhang 1992; Zhang and Beynen 1993a). The serum cholesterol concentrations of rats were slightly lower with fish protein than with casein (Sugano et al. 1984; Iritani et al. 1985; Jacques et al. 1986; Kuyvenhoven et al. 1987; Zhang 1992; Zhang and Beynen 1993a). The serum cholesterol concentrations were lower when pollack or sardine protein was used to replace casein in a low-fat diet of male *Wistar* rats (Sugano et al. 1984). The results were similar in *Sprague-Dawley* rats with a cod-protein diet supplemented by cholesterol and cholic acid (Jacques et al. 1986), whereas serum cholesterol concentrations were higher with a hyperlipidic diet in male *Wistar* rats (Iritani et al. 1985). The enhanced [^{14}C]cholesterol turnover observed by Iritani may well be due to the large amount of fish oil in the diet (West et al. 1990). Cod protein is hypocholesterolemic. This effect is, however, more pronounced when the cod-protein content or the cholesterol content of the diet is high (Zhang and Beynen 1990; Zhang 1992). In these studies on rabbits and rats, the results relating to neutral steroids and bile acid excretion are discordant (Zhang and Beynen 1990; Zhang 1992), and since the effect on bile acid absorption is delayed, it is of secondary importance (West et al. 1990).

In contrast to casein, fish protein did not increase the liver cholesterol concentrations in *New Zealand white* rabbits and male *Wistar* rats (Lapré et al. 1989; West et al. 1990; Lovati et al. 1990). They were nevertheless higher than with soybean protein or wheat gluten in *New Zealand white* rabbits (Kuyvenhoven et al. 1987). The changes in hepatic cholesterol metabolism induced by increased fish protein intake would appear to be less important than with casein because there is no associated increase in hepatic cholesterol levels.

The differences in the digestibility of casein, fish, soybean protein, and wheat gluten do not seem to have a significant role in the different effects of these proteins (Kuyvenhoven et al. 1987).

2.5.2.2 Milk Protein

Milk proteins are the different forms of casein and various whey proteins such as β-lactoglobulin, α-lactalbumin, and lactoferrin. Studies on the effects of whey proteins have been conducted either with whey proteins in general or with β-lactoglobulin.

2.5.2.2.1 Whey Protein

In *New Zealand white* rabbits, whey protein versus casein caused a slight reduction in plasma cholesterol concentrations (Yoshida et al. 1988; Lovati et al. 1990), and likewise in the fecal excretion rates of neutral steroids and bile acids (Lovati et al. 1990). The same results were obtained with lactalbumin versus casein (Carroll and Hamilton 1975). However, comparisons between the respective effects of milk and whey-milk protein are contradictory. Indeed, in the study by Vrecko et al. (1988) on *New Zealand white* rabbits, a milk diet produced either a slight increase or a reduction in serum cholesterol concentrations depending on whether it came before or after the whey diet. The same progression was observed for the reduction in HDL cholesterol and increase in LDL- and VLDL-cholesterol levels, or the opposite, depending on whether the milk diet came before or after the whey diet (Vrecko et al. 1988). In male weanling *New Zealand white* rabbits fed on diets with different casein/whey ratios (100/0, 80/20, 40/60), the serum concentrations of cholesterol, LDL cholesterol, HDL cholesterol, and liver lipids were higher when the casein/whey ratio is 40/60. The differences disappeared, however, when the diet was supplemented by cholesterol (Larson et al. 1992; Wilson et al. 1992; Larson et al. 1994). The serum triacylglycerol concentrations were highest when the casein/whey ratio was 100/0 (Larson et al. 1994).

In *Wistar* and *Brown-Norway* rats fed on cholesterol-free diets, serum cholesterol levels were higher with casein than with whey or sunflower protein, pea, fava, or soybean protein diets (Sautier et al. 1983, 1990). Likewise, in the same strain of rats, serum cholesterol concentrations were lower with whey protein than with casein when the diet contained either no or very little free cholesterol (Park and Liepa 1982).

In normotensive *Wistar* rats, plasma triacylglycerol and total cholesterol levels were similar with the following diets — casein, whey protein concentrates, skimmed milk protein concentrates, and soybean protein isolates — and higher than with dried yogurt or a chow diet. Hepatic total lipids and cholesterol were not significantly dissimilar between the different groups (Yuan and Kitts 1993). In both young and adult male *Sprague-Dawley* rats, whey protein in a cholesterol-free diet was hypocholesterolemic irrespective of the age of the animals (Choi et al. 1989a). However, in another experiment with the same strain of rats, the serum cholesterol level of young and adult rats was similar with a whey diet or a casein diet, both cholesterol-free diets containing 5% sardine oil. In young rats on a cholesterol-free whey protein or soybean protein diet the specific activities of HMG-CoA reductase were more pronounced than if they were fed a casein diet (Choi et al. 1989b).

In *Wistar* rats fed either a cholesterol-free or a cholesterol-rich diet, the hypo-cholesterolemic effect was greater with whey protein than with soybean protein (Nagaoka et al. 1991, 1992). However, in another experiment on *Sprague-Dawley* rats the differences were inconsistent (Choi et al. 1989b). As was demonstrated by Vrecko et al. (1988) in their study on *New Zealand white* rabbits, the chronology and the duration of successive diets can modulate the effects on total serum cholesterol levels since whey protein diet can increase, decrease, or have no effect at all on serum cholesterol concentrations.

Whey protein did not modify fecal excretion of neutral steroids or bile acids in *Wistar* and *Brown-Norway* rats (Sautier et al. 1983, 1990). Plasma free cholesterol, phospholipids LDL-, HDL$_1$-, HDL$_2$-cholesterol, apo A-1 of HDL$_2$, and apo E levels were lower with whey protein than with casein and varied according to the species of rats (Sautier et al. 1990). However, when the whey protein level was high, plasma cholesterol, VLDL-cholesterol, and triacylglycerol concentrations and liver cholesterol levels were significantly decreased and the fecal excretion of bile acids was reduced compared to that observed with casein, whereas in another study, the total serum cholesterol, HDL-, and LDL-cholesterol concentrations of male weanling *Sprague-Dawley* rats were not modified by casein, whey, or soybean proteins, and VLDL cholesterol was only lower with soybean protein. Fecal output was higher with soybean protein during week 1, but reached a peak during week 7 with a whey protein diet (Aljawad et al. 1991). The cholesterol-lowering effect of whey protein is due to the inhibition of hepatic cholesterol synthesis (Zhang and Beynen 1993b). The different distribution of cholesterol in the lipoproteins and tissues of rabbits and rats may well account for these conflicting results (Park and Liepa 1982).

A diet containing fermented whey (from cultured skimmed milk with *Bifido-bacterium longum, Lactobacillus acidophilus, Streptococcus thermophilus*) lowered serum cholesterol concentrations of *Sprague-Dawley* rats and increased the activities of superoxide dismutase and glutathione peroxidase in red blood cells, and catalase in liver. Lipoprotein fractions from rats fed with these products were resistant to the oxidative stress induced by a transition metal ion. In contrast, a diet containing nonfermented whey was not effective in lowering plasma cholesterol levels in rats or in increasing antioxidant systems (Zommara et al. 1996).

In male *Wistar* rats fed for a 6-week period on a cholesterol-free diet containing whey protein isolates or casein, the plasma and liver cholesterol and triacylglycerol concentrations were similar, but the percentage of esterified liver cholesterol was lower with the casein diet and VLDL triacylglycerols lower with the whey diet. Serum apo A-1, A-1V and E levels are similar in plasma and apo B mRNA concentrations are similar in the liver and intestinal mucosa (Marquez-Ruiz et al. 1992).

In calves, serum cholesterol concentrations were not significantly different after 15 weeks of skimmed milk powder or soybean protein concentrates diets. In contrast, in rabbits, serum cholesterol concentrations were higher with skimmed milk powder. These inconsistent results are the consequence of the different regulation of cholesterol metabolism in the two species (Beynen et al. 1983e).

In *Yorkshire/Duroc* 2-day-old piglets fed on one of three diets — 100% casein, 80% casein, and 20% whey or 40% casein and 60% whey — results were comparable to those obtained by the same authors in weanling rabbits using the same protocol as previously reported. The higher the level of dietary casein, the higher the serum concentrations of free and esterified cholesterol, HDL cholesterol, and LDL cholesterol. There was a positive correlation between total serum and free cholesterol levels and the casein/whey ratio. Serum glucagon and cortisol concentrations were high in piglets fed 100% casein. However, these results and those concerning HMG-CoA reductase were only significant when the casein content of the diet was 100%. The VLDL-cholesterol rate was lowest with a 60% whey content. Bile acid excretion and hepatic lipid concentrations remained similar despite these differing diets (Larson et al. 1996).

In pigs fed for a 4-week period with a diet in which dried whey content was 56% of the energy intake, serum cholesterol and HDL-cholesterol concentrations were reduced by −20% and −20.4%, respectively. The reduction in triacylglycerol levels was not significant (Stähelin et al. 1980). Likewise, in *Yorkshire barrow* pigs fed on four successive different diets — basal diet without whey and with (5%) or without cholesterol, 40% dried whey with (5%) or without cholesterol — with each period lasting 14 days followed by a 7-day interval period, serum cholesterol concentrations were low with both diets. When cholesterol was added to the diets, the serum cholesterol levels increased although the concentrations were 15% lower and HDL cholesterol was 16% higher with the whey diet (40%) than with the basal diet (Norton et al. 1987).

2.5.2.2.2   β-Lactoglobulin

β-Lactoglobulin, which is richer in lysine than casein, significantly decreased the serum cholesterol and HDL-cholesterol concentrations and resulted in a nonsignificant, weak reduction in the liver cholesterol concentrations of *Wistar* and *Brown-Norway* rats (Sautier et al. 1990).

2.5.2.3   Egg Protein

A low-cholesterol diet containing ovalbumin does not increase serum cholesterol concentrations in *New Zealand White* rabbits. However, the same experiment has not been carried out with a high-cholesterol diet (Lovati et al. 1990).

Ovalbumin, which is rich in methionine compared to casein, significantly reduced the serum cholesterol and HDL-cholesterol concentrations in *Wistar* and *Brown-Norway* rats, but its lowering effect on liver cholesterol concentrations was not significant (Sautier et al. 1990). In rats (over a period of 3 weeks) or in mice (over 2 weeks), egg-white protein was hypocholesterolemic in comparison with a casein diet. This hypocholesterolemic effect was observed in rats, but not in mice fed on a diet containing soybean protein isolates or egg-white protein hydrolysates.

In contrast to soybean protein, egg-white protein prevented the reduction of HDL cholesterol in male *Wistar* rats (Yamamoto et al. 1993).

Serum cholesterol and triacylglycerol concentrations, but also lipid peroxidation were higher with casein than with egg albumin in male *Golden Syrian* hamsters (Kubow et al. 1997). Hamsters, belonging to the same strain fed on egg albumin, had a lower serum concentration of total and HDL cholesterol than those fed on various other dietary proteins: animal (casein, bovine albumin) or vegetable (soybean, cottonseed, peanut) (Sullivan et al. 1985).

In young male *Yorkshire* swine, the serum cholesterol level was high with casein, but low with egg albumin or soybean protein (Kim et al. 1983).

2.5.2.4 Beef Protein

In rabbits, on five types of diet — beef protein, textured vegetable proteins, casein, beef protein and spen flakes, or beef protein and textured vegetable proteins — for an 8-month period, serum cholesterol concentrations were significantly higher and those of HDL cholesterol lower with casein or beef protein than with the other three diets. The serum cholesterol concentrations were lowest with spen flakes (Kritchevsky et al. 1981). In male *Sinclair* miniature swine, cooked minced beef covering 40% of the protein requirements in a basal diet fed for a 10-week period increased total serum and HDL-cholesterol concentrations. Replacing beef protein with tallow plus cholesterol in a soybean protein diet increased total serum cholesterol and LDL-plus VLDL-cholesterol levels without any effect on HDL cholesterol (Williams et al. 1985). When young crossbred castrated male pigs were liberally fed on beef-based, soybean-based, and conventional diets, plasma free fatty acids, triacylglycerol, and cholesterol concentrations were observed to be greater with the soybean protein and beef diets than with conventional diets. However, these results and those concerning HMG-CoA reductase were only significant when the casein concentrations were greater with soybean protein and beef diets than with conventional diets (Diersen-Schade et al. 1985, 1986). When 8-week-old castrated pigs were fed on a high-fat diet and ground beef or soybean protein isolates, plasma cholesterol, phospholipid, triacylglycerol, VLDL, LDL, and HDL concentrations were unaffected by the different types of dietary protein. Kinetic measurements *in vivo* of LDL metabolism did not show any effect of dietary protein sources on their half-life, fast equilibrating pool size, or fractional catabolic rate (Johnson et al. 1987). Tissue LDL-cholesterol concentrations (muscle, heart, adipose tissue, and kidney) of young castrated male *Yorkshire* pigs were higher in the sartorius muscle with a 6-week beef protein diet and in the heart with a 6-week soybean protein diet (Johnson et al. 1989). In pigs fed on beef tallow or soybean oil as a fat source and minced beef or soybean protein isolates as a protein source, the dietary cholesterol content being similar, the plasma total cholesterol and LDL- and HDL-cholesterol levels were higher with beef tallow than with soybean oil. In the heart and longissimus muscle, cholesterol concentrations, but not those of lipids, were greater in pigs fed soybean oil than in those fed beef tallow (Baldner et al. 1985).

2.5.2.5 Carnitine

Carnitine plays an important role in the regulation of lipid metabolism and fatty acid oxidation in the liver and extrahepatic tissues (Bremer 1983).

In hyperlipidemic male *New Zealand white* rabbits fed over an 8-week period on a high-fat diet containing 0.5% cholesterol, a supplementation with L-carnitine (170 mg/kg of body weight) for 4 weeks reduced the extent of liver steatosis, lowered plasma total cholesterol and triacylglycerol concentrations, and increased acylcholesterol acyltransferase (ACAT) and 7-α-hydroxylase activities (Seccombe et al. 1987). With the same experimental protocol in male *New Zealand white* rabbits, tryptophan supplementation had no effect on the fractional catabolic rates of VLDL triacylglycerols and VLDL apo B, but did significantly lower the VLDL-triacylglycerols transport (James et al. 1995). In spite of these data, the mechanism behind the hypolipidemic effect of carnitine is unknown.

2.5.3 ANIMAL AND VEGETABLE PROTEINS

In rabbits, serum cholesterol concentrations increase to different degrees with vegetable or animal protein diets and also according to the presence or absence of cholesterol. If they are fed on a cholesterol-rich diet, serum cholesterol concentrations increase with different protein sources in the following increasing order: soybean protein, whey protein, casein, and fish protein. In male *New Zealand white* rabbits fed on cholesterol-free, isonitrogenous (25% protein) semipurified diets for a 28-day period, serum cholesterol concentrations increased according to content in following order: fababean, pea, sunflower seed, soybean isolate, alfalfa, sesame seed, cottonseed, oat, wheat gluten, rapeseed, egg white, pork, chicken, beef, fish, whole egg, casein, lactalbumin, turkey, skimmed milk, and egg yolk (Carroll et al. 1979; Carroll 1982).

The respective effects of proteins are different when the diet is low or high in cholesterol. They have been investigated in male outbred *Wistar* rats fed on well-balanced semipurified diets low (8 mg/100 g diet) or high in cholesterol (150 mg/100 g diet) and containing various types of proteins. When the low cholesterol diet contained soybean protein or casein or hemoglobin/casein or ovalbumin, serum cholesterol concentrations were similar. When the diet was high in cholesterol, serum cholesterol concentrations were increased in the following order: first fish protein, and then equally with whey protein, soybean protein, plasma proteins, and beef proteins. Casein, egg-yolk protein, and chicken-meat protein had similar high serum cholesterol levels. Nevertheless, the variations in serum cholesterol concentrations were not significant except for soybean protein and casein, and fish protein and casein with a high-cholesterol diet. The rate of fecal bile excretion was reduced and liver cholesterol concentrations increased with soybean protein (Lapré et al. 1989). According to Lapré (1989), the discrepancy between these results and those of other authors could well be explained by the fact that the different components of the semipurified diet used in the other experiments were not well balanced for residual fat and cholesterol in the protein preparations. Likewise, total plasma cholesterol levels were not different in male *Wistar* rats fed on either beef protein or casein, soybean protein, and zein, with essential amino acids being added to improve the respective chemical score. After 4 weeks of these diets, total plasma cholesterol levels were comparable in the different groups although those of the rats fed on beef protein and casein diets were slightly higher. HDL cholesterol was 30% lower than in the other groups. Although apo A-1 levels were similar in all four groups, apo A-1V concentrations were 20% lower in the beef-protein group. Apo E levels were 20% higher in the group fed on casein and beef (Critchfield et al. 1990).

2.5.4 SUMMARY

Several animal proteins including fish and whey proteins, β-lactoglobulin, egg and beef proteins, and carnitine have been studied. Their effects depend on the animal species, the nature of the fats, and the amount of fats and cholesterol in the diet. It is therefore difficult to suggest any conclusion. In rabbits, serum cholesterol concentrations increase differently with vegetable or animal proteins according to the presence or absence of cholesterol in the diet. The effects of these dietary proteins on lipoproteins are different in rabbits and rats. In rabbits, but only if they are fed on a cholesterol-rich diet, serum cholesterol concentrations increased with the following proteins in the following increasing order: soybean protein, whey protein, casein, and fish protein. In piglets and pigs, casein is more hypercholesterolemic than whey protein and in calves soybean protein and whey protein have similar effects. β-lactoglobulin and ovalbumin are more hypocholesterolemic than casein. Ovalbumin decreases lipid peroxidation in rat and pigs. Lastly, carnitine has a hypolipidemic effect. Although it is widely accepted that vegetable proteins are hypocholesterolemic and animal proteins hypercholesterolemic it is still difficult to rank animal proteins according to the extent of their effects on cholesterol and lipid metabolisms. However, it is clear that the different effects of various food proteins are related to their composition in amino acids.

2.6 EFFECTS OF AMINO ACID MIXTURES AND AMINO ACIDS

As described in previous sections, lipid metabolism may be affected differently according to the amino acid composition of the diet. It has therefore been useful to investigate the influence of amino acid mixtures or of supplementation by each amino acid separately on lipid metabolism.

2.6.1 AMINO ACID MIXTURES

Administration of complete amino acid mixtures produces rapid stimulation of hepatic protein synthesis in fasted young rats (Sidransky 1976). The studies on the effects of amino acid mixtures have been chiefly performed in rabbits and rats.

2.6.1.1 Rabbits

The effects of soybean protein mixtures and soybean protein are similar in rabbits (Huff et al. 1977; Hermus and Stasse-Wolthuis 1978; Hermus et al. 1979; Huff and Carroll 1980a).

The study by Kurowska and Carroll (1989, 1990) on male *New Zealand white* rabbits fed on a cholesterol-free semipurified diet shows that casein and amino acid mixtures corresponding to casein have similar effects on total serum and LDL-cholesterol levels, and on other lipoprotein components. In male *New Zealand white* rabbits fed on a low-fat, cholesterol-free semipurified diet, the effects are also similar with amino acids corresponding to either casein or egg yolk, or with casein or egg yolk protein (Huff and Carroll 1980a; Carroll 1981b). In a later review of these observations, Carroll and Kurowska (1995) suggested that these effects are due to essential amino acids and to lysine and methionine in particular. In young male *New Zealand white* rabbits fed for a 3-week period on a low-fat, cholesterol-free, semi-purified amino acid diet in which lysine and methionine versus lysine and leucine were selectively increased at levels corresponding to 45% casein amino acid diets, the serum cholesterol, LDL-cholesterol, and apo B levels were elevated in the rabbits fed on the lysine and methionine diet and were higher than those of rabbits fed on lysine and leucine. These effects are partially prevented by the addition of a high proportion of arginine (Kurowska and Carroll 1996).

Serum cholesterol concentrations increase with the increase of dietary casein or casein amino acid concentrations in the diets of rabbits (Terpstra et al. 1981; Kurowska and Carroll 1990). In male *New Zealand white* rabbits the essential amino acids of casein are more hypercholesterolemic than nonessential amino acids (Kurowska and Carroll 1990). An amino acid mixture corresponding to casein raised total serum and LDL-cholesterol concentrations when rabbits were fed at levels of 20-30% in a low-fat cholesterol-free semipurified diet (Kurowska and Carroll 1993).

The serum cholesterol variations observed in rabbits fed on different levels of amino acid mixtures are not associated with any changes in fecal excretion of cholesterol or bile acids. According to Kurowska and Carroll (1991), there is no correlation between the plasma amino acid levels in either the fasting or postprandial state and serum thyroid hormone levels, activities of hepatic and intestinal microsomal HMG-CoA reductase, cholesterol esterifying enzymes of intestinal mucosa, or the degree of esterification of VLDL or LDL cholesterol.

When all essential amino acids except arginine, or all ketogenic essential amino acids (lysine, leucine, isoleucine, threonine, phenylalanine, tryptophan, and glycine) are fed at three times the normal level, the hypocholesterolemic response was higher and LDL receptors are down-regulated. Mixtures of lysine, leucine, methionine, isoleucine, and valine or lysine, leucine and methionine induce the same levels of hypercholesterolemia, whereas a mixture containing histidine, phenylalanine, tryptophan, and glycine has only a moderate effect. The serum insulin level is similar with both mixtures (Kurowska and Carroll 1993). Hypercholesterolemia is induced in young male *New Zealand white* rabbits by the same high levels of lysine, leucine, and methionine, but is greater with a combination of lysine and methionine than with one containing either lysine and leucine, or leucine and methionine (Kurowska and Carroll 1994). A significant increase in cholesterol, triacylglycerol, total lipids, and β-lipoprotein serum levels was observed in young *New Zealand white* rabbits fed by stomach intubation for 20 consecutive days, on a mixture containing only two amino acids (isoleucine, methionine or leucine, phenylalanine or lysine and tryptophan), whereas all the lipid parameters were increased by a mixture containing isoleucine and methionine or, and more strongly, leucine and phenylalanine. A mixture containing lysine and tryptophan only enhanced serum triacylglycerol concentrations and a mixture containing six amino acids (isoleucine, leucine, lysine, methionine, phenylalanine, and tryptophan) caused a greater increase in serum cholesterol, total lipid, β-lipoprotein, and triacylglycerol concentrations than did a mixture containing only three amino acids (isoleucine, leucine, and lysine, or methionine, phenylalanine, and tryptophan) (Mahgoub and Abu-Jayyab 1984, 1987).

2.6.1.2 Rats

In rats, amino acid mixtures simulating the composition of casein or soybean protein have similar effects to those of casein and soybean protein (Huff et al. 1977; Yadav and Liener 1977; Nagata et al. 1981a; Muramatsu and Sugiyama 1990; Saeki et al. 1990). However, the effects of amino acid mixtures are sometimes less hypercholesterolemic than casein (Yadav and Liener 1977). When normal or obese female *Zucker* rats were fed on casein (20.8%), serum cholesterol concentrations were higher, especially in LDL and VLDL, than when they were fed on an animal protein mixture (casein 8%, fish proteins 8%, and gelatin 5.5%) (Guigoz et al. 1979). Zhang and Beynen (1993b), however, showed that in weanling female *Wistar* rats the differential effects of casein and whey protein on plasma and liver cholesterol do not depend on their amino acid combinations, but on their different structure or their nonprotein components.

In isolated perfused liver from male *Wistar* rats fed on either soybean protein isolates or casein the secretion of cholesterol, triacylglycerols, and apo A-1 was reduced by almost half with soybean protein isolates. However, these differences disappeared when the same rats were fed on an amino acid mixture simulating these proteins though serum cholesterol and apo A-1 concentrations were decreased in rats fed on soy simulating amino acid mixtures. These data suggest that the different effects of soybean protein might not only be due to its amino acid profile, but also to the increased fecal excretion of steroids and principally to the reduction of liver cholesterol secretion (Sugano et al. 1982a).

In male *Wistar* rats soybean protein isolates diet compared to casein decreased cholesterol absorption, increased fecal steroid excretion, enhanced cholesterol turnover, reduced the rapidly exchangeable cholesterol pool (due to an increase in the removal rate in pool A), without any modification of the production rate, and increased liver steroidogenesis. In contrast, the amino acid mixtures equivalent to soybean protein, compared with casein-type mixtures, did not change cholesterol absorption, fecal steroid excretion, or serum cholesterol turnover; reduced the pool A size, decreasing the production rate; and reduced hepatic steroidogenesis *in vitro*, but not *in vivo* (Nagata et al. 1982). Several similar studies are described in Section 2.3.1 on soybean protein isolates.

Increasing cystine intake, but not that of methionine, reduced the plasma cholesterol levels of male *Wistar* rats fed on the amino acid mixture of casein. Suppression of cystine or glycine from an amino acid mixture such as is found in gluten, increased the plasma cholesterol concentrations of rats (Sugiyama and Muramatsu 1990; Muramatsu and Sugiyama 1990).

The same effects were observed in rats with casein or soybean protein and with their partial hydrolysates. Indeed, an equal mixture (50%/50%) of casein and soybean protein did not increase the serum cholesterol concentration in rabbits (Tanaka and Nozaki 1983). Casein and its hydrolysate peptides had the same effects on plasma cholesterol concentrations in both male *Wistar* rats and male *ICR* strain mice. However, in mice, although HDL cholesterol was not affected, total and non–HDL-cholesterol levels were lower with hydrolysate peptides. After intravenous injection of an amino acid mixture or of short peptides in mice the total plasma cholesterol concentrations were lower with short peptides (Asato et al. 1994).

Hypercholesterolemia was reduced in growing rats fed on an 8.1% soybean protein isolates diet containing 0.5% cholesterol and 0.25% sodium cholate when the diet was supplemented with methionine, cystine, cysteine, or homocystine. In contrast, supplementation with S-methyl-L-cysteine, cysteic acid, or taurine had little effect. These results suggest that hypercholesterolemia due to a low-soybean protein isolates diet containing cholesterol may result from a deficiency in dietary methionine (Mizuno et al. 1988).

Plasma cholesterol concentrations were approximately twofold higher when male albino *Wistar* rats were fed on an amino acid mixture corresponding to casein compared with feeding the amino acid mixture corresponding to wheat gluten. The plasma cholesterol concentrations were reduced or increased, respectively, by increasing the proportion of cystine in the total sulfur amino acids of the amino acid mixture corresponding to casein, or by deprivation of cystine in the gluten type of amino acid mixture. A significant negative correlation was observed between plasma cholesterol levels and the content of cystine in intact dietary proteins (Sugiyama et al. 1986a).

Total serum cholesterol concentrations were lower in *Sprague-Dawley* rats fed diets containing amino acid mixtures simulating rice, potato, or soybean proteins than in rats fed on amino acid mixtures simulating casein; however, the total fecal steroid excretion was the same in all groups. A strong positive correlation was observed between serum cholesterol concentrations and dietary methionine concentrations or the methionine/glycine ratio (Morita et al. 1997).

The addition of a large amount of cystine to a bovine milk-simulated amino acid mixture produced a significant reduction in the plasma cholesterol levels of young male *Sprague-Dawley* rats. On the other hand, the addition of arginine or glycine had no effect. Serum HDL-cholesterol levels and fecal excretion of acidic steroids were higher with cystine than with any addition of arginine or glycine. The liver content of cholesterol was not modified, but triacylglycerol concentrations were elevated with arginine and cystine diets (Yoshida et al. 1988).

Feeding growing male rats of the *Donryu* strain excessive amounts (50%) of individual amino acids did not modify the liver lipid content except when excessive amounts of methionine plus cystine were used. The liver lipid content was raised significantly by threonine- or lysine-deficient diets, whereas it was reduced by a phenylalanine plus tyrosine-deficient and sulfur-containing amino acid-deficient diets. Histidine deficiency also decreased the liver lipid content. An increase in liver lipids was induced by excessive amounts of sulfur amino acids and was not prevented by the addition of threonine or tryptophan (Aoyama and Ashida 1972).

Replacing casein or wheat gluten with amino acid mixtures that are similar to their own composition did not modify serum cholesterol concentrations in young male *Wistar* rats fed on a high-cholesterol diet. However, these same concentrations were reduced if the cystine level was higher than that of methionine and inversely. Cystine or glycine deprivation enhanced serum cholesterol concentrations. These results show that the proportion of sulfur amino acids (cystine, methionine, and glycine) in the diet, are important for the regulation of serum cholesterol concentrations in male *Wistar* rats (Sugano et al. 1982a; Muramatsu and Sugiyama 1990; Sugiyama and Muramatsu 1990) and in weanling female *Wistar* rats (Zhang and Beynen 1993b). In contrast to the effects of soybean protein and casein, the secretion of cholesterol, triacylglycerols and apoprotein A-1 are unchanged by the mixtures of their amino acids.

2.6.1.3 Monkeys

In restrained female baboons, amino acid mixtures simulating the composition of casein or soybean protein have similar effects to those of casein and soybean protein (Wolfe and Grace 1987).

2.6.1.4 Summary

In rabbits and rats, amino acid mixtures simulating the composition of casein or soybean protein or wheat gluten have the same effects as casein, soybean protein, or wheat gluten, respectively. The variations in the serum cholesterol levels of rabbits fed on different levels of amino acid mixtures are not associated with any changes in fecal excretion of cholesterol or bile acids. There is no correlation between plasma amino acid levels, in either the fasting or postprandial state, and serum thyroid hormone levels, activities of hepatic and intestinal microsomal HMG-CoA reductase, activities of cholesterol esterifying enzymes of intestinal mucosa, and the degree of esterification of VLDL or LDL cholesterol. Compared with a casein-type mixture, the amino acid mixture that is equivalent to soybean protein does not change cholesterol absorption, fecal steroid excretion, or serum cholesterol turnover; in addition, it reduces the pool A size and decreases the production rate, as well as hepatic steroidogenesis *in vitro*, but not *in vivo*.

When all essential amino acids are included in the diet, with the exception of arginine, there is a greater reduction in serum cholesterol level and the LDL receptors are down-regulated. The effects of amino acids vary according to the composition of the mixtures. A mixture of leucine, isoleucine, lysine, methionine, phenylalanine, and tryptophan increases serum cholesterol concentrations, total lipid, β-lipoprotein, and triacylglycerol concentrations to a greater extent than a mixture containing only three amino acids (leucine, isoleucine, and lysine, or methionine, phenylalanine, and tryptophan). Partial hydrolysates of casein and soybean protein have similar effects to casein or soybean protein. These results prove that amino acids, used alone, can modify serum cholesterol concentrations.

2.6.2 Amino Acids

High levels of dietary amino acids induce hypercholesterolemia and several metabolic changes (Kurowska and Carroll 1990, 1991, 1992, 1993). The effects of
excessive intakes of individual amino acids, and also those due to amino acid toxicity
or antagonism, and the adverse effects of amino acid imbalance already observed
in chickens (Johnson et al. 1958; Kokatnur et al. 1959; Kokatnur and Kummerow
1961); rats (de Groot 1958, 1959, 1960; Hevia et al. 1980a, 1980b); and rabbits
(Huff and Carroll 1980a) have all been extensively reviewed by Harper et al. (Harper
et al. 1970).

An imbalance between amino acids causes significant changes in the serum
amino acid profile (Harper 1958; Harper et al. 1970); the plasma concentrations of
amino acids vary according to the nature and the amount of dietary proteins. For
example, in adult female *Göttingen* miniature pigs fed on a cholesterol diet, the
plasma concentrations of arginine, cystine, leucine, lysine, methionine, tryptophan,
tyrosine, and valine were higher with animal proteins (casein or lactalbumin) than
with vegetable proteins (soybean protein or proteins from maize or wheat) (Barth
et al. 1990c). The serum concentrations of arginine, aspartic acid, asparagine,
glutamine, histidine, lysine, ornithine, threonine, and serine were not different in
male *Wistar* rats fed casein (20.0%) or soybean protein (22.5%) diets, whereas the
concentrations of alanine, glutamic acid, isoleucine, leucine, methionine, phenylalanine, proline, tyrosine, and valine were significantly lower in the soybean protein-
fed group than in the casein-fed group. Glycine is the only amino acid with a higher
serum concentration in the soybean protein-fed group and in the casein-fed group.
Cysteine and tryptophan are not detectable in the serum of either group (Horigome
and Cho 1992).

The increase, decrease, or absence of amino acid effects on serum cholesterol
concentrations have been investigated in different species, although not in all species
used in laboratory experiments (Terpstra et al. 1983a). In adult male *Sprague-Dawley*
rats fed on a protein-free ration for a 100-day period, the addition of either cystine
(0.24%) or methionine (0.30%) to the diet produced hepatic steatosis. Addition of
cystine (0.24%), methionine (0.30%), or valine (0.24%) increased the liver neutral
glyceride and cholesterol contents, whereas that of isoleucine (0.20%), leucine
(0.26%), and phenylalanine (0.33%) enhanced their reductions resulting from to the
protein-free diet. In contrast, the addition of any one of the following amino acids
has no effect: arginine (0.42%), glutamine (0.30%), histidine (0.42%), lysine
(0.37%), threonine (0.24%), or tryptophan (0.41%) (Williams and Hurlebaus 1965a,
1965b).

The sulfur-containing amino acids have the most potent effects on serum cholesterol concentrations (Seidel et al. 1960; Léveillé and Sauberlich 1964; Fujiwara
et al. 1972; Kato et al. 1982; Terpstra et al. 1983b; Sugiyama et al. 1984; 1985a,
1985b, 1986b; Tanaka and Sugano 1989a; Sugiyama 1989; Muramatsu and Sugiyama 1990; Sugiyama and Muramatsu 1990). In hypercholesterolemic rats, however, cysteine, *S*-methylcysteine sulfone and *S*-methylmethionine sulfonium chloride
have little effect on hypercholesterolemia (Itokawa et al. 1973). A diet that was low
in sulfur amino acids induced hypercholesterolemia and hyper-β-lipoproteinemia in

rats, *white Swiss* mice (Fillios and Mann 1954) and in *Cebus fatuella* monkeys (Mann et al. 1953). The same diet resulted in atherosclerotic lesions in monkeys and rats (Fillios et al. 1956). Serum cholesterol concentrations were increased in cysteine-deficient monkeys (Mann 1960).

The effects of amino acids are related to their concentrations in the dietary protein. Indeed in male *albino Wistar* rats, when the basal diet enriched in cholesterol (1%) was supplemented with one amino acid at a 5% level, the plasma cholesterol levels were enhanced with arginine, histidine, and tryptophan, and reduced with alanine, glycine, leucine, lysine, methionine, and threonine, whereas aspartic acid, glutamic acid, isoleucine, phenylalanine, proline, serine, tyrosine, and valine had no effect. At the cysteine level of 5%, all the animals died within 1 week. However, when sulfur-containing amino acids alone (methionine and cystine) were added at a 1% or 0.5% level, they respectively increased or decreased serum cholesterol concentrations in male *albino Wistar* rats (Sugiyama et al. 1986b; Sugiyama and Muramatsu 1990; Muramatsu and Sugiyama 1990).

The liver content of cholesterol and total lipids was lower in male *albino Wistar* rats fed on methionine and histidine diets, but the plasma triacylglycerol levels were lower and higher, respectively, with methionine and histidine. The plasma triacylglycerol levels were lower when 1% methionine was added to the diet and higher with the addition of tryptophan (1%). The level of cholesterol and total lipids in the liver of male *albino Wistar* rats were significantly lower with the addition (1%) of methionine or cystine (Sugiyama et al. 1986b).

The effects on serum cholesterol concentrations and liver lipids of the addition of amino acids to the diet of chicks, rats, mice, rabbits, pigs, monkeys, and humans fed on a casein and cholesterol diet vary according to the nature and amount of amino acids in the diet. With the exception of arginine and lysine that are assessed elsewhere in this review, the available data relating to the effects on animals of each amino acid are summarized in Section 2.6.2.1 through Section 2.6.2.15. The numerous authors who have investigated the effects of each amino acid on plasma lipids and atherosclerosis in animals and humans are listed in the Amino Acids Index.

2.6.2.1 Alanine

When male *Wistar* rats were fed on a cholesterol-free diet containing casein, whey protein, soybean protein, and sunflower protein, serum cholesterol concentrations were significantly and negatively correlated with alanine (Sautier et al. 1983). At a 5% concentration, alanine, glycine, lysine, leucine, methionine, taurine and threonine were all hypocholesterolemic in male *Wistar* rats fed on a high-cholesterol diet. They reduced total serum cholesterol, LDL-, and VLDL-cholesterol, and triacylglycerol concentrations and also liver cholesterol and triacylglycerol levels (Sugiyama et al. 1989b). There was a significant positive correlation between the plasma total cholesterol concentration and the plasma concentration of methionine and valine and the hepatic concentration of valine and alanine in adult male *Wistar* rats fed with one or other of seven various dietary protein sources (12.3 to 14.4 g/100 g): casein, lactalbumin, whole-egg protein, egg albumin, sardine protein, soybean protein, or wheat gluten (Sugiyama et al. 1996).

In adult male *Hartley white* guinea pigs fed for 7 weeks on a casein diet (227 g/kg diet) that was well balanced in fatty acids (30%), supplementation with alanine decreased cholesterol levels in the LDL sub-fraction with a greater molecular weight (Atwal et al. 1997). The serum cholesterol level of rabbits and rats fed on casein (20%) semipurified diets was reduced after supplementation with 0.35% arginine plus 0.54% alanine for a 48-week period (Katan et al. 1982).

2.6.2.2 Cysteine

The experiments that have investigated the effects of cystine on serum cholesterol concentrations have been chiefly carried out in rats and the results are conflicting. Although cystine has been shown to have either no influence or a cholesterol-elevating effect (Aoyama et al. 1977, 1988), other studies, however, have reported the opposite. The growth retardation due to a low-casein diet can be alleviated by supplementation with cystine and threonine (Fujisawa et al. 1994).

In male weanling albino rabbits, cystine may be hyper- or hypocholesterolemic depending on the level of supplementation. Cystine at the 0.3% dietary level caused a significant increase in both plasma and liver cholesterol concentrations. However, when its concentration in the diet was increased to 2.4%, it caused a significant decrease in plasma and liver cholesterol and a significant increase in the concentration of taurine conjugates of the bile (Burns and Self 1969). Likewise, in male quail, *Coturnix coturnix japonica*, fed on a soybean protein (40%), corn meal (46%), cholesterol-rich diet (1%), the supplementation with cystine (2% or 4%) significantly reduced the serum and liver cholesterol concentrations when compared to a cholesterol control group without cystine supplementation (Jackson and Burns 1974).

Adding L-cystine (0.24%) to the diet of adult male *Sprague-Dawley* rats, maintained on a protein-free ration for 100 days, strongly increased the liver neutral glyceride and cholesterol concentrations and partially prevented the reduction of liver total phospholipid and plasmalogen concentrations (Williams and Hurlebaus 1965a, 1965b).

In *Sprague-Dawley* rats fed a diet containing 0.1% of inorganic sulfate, after stomach-tube feeding of [24-^{14}C]cholic acid the glycocholic/taurocholic ratio (G/T ratio) was lowest and highest, respectively, when cysteine (0.4%) was added or not. A similar trend was observed in the serum cholesterol levels of rats fed on these two diets (Feland et al. 1973).

The negative correlation between the cystine content of dietary proteins and serum cholesterol concentrations is significant in male *Wistar* rats (Sautier et al. 1983; Sugiyama and Muramatsu 1990; Muramatsu and Sugiyama 1990). When male *Wistar* rats were fed on a cholesterol-free diet containing casein, whey protein, soybean protein, and sunflower protein, serum cholesterol concentrations were significantly and negatively correlated with cystine (Sautier et al. 1983). *S*-methylcysteine sulfoxide and *S*-allylcysteine sulfoxide from plants of the Liliaceae family, an important source of nonessential sulfur-containing amino acids in the diet of the Japanese, have little effect in young hypercholesterolemic male *Wistar* rats (Itokawa et al. 1973).

The reduction of hyperlipidemia of male *Wistar* rats with nephritis due to a nephrotoxic agent, when they were fed a diet low (8.5%) in soybean protein isolates, was partially due to decreased liver cholesterol synthesis. The growth retardation could be alleviated by the addition of methionine (0.3%) (Fujisawa et al. 1995). The same result was obtained in the same strain of male rats with a low-casein diet supplemented with cystine and threonine (Fujisawa et al. 1994) and with a low-meat-protein diet (8.5%) or if this diet was supplemented by 0.5% L-valine (Yagasaki et al. 1994).

In male *Donryu* hepatoma-bearing rats the dietary addition of 1.2% cystine plus methionine (1.2%) to casein (20%) free-cholesterol diet suppressed the hepatoma-induced increase in VLDL and LDL cholesterol, but did not modify the hepatoma-induced decrease in HDL cholesterol (Yagasaki et al. 1986b).

Cystine is hypocholesterolemic in mice of the *White Swiss* strain (Fillios and Mann 1954) and in *Cebus fatuella* monkeys (Mann et al. 1953, 1960). Hypercholesterolemia is caused by cystine deficiency in these monkeys (Mann et al. 1960).

The proportionality of sulfur-containing amino acids is one the main differences between the amino acids composition of casein and soybean protein. The cysteine/methionine ratios in casein and soybean protein isolates are 0.34/2.9 and 1.3/1.3, respectively (Tasker and Potter 1993). Their respective effects can therefore be explained by the lower content of cysteine in casein than in soybean protein (0.4% and 1.2%, respectively) and the higher content of methionine in casein than in soybean protein (2.6% and 1.1%, respectively). In rats fed on 8.1% soybean protein isolate diet containing 0.5% cholesterol and 0.25% sodium cholate supplementation with cystine or cysteine decreased plasma cholesterol concentration (Mizuno et al. 1988). Hypocholesterolemia induced by soybean protein may well be due to the higher cystine content, which enhances the production of glutathione, reduced glutathione (GSH) — a tripeptide containing cysteine — being a cofactor in cholesterol metabolism (Hagemeister et al. 1990; Potter and Kies 1990). Indeed, dietary cysteine increases hepatic GSH synthesis and content (Tateishi 1981; Cho et al. 1984; Suberville 1987). The activity of hepatic cholesterol 7-α-hydroxylase, the rate-limiting enzyme in bile acid formation (Myant and Mitropoulos 1977), depends on the hepatic GSH content (Hassan et al. 1984; Hassan 1986; 1989). However, as has been previously described with regard to the effects of soybean protein isolates on cholesterol metabolism in male *Mongolian Meriones unguiculatus* gerbils, the GSH mediation of cholesterol biosynthesis would not appear to be the factor behind the lipid metabolism modifications, at least not in this animal species (Tasker and Potter 1993).

Hypercholesterolemia due to a diet containing choline is mitigated by the addition of cystine in male *Holtzman* rats (Seidel et al. 1960). The effects of cystine could depend on the protein content in a cholesterol-free diet, but also on the level of its supplementation. Indeed, the serum cholesterol concentrations of male *Wistar* rats fed on a 10% casein diet remained unchanged whether the level of cystine supplementation was 0.3% or 0.6%; in contrast, this level increased when the supplementation level reached 1.2%. However, serum cholesterol levels increased, albeit not significantly, when the casein content of the diet was 20%, and cystine supplementation 0.6%, 1.2%, or 2.4%. When the casein level was 10%, serum triacylglycerol concentrations increased with the addition of cystine at 0.6% and 1.2%; this did not apply, however, when the casein level was 20%. The liver cholesterol content was unchanged and that of triacylglycerol increased gradually with a supplement of 0.3% or 0.6% of cystine in the diet (Yagasaki et al. 1986c). In male *Donryu* rats with hepatoma, the addition of methionine (1.2%) and glycine (2.5%) to a 20% casein diet significantly suppressed the hepatoma-induced increase in VLDL and LDL cholesterol, but did not change the HDL-cholesterol level (Yagasaki et al. 1986b).

Supplementing a soybean protein isolates diet with cystine significantly lowers the total serum cholesterol and HDL-cholesterol levels in *Wistar Kyoto* inbred rats (Potter and Kies 1988). Cystine is hypocholesterolemic in rats and mice fed on casein and increases serum HDL-cholesterol levels, fecal excretion of acidic steroids and liver triacylglycerol levels, but does not raise the liver cholesterol content (Fillios and Mann 1954, Seidel et al. 1960, Sugiyama et al. 1984, 1985a, 1985b, 1986b; Yoshida et al. 1988). Compared to arginine or glycine diets, a cystine diet lowers serum cholesterol concentrations of male *Sprague-Dawley* rats and increases both HDL-cholesterol levels and fecal excretion of acidic steroids. Liver cholesterol levels are similar with each of these three diets. Liver triacylglycerol concentrations increase, whereas liver phospholipid concentrations decrease (Yoshida et al. 1988).

The effects of different protein sources with regard to their content in cystine were investigated in male *Wistar* rats fed for a 3-week period on a high-cholesterol diet containing one of various proteins such as casein, egg albumin, pork proteins, cod proteins, corn gluten, wheat gluten, or soybean protein at a 25% concentration The corn-gluten and soybean protein diet were fortified with lysine hydrochloride (0.5% and 0.7%, respectively) to avoid any effects on growth retardation. Plasma cholesterol levels were lower with vegetable proteins and egg albumin. A significant negative correlation ($p < 0.05$) was observed between plasma cholesterol levels and the cystine contents of the diet (Muramatsu and Sugiyama 1990).

As with a cholesterol-free diet, the protein level of a diet influences the effects of cysteine supplementation of a cholesterol-rich diet. In male weanling *Sprague-Dawley* rats fed a high-fat cholesterol-enriched (1.2%) diet, the addition of cystine (1.31%) to the casein (26.12%) diet decreased serum VLDL-, but not HDL- or VLDL-cholesterol concentrations (Aljawad et al. 1991), whereas cysteine supplementation (0.33%) of the casein diet (10%) did not change the total serum cholesterol, LDL plus VLDL-cholesterol, HDL-cholesterol, triacylglycerol, or phospholipid levels in male weanling *Wistar-Kyoto* rats. In contrast, the same supplementation of a soybean protein isolates diet (10%) significantly reduced the total serum cholesterol, LDL plus VLDL-cholesterol, and HDL-cholesterol levels, but did not modify serum triacylglycerol or phospholipid levels. Total liver and intestine cholesterol and lipid contents were unchanged with casein cysteine-supplemented diets, but cholesterol and lipid liver contents were increased with soybean protein cysteine-supplemented diets (Potter and Kies 1990).

When male *Wistar* rats were fed on a base line cystine-enriched (5%), casein (23%) cholesterol-enriched (0.05%) diet, the plasma cholesterol level increased. However, both plasma cholesterol levels and cholesterol secretion decreased when this diet was enriched in cholesterol (1%). Whatever the diet, cystine supplementation reduced the chylomicron and VLDL-cholesterol levels and increased those of LDL (particularly LDL_2) and HDL (Sérougne and Rukaj 1983; Rukaj and Sérougne 1983; Sérougne et al. 1984). The addition of cysteine (5%) to a casein (23%) diet of adult male *Wistar* rats for 2 months increased or decreased the plasma cholesterol level if the cholesterol content of the diet was 0.05% or 1%, respectively. Cholesterol concentrations decreased in chylomicrons and VLDL, but increased in LDL_2 and HDL. The plasma apo A-1, B, E contents were also enhanced in LDL_2 and apo A-1 and E in HDL. Serum triacylglycerol concentrations decreased when *Wistar* rats were fed on a casein diet with excessive levels of cystine (Rukaj and Sérougne 1983; Sérougne and Rukaj 1983; Sugiyama et al. 1984; Sérougne et al. 1984, 1987, 1988). However, the addition of methionine (0.8%) to a casein (25%) high-cholesterol diet of male *Wistar* rats increased the total serum cholesterol, HDL-cholesterol, and phospholipid concentrations, and enhanced fecal and bile acid excretion and 7-α-hydroxylase activity, but caused a slight reduction in the liver cholesterol content (Sugiyama et al. 1984, 1989b). In hypercholesterolemic young male *Wistar* rats, cysteine, *S*-methylcysteine sulfon and *S*-methylmethionine sulfonium chloride had little effect on hypercholesterolemia (Itokawa et al. 1973).

In male *Wistar* rats fed for 8 weeks on a casein diet containing an excess of either cholesterol (1%) or cystine (5%), the plasma cholesterol, triacylglycerol, apoprotein concentrations, and HMG-CoA reductase activity have been studied. With both diets, plasma cholesterol and apo B concentrations and liver apo B mRNA levels increased similarly and significantly compared to the control diet. Plasma apo E levels were higher with the cysteine diet and lower with the cholesterol diet compared to the control diet, and plasma apo A-1V values were lower with the cysteine diet or similar with the cholesterol diet to those of the control diet. Apo E and apo A-1 mRNA levels were similar with both diets, but apo A-1V mRNA levels were higher with the cholesterol diet and lower with the cystine diet compared with the control diet. The plasma apo A-1 and phospholipid concentrations were not significantly different with either cholesterol or cystine or with the control diet. Whereas the liver total cholesterol and triacylglycerol contents were similar with cystine and the control diet, total HMG-CoA reductase activity in liver microsomes was significantly higher with the cystine diet than the control diet (Sérougne et al. 1995).

As mentioned at the beginning of this section, the effects of cysteine supplementation on tissue lipids depend on the nature of the proteins in the diet. Cysteine (0.33%) supplementation of a soybean protein isolates cholesterol-free diet increased liver total lipid and cholesterol concentrations in male weanling *Wistar-Kyoto* rats (Potter and Kies 1990) and in male *Wistar* rats (Aoyama et al. 1992a) in contrast to the same supplementation of a casein-based cholesterol-free diet. When cystine was added to casein diet or a soybean protein isolates diet, the intestinal cholesterol concentration significantly increased or decreased, respectively. Excessive amounts of individual essential amino acids did not affect liver lipid contents unless excessive quantities of methionine plus cystine were added to the diet. In rats, the total liver lipid content produced by an excess of cystine is higher with a soybean protein diet than with casein, egg protein, or wheat gluten diet, whereas it is similar with excess levels of cystine. However, supplementation of this cystine-enriched diet with lysine and threonine increased the serum and liver cholesterol, triacylglycerol, and phospholipid concentrations (Aoyama et al. 1992a). Supplementation with lysine (12.5 g/kg diet) and threonine (5 g/kg diet) of a cystine-enriched wheat-gluten diet in male *Wistar* rats enhanced the liver cholesterol, triacylglycerol, and phospholipid concentrations, but this effect could be prevented by further addition of methionine (0.3 g or 0.6 g/kg diet) (Aoyama et al. 1998). In a short-term experiment in weaning rats fed for a 10-week period on a cholesterol-rich (1%) casein (15%) control diet, the effects of supplementing this diet with egg-albumin (15%) or methionine (15%) or cystine (15%) have been investigated. Methionine supplementation had a slightly more liver lipotropic effect, whereas L-cystine improved liver cholesterol storage (Okey and Lyman 1954, 1956, 1957). Consumption of a cystine-enriched diet (5%) increased cholesterolemia and hepatic, but not intestinal, cholesterogenesis in *Wistar* rats (Rukaj and Sérougne 1983; Sérougne et al. 1983, 1984). A significant positive linear correlation was observed between individual values of plasma cholesterol and those of internal secretion of cholesterol. The plasma cholesterol level of *Wistar* rats varies according to internal cholesterol secretion, depending on the organ that determines the variations of this secretion; it decreases when intestinal cholesterogenesis increases, but increases when hepatic cholesterogenesis is raised (Sérougne et al. 1987).

Hyperlipidemia and proteinuria were reduced when, after an injection of nephrotoxic serum, male nephritic *Wistar* rats were fed for a 14-day period on a diet containing 8.5% or 20% casein. Supplementing this diet with cystine (0.3%) induced hepatic steatosis. The liver fatty acid level was reduced by adding threonine (0.36%), but not with a supplement of glycine (2%). Cystine-threonine supplementation of a low-casein diet has also been shown to have beneficial effects on hyperlipidemia (Fujisawa et al. 1994, 1995). The addition of cystine to the diet of hypercholesterolemic rats fed on polychlorinated biphenyls (PCB) caused an increase in serum cholesterol levels. The higher the addition of sulfur amino acids to PCB, the stronger the metabolic response (Oda et al. 1986).

2.6.2.3 Ethionine

The incorporation of glycine and methionine into the proteins of female *Long Evans* rats and mice is inhibited by ethionine (Simpson et al. 1950). Ethionine is hypocholesterolemic in dogs (Feinberg et al. 1954; Furman et al. 1957) and in male weanling *Holtzman* rats fed on a cholesterol diet (Seidel and Harper 1962, 1963). However, serum triacylglycerol concentrations of rats fed on the ethionine-supplemented diet were increased 7- to 15-fold over those of rats fed on the unsupplemented diet. This rise in triacylglycerols was limited to the low-density-lipoproteins, but the increase in cholesterol and triacylglycerol levels was prevented by adding an equal amount of methionine to the diet (Seidel and Harper 1962). Ethionine causes fatty liver in mice and female *Long Evans* rats (Farber et al. 1950).

2.6.2.4 Glutamic Acid

The addition of L-glutamic acid (0.30%) to the diet of adult male *Sprague-Dawley* rats maintained on a protein-free ration for a 100-day period did not prevent the increase in liver neutral glyceride or the decrease in liver phospholipid and plasmalogen concentrations, but did reduce the liver cholesterol concentrations (Williams and Hurlebaus 1965a, 1965b). Serum cholesterol concentrations were significantly and positively correlated with glutamic acid in male *Wistar* rats fed on a cholesterol-free diet containing casein, whey protein, soybean protein, and sunflower protein (Sautier et al. 1983). Glutamic acid is hypocholesterolemic in chickens and *Mongolian* gerbils; it is hypercholesterolemic in rats and without effect in rabbits (Bazzano 1969; Bazzano et al. 1970). In *Mongolian* gerbils, α-ketoglutarate produced from glutamic acid was more hypocholesterolemic than glutamic acid (Bazzano et al. 1972).

2.6.2.5 Glycine

Herrmann (1959) reported no significant hypocholesterolemic effect of glycine in rabbits and rats in contrast to taurine.

In rabbits fed a casein (20%) semipurified diet for 48 weeks, the serum cholesterol level decreased from 15.7 mmol/L to 12.0 mmol/L after the supplementation of 0.35% L-arginine plus 0.54% L-alanine and then to 8.8 and 8.1 mmol/L, respectively after the addition of 1.40% or 3.15% glycine to the previous diet already supplemented with L-arginine and L-alanine (Katan et al. 1982). Likewise, supplementing a casein diet (20%) with glycine (1.38%, 2%, 3%) reduced the serum cholesterol level in rabbits (Hermus and Dallinga-Thie 1979; Ryzhenkov et al. 1984; Sugiyama et al. 1986a, 1986b, 1986c, 1989b, 1993; Park et al. 1999). In male *New Zealand White* rabbits supplementing a semipurified cholesterol-free casein diet (20.8%) with arginine (0.35%), alanine (0.54%), and three levels of glycine (0.65% or 1.40% or 3.15%) for a 48-week period, reduced the hypercholesterolemic effect of casein, but the effects of the three levels of glycine were not significantly different (Hermus and Dallingha-Thie 1979; Ryzhenkov et al. 1984; Sugiyama et al. 1986a, 1986b, 1986c, 1989b, 1993; Park et al. 1999).

Glycine is hypocholesterolemic and hypotriacylglycerolemic in rats regardless of whether the diet contains cholesterol or not. A low glycine level may be responsible for the hypercholesterolemia observed in rats fed on casein since casein contains about 1.8% glycine and soybean protein, 3.6%. The addition of large quantities of glycine to a semipurified diet had no effect on serum cholesterol concentrations of rats but reduced the level of triacylglycerol concentrations (Aust et al. 1980). In contrast, in another experiment the addition of glycine (0.8/100 g) to a 20% casein, cholesterol-free, low-fat diet in male *Wistar* rats caused a weak but significant reduction not only in triacylglycerol but also in total serum cholesterol concentrations. For the most part the serum levels of amino acids, with the exception of arginine and aspartic acid, were decreased (Horigome and Cho 1992).

The addition of between 0.2% and 1.6% glycine to a semipurified casein or soybean protein diet containing 1.2% cholesterol did not affect serum cholesterol concentrations in male *Wistar* rats. Beynen and Lemmens therefore suggested that the low proportion of glycine in casein had no role in casein-induced hypercholesterolemia (Beynen and Lemmens 1987). However, at 5% concentration, glycine as well as alanine, leucine, lysine, methionine, taurine, and threonine were all hypocholesterolemic in male *Wistar* rats fed high-cholesterol diet. They reduced total serum cholesterol, LDL- and VLDL-cholesterol, and triacylglycerol concentrations, and also liver cholesterol and triacylglycerol levels (Sugiyama et al. 1989b). Likewise supplementing a semipurified casein (20%) diet with cholesterol (1.2%) and glycine (2%) significantly reduced the serum cholesterol levels of female *Zucker* rats (lean phenotype) compared to a casein cholesterol (1.2%) diet unsupplemented with glycine (Katan et al. 1982). The addition of glycine (2%) to a cholesterol-rich (1%) diet of male *Sprague-Dawley* rats significantly reduced the serum and liver cholesterol levels only with a casein diet; the liver triacylglycerol content was only reduced with the soybean protein diet (Tanaka and Sugano 1989a). In male *Wistar* rats fed a casein-based cholesterol-rich (1%) diet, the addition of glycine (5%) was more hypocholesterolemic than taurine (5%) when the level of casein in the diet was 10%, but had the opposite effect when the level of casein corresponded to 25% of the diet. The increase in fecal bile excretion is extremely weak with glycine and can therefore not explain the hypocholesterolemic effect. When the casein level reaches 25%, but not at 10%, glycine increases the cholesterol 7-α-hydroxylase activity. The plasma triacylglycerol level was slightly but significantly decreased by glycine in rats fed on the 10% casein diet and unaffected by a diet containing 25% casein, whereas the plasma phospholipid concentrations were reduced at both casein levels (Sugiyama et al. 1989a).

The addition of glycine (3%) to a casein (25%) high-cholesterol (1%) diet of male *Wistar* rats decreased the total serum cholesterol and phospholipid concentrations without significant modification of fecal and bile acid excretion, 7-α-hydroxylase activity, or liver cholesterol and lipid content (Sugiyama et al. 1984, 1989b). The change in the phospholipid composition of liver microsomes (increased phosphatidylethanolamines, decreased phosphatidylcholines) preceded the decrease in serum cholesterol levels in male *Wistar* rats suggesting that the plasma cholesterol-lowering effect of dietary glycine could be associated with the alteration of the microsomal phospholipid composition (Sugiyama et al. 1993).

Hypercholesterolemia induced by the addition of methionine is almost completely prevented by glycine supplementation. The addition of glycine to a diet prevents the methionine-induced enhancement of cholesterol levels (Sugiyama et al. 1989a, Sugiyama and Muramatsu 1990), as do all methyl-group acceptors, which also reduce plasma cholesterol levels when they are added to make up 25% of a casein diet in male *Wistar* rats. This effect may be due, at least in part, to the depressed phosphatidylcholine biosynthesis via the phosphatidylethanolamine *N*-methylation pathway (Sugiyama et al. 1989b). In male *Wistar* rats with nephrotoxic serum nephritis fed on a casein (8.5%), cholesterol-free diet supplemented with cystine (0.3%), the addition of glycine (2%) to the diet failed to reduce the cystine-induced fatty liver (8.5%) (Fujisawa et al. 1994).

In male *Donryu* rats, with or without hepatoma, the supplementation of a casein diet (20%) with 1.2% methionine, 1.2% cystine, and a combination of 1.2% methionine and glycine (2.5%) significantly suppressed the hepatoma-induced increase in serum VLDL- and LDL-cholesterol levels without any changes in HDL cholesterol or neutral sterol fecal excretion, but with an increase in acidic sterol fecal excretion. Supplementing the diet with methionine (1.2%) and glycine (2.5%) enhanced the liver cholesterol metabolism and reduced VLDL- and LDL-cholesterol levels (Yagasaki et al. 1986b, 1990; Yagasaki and Funabiki 1990). In male *Wistar* rats glycine had a more moderate enhancing effect than taurine on fecal bile excretion (Sugiyama et al. 1989a, 1989b) and a weak or no effect on the activity of hepatic cholesterol 7-α-hydroxylase, the rate-limiting enzyme in bile acid synthesis from cholesterol (Murakami et al. 1996b). The relative conjugation of cholic acid with glycine and taurine (G/T ratio) is also related to the regulation of serum cholesterol levels (Feland et al. 1973).

In adult male *Hartley white* guinea pigs fed for 7 weeks on a casein diet (227 g/kg diet) well balanced in fatty acids (30%), supplementation with glycine decreased cholesterol in the sub-fraction of LDL with larger molecular weight (Atwal et al. 1997).

The mechanisms of the cholesterol-lowering effect of glycine are not yet clearly understood.

2.6.2.6 Histidine

The addition of histidine (0.42%) to the diet of adult male *Sprague-Dawley* rats, maintained on a protein-free ration for 100 days, did not prevent the increase of liver cholesterol and neutral glyceride concentrations or the decrease in liver total phospholipids and plasmalogen concentrations (Williams and Hurlebaus 1965a,b). Liver lipid levels declined when growing male *Donryu* rats were fed on a histidine-deficient diet (Aoyama and Ashida 1972).

Histidine is hypercholesterolemic in young *New Zealand* rabbits (Geison and Waisman 1970), male albino rats (Qureshi et al. 1978), and male *Wistar* rats (Nagaoka et al. 1985). This hypercholesterolemia persists in male *Wistar* rats even during a period of starvation (Ohmura et al. 1986; Aoyama et al. 1991). A high-histidine diet (3 g/kg/day) for a 3- to 4-month period, also induces hyperlipemia and hypercholesterolemia in infant *Macaca mulatta* monkeys without any fatty infiltration of the liver (Kerr et al. 1965, 1966).

In both young and mature *Wistar* rats, excessive quantities of dietary histidine (5%) induced hepatomegaly and hypercholesterolemia (Harvey et al. 1981; Aoyama et al. 1983a). However, liver lipid and cholesterol contents and serum triacylglycerol concentrations were not enhanced (Aoyama et al. 1983a). In male weanling *albino Holtzman* rats fed on a chow diet, supplementation with histidine (5%) for a 4-day period increased the incorporation of [2-^{14}C]acetate or [1-^{14}C]octanoate into cholesterol by 100% in liver samples and decreased incorporation into triacylglycerols by 38% (Solomon and Geison 1978a, 1978b). Likewise, hypercholesterolemia was observed in male albino rats fed on a chow diet supplemented with histidine (5%) for a 3-day period. There was a nine-fold increase in the incorporation of [^{14}C]acetate into the hepatic nonsaponifiable fraction of histidine-supplemented chow-fed rats compared to controls. Thus, histidine facilitates cholesterol biosynthesis in rats (Qureshi et al. 1978).

2.6.2.7 Isoleucine

The addition of L-isoleucine (0.20%) to the diet of adult male *Sprague-Dawley* rats, maintained on a protein-free ration for 100 days, caused a slight inhibition of the increase in liver neutral glyceride and cholesterol concentrations, but did not prevent the reduction of liver total phospholipid or plasmalogen concentrations (Williams and Hurlebaus 1965a, 1965b).

2.6.2.8 Leucine

A 5% leucine concentration in a low fat cholesterol-free semipurified diet is hypo-cholesterolemic in male *New Zealand white* rabbits (Kurowska and Carroll 1994). The addition of L-leucine (0.26%) to the diet of adult male *Sprague-Dawley* rats, maintained on a protein-free ration for 100 days, caused a slight inhibition of the increase in liver neutral glyceride and cholesterol concentrations, but not in the reduction of total phospholipid and plasmalogen concentrations (Williams and Hurlebaus 1965a, 1965b). At 5% concentration, leucine as well as alanine, glycine, lysine, methionine, taurine, and threonine were all hypocholesterolemic in male *Wistar* rats fed the high-cholesterol diet. They reduced total serum cholesterol, LDL- and VLDL-cholesterol, and triacylglycerol concentrations, and also liver cholesterol and triacylglycerol levels (Sugiyama et al. 1989b).

2.6.2.9 Methionine

The effects of methionine depend on the animal species but also, as will be described later, on the levels of protein and methionine supplementation in the diet. Methionine can therefore induce hypercholesterolemia or hypocholesterolemia and the results of experiments have sometimes been conflicting. In rats, depending on the dietary methionine/protein ratio, methionine-enriched diets may be hypercholesterolemic, hypocholesterolemic or without any influence on plasma cholesterol (Yagasaki et al. 1986a, 1986b, 1986c; Sugiyama et al. 1986a, 1986b, 1986c; Toborek and Hennig 1996). The addition of methionine (0.30%) to the diet of adult male *Sprague-Dawley* rats, maintained on a protein-free ration for 100 days, increased liver cholesterol and neutral glyceride concentrations, but only partially prevented the reduction in liver total phospholipid and plasmalogen concentrations (Williams and Hurlebaus 1965a, 1965b).

The metabolism of methionine is accelerated by dietary glycine, especially if the diet is high in methionine (Benevenga and Harper 1970). The effects of methionine and glycine, given simultaneously to rats, are described in Section 2.6.2.5 on glycine.

Methionine is hypocholesterolemic in chicks (Léveillé et al. 1962a; Hill 1966); rats (Fillios and Mann 1954; Shapiro and Freedman 1955; Passananti et al. 1958; Seidel et al. 1960; De Groot 1960; Nath et al. 1961; Seidel and Harper 1962, 1963; Bagchi et al. 1963; Sugiyama et al. 1984, 1985b, 1986c, 1988, 1997); mice (Fillios and Man 1954); rabbits (Kurowska and Carroll 1994; Carroll and Kurowska 1995; Giroux et al. 1999a, 1999b); and monkeys (Mann et al. 1953, 1960).

At 5% concentration, methionine as well as alanine, glycine, leucine, lysine, taurine, and threonine were all hypocholesterolemic in male *Wistar* rats fed high-cholesterol diet. They reduced total serum cholesterol, LDL- and VLDL-cholesterol, and triacylglycerol concentrations and also liver cholesterol and triacylglycerol levels (Sugiyama et al. 1989b).

Methionine has also been shown to be hypocholesterolemic with a low soybean protein diet in mice and rats (Fillios and Mann 1954). However, with a low-protein or a soybean protein diet, with either a low or a high cholesterol content, methionine was hypercholesterolemic in rabbits (Carroll and Hamilton 1975; Hermus and Dallinga-Thie 1979; Terpstra et al. 1983b) and rats (Roth and Milstein 1957; Bagchi et al. 1963; Terpstra et al. 1983b; Sugiyama et al. 1985a, 1985b, 1986a, 1986b, 1986c; Tanaka and Sugano 1989a; Moundras et al. 1995; Kurowska and Carroll 1996). In other experiments, this supplementation was without effect in rabbits (Hamilton and Carroll 1976), rats (Jones et al. 1957), and young male *Yorkshire* swine fed on a high-fat, high-cholesterol diet (Kim et al. 1978). In rats fed on 8.1% soybean protein isolate diet containing 0.5% cholesterol and 0.25% sodium cholate, supplementation of methionine decreased plasma cholesterol concentration (Mizuno et al. 1988). Hypercholesterolemic in mice with a high casein cholesterol-rich diet (Fillios and Mann 1954), methionine is hypocholesterolemic in mice and rats (Fillios and Mann 1954; Sugiyama et al. 1985b) when the diet is low in casein.

Methionine supplementation of a casein diet in rats resulted in significantly higher serum cholesterol and triacylglycerol levels, but this effect depends on the level of supplementation (Kurup et al. 1983; Sugiyama et al. 1986a, 1986b; Potter and Kies 1988) and on the amount of protein and cholesterol in the diet (Sugiyama et al. 1986a, 1986b, 1986c). If the addition of methionine to a casein diet (20%) was in the proportion of 0.2%, the serum cholesterol level increased; it decreased, however, if the amount added was equivalent to 0.8% (Hermus and Dallinga-Thie 1979). The addition of methionine (0.8%) to a casein (25%) high-cholesterol diet of male *Wistar* rats increased the total serum cholesterol, HDL-cholesterol and phospholipids concentrations, fecal and bile acid excretion, and 7-α-hydroxylase activity, but caused a slight reduction in the liver cholesterol, but not in liver lipid contents (Sugiyama et al. 1984, 1989b).

The effects of methionine supplementation of a casein diet also vary according to the amounts of casein and methionine in the diet of male *Wistar* rats. When a casein diet (10%) was supplemented by 0.3% methionine, serum cholesterol concentration increased and then returned to the control value if the level of supplementation was 0.6% or 1.2%. However, serum HDL-cholesterol concentrations increased very significantly when between 1.2% and 10% methionine was added, but not with a 20% casein diet. In contrast, when the casein diet was increased to 20%, the serum cholesterol concentration was similar to the control value if the level of supplementation was 0.6%, but decreased progressively with 1.2% and then 2.4% methionine supplementation. At the casein level of 10%, supplementation with methionine at 0.3% or 0.6% was hypertriglyceridemic, but less at 1.2%, whereas at the casein level of 20%, the addition of methionine was hypertriglyceridemic only at 1.2%. The liver cholesterol content was not affected by the different supplementations of both casein diets (Yagasaki et al. 1986c). Methionine supplementation

(0.8%) of casein or soybean protein isolate high-cholesterol diets at different protein levels (10%, 15%, 20%, 25%, 40%) has different effects in rats. The serum cholesterol concentrations decreased with the addition of methionine to a casein diet (10%), but increased with casein levels of 20% or more. In contrast, regardless of the proportion of soybean protein isolates a methionine supplement did not increase serum cholesterol concentrations in rats. Fecal excretion of bile acids was higher with soybean protein isolates, than with casein diets and tended to increase with methionine supplementation. The difference in glycine content of these two proteins may well account for these contrasting effects (Sugiyama et al. 1988).

The supplementation of casein (10% by weight) diets of *Wistar-Kyoto* rats with 0.33% methionine or cystine did not change the total serum cholesterol, LDL- plus VLDL-cholesterol, HDL-cholesterol or triacylglycerol concentrations. In contrast, the supplementation of a soybean protein isolates (10% by weight) diet with this level of methionine caused a weak increase in total serum cholesterol concentrations, but a nonsignificant rise in the serum LDL-, VLDL- and, HDL-cholesterol levels, whereas supplementation of the same level of cystine decreased total serum cholesterol, HDL-cholesterol, and phospholipid concentrations without any changes in LDL- plus VLDL-cholesterol levels (Potter and Kies 1990).

The addition of methionine to soybean protein and whey diets produced a weak increase in the HDL-cholesterol concentrations in rats. Total serum cholesterol and LDL cholesterol were unchanged, as were liver total lipid or cholesterol concentrations (Aljawad et al. 1991). In *Wistar* rats with hypothyroidism, the addition of methionine (1.2%) suppressed the rise in VLDL plus LDL cholesterol (Yagasaki and Funabiki 1990). In rats fed on a high cholesterol diet containing 25% of one or other different proteins, serum cholesterol levels have been shown to increase to progressively greater extents in the following order: wheat gluten, lactalbumin, soybean protein isolates, casein. Dietary addition of 0.8% methionine resulted in an approximately 2-fold increase in plasma cholesterol concentrations of rats fed on casein or lactalbumin diets. However, this addition caused a mild reduction or was without effect on the plasma cholesterol levels of rats fed on soybean protein isolates and wheat gluten diets. A significant negative correlation was observed between plasma cholesterol levels and the cystine contents of these proteins (Muramatsu et al. 1987). The hypocholesterolemic effects of supplementation of a 20% casein diet with an association of dietary methionine and cystine or glycine in male *Donryu* rats with hepatoma has been already described in Section 2.6.2.2 and Section 2.6.2.5 on cystine and glycine (Yagasaki et al. 1986b).

In adult male *Wistar* rats fed with one or other of seven various dietary protein sources (12.3 or 14.4 g/100 g): casein, lactalbumin, whole egg protein, egg albumin, sardine protein, soybean protein, and wheat gluten, there was a significant positive correlation between the plasma total cholesterol concentration and the plasma concentration of valine and methionine, and the hepatic concentration of valine and alanine. In contrast, the plasma cholesterol concentration and hepatic-free ethanolamine were negatively correlated. Hepatic-free ethanolamine, which is a precursor for phosphatidylethanolamine, can be considered as reflecting the rate of synthesis or the amount of phosphatidylamine in the liver. The phosphatidylcholine/phosphatidylethanolamine ratio in liver microsomes is positively and significantly correlated with plasma cholesterol concentrations and with the methionine content of dietary proteins (Sugiyama et al. 1996). In male *New Zealand white* rabbits, the liver total phospholipid levels and the phosphatidylcholine/phosphatidylethanolamine ratio were higher with methionine or lysine supplements than with arginine. This alteration of liver phospholipid levels may well constitute an additional mechanism in the cholesterol metabolism modifications observed in rabbits (Giroux et al. 1999b).

The addition of methionine (0.6 g/kg diet) to a diet supplemented with cystine, lysine and threonine did not change the liver cholesterol level, decreased liver triacylglycerol and phospholipid content and serum triacylglycerol concentrations, and increased serum cholesterol and phospholipids levels (Aoyama et al. 1998).

In adult male *Wistar* rats fed with one or other of seven various protein dietary sources (12.3 or 14.4 g/100 g) — casein, lactalbumin, whole egg protein, egg albumin, sardine protein, soybean protein, and wheat gluten — there was a significant positive correlation between the plasma total cholesterol concentration and the plasma concentration of methionine and valine, and the hepatic concentration of alanine and valine. In contrast, the plasma cholesterol concentration and the hepatic-free ethanolamine were negatively correlated. Hepatic-free ethanolamine, which is a precursor for phosphatidylethanolamine can be considered as reflecting the rate of synthesis or the amount of phosphatidylamine in the liver.

The differences in nutritional quality between a casein (8%) diet and a soybean protein isolates (10%) diet both supplemented with oligo-L-methionine (a mixture of hexa- and hepta-peptides), are due to the different rates of luminal digestion of this mixture, which, in nutritional terms, is not the same with regard to free amino acids (Chiji et al. 1990). Methionine alone would appear to be hypocholesterolemic, whereas its methyl group would appear to be hypercholesterolemic (Sugiyama et al. 1986c). The factors promoting demethylation and transsulfuration of methionine may protect against the hypercholesterolemic effect of this amino acid. Glycine facilitates the use of methionine via the transsulfuration pathway and lowers serum cholesterol levels in rats fed on methionine (Sugiyama et al. 1986b). However, methionine may be hypercholesterolemic via an effect of down-regulation of hepatic LDL (Kurowska and Carroll 1992).

The reduction of hyperlipidemia of male *Wistar* rats with nephritis due to a nephrotoxic agent, when fed a diet with a low (8.5%) soybean protein isolates level, was partially due to decreased liver cholesterol synthesis. Growth retardation was alleviated by the addition of methionine (0.3%) (Fujisawa et al. 1994, 1995). An identical result was obtained in the same strain of male rats on a low-casein diet supplemented with cystine and threonine (Fujisawa et al. 1994) and with a low-meat-protein diet (8.5%) or if this diet was supplemented by 0.5% L-valine (Yagasaki et al. 1994). In male *Wistar* rats treated with 300 ppm of PCB, serum cholesterol concentrations were higher with casein than with soybean protein isolates. The addition of methionine (0.5%) and cholic acid (0.25%) to the diet greatly increased serum cholesterol concentrations of rats fed on soybean protein isolates, but only a weak increase was observed if they were fed on a casein diet. HMG-CoA reductase activity increased when methionine was added to soybean protein isolates, but the hepatic content of cholesterol was not affected. PCB and methionine act synergistically. Although the cholesterol level was increased in all serum lipoprotein fractions by the addition of PCB, a dietary methionine supplement increased the HDL cholesterol, mainly HDL_1 cholesterol, but did not modify the secretion rate of VLDL cholesterol (Oda et al. 1986, 1989, 1991). These results confirm those obtained in similar conditions by Kato et al. using a diet supplemented with methionine at three different doses (0.2%, 0.5%, 1.2%) (Kato et al. 1982). Likewise, in rats with PCB-induced hypercholesterolemia and fed with a nonprotein diet, methionine and threonine supplement accelerated the rise in plasma cholesterol levels and produced a greater increase in liver HMG-CoA reductase activity (the main cause of hypercholesterolemia) than PCB alone (Hitomi and Yoshida 1989). This effect is similar to that of taurine, which will be described later (Mochizuki et al. 2001).

The effect of methionine on serum cholesterol concentrations is influenced by the type of dietary fat (Shapiro and Freedman 1955). L-Methionine increases the apparent VLDL secretion by the liver in preruminant calves when it is associated with a lipid-restricted diet (Auboiron et al. 1995). A low-fat, cholesterol-free, semipurified amino acid diet enriched with lysine plus methionine caused a notable increase in total serum and LDL cholesterol but also in apo B levels of male *New Zealand white* rabbits, whereas a similar diet enriched in essential ketoamino acids only enhanced these parameters to a moderate degree (Giroux et al. 1999b).

Methionine supplementation of a soybean protein diet in rats increases total serum cholesterol levels and produces a significant reduction in total liver cholesterol concentrations. In rats fed with a cholesterol-free diet and 15% alpha protein with or without the addition of methionine (0.3%) the rate of synthesis and elimination of [^{14}C]cholesterol in all tissues, remained similar, as did the cholesterol/fatty acids ratio, whereas in the liver, the incorporation of [^{14}C]acetate into cholesterol was lower in the rats on a nonsupplemented diet (Portman 1956). This increase in serum cholesterol concentrations was also observed in male *Sprague-Dawley* rats receiving a 25% soybean protein cholesterol-free diet (Tanaka and Sugano 1989a). The liver total lipid and cholesterol content did not change with a casein diet supplemented with methionine or cysteine. In contrast, although the supplementation of a soybean protein isolates diet with methionine did not change the liver lipid content but decreased liver cholesterol concentrations, cysteine supplementation increased both liver lipid and cholesterol content levels (Potter and Kies 1990).

The liver lipid content of adult male rats of the *Donryu* or *Sprague-Dawley* strains was increased when they were fed a protein-free diet supplemented with methionine (Williams and Jasik 1963; Aoyama et al. 1973). The addition of methionine to a protein-free or low-casein or low-soybean protein or soybean infant formula diet resulted in hepatic steatosis (Harper 1958; Yoshida et al. 1966; Theuer and Sarett 1970; Noda 1970, 1973). In female *Wistar* rats fed on a low-soybean protein diet (8%), methionine supplementation of 0.6% (but not with 0.3%) increased liver triacylglycerol concentrations without any change in liver phospholipids or protein concentrations (Ponzio de Azevedo et al. 1994). Supplementation with 0.3% methionine in a low-soybean protein diet (8%), which is deficient in sulfur-containing amino acids, induced an accumulation of triacylglycerols in the liver of young female *Wistar* rats. *In vitro,* compared with animals fed on a soybean diet (20%), the rats fed on the methionine-supplemented diet showed a higher incorporation of [1-^{14}C]acetate into the liver lipid fraction. *In vivo,* incorporation of ^{32}P into the phospholipid fraction was lower in rats supplemented with methionine. Since phospholipid synthesis is relatively reduced triacylglycerol transport from the liver was diminished The relative increase in triacylglycerol synthesis, which enhances the triacylglycerol/phospholipid ratio in the liver of rats fed on methionine, may cause an accumulation of triacylglycerols in the liver (Noda 1971; Noda and Okita 1980).

In a short-term experiment in weaning rats fed for 10 weeks on a cholesterol-rich (1%) casein (15%) control diet, the effects of this diet supplemented with egg albumin (15%), methionine (15%), or cystine (15%) have been investigated. Methionine supplementation had slightly greater liver lipotropic effect, whereas L-cystine improved liver cholesterol storage in adolescent rats (Okey and Lyman 1954, 1957). The addition of methionine (0.3 or 0.6 g) prevented the increase of serum cholesterol concentrations and liver triacylglycerol, cholesterol, and phospholipid contents due to the addition of lysine (12.5 g/kg diet) and threonine (5 g/kg diet) to a wheat gluten (271 g/kg diet) cystine-excessive (35 g/kg diet) cholesterol-free diet of male *Wistar* rats (Aoyama et al. 1983a, 1983b).

Methionine has two opposite effects on serum cholesterol concentrations in rats fed on a hypercholesterolemic choline-deficient diet: firstly, a cholesterol-raising effect that is attributable to its ability to spare choline by providing a supply of preformed methyl groups and a cholesterol-lowering effect common to all sulfur-containing amino acids and not dependent on the provision of methyl-groups (Seidel et al. 1960).

A soybean protein diet supplemented with methionine potentiates the susceptibility of lipoproteins to peroxidation in rats (Moundras et al. 1995). Methionine supplementation increased hepatic lipid peroxidation as measured by the level of thiobarbituric acid-reactive substances and iron concentrations. Thus, methionine toxicity increases oxidative stress (Lynch and Strain 1989) and lipid peroxidation (Toborek et al. 1995). However, the blood lipid peroxidation in vitamin B6–deficient rats is counteracted by methionine supplementation, which restores the levels of antioxidants to near normal (Selvam and Ravichandran 1991).

2.6.2.10 Phenylalanine

A phenylalanine, tyrosine-deficient and sulfur-containing amino acid–deficient diet reduced the liver lipid content in growing male *Donryu* rats (Aoyama and Ashida 1972). The addition of phenylalanine (0.30%) to the diet of adult male *Sprague-Dawley* rats, maintained on a protein-free ration for 100 days, limited the increase in liver neutral glyceride and cholesterol concentrations, but did not prevent the reduction of liver total phospholipid and plasmalogen concentrations (Williams and Hurlebaus 1965a, 1965b). The supplementation of a casein diet (20%) with phenylalanine (8%) did not modify serum cholesterol concentrations in normocholesterolemic male *Wistar* rats (Nagaoka et al. 1985).

2.6.2.11 Taurine

In hamsters and humans, taurine is primarily of dietary origin (Gaul et al. 1985). The effects of supplementation with taurine are species- and age-dependent. The hepatic taurine conjugation of bile acids accounts for about 30-35% of the total bile acid pool in the taurine-sensitive.

The hypocholesterolemic action of taurine has been proven by several studies in rats, mice, and hamsters with cholesterol-free or cholesterol-enriched diets (Herrmann 1959; Tsuji et al. 1983; Sugiyama et al. 1984; Bellentani et al. 1987a, 1987b; Gandhi et al. 1992; Mochizuki et al. 1999a, 1999b; review in Yokogoshi et al. 1999) although it has not been observed in rabbits (Herrmann 1959). Taurine is hypocholesterolemic in rats (Herrmann 1959; Seidel et al. 1960; Yamanaka et al. 1986; Sugiyama et al. 1989a), although to a lesser degree than methionine (Herrmann 1959; Seidel et al. 1960), in *SHR* rats (Murakami et al. 1996a, 1996b), and in monkeys (Mann 1960; Mann et al. 1960). In *Sprague-Dawley* rats fed on a choles-terol-free diet (Park et al. 1998, 1999) and in streptozotocin-induced diabetic rats belonging to different species taurine was hypocholesterolemic and hypotriacyl-glycerolemic (Goodman and Shihabi 1990; Nanami et al. 1996; Mochizuki et al. 1999b). At 5% concentration, taurine as alanine, glycine, leucine, lysine, methionine, taurine, and threonine were all hypocholesterolemic in male *Wistar* rats fed high-cholesterol diet. They reduced total serum cholesterol, LDL- and VLDL-cholesterol, and triacylglycerol concentrations, and also liver cholesterol and triacylglycerol levels (Sugiyama et al. 1989b). Nevertheless, the supplementation with taurine (0.5%, 1.3%, 5%) of a standard diet of male *Wistar* rats for 12 or 14 days, increased HDL-cholesterol concentrations in a dose-dependent manner, but without any change in total cholesterol levels (Mochizuki et al. 1998b). In contrast, with cysteine or methionine, taurine supplementation did not decrease plasma cholesterol concentra-tion in rats fed on 8,1% soybean protein isolate diet containing 0.5% cholesterol and 0.25% sodium cholate (Mizuno et al. 1988).

The addition of taurine (1.5%) to the diet of male *Sprague-Dawley* rats reduced the serum concentrations of total cholesterol (−31%), LDL plus VLDL cholesterol (−38%), triacylglycerols (−43%), and those of hepatic cholesterol (−49%) and tria-cylglycerols (−30%) (Park et al. 1998). When a high cholesterol (10 g/kg) diet of male *Wistar* rats was supplemented with various amounts of taurine (0.25 to 50 g/kg diet) for 2 weeks, a dose response was observed and the serum HDL-cholesterol concentration increased. At the dose of 10 g taurine/kg, serum cholesterol concen-trations were similar to those observed with a cholesterol-free diet. A high-choles-terol diet reduced the taurine concentrations in the serum, liver, and heart and the effective dose of taurine as a supplement capable of improving this reduction is 2.5 g/kg diet. The taurine supplementation significantly increased the excretion of fecal bile acids, hepatic cholesterol 7-α-.hydroxylase (CYP7A1) activity and its mRNA level, indicating an enhancement in cholesterol degradation (Yokogoshi et al. 1999).

In normocholesterolemic *SHR-SP* rats, taurine supplementation (3% in tap water) for 6 weeks produced a significant increase in total serum cholesterol, par-ticularly LDL-cholesterol, phospholipids and apo E-LDL concentrations, whereas serum triacylglycerol levels remained unchanged. In the HDL-fraction, serum con-centrations of apo A-1V were significantly reduced and apo E nonsignificantly. The decrease in apo A-1V may be due to the increased LPL activity since apo A-1V is one of the major components of chylomicrons. Microsomal 7-α-hydroxylase activity was significantly enhanced in the liver, suggesting that taurine may promote hepatic taurine-conjugated bile acid synthesis, leading to a reduction in cholesterol content when an excess amount of cholesterol is taken up in the liver, as in the case of cholesterol feeding. In hypercholesterolemic *SHR-SP* rats on a cholesterol-rich diet, taurine suppressed the increase in total serum cholesterol and triacylglycerol concentrations in the VLDL and IDL fractions, as well as the decrease in serum apo A-1 and the increase in apo B serum concentrations. In the liver, taurine produced a marked reduction in the cholesterol content (Ogawa et al. 1988; Ogawa 1996). In *SHR-SP* rats fed on a hypercholesterolemic diet (cholesterol 5%, cholic acid 2%) supplementation with 3% taurine for a 50-day period, prevented the increase in serum cholesterol levels, enhanced cholesterol 7-α-hydroxylase activity, and stimulated bile acid production (Murakami et al. 1996a, 1996b). When the level of casein is 10% in a cholesterol-rich (1%) diet, the addition of taurine (5%) is less hypocholesterolemic in male *Wistar* rats than the addition of glycine (5%), but it was the reverse when the level of casein in the diet was 25%. The increase in fecal bile excretion with taurine may well explain its hypocholesterolemic effect. The hypercholesterolemia induced by the addition of methionine was insufficiently counteracted by taurine supplementation. At a casein level of 10% or 25%, taurine increased the cholesterol 7-α-hydroxylase activity. The plasma triacylglycerol level was slightly, but significantly decreased by taurine in rats fed on the 10% casein diet and not affected with a level of 25% casein in the diet, whereas the plasma phospholipid concentrations were reduced with both casein levels (Sugiyama et al. 1989a).

In *C57BL/6J* mice fed on a high-fat diet containing 15% fat and 1.25% cholesterol for a 6-month period, serum LDL plus VLDL cholesterol was lowered (−44%), HDL cholesterol increased (+25%), liver cholesterol content reduced (−19%), and liver cholesterol hydroxylase activity was doubled in the group supplemented with taurine dissolved in the drinking water (1% w/v). Murakami et al. have suggested that the cholesterol-lowering action of taurine may be related to the increased conversion of cholesterol to bile acids due to the enhanced cholesterol 7-α-hydroxylase activity (Murakami et al. 1999). In mice of the same strain fed a high-fat (15%) high-cholesterol (1.25%) diet supplemented with taurine dissolved in the drinking water at 1%(w/v), given ad libitum over a 6-month period, taurine doubled the liver activity of cholesterol 7-α-hydroxylase and increased the conversion of cholesterol to bile acids. The cholesterol-lowering action of taurine may well be explained by the increased activity of cholesterol 7-α-hydroxylase (Murakami et al. 1999).

In *Golden Syrian* hamsters, which have a sterol and taurine metabolism that is comparable to that of humans (Bellentani et al. 1987a), and in *Wistar* rats (Cantafora et al. 1994), a diet supplemented with taurine enhanced the hepatic activity of cholesterol 7-α-hydroxylase, the rate limiting enzyme in bile acid synthesis from cholesterol, and of cholesterol ester hydrolase, whereas that of HMG-CoA reductase and ACATase in the intestine, usually activated by a cholesterol-rich diet, was reduced. The bile acid pool size was increased, and the bile saturation index was decreased

In male quail, *Coturnix coturnix japonica*, fed on a soybean protein (40%), corn meal (46%), cholesterol-rich diet (1%), supplementation with taurine (2% or 4%) significantly reduced the serum and liver cholesterol concentrations when compared to a cholesterol control group without taurine supplementation (Jackson and Burns 1974).

Taurine supplementation of a cholesterol-rich diet or a cholesterol- and cholate-rich diet reduced the serum and liver cholesterol levels in rats. The addition of methionine, cysteine, or cystine had a greater hypocholesterolemic effect than taurine, but the growth of the rats was retarded (Herrmann 1959; Tsuji et al. 1983). Bile acid synthesis was stimulated by dietary taurine in cultured HepG2 cells (Stephan et al. 1987), guinea pigs (Kibe et al. 1980), *Wistar* rats (Yan et al. 1993), hamsters (Bellentani et al. 1987a), and mice (Yamanaka et al. 1985). Bile acid conjugation and synthesis, bile flow, biliary cholesterol secretion, and lipid solubility were increased by dietary taurine supplementation in guinea pigs and mongrel dogs (Kibe et al. 1980; Batta et al. 1982; Strasberg et al. 1983). Dietary taurine increased the bile acid pool size and reduced the bile saturation index in hamsters (Bellentani et al. 1987a, 1987b), but was without effect in humans (Truswell et al. 1965).

The conjugation of cholic acid with taurine is related to the regulation of serum cholesterol levels (Mann et al. 1953, 1960). The relative conjugation of cholic acid with glycine and taurine (G/T ratio) is also related to the regulation of serum cholesterol levels (Feland et al. 1973). In *Golden Syrian* hamsters treated for an 8- or 15-day period by tauroursodeoxycholic acid, with or without taurine supplementation, each at the concentration of 0.05 g/100 ml drinking water, the percentage of ursodeoxycholic acid and chenodeodeoxycholic acid in the bile was significantly increased, whereas the percentage of cholic acid was reduced. The activities of HMG-CoA reductase and 7-α-hydroxylase were not affected. The bile acid glycine to taurine conjugation ratio (G/T ratio) was significantly higher in treated hamsters than in control animals. In contrast, in the group of *Golden Syrian* hamsters receiving the taurine supplement, the bile acid G/T ratio was significantly decreased (Bellentani et al. 1987b). The serum cholesterol level of dogs and rats, two species with a low G/T ratio, can be controlled when cholesterol is added to the diet. The percentage of taurine and glycine conjugated with bile acids in the liver is species dependent and is higher for taurine than for glycine in rats (Bremer 1956) and humans (Gottfries et al. 1966). The proportion of either cholesteryl ester in hepatic lipids or taurochenodeoxycholate in biliary bile salts is inversely correlated with hepatic taurine levels (Chao et al. 1983). The changes in hepatocellular levels of taurine influence the liver lipid composition in guinea pigs, cats, and rats.

Taurine has an important role in lipid metabolism for the production of bile acid conjugates in the liver since cholesterol is catabolized to bile acids that are excreted in the bile after conjugation with taurine or glycine. The excretion of fecal bile acids, the activity of hepatic cholesterol 7-α-hydroxylase and its mRNA levels, which are already significantly increased by a cholesterol-rich diet in young male *Wistar* rats, were further enhanced by a supplement of taurine that increases cholesterol degradation and the excretion of bile acids (Yokogoshi et al. 1999).

In male *Holtzman* rats, a strain with endogenous hypercholesterolemia induced in normal rats by a diet containing polychlorinated biphenyls (PCB), this condition was amplified by taurine, as was the accumulation of liver cholesterol (Mochizuki et al. 1998a, 1999a). In *Wistar* rats, taurine also increased

PCB-induced hyper-α-cholesterolemia, total cholesterol, HDL-cholesterol, and apo A-1 serum concentrations. The increase in liver cholesterol concentrations was further enhanced. The effect was similar to that of a methionine and cystine supplement with PCB as previously described (Oda et al. 1986, 1989; Mochizuki et al. 2001). PCB suppresses hepatic cholesterol 7-α-hydroxylase (CYP7A1) gene expression and taurine-induced CYP7A1 gene expression (Mochizuki et al. 2001). Although a taurine supplement did not affect serum cholesterol concentrations in male *Wistar* rats with hypercholesterolemia induced by a diet containing phenobarbital, it did increase liver cholesterol concentrations (Mochizuki et al. 2001).

Depending on the amount of taurine in the diet, different modifications are observed with regard to cholesterol lipoprotein distribution, the phosphatidylethanolamine/phosphatidylcholine ratio, and the fatty acid profile of the major lipid classes in female *Golden Syrian* hamsters (Bellentani et al. 1987a), guinea pigs (Kibe et al. 1980), and mice (Yamanaka et al. 1985). Taurine doubled the number of LDL receptors without affecting receptor affinity in a culture of HepG2 cells (Stephan et al. 1987).

The liver lipid composition of guinea pigs, cats, and rats varies according to the hepatocellular levels of taurine. A taurine-supplemented diet increases the liver triacylglycerol concentrations in guinea pigs and cats, which have a limited endogenous synthesis of taurine, whereas it decreases them in rats in which the endogenous synthesis of taurine is active (Cantafora et al. 1986, 1991, 1994; Yan et al. 1993). The formation of low-affinity charge complexes between taurine and neutral membrane phospholipids accounts for the lipid alterations induced by taurine. The modifications in the cell membrane microenvironment influence the liver biosynthesis of glycerolipids, glycero-phospholipids, and steroids (Cantafora et al. 1994; Murakami et al. 1996a, 1996b, 1999).

The studies on amino acids have shown that methionine, cystine, and glycine have the greatest effects on plasma cholesterol levels (Muramatsu and Sugiyama 1990), but taurine could also be added to this group.

2.6.2.12 Threonine

In male *albino Wistar* rats fed on a casein diet (20%), 1% threonine is hypocholesterolemic, whereas 5% threonine is not (Sugiyama et al. 1986b). However, at 5% concentration, threonine as well as alanine, glycine, leucine, lysine, methionine, and taurine were all hypocholesterolemic in male *Wistar* rats when fed on high-cholesterol diet. They reduced total serum cholesterol, LDL- and VLDL-cholesterol, and triacylglycerol concentrations, and also liver cholesterol and triacylglycerol levels (Sugiyama et al. 1989b). Supplementation of a wheat gluten cholesterol-free diet with threonine, which is a limiting amino acid of this protein source, did not reduce the hypocholesterolemic effect of wheat gluten in male weanling rats in comparison with a casein diet (Bassat and Mokady 1985). However, serum cholesterol concentrations and the liver triacylglycerol, cholesterol, and phospholipid contents were increased in male *Wistar* rats by the addition of lysine (12.5 g/kg diet) and threonine (5 g/kg diet) to a wheat gluten (271 g/kg diet) cystine-excessive (35 g/kg diet) cholesterol-free diet. The addition of methionine (0.3 g or 0.6 g) prevented this effect (Aoyama et al. 1998).

Compared to an 8% casein diet, a threonine-imbalanced diet (8% casein supplemented with 0.3% methionine) resulted in an enlargement of the liver and an increase in serum and liver triacylglycerol concentrations without any differences in the lipid components of the serum or liver. The ketone body production decreased and the secretion rate of triacylglycerols increased when the isolated liver was perfused in the presence of an exogenous oleate substrate. The triacylglycerol accumulation in the liver was partly due to an alteration in the hepatic metabolism of long-chain free fatty acids between the pathways of oxidation and esterification (Fukuda et al. 1990).

A casein diet (8%) increased liver fatty acid synthesis but not cholesterol synthesis, reduced hyperlipidemia, proteinuria, and fatty liver induction after supplementation with cystine (0.3%) and threonine (0.36%). The fecal excretion of both neutral and acidic steroids was significantly higher than that in the 20% casein diet-fed nephritic rats (Fujisawa et al. 1994, 1995).

Addition of threonine (0.24%) to the diet of adult male *Sprague-Dawley* rats, maintained on a protein-free ration for 100 days, reduced the liver neutral glyceride and liver plasmalogen concentrations, and partially prevented the reduction in liver cholesterol concentrations but not that of liver phospholipids (Williams and Hurlebaus 1965a, 1965b). The increase in liver lipids caused by an excessive amount of sulfur amino acids in the diet of male *Donryu* rats was not prevented by the addition of threonine, but was decreased by the reduction in dietary sulfur amino acids. Threonine-deficient diet enhanced the liver lipid content of growing male *Donryu* rats (Aoyama and Ashida 1972), induced hepatic steatosis in *Wistar* rats (Singal et al. 1953), and altered the metabolism of fatty acids in the fatty liver of rats fed on low-rice protein diets (Viviani et al. 1964).

Addition of threonine (0.36%) and cystine (0.3%) to an 8.5% casein diet diminished the cystine-induced fatty liver in male *Wistar* rats with nephrotoxic serum nephritis (Fujisawa et al. 1994, 1995). Hypercholesterolemia and elevation of liver microsomal HMG-CoA reductase activity induced by polychlorinated biphenyls (PCB) were increased in young male *Wistar* rats by methionine and threonine supplementation of a nonprotein diet (Hitomi and Yoshida 1989). The data available on the effects of threonine with and without a choline deficiency (review in Sidransky 1990) are insufficient and require confirmation through further studies.

2.6.2.13 Tryptophan

The effects of tryptophan on liver lipid concentrations vary according to the animal species. In male broiler chicks, liver lipid concentrations significantly decreased as the level of dietary tryptophan increased at each protein level (16%, 20%, 24%, and 28%), but the concentration of total plasma lipids did not vary (Rogers and Pesti 1990). Addition of tryptophan (0.41%) to the diet of adult male *Sprague-Dawley* rats, maintained on a protein-free ration for 100 days, did not prevent the reduction of the liver neutral glyceride, phospholipid, and plasmalogen concentrations, but increased the liver cholesterol concentration (Williams and Hurlebaus 1965a, 1965b).

Administration of tryptophan alone to young fasted rats produced a rapid stimulation of hepatic protein synthesis (Sidransky 1976).

The increase of liver lipids induced by excessive amounts of sulfur amino acids was not prevented by the addition of 1.87% tryptophan to the control diet of male *Donryu* rats (Ayoama and Ashida 1972).

In female weanling rats, an excess of tryptophan in control and atherogenic diets had no further effect on hypercholesterolemia. However, dietary tryptophan increased plasma lipid peroxidation by 9% and 21% in the rats fed on the control diet containing soybean oil or on the atherogenic diet. Plasma lipid peroxidation was enhanced by 9% and 21% with the control and atherogenic diets, respectively and the macrophage cholesterol esterification by 40% and 38%, respectively. Tryptophan, the precursor of serotonin, and the serotonin metabolite, 5-hydroxyindoleacetic acid, were also enhanced by 22% and 118%, respectively. Although tryptophan has no effect, serotonin increases LDL peroxidation as measured by incubation with copper ions (Aviram et al. 1991).

In *Single Comb White Leghorn* laying hens, serum cholesterol, triacylglycerol and nonesterified fatty acid concentrations increased when maize or soybean were supplemented with 1.0 g/kg diet of tryptophan, and decreased with the addition of 3.0 or 4.0 g/kg (Rogers and Pesti 1992). A number of studies have been carried out to determine the effects of tryptophan with and without a choline deficiency (review in Sidransky 1990), but there are still too few data available and further research is necessary.

2.6.2.14 Tyrosine

When male *Wistar* rats are fed on a cholesterol-free diet containing casein, whey protein, soybean protein, and sunflower protein, serum cholesterol concentrations are significantly and positively correlated with tyrosine (Sautier et al. 1983). Tyrosine supplementation (8%) of a casein diet (10% or 20%) of male *Wistar* rats for a 28-day period, increased total serum cholesterol, HDL-cholesterol, and LDL plus VLDL-cholesterol levels without any modification of fecal steroid excretion. This effect is probably due to stimulation of cholesterol synthesis (Nagaoka et al. 1985, 1990). As tyrosine is an amino acid precursor of thyroid hormones, the effects of a cholesterol-enriched diet (containing fish or peanut protein) supplemented (2%) or not with tyrosine, have been investigated in male *Sprague-Dawley* rats in comparison with casein. The serum cholesterol concentrations did not change if tyrosine was added to a peanut diet but increased with a fish diet. The lower release of tyrosine by proteolytic enzymes from fish than from peanut protein explains this different effect. Since plasma triiodothyronine and thyroxine levels are unchanged the thyroid hormones are not responsible for the hypercholesterolemic action of tyrosine (Jacques et al. 1988a; Jacques 1990).

Tyrosine is a precursor of catecholamines; an excess of dietary tyrosine increases urinary excretion of norepinephrine and epinephrine in male *Wistar* rats (Julius et al. 1982; Nagaoka et al. 1985). The mechanism by which excess dietary tyrosine produces an increase in serum cholesterol levels in rats not yet clearly understood.

2.6.2.15   Valine

Addition of valine (0.24%) to the diet of adult male *Sprague-Dawley* rats, maintained on a protein-free ration for 100 days, did not prevent the reduction of liver phospholipids and plasmalogen concentrations, but increased the liver cholesterol and neutral glyceride concentrations (Williams and Hurlebaus 1965a, 1965b). There is a significant positive correlation between plasma total cholesterol concentrations and the plasma concentration of methionine and valine and the hepatic concentration of valine and alanine, in adult male *Wistar* rats fed on one or other of the seven following various protein dietary sources (12.3 to 14.4 g/100 g): casein, lactalbumin, whole egg protein, egg albumin, sardine protein, soybean protein, and wheat gluten (Sugiyama et al. 1996).

In male *Wistar* rats with nephritis, caused by a nephrotoxic agent, the reduction of hyperlipidemia by a diet low (8.5%) in soybean protein isolates is partially due to decreased liver cholesterol synthesis. Growth retardation can be alleviated by the addition of methionine (0.3%) (Fujisawa et al. 1994, 1995). The same result is obtained in the same species of rats with a low-meat protein diet (8.5%) if this diet is supplemented by 0.5% L-valine (Yagasaki et al. 1994).

2.6.2.16   Summary and Conclusion

Amino acids have various effects on plasma and liver lipids, but these are difficult to summarize because studies have often shown conflicting results. They vary according to the species, diet, amount of each amino acid, and whether the animals are normo- or hyper-cholesterolemic. Moreover, although numerous studies have been conducted, most focused on rats. Far fewer have been carried out in hens, gerbils, hamsters, rabbits, or guinea pigs, and those on mice, cats, pigs, and monkeys are particularly rare.

Soybean protein and casein are the most widely studied proteins although several other vegetable and animal proteins have also been investigated. Although it is widely accepted that vegetable proteins are hypocholesterolemic in comparison with animal proteins, it is still difficult to rate the effects of animal proteins on cholesterol and lipid metabolisms. Several factors including animal species, age of animals, amount of proteins, diet composition (particularly the nature and amount of fats and cholesterol), and also study duration are known to modify the results of experiments. There have also been too few studies in animal models such as pigs and monkeys for any valid extrapolation to human use to be made of the results. They do, however, provide several interesting indications. It is obvious that the different effects of various food proteins are related to their amino acid composition.

The data concerning the influence of amino acids on cholesterol and lipid metabolisms are often inconsistent since they too are modified by the same factors as those described for proteins. Moreover, the great majority of experiments have been carried out in rats and too few on other animals.

Sulfur amino acids have the most potent effects. On the whole, cystine, glycine, leucine, and taurine are hypocholesterolemic, whereas histidine is hypercholesterolemic. Methionine may be hyper- or hypocholesterolemic according to the species and the composition of the diet. The effects of glutamic acid differ according to the species and tyrosine-induced hypercholesterolemia varies according to the nature of the proteins in the diet. Tryptophan enhances lipid peroxidation in chickens. The increase in liver lipids caused by cystine can be prevented by methionine, as well as by taurine depending on the endogenous synthesis of taurine that is specific to the animal species studied. HMG-CoA reductase activity is increased by cystine and methionine. The effects of lysine and arginine will be studied in the next section.

Amino acid mixtures simulating the composition of casein, soybean protein, or wheat gluten have, respectively, the same effects as casein, soybean protein, or wheat gluten. When all essential amino acids, except arginine, are included in the diet, the reduction in serum cholesterol levels is greater and LDL receptors are down-regulated. According to the composition of different amino acid mixtures, the effects are different. A mixture of isoleucine, leucine, lysine, methionine, and valine results in the same type of hypercholesterolemia as a mixture with lysine, leucine, and methionine, whereas one containing histidine, phenylalanine, tryptophan, and glycine has only a moderate effect. In rabbits a mixture of isoleucine, leucine, lysine, methionine phenylalanine, and tryptophan produces a greater increase in serum cholesterol levels, total lipid, β-lipoprotein, and triacylglycerol concentrations than a mixture with only three amino acids (leucine, isoleucine and lysine, or methionine, phenylalanine and tryptophan). Partial hydrolysates of casein or soybean protein have similar effects to casein or soybean protein.

2.7 ACTION MECHANISMS OF SOYBEAN PROTEIN, CASEIN, AND AMINO ACIDS

The mechanism of action behind the effects of soybean protein, casein, and amino acids is not yet clearly understood. In addition, it may well vary according to numerous previously described factors. These effects must therefore be investigated under various nutritional conditions. As Wolfe and Grace (1987) demonstrated, in fasting baboons, there is no difference in lipid serum levels whether the diet is based on soybean protein or casein over a period of 4 to 5 days, or if the daily diet is administered rapidly by constant intraduodenal infusion over 7 hours. The diverse effects of soybean protein and casein were observed with a slow, constant, isocaloric intraduodenal infusion.

Several mechanisms have been suggested to explain the various effects of soybean protein and casein on cholesterol metabolism and serum cholesterol levels (Kritchevsky 1979; Carroll 1981b; Terpstra et al. 1983a; Barth and Pfeuffer 1988; Barth et al. 1989; Pfeuffer 1989; Beynen 1990b, 1990c; Beynen and Sugano 1990; West et al. 1990; Pfeuffer and Barth 1990; Kritchevsky 1993a; Carroll and Kurowska 1995; Fox and Flynn 1997; Hambraeus 1997).

2.7.1 Effects on Digestive Absorption of Lipids, Cholesterol, and Steroids and Fecal Excretion of Steroids

2.7.1.1 Digestive Absorption of Lipids, Cholesterol, and Steroids

Gastric emptying of vegetable proteins is faster than that of casein, although the transit and digestive absorption in the first part of the small intestine of rats are lower than those of casein (de Schriver 1990). Casein is more soluble with an alkaline pH; soybean protein has an acid pH. Heat treatment of these proteins reduces their solubility and digestibility. The hypocholesterolemic effect of soybean protein in rabbits may be partly due to the low solubility and digestibility in alkaline conditions (Woodward and Carroll 1985).

The rates at which individual amino acids are absorbed from a mixture of amino acids are particularly unequal in humans (Adibi et al. 1967; Adibi 1971) and in animals (Delhumeau et al. 1962). The characteristics of digestive absorption of amino acid mixtures are not representative of those of intraluminal digestion of physiological products, such as oligopeptides and amino acids (Silk et al. 1973; Gardner 1975). Studies on the intestinal transport of individual oligopeptides and equivalent amino acid mixtures have shown that amino acids are particularly slowly absorbed when used alone; this process is far more rapid when they are absorbed from peptides (Matthews 1972; Burston et al. 1972). In contrast, the competition for intestinal transport among free amino acids is avoided when peptides are absorbed (Matthews et al. 1969; Adibi 1971; Matthews 1972). Thus, the intestinal absorption of intact oligopeptides (Silk et al. 1973) or an interaction of the lipid absorption process with intact proteins (van der Meer et al. 1985a, 1985b) may well explain the modification in cholesterol metabolism resulting from intestinal absorption of various dietary proteins (Vahouny et al. 1985).

Food proteins containing the greatest quantity of hydrophobic peptides after intraluminal digestion absorb far more bile acids in the gut. Intestinal absorption is therefore disturbed in male *Wistar* rats (Nagata et al. 1981a; Iwami et al. 1990). Although bile acids bind more easily to indigestible components of vegetable proteins (Iwami et al. 1987), the hypocholesterolemic effects of soybean protein do not appear to be due only to changes in the bile acid and biliary salt enterohepatic cycle. Although jejunum or ileum resection and ileum bypass increase the elimination of steroids into the feces, the enhancement of serum cholesterol concentrations induced by casein is not reduced by this operation in the rat. The same results were obtained in adult male *Sprague-Dawley* rats after administration of cholestyramine or β-sitosterol (Saeki et al. 1987; Saeki and Kiriyama 1990; Saeki et al. 1990) as a result of increased endogenous cholesterol synthesis (Weiss and Dietschy 1974).

Intestinal concentrations of bile acids are higher in *Syrian* hamsters if they are fed on a cholesterol-free diet containing soybean, cottonseed, or peanut proteins than if they are fed on casein, bovine albumin, or egg albumin (Sullivan et al. 1985). The concentration of free bile acids is increased by the reduced number of binding sites of bile on the calcium phosphate sediment since calcium is removed from the calcium-phosphate intestinal sediment by casein and its phosphopeptides (van der Meer 1983; van der Meer et al. 1985a, 1985b). The enhancement of intestinal bile and steroid absorption in adult male *albino Wistar* rats fed on casein in comparison with soybean protein could be related to the differential phosphorylation state of these two proteins. The increase in bile acid absorption that occurs with a casein diet persists over the first 8 hours (Vahouny et al. 1984, 1985). Nevertheless, this mechanism is only valid for casein and does not account for the different effects of other proteins (Beynen 1990b).

Cholesterol absorption is greater in male *New Zealand white* rabbits (Huff and Carroll 1980b) or male *Wistar* rats (Nagata et al. 1982) fed on casein than in those fed on soybean protein. In contrast, an amino acid mixture similar to soybean protein does not modify cholesterol absorption as much as a casein mixture in male *Wistar* rats (Nagata et al. 1982). In rats (Chang and Johnson 1980) or in male *white Leghorn* chicks (Kenney and Fisher 1973), when casein was substituted for soybean protein or when the amount of proteins was increased, the influx of cholesterol and bile acids from the gut to the liver and the amount of cholesterol in the liver were enhanced, thus inducing a reduction in the number of apo B/E receptors. The output of lipoprotein cholesterol was increased, the biosynthesis of cholesterol and bile acids was inhibited, and cholesterol turnover was reduced.

Although as of this writing no experiments have confirmed the soybean protein-induced reduction in bile acid concentrations in the portal vein and the liver, the stimulation of 7-α-hydroxylase, which catalyzes the first step in the conversion of cholesterol to bile acids, has been demonstrated indirectly in male *New Zealand white* rabbits (Huff and Carroll 1980b) and in male *Wistar* rats (Nagata et al. 1982) fed on soybean protein. In male *Wistar* rats (Nagata et al. 1981a) and in male *New Zealand white* rabbits (Huff and Carroll 1980b) fed on cholesterol-free semipurified diets, intestinal absorption of cholesterol and bile acids decreases, and in mature male *Sprague-Dawley* rats (Reiser et al. 1977), the hepatic production increases. The addition of cholesterol to the diet does not increase digestive cholesterol absorption in male *Wistar* rats (Vahouny et al. 1985). Soybean protein, compared to casein, lowers cholesterol absorption in male *Wistar* rats (Nagata et al. 1982). The rates of cholesterol absorption and plasma cholesterol production were similar with casein or soybean protein diets in male weanling *Sprague-Dawley* rats fed a high-cholesterol (1.2%) diet, but the plasma cholesterol fractional catabolic rate was significantly lower with casein (Cohn et al. 1984).

In barrow pigs derived from a cross between *Dutch Landrace* and *Large white* swine, a casein diet, compared to a soybean diet, increased the absorption of cholesterol and the apparent ileal absorption of proteins associated with a reduced rate of chyme flow through the ileum (Beynen et al. 1990). However, in young male *Yorkshire* swine fed on a high-fat (41.5% calories), high-cholesterol (1,055 mg/day) diet, cholesterol absorption and whole-body cholesterol synthesis were similar with a casein diet or a soybean protein diet (Kim et al. 1978). These data confirm those obtained by Cohn et al. (1984) in male weanling *Sprague-Dawley* rats and previously reported.

Supplementing a diet with amino acids modifies lipid absorption. The lipid absorption is more rapid in adult male *Wistar* rats fed on casein than in those fed on soybean protein. The rate of lipid absorption was slowed down by arginine supplementation of a casein diet and increased by lysine supplementation of a soybean protein diet (Vahouny et al. 1984).

In male *Wistar* rats, the intestinal HMG-CoA reductase activity was higher in animals fed on soybean protein and 1% fat than in those on casein, whereas lymph cholesterol levels were comparable. Apo A-1 concentration in the lymph and *de novo* synthesis of apo A-1 in the small intestine segment were low in animals fed on a soybean protein diet as compared to a casein diet (Tanaka et al. 1983a).

Hypolipidemic substances such as cholestyramine or β-sitosterol do not reduce casein-induced hypercholesterolemia in adult male *Sprague-Dawley* rats even though their site of action is within the gut (Saeki and Kiriyama 1988, 1989, 1990). Neither compactine nor probucol is efficient in contrast to clofibrate and eritadenine. Likewise, they do not increase the hypocholesterolemic effect of soybean proteins. The chief mechanism of action of soybean protein is very likely related to lipoprotein metabolism (Saeki and Kiriyama 1989, 1990).

2.7.1.2 Fecal Excretion of Steroids and Bile Acids

In male crossbred chicks, reduced protein intake induces hypercholesterolemia and a reduction in fecal cholesterol excretion (Yeh and Léveillé 1973). However, if *New Zealand white* rabbits were exposed to dietary casein in early life, no harmful effects on cholesterol and bile acid metabolism were observed in adulthood (Hassan et al. 1985). In chickens, mice, rats, rabbits and pigs fed on a low-cholesterol or a cholesterol-free diet, the fecal excretion of neutral and acidic steroids was always higher with soybean protein than with casein (Howard et al. 1965; Howard and Gresham 1968; Kenney and Fisher 1973; Fumagalli et al. 1978; Kim et al. 1978; Sautier et al. 1979; Huff and Carroll 1980a, 1980b; Huff et al. 1982; Nagata et al. 1980, 1981a, 1982; Sautier et al. 1983; Beynen et al. 1983c; Terpstra et al. 1983b; Tanaka et al. 1983a, 1983b; Cohn et al. 1984; Vahouny et al. 1984; Hassan et al. 1985; Iritani et al. 1985; van der Meer et al. 1985a, 1985b; Kuyvenhoven et al. 1986; Sautier et al. 1986; Beynen et al. 1986b; Park et al. 1987; Lapré 1989; Choi et al. 1989a; Okita and Sugano 1989, 1990; Beynen et al. 1990; Sugano et al. 1990b; Yoshida et al. 1990b; Yamashita et al. 1990; Kritchevsky 1990; review in Potter 1996; Madani et al. 1998). However, in one study of male *New Zealand white* rabbits, replacing casein with soybean protein increased the elimination of neutral steroids but not of bile acids (Fumagalli et al. 1978). In contrast, compared with casein, an amino acid mixture equivalent to soybean protein had no effect on fecal steroid excretion in male *Wistar* rats (Nagata et al. 1982). The increase in fecal excretion of acidic but not neutral steroids is proportional to the level of protein, and is higher with soybean protein than with casein. These effects of soybean protein are not due to nonprotein components since when young rats were fed on a cholesterol-free diet containing highly purified soybean protein (to eliminate the nonprotein components), fecal neutral and acidic steroid excretions were increased (Madani et al. 1998). The amount of fecal steroid excretion, possibly due to soybean saponins, is not correlated with the level of their hypocholesterolemic capacity (Oakenfull et al. 1979; Raheja and Linscheer 1982; Doucet et al. 1987; Lapré et al. 1989).

In young male *Yorkshire* swine fed on a high-fat, high-cholesterol diet, fecal neutral and acidic steroid excretions, dietary cholesterol absorption, and whole-body cholesterol synthesis were similar regardless of whether the diet contained casein or soybean protein (Kim et al. 1978). However, in another experiment with a similar protocol and the same animal species, fecal steroid excretion was shown to be increased and not counterbalanced by a parallel increase in cholesterol synthesis, which could explain the cholesterol-lowering effect of soybean protein (Kim et al. 1980a).

When the amount of casein or soybean protein was increased in the diet of male *Wistar* rats, neutral steroid levels but not acid steroid excretion was enhanced (Okita and Sugano 1989, 1990). In contrast, however, in another experiment in male *Wistar* rats, a lower rate of total steroid excretion was observed (Tanaka et al. 1983b). Supplementation with arginine or lysine does not modify the effects of these proteins in male *Wistar* rats (Nagata et al. 1981a). The hypocholesterolemic effect of soybean protein in the same species of rats is mainly due to the stimulation of cholesterol turnover, which results from the reduced absorption and enhanced fecal excretion of steroids (Nagata et al. 1982). Dietary casein increases the free concentration of bile acids and reabsorption of steroids from the gut. Ileal and fecal excretion of neutral steroids and the output of bile acids were reduced in barrow pigs derived from a cross between *Dutch Landrace* and *Large white* swine fed on casein (Beynen et al. 1990). In hamsters, taurine increases the bile acid pool size and reduces the bile saturation index (Bellentani et al. 1987a, 1987b), whereas a soybean protein diet enhances bile acid excretion and reduces cholesterol gallstones (Jonnalagadda et al. 1993).

In the perfused liver of male *Wistar* rats, bile acid production, biliary flow, and bile acid concentrations were similar when they were fed on casein or soybean protein diets (Sugano et al. 1982a). Excretion of neutral and acidic steroids was greater with a soybean protein diet in male *Wistar* rats (Nagata et al. 1981a). The secretion of cholesterol, triacylglycerols, and apo A-1 obtained by the perfusion of isolated livers was lower in male *Wistar* rats fed on soybean protein than in those fed on casein. However, when the rats were fed on amino acid mixtures corresponding to the composition of these proteins, no such differences were observed (Sugano et al. 1982a; Nagata et al. 1982).

The effects of soybean protein and casein on serum cholesterol concentrations of adult male *Sprague-Dawley* rats are the result of modifications in lipoprotein metabolism and not of differences in intestinal steroid absorption (Saeki and Kiriyama 1990). In male rats of the same species, comparison of the effects of various dietary proteins (casein, fish, soybean, peanut meal, rapeseed, oatmeal) on cholesterol and the soluble apoprotein composition of plasma lipoproteins suggests that they are partly affected by the nutritional value of the proteins (Jacques et al. 1988b). In young male *Sprague-Dawley* rats, the peptide fractions of soybean protein produced in the lumen bind steroids and excrete them into the feces (Sugano and Gotto 1990; Sugano et al. 1990a, 1990b; Yamamoto et al. 1996).

Calcium has the capacity to complex with bile acids (especially glycine-conjugated bile acids in rabbits), which then become unavailable for intestinal reabsorption. The rate of excretion of bile acids, as of fats, is therefore increased in young male *New Zealand white* rabbits and *Wistar* rats (van der Meer et al. 1985a, 1985b). In rabbits fed on a casein diet, casein phosphopeptides compete with insoluble calcium phosphate thus inhibiting their binding to bile acids. The capacity of casein for phosphorylation may well account for the considerable species dependency of the casein response (van der Meer 1983). Excretion of bile acids is very likely influenced by the degree of casein phosphorylation (about 40% of its serine residues are esterified with phosphate) in young male *New Zealand white* rabbits and *Wistar* rats (Samman and Roberts 1984; van der Meer et al. 1983, 1985a, 1985b).

The species sensitivity of casein may well be affected by differences either in the conjugation of bile acids with glycine or taurine or in the activity of intestinal alkaline phosphatase that dephosphorylates casein. As has been demonstrated *in vitro,* glycine conjugates dihydroxy bile acids, but not their taurine conjugated counterparts, and binds to insoluble calcium phosphate (van der Meer and de Vries 1985). A cholesterol-free casein diet (210 g/kg diet), in comparison with a soybean protein diet (208 g/kg diet + 2 g/kg diet methionine), did not affect calcium absorption in *New Zealand white* rabbits; it increased phosphate, but not calcium absorption, and decreased fecal excretion of bile acids. Casein gradually enhanced apo B cholesterol, whereas HDL cholesterol remained constant. In contrast, in male *Wistar* rats on the same diets, none of these casein-specific effects were observed. These diverse effects may be explained by the low activity of intestinal alkaline phosphatase in rabbits, in contrast to rats; this effect has the capacity to preserve the high degree of phosphorylation of casein and its peptides in the lumen of the small intestine (van der Meer et al. 1988). A cholesterol-free semipurified diet induces a more severe form of hypercholesterolemia in rabbits than in rats since their intestinal alkaline phosphatase activity is low. The activities of calcium may be limited to inhibition of biliary salt and the acid enterohepatic cycle. Surgical disruption of this cycle in adult male *Sprague-Dawley* rats fails to modify the hypocholesterolemic effect of casein (Saeki et al. 1987). In these rats, the variations in serum cholesterol concentrations cannot therefore be due to an alteration of the enterohepatic cycle of steroids (Saeki and Kiriyama 1990). The decreasing intestinal absorption of cholesterol and increasing fecal steroid excretion in male *Wistar* rats are primarily responsible for the antihypercholesterolemic effect of soybean protein compared with casein (Nagata et al. 1982).

2.7.2 EFFECTS ON SERUM LIPIDS, LIVER CHOLESTEROL, AND LIVER ENZYMES

When compared with casein, soybean protein is responsible for various hypocholesterolemic actions in rats (Nagata et al. 1980, 1981b; Bosisio et al. 1980, 1981; Sugano et al. 1982b; Eklund and Sjöblom 1986; Pfeuffer and Barth 1986a; Park et al. 1987; review in Beynen 1990b, 1990c). Male weanling *Sprague-Dawley* rats fed a high-cholesterol semipurified diet containing casein developed higher levels of serum cholesterol than soybean protein-fed animals. This hypercholesterolemia was due to the accumulation of VLDL. Cholesterol kinetics measurements by [14C]cholesterol showed that casein-fed rats had a similar rate of plasma cholesterol production, but a significantly lower plasma cholesterol fractional catabolic rate compared with the soybean protein–fed rats. Cohn et al. (1984) suggested that the accumulation of VLDL in the plasma of rats fed on dietary casein is not due to excessive VLDL production, but rather to inadequate VLDL removal. This deficiency was also observed for VLDL apo B since the mean fractional catabolic rate for apo B in VLDL was significantly lower in the casein than in the soybean protein–fed animals, whereas the total daily production of VLDL apo B was similar in the two groups. However, in young male *New Zealand white* rabbits, the substitution of soybean protein for casein, which induces hypercholesterolemia, lowered the hepatic production of apo B (Khosla et al. 1989). In the same species of rabbits fed on a low-fat, cholesterol-free, semipurified amino acid diet, in which lysine and methionine were at levels corresponding to 45% of the casein amino acid diet, the serum cholesterol, LDL-cholesterol, and apo B levels were increased. This effect can be partially prevented by the addition of a high proportion of arginine to the diet. The rates of incorporation of [^{14}C]lysine into LDL apoprotein were elevated in rabbits fed on lysine- and methionine-enriched diets compared with normocholesterolemic animals fed on diets enriched with lysine and leucine, suggesting a contribution of the increase in hepatic apo B production in the hypercholesterolemic response. However, in one *in vitro* study using HepG2 cells in cell culture exposed to the same amino acid mixtures as those of rabbits, apo B responses did not correspond to LDL responses observed *in vivo* with the exception of arginine. This type of investigation can therefore not be considered a good model for this subject (Kurowska and Carroll 1996; Kurowska et al. 2000; Kurowska 2001). During the conversion of VLDL into LDL via intermediate density lipoproteins (IDL), these particles lose triacylglycerols, but not cholesterol, and acquire additional cholesterol esters from HDL in exchange for triacylglycerol molecules. This process is catalyzed by cholesterol ester transfer proteins present in rabbits and in human plasma, but not in rat plasma (Norum et al. 1983). In male *Wistar* rats fed a cholesterol-free diet, serum cholesterol and triacylglycerol levels were higher with a casein diet than a soybean protein diet in both the fasted and fed states. Plasma triacylglycerol changes were due to an increase in VLDL lipid secretion (Pfeuffer and Barth 1986c).

The greater effect of dietary casein on hypercholesterolemia in rabbits than in rats may be due to the differences in the exchange of proteins between lipoproteins in these two species. These facts once again highlight the interspecies differences that could explain the greater effect of casein on serum cholesterol concentrations in rabbits than in rats (West et al. 1990).

The changes in LDL-cholesterol levels are the main reason for the different effects of dietary proteins on serum cholesterol concentrations. When the diet is rich in cholesterol, soybean protein, unlike casein, does not increase hepatic cholesterol concentrations in *New Zealand white* rabbits (cholesterol: 1.40 g/kg) (Lovati et al. 1990) or in male *Wistar* rats (cholesterol: 0.15 g/kg) (Lapré et al. 1989). Increased liver cholesterol levels with casein diets have been observed by several researchers in rabbits (Huff and Carroll 1980b; Beynen et al. 1983a; Lovati et al. 1990) and rats (Sautier et al. 1979; Terpstra et al. 1982a; Sugano et al. 1982a; Kritchevsky et al. 1984; Lapré et al. 1989). The hypocholesterolemia in animals fed on soybean protein is associated with several changes in liver lipid metabolism: low liver cholesterol concentrations; increased number of hepatic apo B/E receptors, rates of hepatic cholesterol and bile acid synthesis; and decreased rates of lipoprotein cholesterol output by the liver (review in Beynen 1990b, 1990c). Soybean protein, compared to casein, reduced liver cholesterol concentrations and the rate of hepatic lipoprotein cholesterol flux in the serum of barrows derived from a cross between *Dutch Landrace* and *Large white* swine (Beynen et al. 1990).

A soybean protein diet increases LDL-receptor expression in the liver of female *Sprague-Dawley* rats (Sirtori et al. 1984). In young male *New Zealand white* rabbits, the substitution of soybean protein for casein, which induces hypercholesterolemia, increased receptor-mediated LDL catabolism (Khosla et al. 1989). An increase in hepatic lipoprotein receptor activity, without any variation in VLDL apo B production, has been demonstrated, as well as a decrease in hepatic lipoprotein-cholesterol output (Sugano et al. 1982b; Sirtori et al. 1984; Cohn et al. 1984; Pfeuffer and Barth 1986b). VLDL catabolism was increased in rats on a soybean diet compared with a casein diet (Lovati et al. 1985; Sugano et al. 1990b). The increase in serum cholesterol concentrations attributable to a casein diet could well be a consequence of the decreased VLDL catabolism (Cohn et al. 1984). The increased fecal excretion with a soybean protein diet induces a shift in liver cholesterol metabolism providing cholesterol for the enhancement of bile acid synthesis. Lipoprotein receptor activity and liver cholesterol biosynthesis increase; serum cholesterol concentrations are thereby reduced due to the enhanced removal of cholesterol from the serum by the apo B/E receptor (Beynen 1990c).

When male *Wistar* rats were fed on a cholesterol-free diet, the specific activity of microsomal HMG-CoA reductase of the liver was twice as high in rats fed soybean protein than in the animals fed on casein, but this effect was reversed if intact proteins were replaced with the corresponding amino acid mixtures, and the HMG-CoA reductase activity was significantly higher in rats fed on casein mixtures. In rats fed on soybean protein, serum cholesterol turnover was more rapid, the size of the exchangeable cholesterol pool (pool A) was reduced due to the increase in the removal rate, and hepatic steroidogenesis was enhanced (Nagata et al. 1982). Similar data were obtained in mature male *Sprague-Dawley* rats (Reiser et al. 1977) or male *Wistar* rats (Sugano et al. 1982a) fed on casein or soybean protein cholesterol-free diets or weakly supplemented in cholesterol (0.05%).

The turnover of cholesterol in rabbits and rats fed on casein is significantly slower than in those fed on soybean protein (Huff and Carroll 1980b; Nagata et al. 1982; Kritchevsky et al. 1983). In contrast, an amino acid mixture equivalent to soybean protein compared to a casein mixture has no effect on the turnover of serum cholesterol in male *Wistar* rats (Nagata et al. 1982; Sugano et al. 1982a).

Casein and soybean protein diets induce different changes in hepatic receptor regulation of cholesterol. The activity of HMG-CoA reductase was reduced by both diets, but more so with soybean protein than with the casein diet (Madani et al. 1998). In adult female *Sprague-Dawley* rats fed on a cholesterol-rich (1.2%) casein diet, a significant marked increase of total and VLDL cholesterol was observed. The substitution of soybean protein for casein counteracted these enhancements. The binding of the cholesterol-rich lipoprotein fraction (β-VLDL) to hepatic membranes was normal with a soybean protein diet and reduced with a casein diet. The hepatic receptor regulation of cholesterol metabolism was differently modified by both diets.

HMG-CoA reductase activity was reduced by both diets, but less so with soybean protein than with casein, in contrast to the data of Madani et al. (1998). Animal and vegetable proteins thus had different effects on the hepatic receptor regulation of cholesterol metabolism (Sirtori et al. 1984). These effects are patent in young male *Wistar* rats fed on a cholesterol-free diet and in adult rats when their diet is enriched in cholesterol. Intestinal HMG-CoA reductase activity was higher in rats fed on a soybean protein diet than in others on a casein diet although the lymph cholesterol level was similar (Tanaka et al. 1983a).

However, when the high-fat, high-cholesterol diet of young male *Yorkshire* swine contains either soybean protein or highly purified soybean protein or casein, total hepatic microsomal HMG-CoA reductase activity is not modified (Kim et al. 1980a). These differences in the HMG-CoA reductase activities could be partly due to the glucagon secretion induced by these diets since glucagon reduces the activity of HMG-CoA reductase (Rodwell et al. 1976). Indeed the relative concentrations of insulin, glucagon, and glucocorticoids are important in regulating of the diurnal variation in hepatic reductase activity (Neprokoeff et al. 1974).

Hamsters and guinea pigs have the same response to dietary cholesterol with different soybean protein/casein ratios. Diets with different casein/soybean protein ratios (60/40, 20/80, 0/100) have no effect on the regulatory enzyme of hepatic cholesterol homeostasis in male *Hartley* guinea pigs and male *Golden Syrian* hamsters, and the lower hepatic cholesterol concentrations observed with a diet containing soybean (100%) as the only protein source are not associated with any changes in hepatic enzyme activities: HMG-CoA reductase, cholesterol 7-α-hydroxylase, and ACATase. Other mechanisms unrelated to cholesterol synthesis or catabolism should therefore be investigated (Fernandez et al. 1999b).

In comparison to casein, soybean protein reduces triacylglycerol synthesis and also the concentrations of diacylglycerols in liver microsomes of rats; this effect is probably a consequence of reduced liver fatty acid synthesis (Nagata et al. 1981a; Ide et al. 1992). As has been shown by studies with triacylglycerols marked by tritiated water, the effect of soybean protein is due more to the reduction in triacylglycerol synthesis than to their degradation (Sugano 1983; Iritani et al. 1986, 1996; Ide et al. 1992).

The secretions of cholesterol, triacylglycerols, and apo A-1 from isolated perfused livers of male *Wistar* rats were significantly reduced when the rats were fed on a soybean protein cholesterol-free diet compared to casein (Sugano et al. 1982a). The output of lipids and lipoproteins by isolated perfused livers of male *English shorthair* rabbits differed if they were fed on chow cholesterol-free or cholesterol-enriched (0.5%) diets. In cholesterol-fed animals, the output of cholesteryl esters was very much greater and the VLDL was enriched with cholesteryl esters (MacKinnon et al. 1985). This finding has also been observed in perfused livers of adult *African green Cercopithecus aethiops* monkeys of the *Vervet* subspecies fed on a cholesterol-rich (0.78 mg/kcal) diet (Johnson et al. 1983).

In growing male *Wistar* rats fed a cholesterol-free diet containing casein or highly purified soybean protein, in order to eliminate most nonprotein components, the activity of cholesterol 7-α-hydroxylase was decreased, but this effect was more marked with soybean protein than with casein. Fecal neutral and acidic steroid excretion was stimulated by a soybean protein diet. When cholesterol (1%) was added to the same diet, the plasma cholesterol and tricylglycerol concentrations were not modified, but their liver concentrations were increased. Cholesterol 7-α-hydroxylase activity was reduced only in rats fed on casein (Madani et al. 1998).

With a cholesterol-free diet, the cholesterol 7-α-hydroxylase activity was three to four times greater in male albino *Wistar* rats fed soybean protein isolates than when they were fed on casein (Vahouny et al. 1985); this finding contrasts with those of Madani et al. (Madani et al. 1998). Cholesterol 7-α-hydroxylase activity was shown to increase twofold when a casein diet was supplemented with arginine, but to decrease moderately if the soybean protein diet of male albino *Wistar* rats was supplemented with lysine (Vahouny et al. 1985; Kritchevsky 1990).

In male *Sprague-Dawley* rats fed on a cholesterol-rich (2%) diet, plasma cholesterol was significantly reduced with a soybean protein compared to a casein diet, but cholesterol 7-α-hydroxylase activity was unchanged (Bosisio et al. 1981). In contrast, with these data, Sirtori et al. (1984) observed an increase of cholesterol 7-α-hydroxylase activity with casein but a normal range with a soybean protein diet. The stimulation of bile acid absorption would appear to induce higher concentrations of bile acids in the portal vein and the liver leading to inhibition of 7-α-hydroxylase, which catalyses the first step in the conversion of cholesterol into bile acids (West et al. 1990). Inhibition of bile acid synthesis has been demonstrated experimentally in rats and rabbits fed on casein (Huff and Carroll 1980a, 1980b; Nagata et al. 1982).

In male *Sprague-Dawley* rats fed on a cholesterol-rich (2%) diet, plasma cholesterol was significantly reduced with a soybean protein compared to a casein diet, but LCAT activity was unchanged. Liver cholesterol ester levels and ACATase activity was elevated with a soybean protein diet (Bosisio et al. 1981). However, in female *Sprague-Dawley* rats fed on a cholesterol-rich diet (1.2%), ACATase activity was significantly enhanced by a casein diet, but remained within a normal range with soybean protein (Sirtori et al. 1984).

In old male rabbits, in comparison with soybean protein, casein in a cholesterol-free diet reduced hepatic-triacylglycerol lipase (HTGL), LCAT, LPL, and post-heparin lipolytic (PHLA) activities (Alladi et al. 1989a). Unlike casein, plant proteins significantly reduced plasma total cholesterol and HDL-cholesterol concentrations in immature and mature male *Wistar* rats. LCAT activity was similar with different plant proteins, but the esterification rate is lower in rats fed on casein (de Schriver 1990). Cholesterol 7-α-monooxygenase activities are not dependent on dietary proteins. They are similar regardless of the age of the rats or the nature of proteins in the diet (Choi et al. 1989a).

Intermediate liver metabolism is influenced by dietary protein levels. In male weanling *Sprague-Dawley* rats fed on 10% or 20% soybean protein diets, a reduction in liver pyruvate kinase activity was observed when the level of soybean protein increased in a diet supplemented with 3.5% methionine (Temler et al. 1983). In male *Sprague-Dawley* rats (Ide et al. 1992) and in male *Wistar* rats (Iritani et al. 1986), liver mRNA concentrations and liver glucose-6-phosphate dehydrogenase, malic enzyme, acetyl-CoA carboxylase, and fatty acid synthetase activities were lower when the rats were fed on a soybean protein diet than a casein diet, but these effects on the lipogenic enzymes were not so great with amino acids simulating casein or soybean protein. Liver cholesterol and dolichol concentrations were also reduced in young *Wistar* rats (Ishinaga et al. 1993). The liver phosphatidylcholine concentrations increase proportionally with the rate of protein in the diet. They are higher in male *Wistar* rats fed on casein than on soybean protein. The plasma arachidonate/linoleate ratio and liver phosphatidylcholines are significantly higher with casein than with soybean protein diets and they increase proportionally with the rate of proteins in the diet (Okita et al. 1989, 1990). The major changes in liver lipid composition of *Sprague-Dawley* rats fed on casein compared with soybean protein were the higher level of 5-, 8-, 11-eicosatrienoic acid 20:3n-9 in the various lipid classes (Sjöblom and Eklund 1990).

The lipid-lowering effect of dietary soybean phospholipids added to a saturated fat diet would appear to be due to the alteration in liver fatty acid synthesis (review in Kabir and Ide 1995). The effect of the source and type of protein on lipid metabolism also depends on the level of dietary lecithin. In male weanling *Sprague-Dawley* rats fed on a cholesterol-free diet containing 0.25% or 5.0% soybean lecithin and 10% of one of the following proteins: lactalbumin, soybean protein concentrates, or wheat gluten, regardless of the protein source, soybean lecithin reduced liver cholesterol and triacylglycerol concentrations and overall liver weight with the exception of subjects fed on wheat gluten. However, the rats fed on animal proteins had lower liver concentrations than those fed on plant proteins with 5.0% lecithin levels, whereas plasma cholesterol and liver protein concentrations were higher (Jenkins et al. 1983). The cholesterol/phospholipid ratio was reduced, and membrane fluidity was increased. These effects may have a certain role in the level of enzyme synthesis in rat liver microsomes (Koba et al. 1993).

Dietary proteins affect the synthesis and digestive absorption of polyunsaturated fatty acids (PUFAs) through the effects of the amino acid components that modulate the cholesterol-lowering effects, which are additive and complementary to those of proteins. PUFAs can modify cholesterol metabolism through the action of eicosanoids, which modulate the activity of the enzymes involved in cholesterol metabolism (Huang 1990b).

The modifications in polyunsaturated fatty acid metabolism are responsible for a number of changes in eicosanoid production, especially in aortic tissue (Huang 1990a), but too few studies have been conducted to date for the real importance of this effect to be assessed (Huang et al. 1990, 1993; Sjöblom et al. 1991; Lu and Tang 1996).

Depending on the nature and proportion within the diet, proteins modulate $\Delta 6$-desaturase activity as well as that of $\Delta 5$-desaturase, although the latter is less sensitive. They also have different effects on polyunsaturated fatty acid n-6 metabolism (Huang et al. 1986, 1993; Sugano et al. 1988a; Koba and Sugano 1989, 1990; Choi et al. 1989b; Koba et al. 1990, 1991; Sjöblom et al. 1991; Lu and Tang 1996; Madani et al. 1998).

The fatty acid composition of liver microsomal phosphatidylcholine is dietary-cholesterol and protein-dependent. The proportions of 18:2n-6 and 20:3n-6 were higher and those of 20:4n-6 were lower with soybean protein than with casein or whey diets. $\Delta 5$(n-6)- and $\Delta 6$(n-6)-desaturase activities were higher in rats fed on casein than in those on soybean protein (Choi et al. 1989a; Huang et al. 1986, 1993; Lindholm and Eklund 1991; Sugano and Koba. 1993; Osada et al. 1996). However,

Madani et al. (1998) showed that in male *Wistar* rats, although Δ6(n-6)-desaturase activity was also higher with a casein diet, the activity of Δ5(n-6) was similar with both diets (Madani et al. 1998). In young and adult male *Sprague-Dawley* rats on a cholesterol-free diet, the Δ6-desaturase activity was higher with casein than with soybean protein or whey protein, whereas that of cholesterol 7-α-monooxygenase was similar regardless of the diet (Choi et al. 1989a).

The 20:3n-6+20:4n-6/18:2n-6 ratio in microsomal phosphatidylcholine was lower for young adult male *Sprague-Dawley* rats fed on soybean protein than when the diet was based on casein. Although this ratio decreases with age, no age-related reduction in desaturase activity has been observed (Choi et al. 1989a, 1989b). However, in liver microsomal phospholipids, the 22:5n-6/20:4n-6 ratio decreased significantly with age while the proportion of 22:6n-3 increased and that of 22:5n-6 decreased with age in young and adult male *Sprague-Dawley* rats whatever the nature of dietary proteins used, thus suggesting a reduced capacity for Δ4-desaturation in relation to age (Choi and Sugano 1988; Choi et al. 1989a).

The degree of conversion of linoleate to arachidonate and liver phosphatidyl-choline was greater with casein than with soybean protein in male *Wistar* rats (Okita and Sugano 1990) and it increased with the increasing dietary protein level from 10% to 30% (Okita and Sugano 1989). The values of the plasma arachido-nate/linoleate ratio and the levels of liver and aortic tissue phosphatydilcholine were higher with casein than with soybean protein diets and were dependent on the level and dietary proportion of these proteins (Sirtori et al. 1984; Huang et al. 1986; Sugano et al. 1988a; Okita and Sugano 1989, 1990; Koba and Sugano 1990; Lindholm and Eklund 1991; Terasawa et al. 1994; Osada et al. 1996; Lu and Tang 1996; Ratnayake et al. 1997; Madani et al. 1998). The ratio of the metabolites of linoleic acid to linolenic acid (20:3 + 20:4)/18:2, which is an index for linoleic desaturation, was significantly lower in rats fed on the undigested fractions of soybean protein than in those fed on soybean protein (Sugano and Koba 1993). Microsomal fatty acids of series ω7 and ω9 were present at higher levels in rats on diets containing casein rather than soybean protein (Lindholm and Eklund 1991). In the phospholipids, arachidonic, docosopentaenoic, and docosahexaenoic acid concentrations were higher with casein than with soybean protein diets, especially with fat-enriched diets (Noguchi et al. 1992; Terasawa et al. 1994; Ratnayake et al. 1997). In liver microsomes phospholipids, the conversion of α-linolenic acid to eicosapentaenoic acid and then to docosahexaenoic acid was enhanced with a soybean protein diet in comparison to a casein diet (Noguchi et al. 1992).

2.7.3 Effects of Amino Acids and Lysine/Arginine Ratio

2.7.3.1 Amino Acids

As seen in the following table, the amino acid composition of casein and soybean protein (g/16 g N) is different (Food and Agriculture Organization 1970).

Amino acids	Casein	Soya
Lysine	8.2	6.6
Arginine	4.0	7.5
Methionine	3.0	1.3
Cystine	0.4	1.3
Methionine/cystine	7.5	1.0
Glycine	1.6	4.2
Lysine/arginine	2.05	0.88

The following table shows the serum acid concentrations in growing male *Wistar* rats fed for 2 weeks on a cholesterol-free diet with casein (20 g/100 g) or soybean protein (22.5/100 g) (Horigome and Cho 1992).

Amino acids (µmol/L)	Casein (20.0%)	Soybean Protein (22.5%)
Ornithine	115 ± 7	96 ± 8
Lysine	759 ± 54	644 ± 32
Histidine	90 ± 6	82 ± 4
Arginine	147 ± 10	148 ± 14
Aspartic acid	51 ± 3	41 ± 5
Threonine, glutamine, asparagine	1084 ± 34	1011 ± 89
Serine	402 ± 13	420 ± 30
Glutamic acid	478 ± 17	$361 \pm 17**$
Proline	560 ± 21	$332 \pm 30**$
Glycine	207 ± 28	$314 \pm 30**$
Alanine	852 ± 23	$654 \pm 43**$
Valine	392 ± 15	$280 \pm 21**$
Methionine	122 ± 3	$78 \pm 3**$
Isoleucine	192 ± 8	$139 \pm 10**$
Leucine	306 ± 10	$205 \pm 17**$
Tyrosine	232 ± 5	$154 \pm 6**$
Phenylalanine	104 ± 3	$81 \pm 5**$
Total	6094 ± 168	$5030 \pm 296*$
Lysine: arginine	5.16 ± 0.14	4.35 ± 0.47

Note: Significantly different from the casein-fed group at * $p<0.05$, ** $p<0.01$.

2.7.3.1.1 Arginine

In adult male *Wistar* rats, the absorption of lipids, which is more rapid with casein than with soybean protein diets, was slowed down by the addition of arginine (1.33%) to a casein diet (Vahouny et al. 1984). An arginine-deficient diet consumed for a 17-day period by weanling rats led to lipid accumulation in the liver (Milner and Perkins 1978). The same effect was observed in male *Wistar* rats (Aoyama et al. 1981). This liver lipid accumulation was prevented by the addition of adenine

(0.30%) to the arginine-deficient diet (Milner 1979). Likewise, the lipid accumulation in the liver decreased with the addition of ornithine, citrulline, and adenine to an arginine-deficient diet consumed by rats during a period of 7 days after a starvation period of 3 days (Aoyama and Ashida 1979).

The addition of arginine (0.42%) to the diet of adult male *Sprague-Dawley* rats maintained on a protein-free ration for 100 days did not prevent the increase of liver neutral glyceride and cholesterol concentrations or the reduction in liver total phospholipid and plasmalogen concentrations (Williams and Hurlebaus 1965a, 1965b). In hyperlipidemic guinea pigs, an arginine diet decreased VLDL-cholesterol and increased HDL-cholesterol levels (Ryzhenkov et al. 1984).

Arginine counteracts the hypercholesterolemic effect of several amino acids (Carroll and Kurowska 1995). In rabbits fed on a hypercholesterolemic diet containing high proportions of several amino acids, mainly lysine and methionine, the rate of incorporation of [^{14}C]lysine into LDL apoprotein was elevated in comparison with that observed in normocholesterolemic animals fed on a diet enriched with lysine and leucine. The increase in LDL-cholesterol and apo B levels was partially prevented by the addition of a high proportion of arginine. This increase is due to the down-regulation of hepatic LDL receptors, and the enhanced hepatic apo B production contributes to the hypercholesterolemic response (Kovanen et al. 1981; Chao et al. 1983; Kurowska and Carroll 1996; Kurowska 2001). *In vitro*, the exposure of liver HepG2 cells to amino acid mixtures similar to those used in rabbits induced a number of changes in apo B levels similar to those produced by arginine, but not to those of other hypercholesterolemic essential amino acids (Kurowska and Carroll 1996; Kurowska 2001).

In adult male *Hartley white* guinea pigs fed for 7 weeks on a casein diet (227 g/kg diet) well balanced in fatty acids (30%), supplementation with arginine decreased cholesterol in the subfraction of LDL with larger molecular weight (Atwal et al. 1997).

Supplementation with arginine and alanine reduces serum cholesterol levels. Male *New Zealand white* rabbits fed on a cholesterol-free, semipurified diet were randomized between a control group, a group on a diet supplemented with arginine and alanine, and three other groups on diets supplemented with arginine plus alanine and three increasing levels of glycine (0.65%, 1.40%, 3.15%); each diet lasted 48 weeks. After 10 weeks, serum cholesterol levels were 15.7, 12.0, 8.5, 8.8, and 8.1 mmol/L, respectively, and were significantly lower than in the unsupplemented group. Moreover, after 48 weeks, the extent of aortic sudanophilia was lower in the amino acid-supplemented groups than in the casein control group (Katan et al. 1982).

In male *Wistar* rats, the addition of arginine (8.6/kg) to casein increased the serum triacylglycerols and glucagon concentrations, but did not change the serum cholesterol levels (Sugano et al. 1982b). Likewise, in male *Sprague-Dawley* rats fed on an arginine-rich (3.040 mg/100 g) diet, liver triacylglycerol and phospholipid concentrations increased (Yoshida et al. 1988).

Whether expressed as rates or total enzyme activities, hepatic 7-α-hydroxylase activities were three to four times greater in male *albino Wistar* rats fed on soybean protein than in those fed on casein. They increased twofold if the casein diet was supplemented with arginine, whereas if the protein diet was supplemented with lysine, they decreased moderately (Vahouny 1985).

2.7.3.1.2 Lysine

In adult male *albino Wistar* rats, the absorption of lipids, which is slower with soybean protein than with a casein diet, was increased by the addition of lysine (1.94%) to a soybean protein diet (Vahouny et al. 1984). The addition of lysine (0.37%) to the diet of adult male *Sprague- Dawley* rats, maintained on a protein-free ration for 100 days did not prevent the increase of liver neutral glyceride and cholesterol concentrations or the reduction of liver total phospholipid and plasmalo-gen concentrations (Williams and Hurlebaus 1965a, 1965b). An increase in liver lipids induced by an excessive amount of sulfur amino acids, was not prevented by the addition of lysine. A lysine-deficient diet enhanced the liver lipid content (Aoyama and Ashida 1972).

A lysine deficiency in rats causes an increase in serum and tissue cholesterol and triacylglycerol levels, particularly in the aorta; hepatic steatosis is another consequence. It decreases fecal excretion of neutral sterols and bile acids (Singal et al. 1953; Viviani et al. 1964; Aoyama and Ashida 1972; Kurup et al. 1983). In male *Sprague-Dawley* rats, hepatic steatosis was induced by a casein-based (15%) lysine-excessive (5%) diet, but these effects were dependent on the dietary casein level (Hevia et al. 1980a, 1980b; Hevia and Visek 1980; Aoyama et al. 1983b).

Lysine was hypocholesterolemic at a concentration of 5% in male *Wistar* rats fed a high-cholesterol diet. Total serum cholesterol, LDL- and VLDL-cholesterol, and triacylglycerol concentrations decreased as well as liver cholesterol and tria-cylglycerol levels (Sugiyama et al. 1989b). The addition of lysine (8%) to a casein diet (20%) of male *Wistar* rats decreased total serum, HDL-, and LDL- plus VLDL-cholesterol levels (Nagaoka et al. 1985). This is in contrast to what is observed in chickens where it has been shown to induce marked hypercholesterolemia (Schmeis-ser et al. 1983). At 5% concentration, lysine as well as alanine, glycine, leucine, methionine, taurine, and threonine were all hypocholesterolemic in male *Wistar* rats fed high-cholesterol diet. They reduced total serum cholesterol, LDL- and VLDL-cholesterol, and triacylglycerol concentrations and also liver cholesterol and tria-cylglycerol levels (Sugiyama et al. 1989b). In growing male *Donryu* rats, a lysine supplementation (1.728%) to a diet containing excess levels of sulfur-containing amino acids did not cause a reduction in liver lipid levels, whereas the reduction of sulfur-containing amino acids in a lysine-deficient diet reduced liver lipid levels (Aoyama and Ashida 1972).

A group of pregnant *Sprague-Dawley* rats were fed on a wheat gluten diet, which is naturally deficient in lysine. Near the end of the gestation period, the liver long-chain acylcarnitine content was shown to be slightly reduced, whereas the liver triacylglycerol content was richer. When this diet was supplemented by 7% or 12% lysine, the liver-free-carnitine content was not modified by the lysine or protein levels of the diets (Fernandez Ortega 1989).

In male *Wistar* rats, the addition of lysine to a soybean protein diet increased the triacylglycerol concentrations, but did not change the serum cholesterol and glucagon levels (Sugano et al. 1982b).

Weanling male *Sprague-Dawley* rats fed on casein (20%) had greater serum and HDL-cholesterol concentrations as well as increased LCAT activities than those fed on cottonseed protein (34.6%). Supplementing a casein diet with arginine (2.5%) resulted in a reduction in both serum and HDL-cholesterol levels, whereas these two cholesterol fractions were increased with the addition of lysine (1.58%) to a cotton-seed protein diet (Park and Liepa 1982). In young male *New Zealand white* rabbits, the greater absorption of lysine into LDL apo B may well promote hypercholester-olemia (Kurowska and Carroll 1994).

Lysine and methionine supplements in a low-fat, cholesterol-free diet in male *New Zealand white* rabbits induced a greater increase in total serum cholesterol, LDL-cholesterol, and apolipoprotein B concentrations than that observed with essential ketogenic amino acids. In contrast, a similar diet enriched in essential ketogenic amino acids only produced a moderate increase in these serum concentrations. The effects of lysine and methionine used together in rabbits was partially counteracted by arginine. This contrasts with individual use of either of these two amino acids or that of essential ketogenic amino acids (Giroux et al. 1999a, 1999b). The propor-tion of lysine, methionine, and arginine in dietary proteins can modulate the cho-lesterolemic response in rats and rabbits (Vahouny et al. 1984, 1985; Kurowska and Carroll 1992; Kurowska and Carroll 1994; Kurowska et al. 1997b). Adding lysine and methionine to a casein diet fed to male *New Zealand white* rabbits significantly increased total serum cholesterol, LDL-cholesterol, and LDL-apo B concentrations, liver levels of phosphatidylcholine, and the phosphatidylcholine/phosphatidyletha-nolamine ratio (Giroux et al. 1999a). The liver total phospholipid levels and the phosphatidylcholine/ phosphatidylethanolamine ratio are higher with a lysine sup-plement than with arginine. This alteration of liver phospholipid levels could be an additional mechanism in the cholesterol metabolism modifications observed in rab-bits (Giroux et al. 1999b).

In male weanling rats of the *Charles River* strain, supplementing a wheat gluten, cholesterol-free diet with threonine (2.8 or 0.3 g/kg) and lysine (9 or 6.5 g/kg) (the limiting amino acids of this protein source), did not diminish the hypocholesterolemic effect of wheat gluten in rats, in comparison with a casein diet. Thus, the hypo-cholesterolemic effect of wheat gluten is independent of the low quality of the protein or of its specific deficiency in lysine or threonine (Bassat and Mokady 1985).

In rabbits fed for 8 months on a protein-rich, cholesterol-free diet (25%) con-taining only casein, soybean protein, casein plus arginine, or soybean protein plus lysine, the serum cholesterol and triacylglycerol levels were higher with casein and casein plus arginine than with soybean protein and soybean protein plus lysine. However, they were lower with casein plus arginine than with casein, and higher with soybean protein plus lysine than with soybean protein. Liver cholesterol levels were similar in all four groups. The addition of arginine to casein lowered VLDL and IDL levels and increased LDL and HDL levels. The addition of lysine to soybean protein had the opposite effect. In another identical experiment over a 10-month period, the serum cholesterol and triacylglycerol levels were higher with casein than with soybean protein, but higher with casein plus arginine than with casein. The consequences of adding arginine to casein are equivocal, but the addition of lysine to soybean proteins clearly increases atherogenicity (Czarnecki and Kritchevsky 1979).

Arginine supplementation of a casein diet can therefore be said to induce a reduction in serum triacylglycerol levels of male albino *Wistar* rats and a redistribution of both triacylglycerols and cholesterol from chylomicron-like particles to higher-density lipoproteins, whereas with a lysine supplement of soybean protein, the triacylglycerols are redistributed into the chylomicrons (Vahouny et al. 1985). The effect of lysine can be partly explained by the methionine/lysine ratio, which is considerably higher in casein than in soybean protein.

2.7.3.2 Lysine/Arginine Ratio

The antagonism between lysine and arginine has been demonstrated in chicks (Jones 1964; Jones et al. 1966) and the importance of the lysine/arginine ratio has been highlighted by Kritchevsky, Czarnecky, and Sugano, among others (Kritchevsky 1979; Czarnecky and Kritchevsky 1979; Kritchevsky 1980b; Kritchevsky et al. 1982a, 1984; Sugano et al. 1984). The increase in the plasma cholesterol concentrations in rats fed different protein sources is strongly correlated with the increasing lysine/arginine ratio, and the correlation is negative between the serum cholesterol level and the arginine/lysine ratio of dietary proteins (Sugano et al. 1984). In male albino *Wistar* rats, supplementation of a casein diet with arginine (1.33%) to give an arginine/lysine ratio of soybean protein (0.9) lowered the serum triacylglycerol concentrations, but did not significantly alter total serum cholesterol levels. However, its distribution was comparable to that in the soybean protein–fed animals. When the soybean protein diet was supplemented with lysine (1.94%) to give an arginine/lysine ratio of casein (2.0), the serum cholesterol and triacylglycerol levels were not significantly different from those of animals with soybean protein or with casein supplemented or not with arginine. These supplementations modified the lipoprotein distribution of cholesterol and triacylglycerols. Total activity of hepatic cholesterol 7-α-hydroxylase was increased or decreased, respectively, by the supplementation of casein with arginine and soybean protein with lysine (Vahouny et al. 1985). Likewise, in other experiments in male *Wistar* rats, when the lysine/arginine ratio was adjusted to that of soybean protein by the addition of L-arginine (8.6 g/kg diet), and that of the soybean protein diet adjusted to that of casein by the addition of L-lysine (17.2 g/kg diet), the serum cholesterol and triacylglycerol concentrations were not significantly different. The arginine/lysine ratio is more effective in regulating serum triacylglycerol levels than those of serum cholesterol. Neither the addition of arginine to casein nor of lysine to soybean protein modified the intrinsic effect of these proteins on serum cholesterol. The addition of arginine to casein did not modify the liver cholesterol- and triacylglycerol-increasing effects, whereas the liver phospholipid level was unchanged. The liver cholesterol level, but not that of triacylglycerols and phospholipids, decreased gradually with increasing levels of lysine compared with soybean protein. The increasing amounts of lysine supplementation enhances serum triacylglycerol levels but is without effect on serum glucagon concentrations, whereas arginine decreases serum triacylglycerol concentrations and increases the serum glucagon level. The effects of these two amino acids on serum insulin are unconvincing (Sugano et al. 1982b).

Numerous experiments have questioned Kritchevsky's (1979) theory. In rabbits, the serum cholesterol level rises with increasing amounts of casein in the diet and without any variation in the lysine/arginine ratio (Terpstra et al. 1981). Several experiments investigating the effects of the supplementation of casein with arginine, and soybean protein with lysine, have failed to obtain the effects predicted by the lysine/arginine ratio (Hermus and Dallingha-Thie 1979; Huff and Carroll 1980a, 1980b; Nagata et al. 1981b; Katan et al. 1982; Sugano et al. 1982b; West et al. 1983a; Vahouny et al. 1985; Tanaka and Sugano 1989b). Likewise, in rats, supplementation of an atherogenic wheat gluten diet with lysine and threonine (the limiting amino acids of wheat gluten) has almost identical effects on serum cholesterol concentrations to those of a gluten diet. Thus, the hypocholesterolemic effect of dietary wheat gluten is independent of its low lysine content and low lysine/arginine ratio (Mokady and Einav 1978; Mokady and Liener 1982). Similarly, the addition of yeast to a soybean protein diet in young *New Zealand-California* rabbits raises the plasma cholesterol levels, but does not cause any significant changes in the lysine/arginine ratio (de Abreu and Millan 1994). This observation contrasts with that of Kritchevsky (1979) and Balogun et al. (1982) who suggested a link between a low lysine/arginine ratio and the hypocholesterolemic effect of soybean protein.

According to Kritchevsky (1979) and Bergeron and Jacques (1989), the lysine/arginine ratio of fish proteins is lower than that of casein. Nevertheless, in male *Sprague-Dawley* rats, Jacques et al. (1986, 1990) found no correlation between serum cholesterol levels and the lysine/arginine ratio of nine different sources of proteins — three animal proteins (casein, beef, fish) and six vegetable proteins (soybean, pea, peanut meal, rapeseed, oatmeal, wheat gluten). A positive correlation was observed only in rats fed cholesterol-rich diet between serum cholesterol levels and the tyrosine content of proteins or the leucine/isoleucine ratio (Jacques et al. 1986, 1990). Likewise, upon investigating the effects of casein and soybean protein in male *Wistar* rats, Horigome and Cho (1992) observed that the difference in the lysine/arginine ratios of casein and soybean protein, 5.16 and 4.35, respectively (which are different of those of the Food and Agricultural Organization), were not statistically significant, although the serum concentrations of total, HDL, and LDL cholesterol and triacylglycerols were significantly lower with the soybean protein diet. For these reasons, they and other authors have suggested that it is difficult to support the hypothesis of a predominant role for the lysine/arginine ratio as the only cause of protein effects on cholesterol metabolism (Sugano et al. 1982b; Gibney 1983; de Schriver 1990; Horigome and Cho 1992). According to Sanchez et al. (1988a, 1988b, 1988c, 1990) the metabolic associations with serum cholesterol levels may be more sensitive with branched-chain amino acids/arginine ratio than with the lysine/arginine ratio.

2.7.3.3 Action Mechanism of Amino Acids

Numerous mechanisms have been suggested to account for the effects of amino acids on plasma lipid metabolism (Sugano 1983; Kurowska and Carroll 1990, 1991,

1993, 1994; Kurowska et al. 1997b). The postprandial concentrations of amino acids vary according to the composition of proteins (Hagemeister et al. 1990). Casein essential amino acids are far more effective in raising total serum and LDL-cholesterol concentrations than the nonessential amino acids (Kurowska and Carroll 1990). The increase in LDL cholesterol is due essentially to the relatively high animal protein content of lysine and methionine, two essential amino acids whose effects are counteracted by arginine (Kurowska and Carroll 1992, 1994; Giroux et al. 1999a, 1999b; Kurowska 2001). These amino acids have been shown to down-regulate hepatic LDL receptors (Kurowska and Carroll 1992), increase the production of apo B (Kurowska and Carroll 1996), and modify the phosphatidylcholine liver metabolism without enhancing homocysteine levels (Giroux et al. 1999a, 1999b).

Variation in the dietary content of amino acids does not have a significant influence on bile acid synthesis. Indeed, whereas serum cholesterol levels are noticeably influenced by dietary contents of methionine, cystine, and glycine, fecal steroid excretion and cholesterol 7-α-hydroxylase (the rate-limiting enzyme for bile acid synthesis) are not modified. Methionine is metabolized to taurine, which reacts with cholic acid to form taurocholic acid, an important bile acid, that via its methyl group contributes to phosphatidylcholine synthesis, a component of bile salt micelles. Thus, it may increase bile acid production and decrease cholesterol levels (Toborek and Hennig 1994).

A deficiency or excess of sulfur amino acids, respectively, increases or decreases serum cholesterol levels, and a deficiency has been shown to have atherogenic activities in mice, rats, cockerels, and monkeys. However, the results of different experiments are conflicting (Fillios and Mann 1954; Laurent 1983). Consumption of excessive amounts of methionine induced membrane damage and liver enlargement in rats and also increased hepatic lipid peroxidation (Klavins et al. 1963; Harper et al. 1970). Lipid peroxidation is likely to initiate and promote atherosclerotic lesions by direct damage to endothelial cells and by enhancing the adhesion and activation of neutrophils, as well as the susceptibility of platelets to aggregation (Hennig and Chow 1988).

The methionine content of soybean protein is lower than that of casein. A significant positive correlation has been observed between plasma cholesterol concentrations and the methionine content of dietary proteins (Sautier et al. 1986; Sugiyama et al. 1996). A methionine-enriched diet may be hypercholesterolemic, hypocholesterolemic, or without any influence on plasma cholesterol according to the dietary methionine/protein ratio (Yagasaki et al. 1986c; Sugiyama et al. 1986c). The addition of methionine (0.8%) to a casein diet (25%) enhances fecal bile acid excretion, although this effect is insufficient to limit any increase in plasma cholesterol levels (Sugiyama et al. 1987). When large quantities of methionine were added to a soybean protein diet, with or without cholesterol, the plasma cholesterol level was increased (Carroll and Hamilton 1975; Sugiyama et al. 1986b; Oda et al. 1986, 1989; Tanaka and Sugano 1989a; Saeki et al. 1990). However, although serum cholesterol concentrations were increased with a soybean protein diet supplemented by methionine at the same level as in casein, this rise was less marked than with a casein diet (Sugiyama et al. 1997). These results could possibly be explained by the fact that most of the hypocholesterolemic effect of soybean protein is due to increased steroid excretion in the feces (Huff and Carroll 1980a; Nagata et al. 1981b). Never-theless, the fact that the hypocholesterolemic effect is unaffected by methionine supplementation is probably due to the presence of other amino acids such as glycine, since glycine concentration in a soybean protein diet is more than twice as high as that of a casein diet (Sugiyama et al. 1997). Indeed, in rats and rabbits fed on soybean protein, glycine has a hypocholesterolemic effect (Katan et al. 1982).

The mechanism behind the cholesterol-lowering effect of glycine is complicated (review in Muramatsu and Sugiyama 1990; Sugiyama et al. 1997). Glycine contrib-utes to methionine metabolism as an acceptor of the methyl group from S-adenosyl-methionine via the glycine N-methyltransferase system (Kerr 1972). Thus, this high glycine content may well depress the hypercholesterolemic effect of methionine.

Since phosphatidylcholine (PC) is the primary phospholipid of serum lipopro-teins, its synthesis is necessary for the assembly and secretion of VLDL into liver cells (Vance and Vance 1985; Yao and Vance 1988). As the dietary methionine level influences PC synthesis via the phosphatidylethanolamine (PE) N-methylation path-way (Zeisel 1981), by its action on phospholipid metabolism, methionine may affect plasma cholesterol concentrations (Sugiyama et al. 1996). The PC/PE ratio of liver microsomes in rats fed on a cholesterol-free diet is significantly and positively correlated with plasma cholesterol concentrations and with the methionine contents of dietary proteins (Sugiyama et al. 1996). It is therefore possible that dietary methionine increases serum cholesterol level and thus enhances PC synthesis (Mura-matsu and Sugiyama 1990). Morita et al. (1997) have shown that diets containing soybean, potato, or rice proteins produce a hypocholesterolemic effect in rats. Taking into account the amino acid composition and the fact that the methionine soybean protein content is very low, dietary methionine and methionine/glycine ratio are the most effective predictors of hypocholesterolemia. Lastly, fatty acids and the molec-ular species composition of PC are sensitive to the dietary methionine level and the microsomal PC/PE ratio is correlated with changes in linoleic acid metabolism (review in Sugiyama et al. 1997), but this effect is not observed in mice (Koba et al. 1994). The suppression of linoleic acid metabolism by soybean protein is due to the decrease in liver microsomal Δ-desaturase activity (the rate-limiting step in its metabolism) (Choi et al. 1989a).

Through the process of liver lipoprotein-cholesterol uptake, the phospholipid molecular species composition of plasma lipoproteins may have a role in the regu-lation of plasma cholesterol concentrations and be associated with the effects of methionine observed in rats fed with a cholesterol-free diet (Sugiyama et al. 1997).

Sanchez et al. (1990) highlighted the fact that animal proteins are rich in essential amino acids and hypercholesterolemic, whereas plant proteins are rich in nonessen-tial amino acids and are hypocholesterolemic. Serum concentrations of certain amino acids are strongly associated with hypercholesterolemia (lysine and tyrosine) or hypocholesterolemia (arginine, cystine, and glycine) (Sugiyama et al. 1985a; Sanchez et al. 1985, 1988a, 1988b, 1990). Although the value of the threonine/gly-cine ratio is lower in soybean protein (1.3) than in casein (2.5), and despite the fact that serum glycine concentrations increase with a soybean protein diet, the serum concentrations of threonine were similar with both diets (Mendiola et al. 1987). Sanchez et al. (1990) suggested that more glycine is converted from threonine during consumption of a soybean protein diet. The phenylalanine/tyrosine ratio is higher in soybean protein (1.3) than in casein (0.9) diets, but the phenylalanine serum concentration is similar with both diets, whereas that of tyrosine is lower with a soybean protein diet (Sanchez et al. 1990).

The serum cholesterol-lowering effect of cystine may be partly explained by the action of glutathione and taurine on the metabolism of cholesterol and bile acids since cystine is converted to cysteine, which can be incorporated into glutathione or converted into taurine. Glutathione is only one of the stimulators of cholesterol 7-α-hydroxylase activity, and taurine has a role in bile acid conjugation (Muramatsu and Sugiyama 1990). The branched-chain amino acids may also modify serum cholesterol levels (Adibi 1980).

The hypercholesterolemic effect of casein may also be due to its content of acetate-generating amino acids. Indeed, in rats, an 8-week supplementation of a soybean protein diet with acetate generating (ketogenic) amino acids, at the same rate as their level in casein, increases the plasma total cholesterol and VLDL- and LDL-cholesterol concentrations, which are nonetheless lower than those of the casein group. The ester cholesterol levels are also enhanced in the liver and aorta (Alladi and Shanmugasundaram 1989b).

Stephan et al. (1987) reported that taurine may enhance LDL receptor activity by sparing cysteine, a donor and stimulator of 7-α-hydroxylase activity, which itself is a stimulator of bile acid production. They further observed that this may lead to increased utilization of cellular free cholesterol and enhanced LDL uptake in cultured human hepatoblastoma cell lines (HepG2 cells).

The effects of soybean protein and their respective amino acid mixtures have different effects from those of casein (Nagata et al. 1982), as summarized below.

- Cholesterol absorption is lower and fecal steroid excretion greater with soybean protein but not with its amino acid mixture. As the phosphopeptides from digested casein inhibit the binding of bile acids and insoluble calcium phosphate, digestive resorption of bile acids, cholesterol, and lipids is increased.
- Reduction of bile acid synthesis with casein.
- With soybean protein but not with its amino acid mixture, there is a more rapid turnover of serum cholesterol and net size reduction of the rapid exchangeable cholesterol pool through a significant increase in the removal rate in that compartment, without any change in the production rate.
- Greater hepatic steroidogenesis *in vitro* and *in vivo* with soybean protein but only *in vitro* with its amino acid mixture.

The stimulation of cholesterol turnover, which is due more to the decrease in intestinal cholesterol absorption and the increase in fecal steroid excretion than to the activation of hepatic steroidogenesis, is the primary mechanism of the different effects of soybean protein and casein on serum cholesterol concentrations. However, reduced hepatic cholesterol synthesis would appear to be the cholesterol-reducing mechanism of soybean protein amino acid mixtures. Moreover, the serum concentrations of branched-chain amino acids, phenylalanine, proline, and tyrosine, are significantly lower in rats fed on a soybean protein diet than in rats fed with casein. In addition, the variations in these amino acids and in leucine, tyrosine, and valine levels are in conformity with those of serum cholesterol concentrations (Horigome and Cho 1992). Hagemeister et al. (1990) have suggested that the correlation between these amino acids and the hypocholesterolemic effect of proteins may well be an explanation.

2.7.4 EFFECTS OF NONPROTEIN COMPONENTS

Various substances can be involved in modifying cholesterol metabolism: dietary fibers, phytic acid, trypsin inhibitors, saponins, and isoflavones are known to down-regulate this process (Shutler et al. 1987a, 1987b; Lovati et al. 1991a; Potter 1995, 1998).

2.7.4.1 Dietary Fibers

Experimental research has as yet failed to demonstrate any major role for dietary fibers (Beynen 1990c). The type of fiber is an important criterion. Anderson et al. (1984) observed that although oat bran diets and soybean protein diets reduced plasma cholesterol concentrations, only the oat bran diet increased fecal steroid excretion. However, Nagata et al. (1982) highlighted the increase of fecal steroid excretion with soybean protein.

The effects of dietary fibers have been widely studied (Kritchevsky and Story 1974; Kritchevsky et al. 1974; 1977; Kritchevsky 1978; Kritchevsky and Story 1978; Kay and Truswell 1980; Kritchevsky 1983a; Shutler et al. 1987b; Kritchevsky 1999), and several books have been published on dietary fibers. In male *New Zealand white* rabbits (Lo et al. 1987) and in rats (Moundras et al. 1998), soybean fibers interfered with soybean protein by counteracting their effects on cholesterolemia or reinforcing their triacylglycerol-lowering effect. However, it is difficult to distinguish among the effects of food proteins, fats, and dietary fibers when assessing the correlations between a normal diet and autopsy observations (Moore et al. 1981).

Soybean hull in the diet of *Macaca fascicularis* monkeys decreased the serum cholesterol level when palm oil or cholesterol was added to the diet, but serum triacylglycerol and LDL-cholesterol concentrations were only significantly affected if cholesterol was added (Piliang et al. 1996). Natural non-nutritive fibers (alfalfa, wheat straw, sugar cane pulp, sugar beet pulp, bran, and oat hulls) have a greater capacity for binding bile salts than synthetic non-nutritive fibers. Alfalfa binds significantly more bile salt than any of the other non-nutritive fibers. The amount and type of dietary fibers in a diet must therefore be taken into account in any experiments (Kritchevsky and Story 1974).

2.7.4.2 Phytates

The phytic acid content of soybeans can vary according to their geographic origin and the processes used in their production (review in Anderson and Wolf 1995). Calcium absorption is reduced by the presence of phytates in soybean protein (Heaney et al. 1991).

2.7.4.3 Saponins

Soybean saponins are complex compounds consisting of nonpolar triterpenoid alcohol aglycones linked to one or more polar oligosaccharides resulting in molecules with amphiphilic properties similar to detergents. Five major saponins have been isolated and structurally characterized (Anderson and Wolf 1995). Saponins remain with the products derived from soybeans except with the alcohol-extracted process.

The saponin content of legume varieties expressed in terms of defatted flour varies from 0.1 to 6.5 g/kg (Price et al. 1986). Plant foodstuffs with a high saponin content produce the greatest reduction in plasma cholesterol levels (Oakenfull 1981). The cholesterol-lowering effect is more likely to be due to saponins than to vegetable proteins or dietary fibers (Newman et al. 1958; Potter et al. 1979).

Dietary saponins suppress the effects of diet-induced hypercholesterolemia in chickens (Griminger and Fischer 1958; Newman et al. 1958; Morgan et al. 1972); rabbits (Cookson et al. 1967; Cookson and Fedoroff 1968; Yanaura and Sakamoto 1975); rats (Malinow et al. 1977b, 1977c, 1979; Oakenfull et al. 1979; Oakenfull and Topping 1983; Topping et al. 1980b); mice and quail (Reshef et al. 1978); pigs (Topping et al. 1980a); and monkeys (Malinow et al. 1976, 1977a, 1978a, 1978b, 1981; Malinow 1984). The addition of different types of alfalfa (alfalfa plant, alfalfa sprouts, alfalfa tops, sun-cured, ground alfalfa hay) to a cholesterol-rich diet prevents hypercholesterolemia in rabbits (Cookson et al. 1967; Cookson and Fedoroff 1968; Barichello and Fedoroff 1971); rats (Wilcox and Galloway 1961; Kritchevsky et al. 1974; Malinow et al. 1979; Story et al. 1984); and monkeys (Malinow et al. 1977a, 1978a). The effect of alfalfa is due not only to its ability to form a nonabsorbable complex with cholesterol in the intestinal lumen (Barichello and Fedoroff 1971), but also to the saponin content (Hanson et al. 1963, cited by Malinow et al. 1977b). Alfalfa saponins have been shown to reduce by a factor of approximately five the intestinal absorption of cholesterol in *Macaca fascicularis* monkeys (Malinow et al. 1981), mice (Reshef et al. 1976), rats and numerous other experimental models (Malinow et al. 1977b, 1977c), if the alfalfa saponins are processed by acid hydrolysis (Morris and Hussey 1965). In pigs (Topping et al. 1980a), rats (Topping et al. 1980b), and *Macaca fascicularis* monkeys (Malinow et al. 1981), saponins increased the fecal excretion of endogenous and exogenous neutral steroids and bile acids. However, saponins did not modify the concentration of either total plasma cholesterol or LDL- and HDL cholesterol. Likewise, the absolute and fractional catabolic rate of LDL or HDL apoproteins remained unchanged (Topping et al. 1980a).

The low saponin level in soybean protein isolates prevents them from modifying serum cholesterol levels (Sautier et al. 1979; Pathirana et al. 1980). In addition, according to Gestetner et al. (1972), soybean saponins are unable to bind cholesterol *in vitro* since they are characterized by triterpenoid aglycones with no carboxylic function (Anderson et al. 1984). In one experiment on *New Zealand white* rabbits fed on either soybean protein isolates or casein, supplemented or not with saponins (10 g/kg), there was no evidence that the effect of the dietary protein source on serum lipids and the excretion of total and individual sterols were influenced by saponin supplementation. Soybean saponins had no effect on fecal sterol elimination or plasma cholesterol levels (Pathirana et al. 1981; Calvert et al. 1981).

The results of several experiments have suggested that saponins may reduce serum cholesterol concentrations without any changes in HDL cholesterol (Potter et al. 1993b); this could result from various mechanisms such as reduced intestinal transit time, binding of bile acids in the intestine, and reduced reabsorption, or modifications of bacterial microflora (Barth et al. 1990b). However, the cholesterol-lowering effect of saponins would only be effective if the hypercholesterolemia is the result of a disease or produced experimentally (Oakenful and Topping 1983). The high-molecular-weight fractions of saponin-rich soybean protein may have a role in lowering serum cholesterol concentrations. They are more hypocholesterolemic than intact soybean protein because they stimulate fecal bile acid and neutral steroid excretions (Sugano et al. 1988b).

Further research is still required to improve our understanding of the potential effects of saponins and their different mechanisms of action (review in Shutler et al. 1987b). Indeed, although *in vitro* some saponins form insoluble complexes with cholesterol and they are thought to prevent digestive absorption of cholesterol (Coulson and Evans 1960; Oakenfull 1981), this does not account for this specific activity since a cholesterol-lowering effect is also observed with saponins that do not form insoluble complexes with cholesterol (Cheeke 1976). It has also been suggested that saponins may inhibit digestive absorption by forming large mixed micelles containing saponins, cholesterol, and bile acids. This has been demonstrated *in vitro* (Sidhu and Oakenfull 1986) where it was shown to disrupt the enterohepatic cycle and increase the fecal excretion of bile acids and neutral steroids (Oakenfull et al. 1979; Topping et al. 1980a), although without systematically lowering the cholesterol concentration (Topping et al. 1980a).

2.7.4.4 Isoflavones

Isoflavones present in legumes, particularly in soybean protein, and lignans found in most fiber-rich foods, are the two main classes of phytoestrogens (Reinli and Block 1996). The protective effect of phytoestrogens toward cardiovascular disease has been well demonstrated by the studies in animals and humans (van der Schouw et al. 2000 for review). They have potent antioxidant effects that reduce arterial lipid peroxidation (Hertog et al. 1993; Kurzer et al. 1997; Tikkanen et al. 1998).

In soybean products, the isoflavone content, also known as isoflavonic phytoestrogens, is high (Dwyer et al. 1994). There are two major isoflavones, genistein and daidzein (Naim et al. 1973), and one minor, glycitein. Their glucosides (genistin and daidzin) are present but in different quantities depending on the technological process used (Walter 1941; Wang and Murphy 1994a; Anderson and Wolf 1995; Lusas and Riaz 1995; Sirtori et al. 1997, 1998; Lichtenstein 1998). Isoflavone contents vary greatly according to soybean products, ranging from 1,200 to 4,200 µg/g (Wang and Murphy 1994b). A crude isoflavone extract from bengal gram seeds contains various isoflavonoids such as pratensein, daidzein, formononetin, and biochanin A, and has been shown to lower the plasma total cholesterol levels in rats (Sharma 1978).

The isoflavone content of soybean protein isolates (600 to 1,000 mg/g) is low in comparison with its content in soybean and soybean flours, and that of a concentrate made by aqueous alcohol extraction is very low (73 mg/g). Soybean protein isolates prepared by extraction with water and ethanol are almost completely depleted of their nonprotein components (Anderson and Wolf 1995). Indeed, ethanol extraction removes isoflavones and other compounds, such as saponins, which bind bile acids. Phytosterols and saponins are the only alcohol extractable substances for which there is a rational basis for a potential effect on plasma lipid and lipoprotein concentrations (Anthony et al. 1996a, 1996b; Clarkson et al. 1998). In addition, they have been shown to have no adverse effects on the reproductive systems in either male or female *Rhesus* monkeys (Anthony et al. 1996a) or surgically postmenopausal *Cynomolgus* monkeys (Clarkson et al. 1998). A hot ethanol extract from soybean protein decreases serum cholesterol concentrations and increases LDL receptor activity (Lovati et al. 1991a).

A relatively pure preparation of protein using traditional methods of isolating soybean proteins (dehulling, flaking, and defatting) produces proteins that are low in isoflavonoids (Adlercreutz 1990; Lusas and Riaz 1995; Anderson and Wolf 1995), whereas the technology used to produce textured soybean protein gives a higher level of isoflavonoids (Anderson and Wolf 1995). In textured soybean protein, soybean flour, and soybean granules, the total isoflavonoid concentration (genistein, daidzein, glycitein) varies from 2.0 to 2.4 mg/g, whereas in soybean protein isolates it varies from 0.62 to 0.99 mg/g of total isoflavonoids. The hypocholesterolemic effect of soybean protein therefore depends on the technological process used.

The isoflavones of ingested soybean protein are biotransformed by intestinal microflora, absorbed, and then subjected to enterohepatic recycling. In *in vitro* and *in vivo*, isoflavones are weakly estrogenic (Adlercreutz et al. 1987; Setchell et al. 1987; Whitten et al. 1992; Cassidy et al. 1995; Miksicek 1995; Anthony et al. 1996a, 1996b; Arjmandi et al. 1997). Genistein has a low affinity for and binds weakly to the estrogen receptor ERα, whereas it shows greater affinity (85% of 17β-estradiol's affinity) and binding potential for receptor ERβ (Kuiper et al. 1997, 1998). On reaching the circulatory system, concentrations exceed those of endogenous estrogens (Setchell 1998). Isoflavones are structurally similar to estrogens, which have hypocholesterolemic properties (Bierman and Glomset 1995; Anthony et al. 1994; Potter 1995).

According to Anderson et al. (1995), at least 60% of the effect of soybean protein on cholesterol levels could be due to isoflavones in primates such as *Cynomolgus* or *Rhesus* monkeys. In 6-month-old golden *Syrian* hamsters ovariectomized and fed for 70 days on either a casein diet or an isoflavone-depleted soybean protein isolates diet processed by ethanol extraction, neither diet had any effect on the increase in total serum cholesterol, VLDL- and LDL-cholesterol, or phospholipid concentrations induced by this operation. However, the serum triacylglycerol concentrations were reduced by this processed soybean protein isolates diet (Lucas et al. 2001). The same effects were obtained in 45 ovariectomized *Cynomolgus* monkeys fed for a 24-month period on an atherogenic diet (0.23% cholesterol) with or without genistein (30 mg/day) or with genistein and vitamin E (179 IU/day). In the three groups of animals, the plasma cholesterol, triacylglycerol, and HDL-cholesterol concentrations were similar (Sulistiyani et al. 1998). However, in rats, the results were different. The supplementation of a chow diet with 0.01% or 0.1% of genistein for 14 days decreased both serum and muscle triacylglycerol concentrations and increased the level of serum free fatty acids in ovariectomized *Wistar* rats. Serum free cholesterol was diminished and liver cholesterol enhanced (Nogowski et al. 1998). Dodge et al. (1996) also reported a reduction in serum free cholesterol level in ovariectomized rats.

The independent effects of isoflavonoids on serum cholesterol concentrations have been confirmed in rats and hamsters (Balmir et al. 1996), nonhuman primates (Anthony et al. 1994, 1996a, 1996b; Honoré et al. 1997), and humans (Cassidy et al. 1995; Clarkson et al. 1998), although apo A-1, apo B and lipoprotein plasma concentrations remained unchanged in two studies in female rhesus monkeys *Macaca mulatta* (Anthony et al. 1996a, 1996b) and female *macaques* (Honoré et al. 1997).

In adult *Mongolian Meriones unguiculatus* gerbils fed on casein or alcohol-washed soybean protein isolates with or without the addition of soybean protein ethanol extracts at three different doses of genistein (2.1, 3.6, or 6.2 mg isoflavones/g of protein), total serum cholesterol, LDL plus VLDL-cholesterol, and apo B levels were significantly lower with soybean protein than with casein. The addition of alcohol extract to soybean protein isolates did not produce a further reduction in serum cholesterol levels, and maintained hepatic apo A-1 mRNA concentrations at a low intermediate level. Levels of apo E mRNA were unaffected by this diet (Tovar-Palaccio et al. 1997, 1998b).

In lean or obese male *(fa/fa)* *Zucker* rats fed on either casein or soybean protein with low (38 mg/kg diet) or high (578 mg/kg diet) isoflavone contents, plasma total cholesterol was lower with the low- and high-isoflavone diets (−21% and −29%, respectively) in comparison with a casein diet. Liver triacylglycerol and cholesteryl ester levels were lower with a low isoflavones diet (−24% and −57%, respectively) than with a casein diet. According to Peluso et al. (2000), the hypocholesterolemic mechanism of dietary soybean protein involves a cooperative interaction between the proteins and the isoflavone-enriched fraction. Indeed, in *Cynomolgus* monkeys fed with an isoflavone-rich extract of soybean protein but without soybean protein, no cholesterol-lowering effect was observed (Greaves et al. 1999, 2000), whereas when this extract was given with soybean protein, the cholesterol-lowering effect was obtained in *C57BL/6* mice (Kirk et al. 1998); female *Sprague-Dawley* rats (Arjmandi et al. 1997); *Rhesus* monkeys (Anthony et al. 1996a); *Cynomolgus* monkeys (Anthony et al. 1994, 1997); ovariectomized *Cynomolgus* monkeys (Tumbelaka et al. 1996); and humans (Wong et al. 1998; Crouse et al. 1999; Lucas et al. 2001).

The effects of genistein as a cause of alterations in cholesterol and lipid serum concentrations have been widely studied (Akiyama et al. 1987; Okura et al. 1990; Linassier et al. 1990). The addition of alcohol-washed isolated soybean protein extract, which is rich in isoflavones (2.1 to 3.6 mg of isoflavones/g of protein), to a soybean protein diet in adult *Mongolian Meriones unguiculatus* gerbils did not reduce serum cholesterol concentrations more than a soybean protein diet alone in comparison with a casein diet; however, it did decrease the level of hepatic apo A-1 mRNA but not that of apo E mRNA. This isoflavone-rich extract is therefore capable of regulating gene expression (Tovar-Palacio et al. 1998a, 1998b).

The effects of soybean isoflavones on lipoprotein metabolism have been studied in HepG2 cells (human hepatoma cell). Incubation of HepG2 cells with the phytoestrogens (24 hours) dose dependently reduced apo B secretion by 70% to 80%. In contrast, there was no effect on apo A-1 secretion. HepG2 cell cholesteryl ester, free cholesterol, and triacylglycerol mass were not affected; however, cholesteryl esterification was reduced by 40% to 45% at 200 μM of either genistein or daidzein (Wilcox et al. 1999). The citrus isoflavone naringenin (Borradaile et al. 1999) or tangerin, a flavonoid from dietary orange juice and grapefruit juice (Kurowska et al. 2000), inhibited cholesterol ester synthesis and apo B secretion in human hepatoma HepG2 cells.

It is also possible that, through their estrogen agonist activity, soy isoflavones may up-regulate LDL receptor expression. Indeed dietary soy protein was ineffective in lowering total plasma cholesterol or inhibiting diet-induced atherosclerosis in LDL receptor null mice in which a greatly exaggerated hypercholesterolemia was induced by diet (Kirk et al. 1998). However, according to Sirtori et al. (1998), although soybean products in which isoflavonoids have been eliminated by ethanol extraction have been shown to reduce serum cholesterol concentrations in monkeys (Wang and Murphy 1994a, 1994b), this process can also remove the low-molecular-weight peptides that are potentially responsible for LDL receptor activation (Lovati et al. 1991a). During a follow-up study in male *Cynomolgus* monkeys, the anticholesterolemic and antiatherosclerotic effects of extracted versus unextracted soybean protein were almost identical (Anthony et al. 1997). Ethanol extraction may have altered the structure of the soybean protein. Likewise in *Sprague-Dawley* rats, with ovariectomy-induced hypercholesterolemia, extracted versus unextracted soybean proteins caused only a weak effect on serum cholesterol levels (Arjmandi et al. 1997). A soybean protein, hot ethanol extract, which is rich in isoflavonoids, reduced serum cholesterol levels in male *Swiss CD-1* mice and increased LDL receptor activity (Lovati et al. 1991a). In premenopausal monkeys fed on a moderately atherogenic diet containing soybean protein that was either high or low in phytoestrogens, total serum cholesterol and lipoprotein(a) concentrations were seen to decrease; in contrast, HDL-cholesterol levels increased with the high phytoestrogen diet. In postmenopausal monkeys, on the same diets as the premenopausal monkeys, serum cholesterol concentrations were similar with both diets but HDL-cholesterol levels and the total cholesterol/HDL-cholesterol ratio were lower with the high phytoestrogen diet (Anthony et al. 1994). The same results were obtained by Topping et al. (1980b) in male adult *Hooded Wistar* rats.

Further studies are still necessary to determine whether the decrease in plasma cholesterol concentrations is caused by isoflavones or by other components of soybean protein, by soybean proteins themselves, or by their combination (Lucas et al. 2001).

Flavonoids also inhibit the oxidative modification of LDL by macrophages (de Whalley et al. 1990; Kapiotis et al. 1997; Darley-Usmar 1997; Mitchell et al. 1997) and increase their resistance to oxidation (de Whalley et al. 1990; Kanazawa et al. 1995; Patel et al. 1997), although Nestel et al. (1997) did not observe this effect. This antioxidant activity, which has been demonstrated *in vitro* (Pratt and Birac 1979; Fleury et al. 1992; Wei et al. 1993; Record et al. 1995; Vinson et al.

1995; Hodgson et al. 1996; Teisseidre et al. 1996; Ruiz-Larrea et al. 1997), is due to the free-radical scavenger capacity of isoflavonoids (Sekizaki et al. 1993). *In vitro*, genistein inhibits LDL oxidation due to copper ions or superoxide/nitrite oxide radicals. Genistein also inhibits bovine aortic endothelial cell and human endothelial cell-mediated LDL oxidation, and protects vascular cells against potential damage by LDL-oxidation (Kapiotis 1997; Patel et al. 1997). Supplementation of the basal diet of *Sprague-Dawley* rats with 250 and 500 ppm genistein significantly decreased total serum cholesterol, LDL-cholesterol, and triacylglycerol levels. The activities of three antioxidant enzymes (superoxide dismutase, catalase, and glutathione per-oxidase) were not significantly different with both levels of genistein. The fact that plasma malondialdehyde levels are significantly lower in rats fed on 250 rather than 500 ppm genistein suggests that 500 ppm genistein from dietary supplementation may have a pro-oxidant activity (Chen and Bakhit 1999).

According to Anthony et al. (1996a, 1996b), the effects of ethanol-extractable substances on plasma lipid and lipoprotein concentrations are more likely to be due to phytoestrogens than to saponins. Indeed, in the presence of soybean protein, soybean saponins had no effect on plasma cholesterol concentrations (Calvert et al. 1981; Pathirana et al. 1980; Potter et al. 1993b; Topping et al. 1980b) and soybean protein interacts with saponins to form insoluble complexes (Potter et al. 1993b).

2.7.4.5 Soybean Globulins

Lovati et al. (1991a) have suggested that lipid changes may be due to a globulin, with a molecular weight of 31 kDa, that is present in soybean protein extracts. The 7S globulin, which is an important component of soybean protein (Brooks and Morr 1992) directly up-regulates LDL receptor expression. These effects have been dem-onstrated in a human hepatoma HepG2 cell line that is highly sensitive to factors regulating LDL receptor expression and cholesterol biosynthesis and breakdown. The incubation of HepG2 cells with 7S globulin from soybean induces a high affinity of LDL receptors (Lovati et al. 1992) associated with 7S recognition by a specific uptake and degradation system (Lovati et al. 1996). The 7S globulin is more active than 11S globulin (Lovati et al. 1992, 1998, 2000,) but the $\alpha + \alpha'$ subunits of globulin 7S are more active in LDL receptor up-regulation than either the whole 7S globulin or the β subunit (Lovati et al. 1998). According to Manzoni (1998), the effect induced by $\alpha + \alpha'$ subunits would appear to be due to the α subunit because a mutant soy cultivar devoid of α' has no effect on LDL receptor activity (Manzoni et al. 1998). ^{125}I-LDL uptake in human skin fibroblasts is more greatly enhanced by 11S globulin than by 7S globulin although neither stimulates LDL degradation (Lovati et al. 1992, 1998). Therefore, if one or more peptides can reach the liver after digestion they may elicit a cholesterol-lowering effect (Lovati et al. 2000). Most of these studies have recently been reviewed by Lovati (2001). Recently, Adams et al. (2002) compared the effects of dietary soybean protein isolates in male and ovariectomized females belonging to two genetically engineered mouse models of atherosclerosis (Zhang et al. 1992; Ishibashi et al. 1993; Linton et al. 1993). One transgenic mouse (LDL-receptor -/- + apolipoprotein [apo] B) was devoid of LDL receptors and overproduced apolipoprotein B, whereas the other (apo E-/-) had a normal complement of LDL receptors but did not produce apolipoprotein E. These mice were fed on three diets differing by the source of the protein component: casein/lactalbumin or alcohol-washed soybean protein isolates or intact soybean protein isolates. Relative to the casein/lactalbumin group, atherosclerosis was partially inhibited by both alcohol-washed and intact soy protein isolate in LDL receptor -/- and apo E -/- mice without sex difference. The antiatherosclerosis effect was enhanced in LDL-receptor -/- mice, diminished in mice fed alcohol-washed soybean protein isolates, and unrelated to LDL-, VLDL-, or HDL-cholesterol plasma concentrations. These results show the existence of LDL receptor and plasma lipoprotein-independent pathways by which dietary soybean protein isolates inhibit atherosclerosis (Adams et al. 2002).

2.7.5 EFFECTS ON ENDOCRINE RESPONSES

The influence of a single amino acid on serum cholesterol concentrations does not appear to support the hypothesis than one or several amino acid(s) are responsible for protein-induced hypercholesterolemia. Indeed, the difference in the serum amino acid profiles in *Göttingen* miniature swine consuming a casein or a soybean protein diet is not as notable as could be expected considering the amino acid composition of these proteins. Moreover, a number of studies have reported conflicting results. Hagemeister et al. (1990) have therefore suggested that differences in serum hormone levels induced by amino acids are very likely capable of modulating serum cholesterol concentrations.

Serum levels of insulin, glucagon, somatotropin, thyroid hormones, and cortisol are influenced by the nature and amount of proteins (Cree and Schalch 1985) and by amino acids (Floyd et al. 1966).

2.7.5.1 Insulin and Glucagon

It is widely known that insulin release is stimulated by various proteins and amino acids, including arginine, leucine, and lysine (Reaven and Greenberg 1965; Fajans et al. 1967; Floyd et al. 1966; Floyd et al. 1970a, 1970b; Palmer et al. 1975; Sugano et al. 1982b; Nuttall et al. 1985). It is also well established that branched amino acids, leucine in particular, stimulate insulin release from the pancreas (Milner 1970; Anderson et al. 1977). The ratio of various amino acids (histidine, methionine, phenylalanine, tyrosine) with arginine in the serum is lower with soybean protein than with casein diets (Sanchez and Hubbard 1991).

In female *Wistar* rats, a hyperproteic diet (55%) administered with no further modifications of body weight or food intake, increased the fasting serum glucose and insulin concentrations but did not change that of glucagon (Usami et al. 1982). The fasting levels of circulating insulin were lower, whereas those of glucagon were higher, though not significantly, in male *Wistar* rats fed on vegetable proteins (soybean protein, rice protein, peanut protein) than in subjects fed on animal proteins (casein, pollack protein, sardine protein, egg-yolk protein) (Sugano et al. 1984). Likewise, the fasting plasma insulin concentrations were lower in male *albino Wistar* rats fed on soybean protein instead of casein (Sugano et al. 1982b). In contrast, in male *Mongolian Meriones unguiculatus* gerbils fed on soybean protein, the plasma insulin and glucagon concentrations were, respectively, higher and lower than in those fed on casein (Forsythe 1986). In female lean *Zucker* rats, a diet high in casein did not modify the serum insulin concentrations (Rabolli and Martin 1977). A negative correlation was observed in male *albino* rats between the serum cholesterol level and the arginine/lysine ratio (Sugano et al. 1984). The addition of arginine to casein or lysine to soybean protein diets of male *Wistar* rats did not change the plasma insulin level induced by each protein alone (Sugano et al. 1982b). However, in contrast with the findings of Sugano, another study reported that the addition of arginine to a casein diet lowered the insulin concentrations, whereas the supplementation of soybean protein with lysine increased the plasma insulin levels (Vahouny et al. 1985). It is possible that the discrepancies between these experiments are due to the species or to differences in the diet composition, particularly with regard to carbohydrates.

Although the effects of dietary proteins on insulin and glucagon have been observed in the fasting state, fluctuations in response to meal patterns may be more significant. Such studies are therefore of particular importance and need to be carried out. In adult male *Sprague-Dawley* rats fed on casein, after an adaptation period of 2 weeks, the portal ratio of insulin to glucagon decreased over the 3 hours following a protein meal (3.1 g protein concentrate containing 70% casein, 20% starch, and 10% sucrose for palatability). No correlation could be demonstrated between portal insulin concentrations and the aortic levels of any amino acid, whereas portal glucagonemia was significantly correlated with the aortic level of the three branched amino acids (leucine, isoleucine, and valine) with the aromatic amino acids (phenylalanine and tyrosine) and with asparagine, proline, and arginine. Likewise, no correlation was found with alanine, glutamic acid, serine, threonine, or glycine. In contrast, in an animal model near-significant correlation was observed with arginine in a semisynthetic control diet (Jarrousse et al. 1980). Unfortunately, this experiment has not as yet been conducted with soybean protein.

The increase in glucagon secretion would appear to be associated with metabolic changes that are different with soybean protein and casein diets in male *Wistar* rats (Sugano et al. 1982b). The circadian variations of these hormones have been studied in female *Göttingen* miniature minipigs on diets containing casein or soybean protein. The serum insulin levels were only significantly different at 45 minutes after the meal, and serum glucagon levels were similar with both diets (Scholz-Ahrens et al. 1990). The postprandial peak of serum insulin and glucose concentrations was temporarily higher in barrows from a cross between *Dutch Landrace* and *Large White* pigs fed on casein than in those fed on soybean protein (Beynen et al. 1990). In *Yorkshire/Duroc* male and female piglets on diets differing only in the casein/whey ratio (100:0, 80:20, 40:60), the serum insulin level was not significantly affected. The level of glucagon, however, was elevated in animals fed on 100% casein (Larson 1996). Insulin and glucagon are, respectively, positively and negatively correlated with diurnal variations in the activity of rat hepatic HMG-CoA reductase. The conversion of acetate to cholesterol is also enhanced but its effect is blocked by glucagon (Lakshmanan et al. 1973).

Gibney (1982) suggested the existence of a hormone-mediated effect of insulin and glucagon whereby the release of arginine following soybean protein digestion leads to enhanced stimulation of insulin release, stimulating the HMG-CoA reductase rate-limiting enzyme of cholesterol biosynthesis (Neprokoeff et al. 1974) and increasing the turnover of VLDL (Gibney 1982). When male *Wistar* rats are put on a high-protein diet, both insulin and glucagon secretions and their liver uptake are enhanced. The systemic insulin/glucagon ratio is lower than the portal insulin/glucagon ratio because the hepatic fractional extraction is higher for insulin than for glucagon (Demigne et al. 1985). The effects of amino acids on gut hormones, particularly the gastrointestinal inhibitory polypeptide (GIP), must also be taken into account (Thomas et al. 1976).

2.7.5.2 Growth Hormone

Mean plasma growth hormone values and area under the time-concentration curve are significantly higher in male *Wistar* rats fed on casein than in those fed on soybean protein (Pfeuffer et al. 1988b). Physiologic doses of growth hormone have been reported to lower plasma cholesterol concentrations, although not in all experiments (Friedman et al. 1974; Blackett et al. 1982; Asayama et al. 1984). In *Long Evans* hypophysectomized rats, the injection of growth hormone increased to an above-normal level the liver's capacity for converting acetate carbon to cholesterol. An increase in hepatic cholesterolgenesis was observed as early as 6 hours after a single intravenous injection of the hormone (Bauman et al. 1959). Growth hormone reduces lipoprotein lipase and hepatic lipase activities (Asayama et al. 1984), enhances hepatic cholesterol 7-α-monooxygenase activity (Mayer and Voges 1972), inhibits lipogenic enzymes in cultured rat hepatocytes (Schaffer 1985), and stimulates bile acid synthesis (Heubi et al. 1983). In male and female *mongrel* dogs, infusion of growth hormone synthetic 32-46 fragments increases insulin and glucagon levels under euglycemic conditions (Stevenson et al. 1987).

2.7.5.3 Thyroid Hormones

It is generally accepted that the thyroid gland involutes during severe protein depletion of rats (Deb et al. 1973) or swine (Atinmo et al. 1978). There does, however, appear to be some disagreement as to whether the thyroid/serum iodide accumulation ratio in rats is elevated (Aschkenazy et al. 1961; Ramalingaswami et al. 1965) or depressed (Srebnik et al. 1963; Cowan and Margossian 1966). This lack of consistency could be due to the differences in experimental conditions (Cowan and Margossian 1966).

Several experimental studies in animals and humans with preexisting elevated blood lipids have investigated the effects of food proteins on plasma thyroid hormones. Results are more often consistent in animal models than in humans; in humans no clear relationship between serum thyroid hormone concentrations and soybean protein ingestion can be demonstrated (Balmir et al. 1993; Ham et al. 1993). In female lean *Zucker* rats, a diet high in casein did not modify the serum thyroid hormones (T_3, T_4) concentrations (Rabolli and Martin 1977).

Soybean protein influences serum thyreostimulin concentrations differently according to the animal species. In *Meriones unguiculatus* gerbils, an increase of thyroid stimulating hormone (TSH) and thyroxine was observed (Forsythe 1986), whereas casein and soybean protein had no effect on plasma TSH concentrations in adult *Göttingen* minipigs (Barth et al. 1990b).

In chicks, a diet that is severely deficient in lysine or valine reduced serum concentrations of both triiodothyronine (T_3) and thyroxine (T_4). Serum thyroid hormone levels have been shown to decrease, although only when the growth of the birds was affected (Elkind et al. 1980). Compared with *golden Syrian* hamsters fed on casein, total serum cholesterol concentrations were lower when the animals were fed on isolated soybean protein and soybean protein concentrates. Serum thyroxine and free thyroxine levels, however, were greater only in hamsters fed on isolated soybean protein, whereas triiodothyronine concentrations were higher in hamsters fed on casein than in those fed on soybean protein concentrates. As the hypo-cholesterolemic effect is similar with both soybean protein diets in spite of the different thyroid hormone levels, it appears unlikely that changes in thyroid hormone status are responsible for the cholesterol-lowering effect of soybean protein (Potter et al. 1996a).

In adult *Göttingen* minipigs, total serum triiodothyronine (T_3) and free thyroxine (T_4) levels were enhanced by soybean protein isolates (Barth et al. 1990b). The plasma thyroxine level was higher in laying hens fed on corn-soybean proteins instead of a fish-meal protein diet (Akiba et al. 1982; Akiba and Jensen 1983), but also in *Meriones unguiculatus* gerbils fed soybean protein instead of casein (Forsythe 1986, 1990; Balmir et al. 1996) and rats (Cree and Schalch 1985; Barth et al. 1989; Klein et al. 2000) fed on casein, or rats fed on gluten (Cree and Schalch 1985), or minipigs fed on dietary soybean protein isolates (Barth et al. 1989, 1990b; Scholz-Ahrens et al. 1990). In *Yorkshire/Duroc* piglets fed on a diet differing only in the casein/whey ratio (100/0, 80/20, 40/60) for a 3-week period, the serum levels of thyroid hormones were similar and HMG-CoA reductase activity was lowest in 100% of the casein-fed piglets (Larson 1996). Reiser et al. (1977) reported that the substitution of soybean protein for casein increased the HMG-CoA reductase activity. The activity of this enzyme is induced by thyroxine (Guder et al. 1968). The receptor-mediated catabolism of LDL was impaired and restored by the appropriate treatment, as has been shown after experimental hypothyroidism by surgical removal of the thyroid in male *Sprague-Dawley* rats (Scarabottolo et al. 1986).

The different thyroxine and free thyroxine indexes did not exist in all groups of rats and hamsters fed on various diets (casein, soybean protein isolates, or these diets with the addition of soybean protein ethanol-isolated extracts) with lower serum cholesterol concentrations. The changes in hormone concentrations were not related to those in serum cholesterol concentrations (Balmir et al. 1996). The mild hyper-thyroxinemia can therefore not be due to the soybean protein-lowering factor of serum cholesterol concentration (Forsythe 1986). The reduction observed with soybean protein products could be the result of a number of factors including the protein and minor nonprotein components (Balmir et al. 1996). Plasma thyroxine concentrations precede the changes in plasma cholesterol concentrations (Forsythe 1995).

The main effects of thyroid hormones on lipid metabolism are enhanced utilization of lipid substrates and increased synthesis and mobilization of triacylglycerols stored in adipose tissues. They are also responsible for increasing nonesterified fatty acid concentrations and lipoprotein lipase activity (review in Pucci et al. 2000). Various mechanisms have been suggested to explain the effects on hepatic metabolism of enhanced thyroid secretion in rats fed on soybean protein; these include higher hepatic HMG-CoA reductase and cholesterol 7-α-monooxygenase activities, induction of hepatic apo B, apo E receptor activities, or increased fecal bile excretion (review in Barth et al. 1990b).

Flavonoids may also displace thyroid hormones from their serum transport proteins, increase their serum concentrations, and decrease serum cholesterol concentrations (Köhrle et al. 1989; Lueprasitsakul et al. 1990; Mendel et al. 1992; Balmir et al. 1996).

2.7.5.4 Cortisol and Corticosterone

In lean female *Zucker* rats the corticosterone secretion was significantly higher but only if they are fed on a very high casein diet (60%) (Rabolli and Martin 1977). In *Yorkshire/Duroc* piglets fed on diets differing only in their casein/whey ratio, the serum cortisol level was shown to increase when the animals were fed 100% casein (Larson et al. 1996).

2.7.6 CONCLUSION

The various effects of protein on lipid metabolism have chiefly been investigated with soybean protein or casein diets and more rarely with fish protein. In most cases, although not systematically, animal proteins are more hypercholesterolemic than soybean protein. These effects are still not clearly understood despite numerous studies. They have been well described, particularly by Sugano (1983), Pfeuffer and Barth (1990), West et al. (1990), and Lovati et al. (1991b). It is, however, difficult to propose a schematic summary of these effects because they vary according to animal species, genetic factors, age, sex, the amount of protein in the diet, food environments (particularly cholesterol and fats), and the duration of experiments. It is therefore impossible to generalize any of these effects and further investigation into these mechanisms is still necessary. Consequently, this brief summary focuses exclusively on the differences between soybean protein and casein.

The following factors must be considered:

* Amino acid composition of proteins
  - Arginine, cystine, leucine, methionine, and taurine are hypocholesterolemic, whereas histidine, lysine, and tyrosine are hypercholesterolemic. The differences in the amino acid composition of soybean protein and casein account for their contrasting effects on plasma cholesterol. Methionine can be hyper- or hypocholesterolemic according to the species and diet composition, and particularly the methionine proportion.
* Nonprotein components
  - Dietary fibers and other components with fiber-like effects and/or water-retention capacity reduce intestinal transit time and enhance

bacterial conversion of cholesterol, production of propionate that decreases cholesterol, and morphologic changes of intestinal mucosa.

– Saponins increase the fecal excretion of endogenous and exogenous neutral steroids and bile acids, which counteracts the effects of hypercholesterolemia-inducing diets.

– The 7S and 11S globulins of soybean protein have a hypocholesterolemic effect that up-regulates LDL receptors and increases the resistance of LDL to oxidation.

– Isoflavones shift thyroid hormones from their serum transfer proteins, thus increasing serum concentrations.

• Endocrine response to protein diets

– The responses of hormonal secretion for insulin, glucagon, growth hormones, thyroid hormones, corticosterone, and cortisol depend on the amino acid composition and the amount of proteins in the diet. They modify the activities of several enzymes, including HMG-CoA reductase, β-hydroxy-β-methylglutaryl coenzyme A reductase, cholesterol 7-α-monooxygenase, lipoprotein lipase, hepatic lipase, lipogenic enzymes and also the induction of hepatic apo B and apo E receptor activities.

These mechanisms induce the following changes when soybean protein is substituted for casein:

• Reduced intestinal absorption of cholesterol and/or bile acids and their influx into the liver
• Increased fecal excretion of cholesterol and bile acids
• Stimulation of metabolic turnover of cholesterol in the body
• Decrease in hepatic intracellular cholesterol concentrations
• Reduced hepatic production of lipoproteins and increased number of LDL receptors

West et al. (1990) pointed out that the mechanism behind the effects of fish proteins is not the same as that of casein or soybean protein. There are probably fewer changes in hepatic cholesterol metabolism than with casein or soybean protein because it does not involve an increase in hepatic cholesterol levels. Moreover, with fish proteins, the lipoprotein pattern is different: LDL and HDL concentrations rise with fish proteins, whereas VLDL levels are increased with casein. Nevertheless this field requires further investigation.

3 Experimental Data on Humans

Studies of humans have focused on both healthy and hyperlipidemic men and women.

3.1 HEALTHY HUMANS

In humans as in animals, genetic variation contributes to the basal plasma levels of lipids and lipoproteins (Friedlander et al. 2000).

3.1.1 AMOUNT OF PROTEINS

Serum cholesterol is significantly below normal in infants with severe protein-calorie malnutrition (Schendel and Hansen 1958), and a relationship between clinical condition and the nonessential-to-essential amino acids ratio has been established (Whitehead and Dean 1964a, 1964b, 1964c). Terpstra et al. (1983a) have summarized the results of the first ten experiments investigating the effect of the amount of proteins, highlighting the fact that these data are sometimes conflicting because of the variety of experimental conditions, especially different dietary fat content and fatty acid composition and the presence or absence of cholesterol (Keys and Anderson 1957; Olson et al. 1958a; Furman et al. 1958; Lutz et al. 1959; Albanese et al. 1959; Léveillé et al. 1962b; Beveridge et al. 1963; Wilcox et al. 1964; Prather 1965; Elson et al. 1971). One study reported that, in middle-aged people, supplementing dietary proteins (from 8.6% to 17% of daily energy intake) with skimmed milk powder produced no effect (Keys and Anderson 1957), whereas in another study, if milk concentrates were added to the diet of elderly people, a moderate increase in body weight was observed. Furthermore, a reduction in serum cholesterol concentrations was observed more frequently than any increase (Albanese et al. 1959). In men, a diet containing 25 g of vegetable proteins increases the molar ratio of nonessential to essential amino acids from 1.82 to 2.90. Plasma alanine, glycine, and asparagine-glutamine concentrations are increased, whereas plasma lysine, threonine, valine, and leucine levels are decreased (Garlich et al. 1970), although to a lesser degree than in kwashiorkor (Holt et al. 1963).

In infants with kwashiorkor, clinical conditions are related to the nonessential/essential amino acid ratio (Whitehead and Dean 1964a, 1964b). The quality of protein synthesis has to be sufficient to allow physiologically normal digestive absorption and lipid transport (Lewis et al. 1964). The plasma level of triacylglycerols is low due to reduced circulating VLDL resulting from a reduction in VLDL-apoprotein synthesis and significantly lower than normal serum cholesterol levels (Schendel and Hansen 1958; Truswell and Hansen 1969; Flores et al. 1970a; Seakins and Waterlow 1972; Waterlow 1975).

In adult humans, the effects of a protein-rich diet have not been so clearly demonstrated as in animal models. A hypolipemic effect was observed in four normocholesterolemic and five hypercholesterolemic subjects in a metabolic ward and consuming a low-protein diet containing 0.18 and 0.22 g of choline, whereas the choline content of the control diet was 1.0 and 1.2 g (Olson et al. 1958b). In contrast, in five healthy young men, a diet with proteins (8% including 4% from skimmed-milk proteins) and cholesterol (23 mg/kg/day) for a 2-week period induced a significant increase in total serum and LDL-cholesterol concentrations. The substitution of soybean protein isolates (4%) for skimmed-milk protein produced a significant increase in lipid, cholesterol, and neutral steroid fecal excretion but did not change serum lipid and cholesterol concentrations (Okuda et al. 1987). Nevertheless, the different levels of fecal excretion were not observed in another similar experiment (Okuda et al. 1988). With protein supplements of 8% to 17% calories, such as skimmed milk powder, the serum concentrations of cholesterol did not vary significantly (Keys and Anderson 1957).

When the dietary protein level of students varied from 5% to 10% or 15% or 20% or 25%, serum cholesterol concentrations decreased weakly, only reaching a level of significance with the 25% protein level (Beveridge 1963). In young women, a high-protein diet (25% of daily energy intake) caused a moderate reduction in the serum protein and cholesterol levels, whereas no variation was observed in young men (Beveridge et al. 1963). Soybean protein supplementation (20 g containing 34 mg of phytoestrogen) in the diet of nonhypercholesterolemic, normotensive, perimenopausal women, reduced total cholesterol (–6%) and LDL-cholesterol (–7%) levels but was without effect on plasma HDL-cholesterol and triacylglycerol levels (Washburn et al. 1999).

The dietary protein intake did not significantly modify postprandial lipemia or chylomicron-triacylglycerol clearance. Indeed, in 15 normolipemic young men and women, mean postprandial lipemia was similar after meals containing 100 ml of dairy cream, supplemented or not with 23 g of casein. The rate of disappearance of an intravenous bolus of Intralipid was similar before and after the consumption of casein (23 g) (Cohen 1989).

3.1.2 NATURE OF PROTEINS

In several studies on vegetarians, although lacking in adequate control models, serum cholesterol levels were low (Hardinge et al. 1954, 1962; Sacks et al. 1975; Ruys and Hickie 1976; Burslem et al. 1978). West and Hayes (1968) observed that serum cholesterol levels of 233 vegetarians were significantly lower than those of 233 nonvegetarians, several confounding factors having been taken into account. A longitudinal study in nonstitutionalized adolescents failed to demonstrate any relationship between the consumption of dietary proteins and serum lipid concentrations (Potter and Kies 1989a). However, in 77 healthy nonstitutionalized men, there was a relation between protein consumption and blood lipids as confirmed by 3-day food records. The consumption of animal proteins was positively correlated and that of plant proteins negatively correlated with triacylglycerol, smaller LDL-mass, VLDL-cholesterol, and VLDL-mass levels (Williams et al. 1986).

Studies of the effects of vegetable proteins on cholesterol metabolism, particularly soybean protein, are the most numerous. They have been reviewed by several authors (Meinertz et al. 1988; Pfeuffer and Barth 1990; Carroll 1991a, 1991b, 1992; Carroll and Kurowska 1995; Anderson et al. 1995; Potter 1995, 1996; Sirtori et al. 1995, 1998). As was highlighted by Young et al. in assessing the experiments, it is important to evaluate protein quality in relation to protein requirements (Young et al. 1984a, 1984b; Young 1991).

3.1.2.1 Casein and Soybean Protein

The hypocholesterolemic effect of soybean protein has been clearly observed in some experiments. In young women, after supplementation with a high molecular fraction of soybean protein, the serum concentrations of LDL cholesterol were shown to decrease and those of HDL cholesterol to increase (Wang et al. 1995). Since high HDL/LDL cholesterol ratio is predictive for lower risk for coronary heart disease (Miller and Miller 1975), soybean protein might have a beneficial effect, even when it does not lower the level of total serum cholesterol (Terpstra et al. 1983a, 1983b). However, soybean protein could be without effect on HDL. Indeed in 51 nonhypercholesterolemic, nonhypertensive, perimenopausal women, soybean protein supplementation (20 g containing 34 mg of phytoestrogen) in the diet caused a reduction in total cholesterol (−6%) and LDL cholesterol (−7%) but had no effect on plasma HDL-cholesterol or triacylglycerol levels (Washburn et al. 1999).

Results of studies comparing the respective effects of soybean protein and casein or other animal proteins on serum cholesterol levels are sometimes conflicting. In strict vegetarians, casein did not induce hypercholesterolemia (Sacks et al. 1983). Studies comparing vegetarians with control subjects have shown that plasma triacylglycerol levels were higher with a soybean protein diet (Burslem et al. 1978). The results of several published studies show either a similar effect of casein and soybean protein diets or a hypocholesterolemic effect of soybean protein compared to casein. In healthy humans, casein and soybean protein-rich diets (van Raaij et al. 1979, 1981, 1982; Grundy and Abrams 1983; Wiebe et al. 1984) had similar effects on blood lipids, although in certain cases, soybean protein had a slight beneficial effect on the distribution of cholesterol between the different lipoprotein fractions. Likewise, Meinertz et al. (1984) obtained the same results as Van Raaij et al. (1981, 1982) when they substituted soybean protein for casein, but only in male subjects. LDL-cholesterol levels were lower and HDL-cholesterol levels were higher because of the increase in HDL_2-cholesterol, which meant that the HDL/LDL cholesterol ratio was higher. According to Pfeuffer and Barth (1990), in seven strictly controlled clinical trials performed on healthy humans, serum cholesterol levels were similar with casein or soybean protein diets (Bodwell et al. 1980; van Raaij et al. 1979, 1981, 1982; Grundy and Abrams 1983; Meinertz et al. 1984; Sacks et al. 1983). In other less well-controlled trials (review in Pfeuffer and Barth 1990), the results were conflicting: reduction of serum cholesterol concentrations with textured soybean protein (Carroll et al. 1978) or soybean protein isolates (Shorey et al. 1981), whereas other investigators reported no effect with soybean protein isolates (Goldberg 1982; Mercer et al. 1987). The small but significant cholesterol-lowering effect of soy observed by van Stratum (1978, quoted by Pfeuffer and Barth) is debatable since the fat content of the diet was changed when switching from the control diet to the soybean protein diet. In ten normolipidemic adults (five women and five men) on low-cholesterol (<100 mg/day), low-fat (28% kcal) diets containing for 1 month, 20% kcal from casein and for 1 month, 20% kcal from soybean protein, with a 1-month interval of self-selected food between each diet period, plasma cholesterol and LDL-cholesterol levels decreased during the first days of the experiments with both diets, and then were similar during the experimental periods, as were VLDL, IDL, LDL, HDL_2, and HDL_3 levels. Casein and soybean protein therefore have the same effects (Meinertz et al. 1988).

Nevertheless, in other experiments, the results were slightly different. In 11 normolipidemic male subjects following an identical controlled diet, the effects of supplementation with 20 g/day of soybean protein isolates or casein for 3-week periods in a crossover design, have been investigated. Neither soybean protein isolates nor casein affected the fasting plasma concentration of lipids and apoproteins. However, the area under the incremental curve of remnant-like particles of cholesterol was significantly lower after the diet supplemented with soybean protein isolates (Shighe et al. 1996). In 41 healthy adults, the changes observed in blood lipid levels were weak with two diets containing 39 g or 40 g of soybean protein or casein for 1 year. These changes were, however, greater in hypercholesterolemic than in normocholesterolemic subjects. Total cholesterol and apo A-1I serum concentrations decreased, whereas HDL-cholesterol and apo A-1 levels increased with soybean protein. Apo A-1 and B have been shown to decrease with casein (Thiagarajan et al. 1997). Wong et al. (1998) studied the effect of soybean protein as a complement of the National Cholesterol Educational Program (NCEP) Step 1 diet in 13 normocholesterolemic men aged 20 to 50 years consuming both soybean protein or animal protein diets, each for 5 weeks alternately after a wash-out period of 10 to 15 weeks. The diets provided the subjects' usual energy intake to maintain body weight (20% protein, 20% fat, and 50% carbohydrate; cholesterol 300 mg/day, dietary fiber 25 g/day, soybean or animal protein 75% of the total protein content). The hypocholesterolemic effect, the reduction in plasma LDL-cholesterol concentrations, and the LDL-cholesterol/HDL-cholesterol ratio were independent of age, body weight, or the sequence of dietary treatment. Nine normolipemic men consumed their usual diet and then two liquid-formula diets of identical composition, one containing soybean protein and the other casein for 33-day (for two men) or 45-day (for seven men) periods, respecting an interval of about 53 days between the two dietary periods. Plasma HDL-cholesterol and apo A-1 concentrations were increased by the soybean protein diet and the LDL-cholesterol/HDL-cholesterol ratio was reduced. Total cholesterol, triacylglycerol LDL cholesterol, apo B, and apo A-1I were not significantly modified. However, in five individuals, plasma LDL-cholesterol, LDL_2-cholesterol, and LDL_2-apo B cholesterol concentrations were reduced (26%), as were apo A-1 levels (−16%). The extent of these effects varied by individual (Nilausen and Meinertz 1998). With the same protocol design, the plasma lipoprotein(a) concentration decreased (−50%) after the casein diet compared with both the soybean protein and the self-selected diet in nine normolipidemic men (Nilausen and Meinertz 1999). After a double-blind switch of the usual breakfast for a beverage containing either 60 g of soybean protein isolates or caseinate for a 12-week period the favorable modification in lipoprotein metabolism was greater in 104 postmenopausal women with soybean protein powder than with caseinate. However, the change was more apparent in hypercholesterolemic than in normo-cholesterolemic women (Vigna et al. 2000). Making allowance for several confounding factors, Nagata et al. (1998) observed a significant negative correlation between intake of soybean products and total serum cholesterol concentrations in 1,242 men and 3,596 women in Japan. The addition of an extruder-cooked soybean protein to conventional meals in 17 healthy young subjects for 2 weeks significantly reduced total plasma and free-cholesterol, β-lipoprotein, and phospholipid levels (Kito et al. 1993).

3.1.2.1.1   Effects of Cholesterol

The following studies confirm the importance of the presence or absence of cholesterol in a diet, as has already been demonstrated by experiments described in previous sections. Although the action of casein would appear to be influenced by the presence and quantity of cholesterol and fats in the diet, the data from various studies of both humans and animals are conflicting.

In 12 healthy subjects, the substitution of soybean protein with animal protein in a very low-cholesterol diet for a 2-week period did not modify the blood lipid or plasma concentrations of different lipoprotein classes (Auboiron et al. 1996, 1997, 1998).

One experiment in normocholesterolemic adults investigated the respective effects of the same diets containing either 100 mg/day (five men, five women) or 500 mg/day (five men, six women) of cholesterol in two crossover studies. Each dietary period lasted for 31 days with a 1-month interim period of self-chosen food. On the low-cholesterol diets, the mean plasma levels of LDL cholesterol and HDL cholesterol were similar regardless of whether the dietary protein was casein or soybean protein. In contrast, with cholesterol-enriched diets, the mean plasma levels of LDL cholesterol were significantly lower with soybean protein than casein while those of HDL cholesterol were significantly higher (Meinertz et al. 1990).

The effects of proteins may well vary on an individual basis even in healthy subjects. This was demonstrated by a study of nine normocholesterolemic men who followed three dietary periods. They consumed first their usual diet, and then during the second and third periods, lasting 33 and 45 days according to the subjects, a liquid formula diet with soybean protein or casein (20% of energy) containing cholesterol (236 mg/1,000 kcal). These two periods were separated by an interval of about 1 month. After the soybean protein period, the serum HDL-cholesterol and apo A-1 concentrations increased and the value of the LDL/HDL cholesterol ratio decreased. Total serum cholesterol, LDL-cholesterol, apo B, apo A-1I, and triacylglycerol levels were not affected. The degree of variation, however, did vary from one subject to another and the authors identified three types of lipemic responses (Nilausen and Meinertz 1996, 1998).

The effects of soybean based on texturized vegetable proteins (TVP) (15% to 18% of energy intake) with a standard (190 to 550 mg/day) or a low-cholesterol diet (17 to 30 mg/day) were compared with those of a typical American diet, over 6- to 7-week periods of each. Eight healthy adult subjects, residing in a metabolic ward, were studied in three randomly ordered 6- to 7-week periods. During the standard cholesterol period, each subject ate typical American foods (protein, 15% to 18% of caloric intake; fat, 17% to 22%; and cholesterol, 192 to 550 mg/day). During the second period, the substitution of texturized soybean proteins removed nearly all dietary cholesterol (17 to 30 mg/day) whereas during the third period, eggs were isocalorically substituted for an equivalent amount of protein and fat to bring the dietary cholesterol levels back to the average range (494 to 515). Serum cholesterol and LDL-cholesterol concentrations were weakly but significantly reduced only with the TVP low-cholesterol diet. Serum HDL-cholesterol concentrations were slightly but significantly lower with both TVP diets, but lowest with the TVP low-cholesterol diet. Serum triacylglycerol concentrations were similar with both TVP diets, but higher than with the standard cholesterol diet. Excretion of neutral and acidic steroids was higher with both TVP diets but only reached statistical significance with neutral steroids (Duane 1999).

The effects of soybean protein isolates and soybean protein in a cholesterol-rich diet (1.6 g/day) have been compared with each other and also with a milk diet containing 25 mg/kg/day of cholesterol. Total serum cholesterol and HDL-cholesterol concentrations were unchanged by either soybean protein diet but increased with the milk diet. With the soybean protein diet, the fecal excretion of lipids was 2.4 times higher than with the soybean protein isolate diet. In addition, intestinal digestion of lipids was significantly decreased by the soybean protein diet (Okuda et al. 1988, 1989).

3.1.2.1.2 Effects of Study Duration

The duration of experiments is also a very important factor to consider. Certain effects may appear only at the beginning or near the end of the study. In 1960, Walker et al. (1960) found that in 12 healthy young women, following a 6-week isocaloric diet containing the same fat (95 g/day, 36% of energy) and vegetable or animal protein levels (50 g/day, 8% of energy), serum cholesterol concentrations were significantly lower with the vegetable protein diet at weeks 2 and 5, whereas the difference was not significant at weeks 3 and 4. Indeed, although the reduction in serum cholesterol and lipid concentrations with a soybean protein or casein (20% of calories) low-cholesterol (<100 mg/day) diet was observed for a number of days or even weeks, by the end of a month these levels are similar with soybean protein or casein, the diet being low in cholesterol and low in saturated fat (Meinertz et al. 1988).

In nine healthy subjects receiving a liquid diet containing 20% proteins (soybean protein or casein), 55% carbohydrates, and 25% lipids (oleinate) and cholesterol (55 mg/MJ), the lipoprotein(a) level increased (+20%) and then returned to the initial value with soybean protein, but decreased to 65% of this initial value with casein. Total plasma cholesterol and LDL-cholesterol and triacylglycerol concentrations were similar with both diets after 30 days and lower than with the usual diet. HDL cholesterol was 11% higher after the soybean protein diet than after the casein diet (Nilausen and Meinertz 1999).

3.1.2.1.3 Effects of Body Weight

Excess body weight as well as a hypocaloric diet must also be taken into consideration. In 11 obese patients on a hypocaloric diet (1,000 kcal), the daily substitution of two regular low caloric meals for a soybean formula significantly reduced the total serum and LDL-cholesterol concentrations (Jenkins et al. 1989). In 31 normocholesterolemic or hypercholesterolemic obese patients on a diet containing 1,300 or 1,700 kcal daily, the use of soybean protein isolates in the diet reduced blood cholesterol values by -41% in hypercholesterolemic and by -16% in normocholesterolemic patients; however, it is important to consider the inherent effect of a hypoenergetic diet (Volgarev et al. 1989). In 24 obese subjects following a very low-calorie diet (375 kcal/day for 15 days and 800 kcal/day for 60 days), body weight reduction was the same with casein or soybean protein. However, the reduction in serum cholesterol concentrations was higher with the soybean protein diet than with casein. The percentage decrease in both VLDL and LDL cholesterol was always significantly greater with the soybean protein diet as was that of HDL but only on the 75th day of the study. The percentage reduction of apo A-1 was greater than that of apo B and significantly greater with a soybean protein diet (Bosello et al. 1988).

3.1.2.1.4 Summary

Data relating to the effects of casein and soybean protein diets are somewhat conflicting. Pfeuffer and Barth (1990) have reported the results of several trials, but they do point out that very few of these studies were adequately controlled. According to their analysis, soybean protein induces no or only a very weak reduction in serum cholesterol concentrations of normocholesterolemic subjects (Carroll et al. 1978; van Raaij 1979; Bodwell 1980; van Raaij 1981, 1982, 1983; Grundy and Abrams 1983; Sacks et al. 1983). Likewise, several other authors have observed that in healthy individuals, the results of both casein and soybean protein diets are similar (Walker et al. 1960; Campbell et al. 1965; Anderson et al. 1971; Holmes et al. 1980; Shorey et al. 1981; Goldberg et al. 1982; Grundy and Abrams 1983; Sacks et al. 1983; Meinertz et al. 1988). Later, other authors found the same results (review by Anderson et al. 1995). However, the effects of soybean protein observed in some studies are more beneficial for hypercholesterolemic than normocholesterolemic subjects.

3.1.2.2 Fish, Pork, Beef, Soybean Protein Analogues, and Poultry Proteins

In healthy humans, casein and soybean protein-rich diets (van Raaij et al. 1979, 1981, 1982; Grundy and Abrams 1983; Wiebe et al. 1984), or meat, dairy protein, and soybean protein diets (Giovanetti et al. 1986) had similar effects on blood lipids, although in some cases, soybean protein had a slight beneficial effect on the distribution of cholesterol among the various lipoprotein fractions.

The effects of fish are different. Twenty-six healthy adult men and women following their usual diet for a 6-week period were separated into two groups. The first group replaced all the fatty fish in their diet with red meat, whereas the second group replaced all the red meat with fatty fish, each for a 6-week period. Plasma cholesterol, LDL- and VLDL-cholesterol, triacylglycerol, and VLDL-triacylglycerol concentrations were significantly lower with the fish diet than the red meat diet (Wolmarans et al. 1991). As dietary polyunsaturated to saturated ratios were 0.45 with red meat and 0.93 with fatty fish, and the intake of ω-3 PUFAs was higher with fatty fish, the nature of proteins cannot be the only factor to account for the different effects of the two diets.

However, with lean fish, the results are different. Fifteen postmenopausal (11 normocholesterolemic and 4 hypercholesterolemic type IIA) women aged 50 to 79 years followed in an 8-week crossover experiment an isoenergetic diet containing 19% of energy as protein, of which 70% to 75% was protein from either lean white fish or beef, pork, egg, and milk products, and 29% of energy as fat with a poly-unsaturated/monounsaturated/saturated ratio of 1/1/1. Total plasma cholesterol, and LDL-apo B, HDL-cholesterol, and HDL_3-cholesterol concentrations were significantly higher with the lean white fish diet than with the beef, pork, eggs, and milk products diet (Jacques et al. 1992a, 1995). In a second experiment in 14 premeno-pausal women on a careful isoenergetic diet, similar to that of the first experiment, the substitution of lean white fish for the same diet containing beef, pork, veal, eggs, and milk products significantly reduced the serum cholesterol, LDL-cholesterol, HDL-cholesterol, apo B, HDL-apo A-1, and LDL-apo B concentrations. With the lean white fish diet, serum VLDL triacylglycerol concentrations were lower and those of LDL triacylglycerols and LDL apo B higher. In this experiment, the increased polyunsaturated/saturated fatty acid ratio with fish compared to other sources of animal protein produced only a weak improvement in the lipoprotein profile (Gascon et al. 1996). In 11 normolipidemic young adults following a careful diet recommended by the 1994 NCP — low fat (30%), high polyunsaturated/saturated (P/S) ratio (1/1), and 260 mg cholesterol/day, substitution of lean fish protein with nonfish protein (beef, veal, pork, eggs and milk) corresponding to between 70% and 75% of total protein intake (18% of the diet) — resulted in higher plasma concentrations of total cholesterol and LDL-apo B, higher apo B/apo A-1 ratio and HDL_2-cholesterol levels, and an increased HDL_2/HDL_3 cholesterol ratio. The tri-acylglycerol/apo B and cholesterol/apo B ratios of VLDL were lower. With the lean fish diet, plasma post-heparin lipoprotein lipase activity was negatively correlated with VLDL triacylglycerols and the VLDL triacylglycerol/apo B ratio. The plasma concentrations of sex hormone-binding globulins were enhanced and the positive correlation between these sex hormone-binding globulins and HDL_2-cholesterol levels suggests that they may have an influence on their metabolism or production (Lacaille et al. 2000).

In college students, the inclusion of fish, pork, or beef in the diet increased LDL-cholesterol levels, whereas adding soybean protein analogues or poultry proteins caused them to decrease in comparison to pre-observation values (Chu and Kies 1993). Removing all animal foods (meat and fish) except egg and milk products from the diet of 14 healthy young subjects (ovo-lacto-vegetarian diet) decreased the intake of saturated and mono-unsaturated fats, protein, and cholesterol. After 3 months of this diet, plasma cholesterol was significantly decreased mostly as a result of the HDL-cholesterol reduction. LDL cholesterol was also reduced but not significantly. Body weight and lean body mass were not modified (Delgado et al. 1996). In another study, 13 normocholesterolemic adults enrolled in a randomized, two-part, crossover study were fed an NCEP Step 1 diet with either an isolated soybean protein diet or animal proteins. The nature of the animal proteins were not specified but the content of fat (30%), cholesterol (300 mg/day), and dietary fibers (25 g/day) were similar in both diets, which were followed for a 5-week period each and separated by a 10- to 15-week period of the usual diet. With the soybean protein diet, plasma LDL cholesterol and the ratio of plasma LDL cholesterol/HDL cholesterol were significantly decreased compared with the animal protein diet (Wong et al. 1996, 1998).

The substitution of a soybean protein isolates drink (750 ml) for cow's milk (750 ml), each for a 8-week period, caused a significant although weak reduction (−4%) in the serum cholesterol levels of 21 healthy adults without any changes in serum triacylglycerol and HDL- or LDL-cholesterol concentrations (Laidlaw and Mercer 1985). In another experiment, 33 healthy adults drank 500 ml of 2% cow's milk/day for a 6-week period, and then for a similar duration, an equal volume of a drink containing similar amounts of proteins and fats such as soybean protein isolates and 2% butter fat. During both periods, the daily intake of calories, protein, carbohydrates, fat, and cholesterol were not significantly different and the diet P/S ratios were similar. However, the ratios of animal/plant proteins in the diet were reduced from 2.44 on the milk diet to 1.08 for the soybean protein period. Although the reduction in plasma VLDL-cholesterol and triacylglycerol levels were significantly higher during the soybean protein than the casein period, no effect was observed on total plasma cholesterol concentrations. However, the plasma cholesterol levels were significantly decreased in the subjects with the highest baseline plasma cholesterol concentrations (Mercer et al. 1982, 1987).

Thirty-six premenopausal obese women were enrolled in a 16-week, parallel-design trial and carefully allocated to one of two equienergetic hypocaloric diets (1,500 kcal) designed to produce weight loss. One diet contained meat and the other plant proteins rich in soybean protein. The body weight loss (−9%) and the decrease in plasma total and LDL-cholesterol (−12% and −14%), triacylglycerol (−17%), and leptin (−24%) concentrations were not significantly different in the two groups. However, the plasma lipoprotein(a) level did not change (Yamashita et al. 1998). Two diets were compared in 26 healthy men: one was a modified-fat lacto-ovo-vegetarian diet, and in the other lean meat was substituted to replace 60% plant proteins of the lacto-ovo-vegetarian diet. The cholesterol-lowering effect was weaker with the lean meat diet (−5%) than the lacto-ovo-vegetarian diet (−10%) but blood pressure levels were similar (Kestin et al. 1989). In a crossover study of 42 noninstitutionalized men on two different diets — one containing lean meat (150 g/day) and the other tofu (290 g/day) in an isocaloric and isoprotein substitution, and with a strictly controlled fat intake — for 1 month each, plasma total cholesterol and triacyglycerol levels were significantly lower with tofu than with the lean meat diet. The LDL cholesterol/HDL cholesterol ratio was similar although HDL-cholesterol levels were significantly lower on the tofu diet (Ashton and Ball 2000).

3.1.2.3 Milk and Whey Proteins

In Masaï tribes, the low serum concentration of cholesterol and low incidence of cardiovascular disease, despite a very high intake of fermented milk cannot be explained by a hypocholesterolemic factor but rather by a probable relatively low energy intake in comparison with high energy expenditure (Gibney and Burstyn 1980). According to Gibney and Burstyn (1980), the real cause of this hypocholesterolemia may well be related to a genetic characteristic since in one controlled study of cholesterol metabolism without a high intake of milk but with a diet containing 2,000 mg of dietary cholesterol, young Masaï demonstrated a marked capacity to reduce endogenous cholesterol synthesis. However, the role of fermented milk cannot be excluded since large dietary intakes of yogurt have been shown to lower plasma cholesterol concentrations in humans (Mann 1977), and high milk consumption has been correlated with low serum lipid levels in a survey of 4,500 volunteers in Basel (Stähelin and Ritzel 1979).

In 40 full-term infants fed on either human milk or one of three formula milks containing casein/whey ratios of 82/18, 66/34, or 50/50, those receiving the 82/18 casein/whey ratio had significantly higher plasma cholesterol values at both 4 and 8 weeks compared to the other groups of infants; their plasma triacylglycerol levels were similar to those fed human milk. Plasma triacylglycerol concentrations increased proportionally with the rise in casein concentration (Tseng et al. 1990; Potter et al. 1990).

In five healthy young men studied over two 2-week periods, the substitution of soybean protein isolates for skimmed milk protein with 25 mg/kg/day of cholesterol significantly increased total- and LDL-cholesterol levels as well as the atherogenic index. No differences in fecal excretion of neutral sterols or cholesterol were observed between the two diets. Likewise, just after the last breakfast, serum insulin and glucagon concentrations were similar in the both diets (Okuda et al. 1988).

In 33 healthy volunteers, the 6-week substitution of 500 ml of soybean drink (soybean protein isolates) for cow's milk with similar nutrient content of the diet significantly reduced the plasma VLDL-cholesterol concentrations, whereas the fasting plasma total cholesterol remained unchanged. However, it was lower in five subjects who had the highest baseline plasma cholesterol concentrations (Mercer et al. 1982; Laidlaw and Mercer 1985; Mercer et al. 1987). In ten healthy subjects, serum uric acid decreased significantly 3 hours after ingestion of either casein or lactalbumin (80 g) but increased after ingestion of soybean protein (80 g). Urate clearance was significantly increased after ingestion of each of the three proteins. Multivariate analysis of the results obtained with β-lactalbumin and casein showed an independent correlation between serum alanine and urea concentrations (Garrel et al. 1991).

3.1.2.4 Egg Protein

In a 28-day crossover study of 11 healthy young men on diets differing only in that one contained 83.3 g/day of wheat gluten and the other 74.8 g of egg-white powder, plasma cholesterol and triacylglycerol concentrations were modified from baseline but remained similar in both groups despite the different diets. The amino acid content of gluten is lower than that of egg white in aspartic acid, lysine, methionine, and alanine, but much higher in glutamic acid and proline (Anderson et al. 1971). The differences between these results and those of Olson et al. (1970b) is due to the lower level of glutamic acid in both diets since in another study these authors found no differences in serum cholesterol level in men when glutamic acid was added to a normal diet (Bazzano 1969).

3.1.2.5 Amino Acids

The effects of plasma amino acid patterns on plasma lipid and cholesterol levels are still under discussion. Dietary amino acid composition influences free amino acid patterns in the plasma. Three healthy adult men in a metabolic ward were studied over 2- to 4-week periods. Changes were observed when they were switched from a control diet containing 100 g of protein/day to either a low-protein vegetable-cereal diet (25 g of protein/day) or an amino acid formula containing the eight essential amino acids to give a total of 16 g of nitrogen/day. Serum cholesterol levels decreased 16 mg/100 ml but triacylglycerol concentrations were not significantly altered when the diet was reduced to 25 g protein/day. Plasma alanine, glycine, and asparagine-glutamine concentrations increased, whereas lysine, threonine, and valine levels decreased, and methionine levels remained constant. Supplementation with 122 g of glutamic acid/day produced a further reduction in plasma threonine, histidine, lysine, valine, and isoleucine levels, but these changes varied by individual. A low-protein diet produced an increase from 1.82 to 2.90 in the plasma molar ratio of nonessential/essential amino acids. However, these changes do not explain the hypocholesterolemic action of these diets (Garlich et al. 1970).

In 73 subjects (35 men and 38 women) with cardiovascular disease and obesity or diabetes, who were placed on a cholesterol-free diet containing vegetable protein and skimmed milk as the only source of animal protein for a 4-week period, the plasma amino acid pattern was modified: plasma threonine, serine, glycine, and arginine levels increased significantly and plasma valine, leucine, tyrosine, and histidine concentrations decreased significantly. The mean lysine/arginine ratio decreased significantly from 3.46 to 2.72 (Sanchez et al. 1983).

Supplementation of a low-protein diet (25 g/day) with a single amino acid does not prevent the 20% fall in serum cholesterol resulting from the protein-deficient diet. When the same diet was supplemented for 3 to 4 weeks, with a mixture containing all L-amino acids there was no significant change in serum lipids from control values with an ordinary ration containing 100 g of protein/day. However, if the diet was supplemented with adequate amounts of the eight essential amino acids, plus glutamate as a source of essential nitrogen, a more marked level of hypocholesterolemia was observed (Olson et al. 1958b, 1964).

The results of several experimental trials with amino acid mixtures were not convincing except when they contained glutamic acid (Olson et al. 1970a, 1970b). In three separate 28-day laboratory-controlled feeding studies, 11 healthy adults per study received the basal diet alone and the basal diet plus one of the three study amino acids in capsule form containing 1.2 g of arginine, 1.2 g of lysine, or 1.5 g of tryptophan, each test period lasting 14 days. Compared to the basal diet, arginine lowered serum cholesterol and LDL-cholesterol but not HDL-cholesterol concentrations, whereas lysine had no effect. Tryptophan reduced serum cholesterol levels, and increased HDL-cholesterol concentrations and the value of the HDL/LDL ratio. However, the results were only significant for arginine (Kohls et al. 1985, 1987).

In 40 healthy males, LDL cholesterol was negatively correlated with plasma L-arginine and positively correlated with urine L-arginine excretion (Pentinen 2000). In a controlled crossover study of 30 patients with diabetes mellitus, after 3-month periods of either a placebo or two daily dosages of 1 g of L-arginine, serum malondialdehyde levels were significantly reduced by arginine. Thus, treatment with L-arginine may counteract lipid peroxidation and reduce long-term microangiopathic complications in diabetes mellitus (Lubec et al. 1997).

In ten healthy adults fed on soybean protein isolates alone or supplemented by either L-methionine (0.5%) or L-cystine (0.5%), serum lipid levels, with the exception of HDL cholesterol, increased with methionine. Addition of cystine did not affect serum lipid concentrations. Fecal excretion had a tendency to be reduced with the addition of either amino acid (Potter and Kies 1989b). In other experiments, the addition of cystine (Morse et al. 1966), histidine (Gerber et al. 1971), or leucine (Truswell 1964) had no effect on serum cholesterol concentrations. When the usual diet of young men containing 60 g of protein and an average of 1.3 g of sulfur amino acid was supplemented daily for a 3-week period with 4 g of methionine (five subjects) and 3.24 g of cystine (five subjects), serum lipid levels remained comparable to those of the control group without supplementation (five subjects). However, the mean serum triacylglycerol concentrations were significantly higher after methionine supplementation than in the control groups or in those on glycine (Morse et al. 1966). These results confirm those of Mann et al. (1953). Administration of capsules containing L-tryptophan (69 mg) and L-lysine monohydrochloride (205 mg) three times daily after meals significantly reduced the plasma cholesterol and triacylglycerol levels in men (Raja and Jarowski 1975).

The data concerning the effects of taurine administration are conflicting (Bellentani et al. 1987a). When premature infants were given a taurine supplement (45μmol/kg/day) to a whey-predominant cow's milk formula, the mean plasma taurine concentrations did not change, but total duodenal bile salt concentrations were positively correlated with increases in the taurine status and reduction in that of cholesterol (Okamoto et al. 1984). In another study, however, the rate of bile acid synthesis was unmodified in low-birth-weight infants (Watkins et al. 1983).

In healthy young volunteers on cholesterol-rich diets who received a taurine supplement, hypercholesterolemia was shown to decrease (Mizushima et al. 1996). In ten obese children with fatty liver syndrome due to simple obesity, taurine given at 2 to 6 g/day for 6 months or more caused a reduction in the hepatic lipid content (Obinata et al. 1996). Oral administration of a taurine load increased taurine conjugation and decreased the G/T acid ratio, which has been related to the regulation of cholesterol serum levels (Bremer 1956). In humans, the G/T ratio changes throughout the life cycle (Jacobsen et al. 1968) and can be altered in adults by dietary changes. Administered taurine has been shown to be utilized for bile acid conjugation in humans (Sjövall 1959). In patients with hypothyroidism, oral administration of taurine decreased the glycine-bile acid/taurine-bile acid ratio (Hellstrom and Sjövall 1961), but did not cause a decrease in serum cholesterol (Truswell et al. 1965). In adults, the consumption of 1.5 g/day of taurine for 5 days induces an increase in the conjugation of biliary acids. This contrasts with the results observed with glycine (Sjövall 1959; Truswell et al. 1965; Hamaguchi et al. 1974). In six adult men fed on 0.5 g of taurine six times daily for 2 weeks, the bile acid glycine-to-taurine conjugation ratio was reversed, and the total bile acid pool size decreased, as was chenodeoxicholic acid pool size. However, pool sizes of cholic and deoxycholic acids did not change. Biliary cholesterol saturation and biliary secretion rates of cholesterol, phospholipids, and bile acids were not modified (Hardison and Grundy 1983). An oral taurine supplement (3.2 g/d for 2 weeks) to a diet with or without a cholesterol supplement did not modify the serum and biliary lipid composition, but did increase the taurine-conjugated bile acids. When the diet was supplemented with cholesterol (1 g/day), the serum LDL-cholesterol concentrations and the lithogenic index increased (Tanno et al. 1989).

3.1.2.6 Carnitine

In infants fed on isolated soybean protein–based formula milk unsupplemented with carnitine, plasma carnitine concentrations decreased (Schiff et al. 1979; Novak et al. 1979, 1983; Olson and Rebouche 1987; Olson et al. 1989), plasma triacylglycerol and free-fatty acid concentrations increased (Novak et al. 1983; Olson et al. 1989), and the excretion of all three medium-chain dicarboxylic acids (adipic acid, suberic acid, and sebacic acid) also rose. These changes were not observed in infants on a diet supplemented with carnitine (Olson et al. 1989). Fat is underused as an energy substrate because of inhibition of mitochondrial β-oxidation of the long-chain fatty acid. As a result, serum free fatty-acid concentrations increased, and the metabolism of fat by the carnitine-independent microsomal ω-oxidation pathway of long-chain fatty acids, which produces medium-chain dicarboxilic acids, was enhanced in infants not receiving dietary carnitine (Mortensen 1984; Olson et al. 1989). Exogenous supplies of carnitine to premature infants may have a significant influence on the ability to stimulate optimal fatty acid oxidation (Schiff et al. 1979). Urinary excretion of medium-chain dicarboxylic acids was increased because omega oxidation is not carnitine dependent (Karpatti et al. 1975).

3.1.2.7 Food Environments

As in animal studies, food environments are an important parameter to consider in investigations on the effect of food proteins on cholesterol and lipid metabolisms in humans. This is especially relevant for calcium, which, in healthy men, reduces plasma total cholesterol and LDL cholesterol in particular (Klevay et al. 1979). Individual responsiveness of serum cholesterol to fat-modified diets is different (Katan et al. 1988a, 1988b). In ten normolipidemic adult women, plasma total cholesterol and LDL-cholesterol concentrations were lower after 3 weeks of a low-fat diet containing tofu (soybean curd) instead of cheese; no differences were observed with regard to VLDL- and HDL-cholesterol or triacylglycerol plasma concentrations. However, this effect was not due to the different proteins in the diet but to the low-fat content and high P/S ratio of tofu compared to cheese (Meredith et al. 1989). Similar results were reported by Dunn and Liebman (1986). Hodges et al. (1967) suggested that in humans soybean proteins are responsible for the reduction in levels of serum cholesterol when soybean protein diet replaced a mixed diet, whereas according to Keys (1957), 90% of this decrease could be due to differences in the amount of dietary fat and cholesterol.

The reduction of dietary protein and choline, without altering dietary fat or energy level, caused hypocholesterolemia and hypo-β-lipoproteinemia in humans. A daily supplement of choline (0.87 g) and DL-methionine (1 g) induced a hyper-cholesterolemic response and serum cholesterol levels returned to their previous normal values (Olson et al. 1958b). In contrast, to animal studies, the findings reported in humans on the effects of vitamin E on serum cholesterol and lipids are conflicting (Harman 1960; Nikitin 1962) and unsettled (Chen et al. 1972).

3.2 HYPERLIPIDEMIC HUMANS

In hyperlipidemic humans as in animals, genetic variation contributes to the basal plasma levels of lipids and lipoproteins and to the diet response (Sarkkinen 1994).

3.2.1 SOYBEAN PROTEIN, ANIMAL PROTEIN, AND AMINO ACIDS

Compared to animal proteins, plant proteins lower serum cholesterol, LDL choles-terol, apo B, and triacylglycerol concentrations in hypercholesterolemic patients (Sirtori et al. 1977, 1979; Descovich et al. 1980, Schwandt et al. 1981; Wolfe et al. 1981; Goldberg et al. 1982; Verrillo et al. 1985; Mercer et al. 1987; d'Amico et al. 1992), in hypercholesterolemic children (Widhalm 1986; Gaddi et al. 1987; Widhalm et al. 1993), and in hypercholesterolemic pre- and postmenopausal women (Steinberg and Villablanca 1998). The same results were observed in one study in a metabolic ward (Vessby et al. 1982). Plasma L-arginine concentrations appeared to be reduced in hypercholesterolemic patients (Jeserich et al. 1992), although this result was not confirmed (Oleesky et al. 1982).

The substitution of soybean protein for casein reduces serum cholesterol levels to a greater extent in hypercholesterolemic than in normocholesterolemic subjects. However, the results of several studies are conflicting. Since the first trial by Sirtori et al. (1977), numerous other studies have been performed. The amount of soybean protein required to reduce blood lipid concentrations was evaluated over 6 weeks in 81 moderately hypercholesterolemic men divided into five groups according to the following ratios of casein/soybean protein isolates: 50/0, 40/10, 30/20, 20/30, and 0/50. The consumption of as little as 20 g/day of soybean protein instead of animal protein is sufficient to reduce serum concentrations of non–HDL cholesterol and apo B by −2.6% and −2.2%, respectively (Teixeira et al. 2000).

The substitution of soybean protein or textured soybean protein for animal protein in a diet with or without dietary cholesterol induced a significant decrease in serum cholesterol concentrations, particularly serum LDL-cholesterol concentra-tions, although the reduction in triacylglycerol and HDL-cholesterol levels was not significant (Sirtori et al. 1977, 1979; Descovich et al. 1980; Wolfe et al. 1981; Goldberg et al. 1982). The addition of soybean protein to a standard low-lipid diet gave the same effects (Verrillo et al. 1985). Likewise, plasma triacylglycerol and VLDL-cholesterol levels were reduced and HDL cholesterol increased in children with familial hypercholesterolemia fed two diets successively, each for a 4-week period, containing 20% of energy as protein of which 35% was from cow's milk proteins or soybean protein isolates, 28% of energy as fat with a P/S ratio of 1/3.3, and less than 200 mg/day of cholesterol (Jacques et al. 1992b). In 23 children with familial or polygenic hypercholesterolemia, a soybean diet (20 g of soybean protein isolates) mixed with a low-fat, low-cholesterol standard diet resulted in greater reductions in plasma cholesterol levels (−16% versus −8%) and LDL-cholesterol levels (−22% versus −7%) than those produced by a low-fat, low-cholesterol standard diet (Widhalm 1996, 1998). Reductions in VLDL-cholesterol and triacylglycerol serum concentrations in hypertriglyceridemic patients have also been observed (Grundy and Abrams 1983).

A soybean protein isolates diet lowers not only the serum cholesterol and triacylglycerol levels, but also the atherogenic index in coronary patients and hypertensive subjects (Samsonov et al.1993).

In 20 hypercholesterolemic patients (9 with type IIA and 11 with type IIB hypercholesterolemia), replacing animal protein with textured soybean protein caused a reduction in serum cholesterol concentrations. This effect was more marked in subjects who had higher baseline levels (Sirtori et al. 1977). In a crossover study on hypercholesterolemic patients receiving either animal protein or textured vegetable soybean protein, the decrease in plasma LDL-cholesterol levels was only observed with textured soybean protein; in addition, the LDL particles were strongly degraded by mononuclear cells in spite of the high cholesterol intake (Lovati et al. 1987). After 4 weeks of a traditional hypocholesterolemic diet, 1 homozygous and 20 heterozygous type IIA hypercholesterolemic subjects followed a 4-week diet containing textured vegetable soybean protein instead of animal protein. Whereas no significant changes were observed in plasma lipid levels during the low-lipid diet, total serum cholesterol, LDL-cholesterol, and apo B plasma concentrations decreased by −20.8%, −25.8%, and −14.1%, respectively, with the soybean protein diet. The plasma cholesterol reduction differs according to the type of apo E isoforms since it is very weak in type apo E3/E2 but higher in patients with type apo E3/E3 or E3/E4. This difference could be due to activation of B- and E-receptors by soybean protein (Gaddi et al. 1991). Thus, patients with greater LDL-receptor activity are less likely to benefit from a soybean protein diet (Lovati 2001).

In a group of 24 young men with mildly elevated plasma cholesterol levels, soybean protein isolates of great purity (92% protein diet) or animal protein in low-cholesterol mixed diets with a similar P/S ratio caused a reduction in plasma cholesterol concentrations (−16% and −13%, respectively) in 20 responder subjects who had higher initial plasma cholesterol values than the 4 nonresponding subjects. The protein and fat contents of these diets were lower than in the previous diet of the responders. HDL-cholesterol levels were only moderately reduced but the HDL-cholesterol/total cholesterol ratio remained constant in most individuals (Shorey et al. 1981). According to Carroll et al. (1978a, 1978b), who used similar products and the same mixed diets, the amino acid composition of these animal and vegetable diets are similar, and it is this factor that may explain the similarity in the results (Shorey et al. 1981). Moreover, the soybean protein isolates used in this experiment have greater purity than those used by Sirtori et al. (1977).

In coronary and hypertensive subjects, a diet containing soybean protein isolates lowered serum cholesterol and triacylglycerol levels and the atherogenic index (Samsonov et al. 1993). In 31 normocholesterolemic or hypercholesterolemic obese patients following a diet containing 1,300 or 1,700 kcal daily, the use of soybean protein isolates in the diet reduced blood cholesterol values by −41% in the hyper-cholesterolemic and by −16% in the normocholesterolemic patients; it is therefore important to consider the individual effect of a hypoenergetic diet (Volgarev et al. 1989).

The hypocholesterolemic effect of the undigested high molecular fraction (HMF) of soybean protein is well known in rats. Mildly hypercholesterolemic young female students took part in two trials (one during menstruation) with three diets (casein, soybean protein, undigested HMF). Compared to casein, undigested HMF had the same effects as soybean protein on LDL- and HDL-cholesterol concentrations and also on fecal steroid excretions (Wang et al. 1995). Similar results have been obtained by other authors with soybean protein isolates (Wong et al. 1995; Teixeira et al. 1998) or extruder-cooked soybean protein (Kito et al. 1993).

Compared to casein, soybean protein decreased the serum concentrations of LDL cholesterol but those of HDL cholesterol were unchanged (Raja and Jarowski 1975; Sirtori et al. 1977, 1979). This effect was increased with lecithinated soybean protein (Noseda et al. 1987). The hypocholesterolemic effect of soybean protein was also enhanced by soybean oil (Kurowska et al. 1997a).

However, the results are not always the same, since in one study of healthy young men with mildly elevated plasma cholesterol levels, some did not respond to the experimental diet. Moreover, among the responders the reduction in plasma cholesterol concentrations, compared to those observed with the previous diet, was similar with soybean or animal protein (−13% and −16%, respectively) (Shorey and Davis 1979; Shorey et al. 1981). The differences between the previous and experi-mental diets of responders have to be taken into account. Indeed the protein, carbo-hydrate, fat (particularly saturated fats), and cholesterol contents were significantly higher in the previous diets than in the study diet and this may alter the significance of the results.

In subjects with primary hypercholesterolemia, the substitution of animal protein with an isocaloric amount of soybean protein significantly reduced serum cholesterol concentrations (Goldberg et al. 1982). Similar results were obtained in another clinical trial (Mercer et al. 1987). The substitution of soybean protein with meat and dairy protein in the diets increased the VLDL-apo B pool size and production rates along with a significant increase in the fractional catabolic rate of fasting hyper-cholesterolemic men (Huff et al. 1984). After the double-blind switch, from the usual breakfast to a beverage containing either 60 g of soybean protein isolates or caseinate in powder form for 12 weeks, the favorable modification in lipoprotein metabolism was greater in 104 normolipidemic and 44 hyperlipidemic postmenopausal women with soybean protein powder than with caseinate. The improvement was, however, more apparent in hypercholesterolemic than in normocholesterolemic women. Although plasma apo B concentrations and the LDL-cholesterol/HDL-cholesterol ratio (−6% and 8% from baseline, respectively) were significantly reduced, in contrast lipoprotein(a) plasma levels were unchanged (Vigna et al. 2000). Diets rich in *Vicia* faba protein decreased serum cholesterol concentration in nine hypercholesterolemic subjects. This protein may be the most powerful cholesterol-lowering agent among vegetable proteins (Weck et al. 1983).

Replacing cow's milk with a soybean beverage in a similar diet in 21 hypercholesterolemic adults reduced plasma cholesterol levels by only −4%. However, in this group, the reduction in plasma cholesterol was different in low and high responders, at −3% and −8.5%, respectively. LDL- and HDL-cholesterol levels remained unchanged (Laidlaw and Mercer 1985). In another study, the results were similar (Mercer et al. 1987). Serum triacylglycerol concentrations decreased in hypercholesterolemic, normotriglyceridemic subjects or in hypertriglyceridemic patients when soybean protein beverages were substituted with milk protein (Grundy and Abrams 1983; Laurin et al. 1991). In 34 subjects with moderate hypercholesterolemia, substituting dietary whole soybean products that contain both soybean protein and soybean oils for cow milk products improved the plasma lipid profile, chiefly with soybean protein and only moderately as a result of soybean oil. This effect is particularly important if the initial LDL-cholesterol level is high and the initial cholesterol level low (Kurowska et al. 1996, 1998). However, in hypercholesterolemic subjects, skimmed milk from cows immunized against intestinal bacteria caused an 8% reduction in serum cholesterol concentrations, a 4% reduction in LDL cholesterol, and an 8% reduction in the value of total cholesterol/HDL-cholesterol ratio. The mechanism behind this effect remains unknown (Golay et al. 1990).

In 24 female university students presenting moderate hypercholesterolemia throughout their complete menstrual cycle, 30% of total protein intake was replaced by egg white, tofu, or cheese in a diet containing about 500 mg of cholesterol. In the egg-white group compared to the tofu group, the reduction in total serum cholesterol concentrations were similar although the serum HDL-cholesterol levels were higher. The decrease in total cholesterol and LDL-cholesterol and the increase in HDL-cholesterol levels were greater than in the cheese group (Asato et al. 1996).

However, the results of trials focused on hypercholesterolemic patients are conflicting (Meinertz et al. 1988, 1989). Compared to animal proteins, although plasma cholesterol levels are reduced with a soybean diet, plasma triacylglycerol concentrations remained unchanged (Fumagalli et al. 1982) and plasma levels of VLDL, HDL, and apo A and E are not modified (Goldberg et al. 1982). Six studies reported no change in serum cholesterol concentrations (Holmes et al. 1980; Calvert et al. 1981; Lembke et al. 1981, 1983; Huff et al. 1984; Wolfe and Giovanetti 1985), as did one study in a metabolic ward (Vessby et al. 1982).

The amount of protein in the diet has to be considered. Five subjects with familial hypercholesterolemia treated with resin therapy were put on either a high- or low-protein diet in which meat and dairy protein was substituted for carbohydrates (protein 27%, fat 25%, carbohydrates 48% to protein 10%, fat 25%, carbohydrates

65%). Cholesterol intake varied among the subjects but was always between 10 and 107 mg/1,000 kcal. The high-protein diet induced a significant increase (+17%) of plasma HDL cholesterol and a significant decrease of VLDL-cholesterol (−32%), total triacylglycerol (−23%), and VLDL-triacylglycerol (−28%) levels. The ratios of LDL cholesterol/HDL cholesterol and total cholesterol/HDL cholesterol were also reduced by −19% and −16%, respectively. These results show that increasing protein levels at the expense of carbohydrates may be useful in the treatment of hypercholesterolemia (Wolfe and Giovannetti 1992).

Serum cholesterol and triacylglycerol concentrations and the VLDL apo B pool size were unchanged in five hypercholesterolemic men after 6 weeks of two successive diets — either a high-polyunsaturated fat, low-cholesterol control diet with mixed protein from meat, dairy products, and plant sources, or an all-plant protein experimental diet in which soybean protein and soymilk were used to replace the meat and dairy protein of the former diet. Although the VLDL apo B pool size was similar for both diets, the fractional catabolic rate and the VLDL apo B production rate were increased after the vegetable diet (Huff et al. 1984). These results concord with those of several other experiments (Sirtori et al. 1979; Holmes et al. 1980 Wolfe et al. 1981; Goldberg et al. 1982). The variations in the amounts and components of diets (level of proteins and nature of soybean protein, amount of polyunsaturated fats, value of P/S ratio) could explain the different results of these experiments.

In outpatients with hyperlipoproteinemia of types II and IV, the substitution of meat with soybean protein after 3 weeks of a careful low-fat, low-cholesterol diet, had only a minor additional effect (Holmes et al. 1980). This result did not confirm the observations reported by Sirtori (1977, 1979). These conflicting data could be the result of differences in the two diets (Sirtori: protein 21% and fat 20.8% of calories; Holmes: 15% and 34%, respectively), and provide clear evidence of the importance of carefully highlighting the dietary conditions of experiments and possibly the composition of the processed products used (Holmes et al. 1980).

Two successive experiments, each including two groups of male and female patients, have investigated the effects of either casein or soybean protein in balanced diets (2,230 kcal/day) that vary only in the casein (milk protein) or vegetable protein (mainly soybean protein) contents (16.4 kcal/day). In one 18-month experiment, 197 men and women followed balanced diets (2,230 kcal/day) that varied only in the casein or soybean protein contents (16.4 kcal as percentage of the diet). No changes were observed in the lipid status of 70 normocholesterolemic or 127 hypercholesterolemic subjects (IIa: 30, IIb: 18, IV: 79) (Lembke et al. 1981). In another experiment involving two groups of 100 men and women each, who were followed for a 2-year observation period, the effects of either casein or soybean protein in the diet (2,230 kcal/day) were investigated. Clinical and biological examinations were carried out in 87 and 71 men and women from each of these two groups (normolipemic 75: 36 casein, 30 soybean; type IIa 35: 20 casein, 15 soybean; type IIb 17: 10 casein, 7 soybean; type IV 79: 40 casein, 39 soybean). At the end of the 2-year follow-up, no significant differences were observed between the groups in terms of total plasma cholesterol; triacylglycerol, HDL-, LDL-, VLDL-cholesterol concentrations; LDL-cholesterol/HDL-cholesterol ratio; or apo A, apo B, and apo B/apo A ratio in blood lipid levels (Lembke et al. 1983).

Since these meta-analyses and experiments were performed, Sirtori et al. (1999) have studied 21 severely hypercholesterolemic patients with resistance or intolerance to statins, comparing the effects of a significant percentage of the dietary protein being provided by either cow's milk or high-protein soymilk. These patients followed a low-cholesterol, high polyunsaturated/saturated fatty acid diet for at least 2 years. A soy drink was given, in a crossover design, versus a cow's milk preparation of similar composition and taste. Each dietary supplement was given for 4 weeks, with a 4-week interval between the treatments. The results of this double-blind study confirm a significant cholesterol-lowering effect of partial replacement of the protein in the diet by soybean protein. In their review of the literature and their personal experience of over 1,000 hyperlipidemic patients, Sirtori et al. (1995) have suggested that soybean protein up-regulates LDL receptors that are depressed by hypercholesterolemia or by dietary cholesterol administration.

3.2.2 WHEAT GLUTEN

In 20 hyperlipidemic men and women with elevated LDL-cholesterol serum concentrations, a high-protein wheat gluten diet (27.4% of total energy) for 1 month compared with a bread control diet (15.6%, the other components of the diets being similar), lowered serum triacylglycerol and uric acid concentrations. LDL oxidation, assessed as the ratio of conjugate dienes to LDL cholesterol in the LDL fraction, was also reduced. However, total or HDL-cholesterol serum concentrations and renal clearance of creatinine were not significantly different (Jenkins et al. 2001).

3.2.3 GARLIC PROTEIN

In 50 adult male subjects with moderate hypercholesterolemia, garlic supplementation (900 mg/day) for 12 weeks significantly decreased both total cholesterol and LDL-cholesterol levels and also the ratios of total cholesterol/HDL cholesterol and LDL cholesterol/HDL cholesterol (Adler and Holub 1997). The presence of large amounts of sulfur amino acids in garlic protein, but perhaps also its low lysine/arginine ratio (0.77) compared to soybean protein (0.84) and casein (2), account for the hypolipidemic action of garlic protein (Mathew et al. 1996). These effects have been previously reviewed by Silagy and Neil (1994) and Warshafsky et al. (1993).

3.2.4 FOOD ENVIRONMENTS

The effects of diet cholesterol levels were discussed in Section 2.4.4, but carbohydrate, fat, and dietary fiber composition must also be taken into account. The varying protein and carbohydrate contents in a diet modify the serum lipoprotein concentrations. Indeed, in one crossover study, ten subjects with moderate hypercholesterolemia and five with familial hypercholesterolemia followed two diets in succession. The diets were similar in terms of dietary fibers, cholesterol, and fat contents and also in fat composition. However, they differed in as far as 10%, 11%, or 17% of total energy from proteins was exchanged for carbohydrates. This switch significantly reduced the serum concentrations of LDL cholesterol, increased those of HDL cholesterol, and reduced the total cholesterol/HDL-cholesterol ratio and the serum triacylglycerol concentrations (Wolfe 1995).

Sommariva et al. (1985) compared the effects of two different low-fat diets in hypercholesterolemic patients. Thirty-two subjects followed a conventional low-fat diet (carbohydrates 56%, fats 25%, vegetable proteins 7%, animal proteins 12%, P/S ratio 1.0, cholesterol 300 mg, dietary fiber 2.0 g/1,000 kcal) and 32 other similar outpatients followed the second diet (carbohydrates 69%, fats 19%, vegetable proteins 7%, animal proteins 5%, P/S ratio 1.3, cholesterol 100 mg, dietary fiber 5.6 g/1,000 kcal) for 1 month. Twenty-four similar outpatients followed both diets in a crossover design for a 1-month period each. Both diets reduced total and LDL cholesterol (–9% and –12%, respectively), but only the first diet, with the P/S ratio of 1.0, reduced VLDL cholesterol and HDL_2 cholesterol.

In 58 hypercholesterolemic children who followed for a 12-week period a low-fat-and-cholesterol diet, with or without soluble psyllium dietary fibers (3.2 g per serving), a greater reduction of total and LDL cholesterol, and an increase in HDL cholesterol were observed in the high-fiber group (Williams et al. 1995). However, in six healthy volunteers the supplementation of normal diet by 21 g of dietary fiber from two different soybean seed fiber preparations, either a nonpurified and never-dried soy pulp or a purified soy fiber for 3 weeks each, does not change serum triacylglycerol levels and the HDL-cholesterol/LDL-cholesterol ratio (Schweizer et al. 1983).

3.2.5 SUMMARY

Several authors have reported that in comparison with casein or animal protein, soybean protein decreases serum cholesterol concentrations (Sirtori et al. 1977, Descovich et al. 1980, Wolfe et al. 1981, Goldberg et al. 1982). Other investigators, however, have not confirmed this effect (Holmes et al. 1980, Lembke et al. 1981, 1983, Huff et al. 1984, Wolfe and Giovanetti 1985).

Pfeuffer and Barth (1990) have analyzed several trials. They observed that only 1 of 14 studies on different types of soybean products in hyperlipidemic outpatients was performed under strictly controlled conditions (Grundy and Abrams 1983). The substitution of animal protein with soybean protein in three trials, with good although not strict control criteria, caused a weak reduction in serum and LDL-cholesterol concentrations of –3.5% and –6%, respectively (Goldberg et al. 1982), or –13% and –17% (Wolfe et al. 1981). However, as West et al. (1990) suggested, the difference between the triacylglycerol and cholesterol contents in animal protein and soybean protein diets renders the validity of this comparison questionable.

In their review, Pfeuffer and Barth (1990) point out that no study with strict control conditions has been able to prove that serum cholesterol concentrations increase with a casein diet and decrease with a soybean protein diet in primates and humans. The decreasing effect of soybean protein is only observed in trials on hyperlipidemic patients following a diet with pure soybean protein concentrates and there is no evidence to prove that the possible increase in these levels results from a diet containing animal protein. However, Anderson et al. (1995) have conducted a meta-analysis of 37 experimental controlled studies with crossover or parallel designs. They found that the consumption of soy protein rather than animal protein significantly decreased serum concentrations of total cholesterol, LDL-cholesterol, and triacylglycerols, and that the changes in serum cholesterol and LDL-cholesterol concentrations were directly and very significantly related to the initial serum cholesterol levels.

As in animals, the effect of vegetable protein is dependent on the amount of cholesterol in the diet. According to Sirtori et al. (1977, 1979, 1993, 1995, 1998), the overall conclusion of recent studies is that any reduction of plasma cholesterol in humans is strongly dependent on the baseline level. The addition of soybean protein to a diet may offer a nonpharmacologic approach to the prevention of hyperlipidemia and atherosclerosis but could also constitute a complement to pharmacologic treatment. Several challenges must still be overcome to obtain adequate rationale for the general use of vegetable protein for the prevention and treatment of hypercholesterolemia and atherosclerosis (Kolb and Sailer 1984; Wolfe and Giovannetti 1992; Sirtori et al. 1993; Erdman 1995; Goldberg 1995). According to Lovati et al. (1991b), with the exception of methionine and cysteine levels that are below the recommended requirements, soybean protein is the plant protein with the most appropriate amino acid profile according to the guidelines published by the Food Nutrition Board or the Food and Agriculture Organization. Lovati et al. (1991b) therefore recommend a total protein intake of 60 to 100 g; the intake of vegetable protein should be around 40 to 70 g, and clinical studies suggest that a complete replacement with these proteins may be therapeutic for patients with type II hyperlipoproteinemia.

3.3   MECHANISMS INVOLVED IN SOYBEAN PROTEIN, CASEIN, AND AMINO ACID EFFECTS

Although the hypocholesterolemic response to dietary soybean protein has been proven by several but not all trials, the substitution of animal protein with soybean protein in North American diets has generally had few results. In humans, the mechanisms involved in the effects of protein on cholesterol metabolism are still insufficiently understood, although they may well vary (Carroll 1991a, 1991b). On the basis of their general reviews, Potter (1995, 1996) and Sirtori et al. (1996, 1998) have concluded that the precise mechanism of action and the soybean components involved have not yet been fully established.

3.3.1   Effects on Digestive Absorption of Lipids and Fecal Excretion of Steroids

The rates at which individual amino acids are absorbed from a mixture of amino acids vary widely in humans (Adibi et al. 1967; Adibi 1971). In the human intestine, the interactions among these various proteins, cholesterol, and lipids are not similar to those known in animals, which vary according to species. Indeed, neutral and acid fecal steroid excretions of normolipidemic, hypercholesterolemic, or hypertriglyceridemic individuals are not significantly different with casein, soybean protein, or mixed protein diets. However, the amount of cholesterol in the diets was perhaps insufficient (Fumagalli et al. 1982, Grundy and Abrams 1983). Fecal neutral steroid and bile acid excretions were not significantly different in seven hyperlipoproteinemic (type II) patients fed on a standard low-lipid diet or a textured soybean diet, in spite of the patent hypocholesterolemic effect of the soybean diet (Fumagalli et al. 1982). In five young men on a diet containing soybean protein isolates or skimmed milk as the protein content (0.8 g/kg/day) and cholesterol (23 mg/kg/day), the serum cholesterol, LDL-cholesterol concentrations, and atherogenic index increased only with skimmed milk, whereas fecal excretion of lipid, cholesterol, and neutral steroids was increased only with the soybean protein isolates diet (Okuda et al. 1987) or did not vary (Okuda et al. 1988), with no changes in fecal weight (Okuda et al. 1987, 1988). In five healthy young men subjected to the same dietary conditions, the lipid level in the feces was higher (about 2.4 times) with soybean protein diets than with soybean protein isolates, whereas the total amount of neutral sterols and cholesterol excreted into the feces was the same with both diets (Okuda et al. 1989). With a short (2-day) test meal in ileostomized subjects, daily bile acid and cholesterol excretion were not significantly different when meat proteins were replaced in the diet by soybean protein from soybean flour, soybean protein concentrates, or soybean protein isolates. Ileostomy sterol concentrations were lower when the diet contained soybean products (Bosaeus et al. 1988).

3.3.2 Effects on Hepatic and Lipoprotein Cholesterol

Since dietary casein, compared to soybean protein, increases intestinal uptake of cholesterol and bile acids in rabbits, both LDL-receptor activity and fractional catabolic rates of LDL should be reduced and the plasma LDL-cholesterol level increased (Meinertz et al. 1990). This hypothesis was confirmed by another experiment on rabbits (Samman et al. 1989), but the same effect was not observed in humans because the fractional catabolic rates of both native and modified LDL were similar with both casein and soybean protein diets enriched with 500 mg of cholesterol (Meinertz et al. 1990). Meinertz et al. (1990) have suggested several hypotheses to attempt an explanation for the differences in serum LDL concentrations induced by these two diets. They could be the result of diet-induced differences in LDL-production rates rather than catabolic rates. Soybean protein and casein may also modify the production of small VLDL and IDL fractions, which are precursors of LDL or their transformation into LDL. Lastly, the *de novo* production of hepatic LDL may well be modified. Likewise, according to Meinertz et al. (1990), the increase in serum HDL concentrations observed with a cholesterol-enriched diet may be due to the enhanced synthesis or to the reduced elimination rate. Finally, the increase in HDL with a cholesterol-enriched soybean protein diet may be due to an increase in the production of these particles in the same way as, in hypercholesterolemic patients, the fractional catabolic rate of VLDL apo B is increased when a soybean protein diet is used to replace a meat or dairy protein diet (Huff et al. 1984).

In a 3-week crossover study, 11 normolipidemic male subjects followed a control diet supplemented with 20 g/day of casein or soybean protein isolates. No differences were observed between the fasting lipid and apoprotein serum concentrations or the postprandial areas under the incremental curve of triacylglycerol and remnant-like triacylglycerol particles. Nevertheless, the area under the incremental curve of remnant-like cholesterol particles was significantly lower with the soybean protein isolates (Shighe et al. 1996).

The nature of the proteins could be responsible for regulating the expression of lipoprotein receptors in peripheral cells. In 12 patients with severe type II hypercholesterolemia, the LDL-receptor activity of freshly isolated mononuclear cells was tested after two similar 4-week diets (animal protein or textured soybean protein) in a crossover design. With the soybean diet, total and LDL-cholesterol levels were reduced by −15.9% and −16.4%, respectively, whereas the animal protein diet produced no significant changes. LDL degradation by mononuclear cells was 16 times greater than the basal activity and 8 times that of a standard low-lipid diet with animal protein. Nevertheless, the reduction in total and LDL-cholesterol plasma concentrations was not clearly related to the increase in LDL degradation (Lovati et al. 1987). LDL-receptor activation is the main mechanism behind LDL receptor regulation of hepatocytes. The levels of mRNA for LDL receptors are higher in the mononuclear cells of humans fed on soybean protein isolates than in those of subjects on milk proteins (Teng et al. 1996).

Small amounts of intact peptides, with a molecular weight ranging from 3,000 to 20,000 Da and absorbed by the intestinal wall, have been observed to reach the liver (Warshaw et al. 1974). When absorbed intact, these oligopeptides derived from soybean protein might have a hypocholesterolemic effect (Redgrave 1984). The action of globulins released from the digestion of soybean protein has been investigated by Sirtori et al. in several studies. The 7S globulins and their 7S α + α' subunits are present in soybean protein in large quantities (Brooks and Morr 1992); they up-regulate LDL-receptor expression by over 50% of control levels following prolonged incubation *in vitro* with human hepatoma cell lines (HepG2 cells). With regard to the up-regulation of lipoprotein uptake and the degradation of ^{125}I-LDL in HepG2 cells, 7S globulins are more active than 11S globulins. However, in human skin fibroblast (HSF)[3] cells, the 11S globulins increase the uptake of ^{125}I-LDL more than the 7S β subunits. Degradation, however, is not stimulated by either globulin (Lovati et al. 1992, 1996; Sirtori 1995; Manzoni et al. 1998; Sirtori et al. 1998). Moreover, exposing HepG2 cells to 7S globulins strongly reduces the production of apo B; this effect is dose dependent although weak during exposure to 7S β subunits. Exposure to α + α' subunits or to whole soybean protein has no effect (Lovati et al. 2000). The reduction in apo B is associated with a reduced rate of synthesis of cellular lipids, free cholesterol, cholesteryl esters, triacylglycerols, and cellular free cholesterol (Lovati et al. 2000; Kurowska 2001).

3.3.3 EFFECTS OF NONPROTEIN COMPONENTS

Evidence on the effects of nonprotein components in animals has already been discussed. This section presents selected human studies that have led to a better understanding of the mechanisms involved.

3.3.3.1 Lecithin

The activity of soybean lecithin on lipid metabolism has been investigated in several studies (Knuiman et al. 1989; Sirtori 2001). Lecithin modifies both lipid and lipoprotein metabolism (Kesaniemi and Grundy 1986) and induces a regression of atherosclerosis (Adams et al. 1967; Wilson et al. 1998b). Knuiman et al. (1989) carried out a detailed analysis of 24 studies on the effect of supplementary lecithin intakes ranging from 1 to 54 g/day. According to Knuiman et al. (1989), most of these studies lacked an appropriate control group, had a small sample size, or observed changes in intake of other foods because of increased energy intake from lecithin. There is therefore no evidence for a specific effect of lecithin on serum cholesterol, independent of its linoleic acid content or secondary changes in food intake.

In noninstitutionalized hyperlipidemic men, lecithin treatment has no effect on serum lipoprotein, total cholesterol, triacylglycerol, HDL- and LDL-cholesterol, apo A, apo B, or lipoprotein(a) levels (Oosthuizen et al. 1998).

3.3.3.2 Dietary Fibers

The bulking effect of soybean fibers did not appear to be influenced by heat processing (Slavin et al. 1985). The high fermentability of soybean dietary fibers and their high digestibility (86% to 93% according to the dose used in the Ensure/Enrich study) (McNamara et al. 1986) may well account for some of their positive physiologic effects (Slavin 1991).

The effects of dietary fibers with soybean protein have already been described in animal studies. A supplement of two dietary fibers prepared by extraction from soybeans (addition of 39% dietary fiber, undried soy pulp, and 79% extracted with water and alkaline wash) was added to the diet of six volunteers. Although stool weight was increased by 19% and 38%, respectively, neither diet had any effect on stool frequency or transit time (Schweizer et al. 1983). In hypercholesterolemic adults consuming diets containing either oat bran with β-glucan or soybean protein, plasma cholesterol levels were reduced with both diets but fecal sterol excretion was only increased with oat bran (Anderson et al. 1984). Blumenschein et al. (1991) have also described the effects of oat bran and soybean protein in hypercholesterolemic children.

In 14 healthy students, the addition of 25 g/day of soybean polysaccharides to the diet significantly increased both fecal weight and fecal water content, although the transit time remained unchanged. Serum cholesterol and triacylglycerol concentrations were, however, significantly reduced (Tsai et al. 1983), as they were in patients with diabetes and obesity and consuming 26 to 52 g/day of soybean hulls (Mahalko et al. 1984). In noninstitutionalized men with mild or moderate hypercholesterolemia and on a normal diet, a soybean polysaccharide supplement of 25 g/d reduced serum cholesterol and HDL-cholesterol concentrations by 11% and 8%, respectively, without any change in triacylglycerol concentrations (Shorey et al. 1985).

In 59 moderately hypercholesterolemic patients, a long-term treatment (36 to 51 weeks) with 20 g/day of a mixture of dietary fibers (guar gum, pectin, soybean, pea, corn bran) reduced the levels of total cholesterol (−5%), low density lipoprotein cholesterol (−9%) and the LDL/HDL ratio (−11%), but had no effect on triacylglycerol or HDL-cholesterol serum concentrations (Hunninghake et al. 1984). However, in other hyperlipidemic subjects, a crude fibers extract from soybean did not reduce serum cholesterol concentrations (Sasaki et al. 1985). This type of experiment was continued with similar results in another trial with 42 hypercholesterolemic patients (Sirtori et al. 1979), and later by two studies on 130 and 127 patients (Descovich et al. 1980; Sirtori et al. 1983). When 21 mildly hypercholesterolemic men on a low-fat, low-cholesterol diet given 25 g of protein and 20 g of dietary fibers daily from either soybean protein isolates plus soybean cotyledon fibers, soybean protein isolates plus cellulose, casein plus soybean cotyledon fibers, or casein plus cellulose, the degree of lipemia was not influenced. However, compared with both casein diets, a significant reduction in total and LDL-cholesterol levels without any change in HDL cholesterol was observed with both soybean diets but only in subjects whose initial cholesterol concentrations were higher than 5.7 mol/L. In these subjects, a weak reduction in apo A-1 concentrations was observed but apo B levels remained unchanged (Bakhit et al. 1993). In 26 mildly hypercholesterolemic men, the effects of various sources of proteins and dietary fibers were investigated. Over a 4-week period, patients followed a low-fat, low-cholesterol diet containing 50 g of proteins (soybean flour or isolated soybean protein and cellulose or soybean protein and soybean cotyledon fibers or nonfat dried milk and cellulose). Plasma total and HDL-cholesterol levels were lowest with both soybean protein isolates diets. Serum apo B concentrations were lowest with soybean protein isolates and cellulose. HDL-cholesterol and triacylglycerol serum concentrations were not affected (Potter et al. 1993a).

In hyperlipidemic patients supplementing their diets with 25 g/day of both cellulosic and noncellulose dietary soybean fibers over a 12-week period reduced plasma cholesterol and LDL-cholesterol concentrations by −13 mg/dL and −12 mg/dL, respectively. However, no effects on HDL cholesterol, apo A-1, or A-1I were observed. In type IIA hypercholesterolemia and type IV hypertriglyceridemia, the insulin responses to an oral glucose challenge were significantly reduced by −20% and −16.5%, respectively. These results clearly demonstrate the importance of taking into account dietary soybean fibers in any assessment of the hypocholesterolemic effect of soybean protein (Lo et al. 1986).

3.3.3.3 Saponins

In healthy men, saponins increase fecal bile acid excretion without reducing serum cholesterol concentrations (Potter et al. 1979, 1980). In contrast, in hypercholesterolemic men consuming 22 g/kg/day for 4 weeks, they had no effect on fecal bile acid or neutral sterol excretion, or on fasting plasma cholesterol, triacylglycerol, and plasma lipoprotein fractions (Calvert et al. 1981). Moreover, the reduction in plasma cholesterol concentrations observed with a soybean protein diet, in contrast to oat bran, was not associated with fecal sterol excretion or changes in plasma cholesterol turnover (Fumagalli et al. 1982; Anderson et al. 1984).

In healthy men and postmenopausal women, saponins increased fecal bile acid excretion with no reduction in serum cholesterol concentrations, but with an increase in HDL cholesterol (Potter et al. 1979, 1980).

3.3.3.4 Isoflavones

Isoflavones are structurally similar to estrogens, bind to estrogen receptors, and elicit a weak estrogenic response as has been previously described. A number of studies have associated their consumption with a reduction in the risk of cardiovascular disease; the beneficial effects of soybean isoflavone consumption have been observed in peripubertal *Rhesus* monkeys without any consequences on the reproductive system (Anthony et al. 1996a).

The hypocholesterolemic effects of soybean protein may well depend on the isoflavone content, which varies according to product type (review by Sirtori et al. 1998). Several host-related factors, such as the status of intestinal microflora, can influence the bioavailability of soybean isoflavones (Xu et al. 1995). Intestinal microflora must be intact to allow formation of lignans and isoflavonoids (Setchell and Adlercreutz 1988; Rowland 1991), and high levels of dietary fibers in a diet influence both their development and their activities (Lampe et al. 1998).

Isoflavones can have differential effects depending on their nature, the quantity available, and the food environment. Indeed, the intake of wheat fibers with soybean protein reduced plasma genistein by 55% but had no effect on daidzein concentrations (Tew et al. 1996). In women, daidzein in soymilk shows greater bioavailability than genistein (Xu et al. 1994), and digestive absorption varies according to the nature of the intestinal microflora (Xu et al. 1995) and the composition of the diet. The technology chosen for preparing soybean products is another factor likely to modify their effects. In fermented soybean products such as tempeh, the daidzein and genistein content is increased (40 and 8 times higher, respectively) (Hutchins et al. 1995). However, on the basis of their study of eight adult women, Xu et al. (2000) observed that the bioavailability of isoflavones was not affected by the choice of background diet or food source of isoflavones.

The protein and isoflavone constituents of soybeans have additive and/or synergistic effects on lipid metabolism (Griffin 1999). The role of isoflavones is therefore particularly complex and these factors must be taken into account.

The consumption of isoflavones varies widely according to the food habits of different populations. In one group of Japanese subjects, the mean plasma concentrations of genistein and daidzein were 0.27 μM and 2.24 μM, respectively, and in subjects fed with isoflavonoids or soymilk, they reached 0.74 μM and 2.24 μM after isoflavonoid intake of 0.7 to 2 mg/kg body weight (Xu et al. 1994). In postmenopausal Australian women consuming their traditional diet supplemented with soybean flour (providing a daily dose of 45 g), plasma concentrations of daidzein were increased but only four subjects were able to metabolize daidzein to equol. Daidzein and genistein plasma levels reached 312 and 148ng/mL, respectively (Morton et al. 1994). Urinary isoflavonoid excretion in humans is dose dependent at low to moderate levels of soybean protein consumption (Karr et al. 1997).

Genistein inhibits LDL oxidation to a greater degree than daidzein *in vitro* but not *in vivo*; this effect is time and concentration dependent *in vitro* (Chait 1996, 1998). Soy cream suppresses the production of peroxidized LDL in heavy smokers and patients with myocardial infarction (Kanazawa and Osanai 1998). Lichtenstein (1998) recently reviewed the studies in animal and human models with regard to the effect of isoflavones on lipid metabolism and cardiovascular risk.

3.3.3.4.1 Effects in Normolipidemic Subjects

In normolipidemic subjects, the effects of isoflavones on serum lipids and cholesterol are still under discussion. In several trials, a hypocholesterolemic effect of isoflavones has been observed.

In ten male college students, daily supplementation of their usual diet with 40 mg of high-genistein soybean protein for 13 days only slightly reduced plasma total and LDL-cholesterol levels, whereas malondialdehyde concentrations were significantly lower. Therefore, even during a short period of supplementation, high soybean protein has been shown to possess a potential antioxidant capacity (Bakhit et al. 1999). In nine adult men, consuming two liquid-formula diets of identical composition with the exception of the protein component (soybean protein or casein) for 1 month, plasma HDL-cholesterol and apo A-1 concentrations were significantly increased with the soybean protein diet; the LDL-cholesterol/HDL-cholesterol ratio was reduced, whereas total cholesterol, triacylglycerol, LDL-cholesterol, apo B, and apo A-1I serum levels were not affected. In young women, a significant reduction in total and LDL plasma cholesterol concentrations was obtained with 45 mg of isoflavonoids but not with 23 mg (Cassidy et al. 1995), and numerous authors have observed similar results (Bakhit et al. 1994; Anthony et al. 1996a, 1996b; Balmir et al. 1996; Honoré et al. 1997), even though apo A-1, apo B, and lipoprotein plasma concentrations remained unchanged in two studies (Anthony et al. 1996a, 1996b; Honoré et al. 1997). However, the extent of the response did vary by subject (Nilausen and Meinertz 1998).

In 14 healthy premenopausal, normocholesterolemic women consuming diets containing three levels of soybean isoflavones (2.01, 1.01, and 0.15 mg of isoflavones/kg of body weight daily) over successive periods covering 35 menstrual cycles each, plasma triacylglycerol, total, LDL- and HDL-cholesterol concentrations decreased during the menstrual cycles, but only when the isoflavones were consumed in large quantities. However, the effects of other soybean components cannot be excluded (Merz-Demlow et al. 1998). In 13 healthy normocholesterolemic premenopausal women, total cholesterol and HDL and LDL cholesterol were monitored over a period covering three menstrual cycles during which 10.0, 64.7, or 128.7 mg/day of isoflavones provided by soybean protein isolates were consumed. With the high isoflavone diets, LDL-cholesterol plasma concentrations were lowered (−7.6% to −10%), as were the cholesterol/HDL-cholesterol ratio (−10.2%) and the LDL/HDL cholesterol ratio (−13.8%) (Merz-Demlow et al. 2000). However, no changes in the oxidizability of LDL or in plasma total cholesterol or triacylglycerol concentrations were observed in 14 premenopausal women participating in a randomized crossover trial lasting four menstrual cycles, during which they consumed 86 mg of isoflavones daily for the duration of two menstrual cycles followed by a placebo for an equivalent period or vice versa (Samman et al. 1999). These data are similar to those of Greaves et al. (1999) observed in *Cynomolgus* monkeys. Eighteen postmenopausal women were followed over three diets for 93-day periods separated by 26-day washout periods. During the diet periods, the subjects consumed one, two, or three supplements of soybean protein isolates (powder of different SPI concentrations) daily, providing an average isoflavone intake of 7.1, 65, or 132 mg of isoflavones/day, respectively, expressed as an aglycone units. Plasma LDL concentrations were 6.5% lower during the high isoflavones diet, and the LDL/HDL cholesterol ratio was 8.5% and 7.5% lower during the low- and high-isoflavone diets, respectively (p<0.02). Serum HDL-cholesterol, triacylglycerol, apo A-1, apo B, and lipoprotein(a) levels were not affected (Wangen et al. 2001).

According to Anderson et al. (1995), at least 60% of the effect of soybean protein on cholesterol levels in primates such as *Cynomolgus* or *Rhesus* monkeys could be due to isoflavones. In humans, however, according to Sirtori et al. (1997, 1998), the reduction in serum cholesterol concentrations observed with a soybean diet does not appear to be caused by isoflavones since in the clinical studies carried out by several Swiss and Italian investigators, the soybean products used were almost totally free of isoflavones. The biochemical action of isoflavones on LDL receptors is not clear. Although soybean protein activates cellular LDL receptors, isoflavones inhibit tyrosine kinase and down-regulate LDL receptors. Indeed, genistein in HepG2 cells inhibits the LDL-receptor up-regulation induced by oncostatin-M, a tyrosine kinase activator (Grove et al. 1991). Since they inhibit tyrosine kinase and down-regulate LDL receptors in cells (Anthony et al. 1996b), they should increase plasma cholesterol concentrations (Sirtori et al. 1998).

3.3.3.4.2 Effects in Hyperlipidemic Subjects

The effects of isoflavones in hyperlipidemic patients are more widely understood than in normolipidemic subjects. However, in one recent study (Howes et al. 2000), isoflavone phytoestrogens did not significantly alter plasma lipid levels. Indeed, in 66 moderately hypercholesterolemic postmenopausal women on low-isoflavone diets for 2 weeks, consumption of one and then two tablets per day of a purified extract of red clover (26 mg biochanin A, 16 mg formononetin, 0.5 mg daidzein, 1 mg genistein), each period lasting 4 weeks, did not significantly alter the total plasma cholesterol, LDL-cholesterol, HDL-cholesterol, and triacylglycerol levels. In contrast, the results of several trials support the hypothesis of a hypolipidemic effect of isoflavones. In 31 hyperlipidemic subjects consuming 33 g/day of soybean protein providing 86 mg isoflavones/2,000 kcal/day, the level of oxidized LDL, measured as conjugated dienes in the LDL fraction, and the ratio of conjugated dienes to LDL cholesterol were decreased. Urinary isoflavone excretion was enhanced but urinary estrogenic activity was not modified (Jenkins et al. 2000).

As shown by Merz-Demlow et al. (2000) in their study of premenopausal women, the higher the dose of isoflavones the greater the reduction in plasma LDL-cholesterol concentrations. Patients were fed a diet containing 53 g soybean protein (per day); plasma LDL-cholesterol concentrations were lowered to a greater extent when the isoflavone content was 129 mg than when it was 65 mg. Similar results were observed by Baum et al. (1998) in 66 hypercholesterolemic postmenopausal women on the

National Cholesterol Education Program (NCEP) Step 1 diet for 22 weeks (after 2 weeks of a basal diet) with the protein content (40 g/day) provided by a high amount of isoflavones. Compared to control groups, non–HDL-cholesterol levels were reduced, HDL cholesterol increased, total cholesterol was unchanged, and the total cholesterol/HDL-cholesterol ratio was significantly reduced in both groups with isoflavones. Mononuclear cell LDL-receptor messenger RNA concentrations were also increased in both groups. Baum et al. (1998) suggested that the reduction in apo B-containing lipoproteins could be due to the increase in hepatic LDL-receptor mRNA concentrations and the enhanced LDL-receptor activity. Potter et al. (1996b, 1998) conducted an identical study to that of Baum in 66 noninstitutionalized hyper-cholesterolemic postmenopausal women. Compared with casein and nonfat dried milk, serum LDL concentrations decreased and serum HDL-cholesterol levels increased in the groups on isoflavones. Mononuclear cell LDL-receptor mRNA concentrations were also enhanced. The results obtained by Crouse et al. (1999) regarding the effects of isoflavones in hypercholesterolemic men and women are similar to those of Wangen et al. (2001) in normolipidemic subjects. In a double-blind, randomized parallel trial, 156 mildly hypercholesterolemic men and women received 25 g/day of casein or soybean protein isolates containing 2, 27, 37, or 62 mg/day of isoflavones. After 9 weeks, in the groups receiving 62 mg of isoflavones, the reduction in cholesterol and plasma LDL-cholesterol concentrations were −9% and −10%, respectively, in the patients with highest cholesterol levels, and −4% and −6% in the others. Comparison with the other groups shows the existence of a dose–response effect. Plasma concentrations of triacylglycerols and HDL cholesterol were unaffected by isoflavones (Crouse et al. 1999). Addition of soybean isoflavones to a casein semipurified diet counteracted the increase in VLDL-cholesterol but not that of serum LDL-cholesterol concentrations (Kurowska et al. 1994). In a diet containing 50 g/day of soybean protein with high levels of isoflavones for 12 weeks, total cholesterol and LDL-cholesterol serum concentrations were reduced and the level of HDL cholesterol increased (Fache 1997).

A diet supplemented with either milk protein or soybean protein (42 g/day) containing either ethanol-extracted isolated soybean protein with trace amounts of isoflavones (Soy−) or soybean protein isolates containing 80 mg aglycone isofla-vones (Soy+) was consumed for 12 weeks by 115 hypercholesterolemic postmeno-pausal nonsmoking women who were not on hormone replacement treatment or lipid-lowering drugs. The decrease in total cholesterol and LDL-cholesterol plasma levels was slightly greater in the Soy+ group than in Soy− group, but it was also observed in the milk group so that the reductions were not significantly different among the three groups (Gardner et al. 2001).

Soybean protein reduces plasma levels by LDL-receptor activation, but isofla-vones, which inhibit tyrosine kinase and down-regulate the LDL-receptor in cells, should have the opposite effect (Sirtori et al. 1998). Oncostatin M, a growth regu-latory protein secreted by macrophages increases the number of cell-surface LDL receptors and LDL uptake in HepG2 cells (Grove et al. 1991), but this effect, which is induced by a tyrosine kinase activation, is directly inhibited by genistein (Anthony et al. 1996a, 1996b). Teng et al. (1996) reported one effect on LDL receptors. In 30 hypercholesterolemic postmenopausal women receiving an NCEP Step 1 diet for a 2-week period, and then randomly assigned to three groups consuming for 6 months, 40 g protein/day of casein, nonfat dried milk, or soybean protein isolates (0.8 mg isoflavones/g protein), or soybean protein isolates (1.6 mg isoflavones/g protein), the level of LDL-receptor mRNA was greater in both soybean groups than in the casein group. Thus, a soybean protein diet can influence gene expression in human tissues.

Despite these results, which are more often in favor of a hypocholesterolemic effect of isoflavones in hyperlipidemic than in normolipidemic subjects, their possible contribution to a serum cholesterol–lowering effect remains unclear because their estrogenic effect is less potent than that of synthetic estrogens (Davis 1998). On the other hand, the influence of soybean technology and the food environment on their bioavailability excludes any generalization.

The hypocholesterolemic effect of the isoflavones of soybean protein has therefore been investigated. In their meta-analysis of 38 studies in healthy volunteers and hypercholesterolemic patients, Anderson et al. (1995) estimated that the role of isoflavones represents 60% of this effect. Nevertheless, Sirtori et al. (1997) pointed out that the effect is observed with low isoflavone soybean products. The lack of effect of purified isoflavones could suggest that soybean isoflavones require other components of soybean protein to be able to exert their cholesterol-lowering effects (Wangen et al. 2001). The potential drawback of soybean protein — their insufficient content of sulfur amino acids as postulated from rodent data (Moundras et al. 1995) — is of no significance in humans (Sirtori et al. 1998).

3.3.3.5 Summary

The effects of isoflavones on lipid metabolism are greater in hyperlipidemic than normolipidemic subjects. They would appear to be dependent on the presence of soybean protein. However, according to Sirtori et al. (1997, 1998), in the absence of isoflavones, soybean protein has a hypocholesterolemic effect. On the other hand, several authors failed to observe any improvement in plasma lipid concentrations with purified soybean isoflavones (Nestel et al. 1997; Greaves et al. 1999; Simons et al. 2000). On the basis of these last studies therefore, Sirtori (2001) has affirmed that isoflavones have nothing to do with cholesterol reduction, a fact that can be clearly explained by soybean protein composition.

3.3.4 Effects on Endocrine Response

3.3.4.1 Insulin and Glucagon

The intake of dietary protein or amino acids increases insulin secretion (Fajans et al. 1967; Nuttal et al. 1985). The endocrinologic effects of soybean protein have been investigated in hyperlipidemic humans. In comparison with casein, soybean protein contains greater amounts of arginine and glycine, and induces a low postprandial insulin/glucagon ratio in both normocholesterolemic and hypercholesterolemic subjects. With a casein diet, this ratio is higher in hypercholesterolemic than in normocholesterolemic subjects. The reduction in serum cholesterol levels is associated with arginine and glycine levels, whereas an increase is related to lysine and branched-chain amino acids. Sanchez and Hubbard (Sanchez et al. 1988b, 1990; Hubbard and Sanchez 1990; Sanchez and Hubbard 1991) have therefore suggested that the control of cholesterol levels with insulin and glucagon is regulated by dietary and plasma amino acids.

In five young men on a diet containing soybean protein isolates or skimmed milk as the protein content (0.8 g/kg/day) and cholesterol (23 mg/kg/day), no differences in serum insulin and plasma glucagon concentrations were observed with either diet (Okuda et al. 1988). However, hypercholesterolemic men on a casein test meal had an insulin/glucagon ratio higher than that of normolipidemic subjects. Nevertheless, after a soybean test meal, the values were similar (Hubbard et al. 1989).

In humans, a high soybean protein diet over an 8-week period, enhanced the plasma glucagon concentrations. Moreover, the glucagon release following arginine infusion into the bloodstream was higher in patients on a soybean protein diet (Noseda et al. 1980). In five young men on a diet containing soybean protein isolates or skimmed milk protein (0.8 g/kg/day) and cholesterol (23 mg/kg/day), the serum cholesterol, LDL-cholesterol, and atherogenic index concentrations increased only with skimmed milk (Okuda et al. 1987) or did not vary (Okuda et al. 1988). No differences in serum insulin and plasma glucagon concentrations were observed in subjects consuming either diet (Okuda et al. 1988).

In 15 patients (7 with type IIA and 8 with type IIB hyperlipidemia), after 4 weeks of a hypolipidemic diet with 8 to 9 mg/1,000 kcal of cholesterol and a P/S ratio greater than 1.8, animal proteins were replaced by soybean protein for 8 weeks, with a P/S ratio greater than 2.2. Total and LDL-cholesterol concentrations decreased significantly, and those of HDL cholesterol and triacylglycerols increased slightly. During the soybean period, the plasma insulin/glucagon ratio was lower and the plasma glucagon concentrations increased significantly, whereas those of insulin decreased slightly and nonsignificantly (Noseda and Fragiacomo 1980). In 17 hypercholesterolemic men following four different diets, each for a 4-week period (50 g/day of protein and 20 g/day of dietary fibers from either soybean flour, or soybean protein isolates and soybean fibers, or soybean protein isolates and cellulose, or nonfat dried milk and cellulose), hormone levels were analyzed after an initial baseline period of 10 days and at the end of each period. Mean serum insulin concentrations increased when the subjects were fed soybean flour compared to other diets but only significantly with soybean protein isolates and soybean fibers (Ham et al. 1993).

3.3.4.2 Growth Hormone

A growth hormone deficiency in humans is associated with hypercholesterolemia (several references in Pfeuffer et al. 1988b) and is also responsible for reduced cholesterol synthesis (Friedman et al. 1970). In six hypercholesterolemic and five normocholesterolemic adult subjects, a growth hormone injection (5 mg twice daily) for a 5-day period significantly decreased serum cholesterol and increased triacylglycerol levels in both types of subjects (Friedman et al. 1974).

In 16 children with human growth hormone deficiency, plasma lipid and cholesterol concentrations, biliary lipid composition, and cholesterol synthesis were unchanged after growth hormone therapy. Nevertheless, bile acid synthesis was increased and chenodeoxycholate pool size significantly reduced. These data suggest that growth hormone may indirectly modulate cholesterol metabolism through regulation of hepatic cholesterol 7-α-hydroxylase activity, the rate-limiting enzyme of bile acid synthesis, since it is decreased after hypophysectomy (Tomkins et al. 1952; Heubi et al. 1983). Growth hormone enhances hepatic cholesterol 7-α-monooxygenase activity (Mayer and Voges 1972).

3.3.4.3 Thyroid Hormones

In subjects with hypothyroidism, the receptor-mediated catabolism of LDL is impaired but restored by appropriate treatment (Walton et al. 1965; Thompson et al. 1981). *In vitro*, the modulation of plasma LDL catabolism is due to the regulation of receptor expression by thyroid hormones (Chait et al. 1979; Krul and Dolphin 1982).

In humans, serum T_3 concentrations decrease while serum 3,3′,5′-triiodothyronine (reverse T_3) increases during total energy restriction (Vagenakis et al. 1975) or protein-energy malnutrition (Chopra et al. 1975). In the experiments of Ham et al. (1993) on 17 hypercholesterolemic men previously quoted in Section 2.7.5.3, total serum thyroxine (T_4) concentrations increased with all types of diets compared to the basal diet, but only significantly with soybean protein isolates and soybean fiber or with soybean protein isolates and cellulose. These diets had no effect on triiodothyronine (T_4) or the thyroid-stimulating hormone (TSH). The same results were also obtained by Balmir et al. (1993) in a similar experiment on 21 noninstitutionalized hypercholesterolemic men. There are no data available relating to the effect on thyroid status of substituting soybean protein with casein (Lichtenstein 1998).

3.3.4.4 Cortisol and Corticosterone

The protein content of a meal induces cortisol and corticosterone secretion. Indeed, in 52 healthy young adults, a high-protein diet (4 gm/kg body weight) induced a significant increase in plasma cortisol and ACTH levels at 30 and 60 minutes after the mid-day meal and 30 minutes after evening meal (Slag et al. 1981).

3.4 CONCLUSION

Numerous mechanisms have been put forward in an attempt to explain the effects of food proteins on lipid metabolism in humans and on cholesterol metabolism in particular. No single theory would appear to apply. Further studies are necessary because of the numerous factors presumed to be involved and also because the effect of each would appear to vary according to species and subspecies, genetic factors, and the food environment. However, the hypocholesterolemic action of soybean protein and the absence of side effects have been sufficiently well demonstrated to justify recommending this protein as a drug therapy in the treatment of type II hyperlipoproteinemia (Beynen et al. 1987b).

4 Data on Atherosclerosis

4.1 EXPERIMENTAL DATA IN ANIMALS

4.1.1 Low-Protein Diet

In pigeons, a low-protein diet (10%) reduced body weight and increased plasma cholesterol concentrations and the mortality rate (Little and Angell 1977). Dietary restrictions (40% of usual intake) in *White Carneau* pigeons from the age of 3 to 9 months reduced body weight by about −30%, plasma cholesterol levels by −20%, and the content of both free and esterified cholesterol in the aorta. This diet prevented the development of fatty streaks (Subbiah and Siekert 1977).

In male *Sprague-Dawley* rats, protein (2.6%) undernutrition with a cholesterol-free diet for 4 weeks, decreased cholesterol, triacylglycerol, phospholipid, total protein, and hydroxyproline levels in both plasma and the aorta (Bydlowski et al. 1984). When dietary cholesterol (2%) was combined with a low-protein diet, the effect was greater and aorta hexosamine concentrations were decreased. Thus, the amount of protein consumption may modulate the effect of dietary cholesterol (Bydlowski et al. 1986).

The effects of proteins depend on the animal species. In underfed male adult white *Swiss* rabbits on a cholesterol-rich (2 g/day) diet for 9 weeks, consuming (1) protein 16%, methionine 0.33%, and arginine 1%, or (2) protein 35%, methionine 0.67%, and arginine 2.4%, blood cholesterol, lipoproteins, phospholipids, and fatty acid levels rose considerably in both groups. The aortas of the animals showed a more marked atherosclerotic involvement in the high-protein group. These data show that in underfed rabbits, an adequate protein content in a restricted diet did not exert any protective action against atherogenesis (Loewe et al. 1954).

When male pigs were fed on a diet that was rich in fats (46%) and cholesterol (6 gm/day) and contained a normal level (25%) of protein (vegetable protein plus fish protein) for an 18-month period, Gupta et al. (1974) showed that the extent and severity of lesions in the aorta and coronary arteries were not significantly different from those observed in animals fed on a normal chow diet with the same protein content (25%) but without the addition of fat or cholesterol. In contrast, the pigs fed on the low-protein (5%) diet showed maximal intimal surface area involvement of atherosclerotic lesions and a higher cholesterol content. The cholesterol/phospholipid ratio in the lesions was also higher than in the other groups (Gupta et al. 1974). In pigs, the composition of aortic tissue may be altered by a low-protein diet (Gupta et al. 1974) or remain unchanged (Greer et al. 1966). In monkeys, in some cases aortic tissue composition is unchanged (Deo et al. 1965) by a low-protein diet, whereas other authors have reported highly variable inter-individual effects (Strong and McGill 1967). The atherosclerotic lesions induced in the aorta of cockerels by a high-cholesterol diet have been shown to regress to a lesser degree when the protein content of the diet was low (7.5% or 10%) than when it was high (Pick et al. 1965).

4.1.2 HIGH-PROTEIN DIET

The extent of atherosclerosis was less in rabbits when a high-protein diet with cod liver oil was composed of oats, tomatoes, and alfalfa instead of liver and casein. Moreover, a diet containing soybean protein instead of oats did not produce arterial lesions (Nuzum et al. 1926). A high level of animal proteins in the diet increased the plasma cholesterol levels and the development of atherosclerosis, whatever the origin of the dietary animal proteins (for milk, see Lee et al. 1981; for fish, see Goulding et al. 1983). The effects can, however, vary according to species since, in pigeons, a high-protein diet (20% versus 40%) did not increase blood cholesterol, aortic cholesterol, or the aortic atherosclerosis index (Little and Angell 1977). Numerous experiments and general reviews have dealt with this particular aspect (Newburgh and Clarkson 1923a; Hermus 1975; Hamilton and Carroll 1976; Huff and Carroll 1980a; 1980b, Kritchevsky 1980b; Carroll 1981a, 1981b; Lee et al. 1981; Terpstra et al. 1983a, 1983b, 1983d; Sugano 1983; Kritchevsky and Czarnecki 1983; Kritchevsky et al. 1983a, 1983b; Goulding et al. 1983).

4.1.3 NATURE OF PROTEINS

In pigeons, different proteins (casein/lactalbumin 85/15 from 8% to 30% in comparison with gluten 8% to 30%) in a diet with cholesterol (30 mg/100 mg of fats from different sources) have similar effects on plasma cholesterol concentrations and the development of atherosclerosis (Lofland et al. 1961, 1966).

Casein is the animal protein that has been the most extensively investigated, often in comparison with soybean protein: mice (Ni et al. 1998); rats (Nagata et al. 1980; Terpstra et al. 1982a, 1982b); rabbits (Knack 1915; Newburgh 1919; Newburgh and Squier 1920; Clarkson and Newburgh 1926; Howard et al. 1965; Kritchevsky et al. 1978; Lacombe and Nibbelink 1980; Kritchevsky 1980b, 1981; Terpstra et al. 1982c; Kritchevsky 1983a; Laurent 1983; Hassan et al. 1985; Kritchevsky 1987; Kritchevsky et al. 1988b, 1989; Sjöblom et al. 1989; Kratky et al. 1993; Daley et al. 1994a, 1994b; Richardson 1994); hamsters (Beynen and Schoulten 1983); guinea pigs (Terpstra et al. 1982d; Haban and Stanova 1989); and monkeys (Terpstra et al. 1984; Barth et al. 1984; Anthony et al. 1997). These studies have clearly established that the prevalence of atherosclerosis lesions is lower with a soybean protein than with a casein diet and is even lower with a soybean protein diet enriched with phytoestrogens (Anthony et al. 1997). In male *Sprague-Dawley* rats fed on soybean protein or casein diets for 9 months, the serum cholesterol concentrations were lower with soybean protein than with casein and no evidence of arteriosclerosis of the aorta was observed in either group. Varying degrees of lipid staining in coronary arterial branches were observed in 60% of the hearts (Lindholm et al. 1993).

In male *C57BL/6J* apo E-deficient mice fed on a purified diet containing soybean protein isolates or casein, cholesterol (1/100 g), and cholate (0.25 g/100 g) for

6 weeks, the lesion surface area in the thoracic aorta was lower in the soybean group than the casein group, although the serum total cholesterol levels did not differ between the two groups. With the same diet but minus supplementation with cholesterol and cholate for 9 or 24 weeks, similar results were obtained and serum homocysteine concentrations did not differ between the two groups. These data indicate that the antiatherogenic effect of native soybean protein isolates cannot be explained by their effect on serum lipids or homocysteine (Ni et al. 1998).

Young animals are more susceptible than adults to hypercholesterolemia induced by a casein-rich diet (West et al. 1982), although exposing rabbits to dietary casein in early life has no detrimental effect on atheroscrosic lesions or on cholesterol and biliary acid metabolism (Hassan et al. 1985). Inbred rabbits that are either hyper- or hyporesponsive to dietary cholesterol are also hyper- or hyporesponsive to the type of protein in the diet. Casein has a similar effect to saturated fats on the plasma cholesterol response to dietary cholesterol in rabbits (Beynen et al. 1986a) and can lead to hypercholesterolemia and the development of atheroma. This reaction is independent of cholesterol or saturated fat in the diet (Carroll and Hamilton 1975; Terpstra et al. 1983a; Beynen et al. 1986a). Searching for a possible role of the arginine/lysine ratio, Kritchevsky et al. (1978) investigated this hypothesis in rabbits in two similar experiments. The animals were fed for an 8-month period on a semipurified cholesterol-free diet with protein (25%, either casein or soybean protein) and a lysine arginine/ratio of 0.49 and 1.13, respectively, or casein plus arginine and soybean protein plus lysine. At the end of the studies, serum cholesterol levels (mg/dL) were casein 174 and 283, soybean protein 59 and 234, casein plus arginine 129 and 343, and soybean protein plus lysine 106 and 242. Liver cholesterol contents were similar. Serum triacylglycerol levels (mg/dL) were casein 133 and 81, soybean protein 95 and 53, casein plus arginine 186 and 59, and soybean protein plus lysine 101 and 70. Average atheromata were expressed as arch plus thoracic atheromata/2 for two experiments: casein 1.86 and 0.94, soybean protein 0.67 and 0.41, casein plus arginine 1.9 and 1.11, and soybean protein plus lysine 1.33 and 0.62. Although the addition of lysine to soybean protein increased the atherogenicity by 100% and 50% in two experiments, the consequences of the addition of arginine to casein were unclear: −41% and +13% (Kritchevsky et al. 1978).

Since soybean protein decreases the production of oxidized LDL and deformed LDL in rabbits, it may have a genuinely protective effect against the development of atherosclerosis (Kanazawa et al. 1993, 1995). In contrast, the peptides produced by bovine casein hydrolysis induced oxidation of human LDL independently of peroxidases and metal ions. They are influenced by the presence of tyrosyl residues in these peptides, which carry the oxidative potential from the enzyme active site to the lipids of LDL (Torreilles and Guerin 1995).

The results of experimental studies on male *New Zealand white* rabbits fed on a casein-free cholesterol diet or chow supplemented with low levels of cholesterol (0.125% to 0.5% of body weight) or a chow diet for 24 weeks showed that the two first diets had different effects on lipoprotein levels and atherosclerosis. The casein-fed rabbits had a mainly low-density lipoprotein hypercholesterolemia while the cholesterol-fed rabbits had approximately the same levels of VLDL-, IDL- and LDL-cholesterol fractions. The luminal surface area and the total volume of lesions were, respectively, two and three times greater in the cholesterol-fed animals than in casein-fed animals (Daley et al. 1994a). In male *New Zealand white* rabbits fed for 3 months on a semipurified, low-fat, cholesterol-free diet containing casein, the plasma total cholesterol and LDL levels were higher compared to the chow-fed or soybean-fed rabbits. In casein-fed but not in soybean protein-fed rabbits, endothelial cell injury in the aortas was evident. Macrophages, T-lymphocytes, and smooth muscle cells were identified in the lesion, as well as an expression of leukocyte adhesion molecules. The endothelial fatty lesions and leukocyte and lymphocyte adhesions were similar to those observed in human atherosclerosis (Richardson et al. 1994). In male *New Zealand white* rabbits fed on a casein atherogenic diet for 6 or 10 months advanced atherosclerotic plaques were seen to develop in the same location as the fatty streak observed in shorter experiments (Kratky et al. 1993). The male *New Zealand white* rabbits fed a low-cholesterol–supplemented chow for 24 weeks had more advanced atherosclerotic lesions than those fed on a cholesterol-free diet, although their plasma cholesterol levels were similar (Daley et al. 1994a, 1994b). In male and female *ExHC* rats (*F55-1/2*) initially treated with vitamin D_2 (200 IU/kg body weight) for a 4-day period, and fed on a casein or soybean-protein-isolates (20%) purified diet supplemented with cholesterol (1%), methionine (0.3%) and choline bitartrate (0.2%) for 180 days, the development of atherosclerosis was, however, weaker with soybean protein than with the casein diet. Cholesterol was distributed in low-cholesterol lipoproteins whereas the LDL particles were enriched in cholesterol with casein (Sakono et al. 1997). Because LDL-receptor activities are reduced with casein diets, LDL uptake and LDL-apo B catabolism are diminished (Khosla et al. 1989, 1991; Samman et al. 1990c).

Compared with casein, soybean protein diets significantly reduced serum cholesterol concentrations and the rate of Nile fluorescence intensity in the wall of the aortic arch in guinea pigs (Haban and Stanova 1989). In ovariectomized *Cynomolgus* monkeys, a soybean protein isolates diet with an isoflavone dose of 148.4 mg/day and cholesterol (0.2 mg/kcal) for a 7-month period induced an improvement in various coronary heart disease risk factors. Total plasma cholesterol concentrations were reduced without changes in HDL cholesterol or triacylglycerol levels, and the arterial cholesteryl ester content was decreased (Wagner et al. 1997). The concentration in LDL cholesterol is associated with cholesterol deposits in the peripheral tissue and the development of premature atherosclerosis (Brown et al. 1981), whereas the HDL-cholesterol fraction is associated with cholesterol flux from peripheral tissues and protection against atherosclerosis (Gordon et al. 1977). The accumulation of cholesterol esters by macrophages was inhibited by lactotransferrin, which prevented the oxidation of LDL that is bound to macrophages (Kajikawa et al. 1994).

When a sample of serum taken 2 or 4 hours after a single intake of 50 g of soybean-protein isolates was added to a culture medium, the activity of lysosomal hydrolases in blood platelets, cholesterol content in lipoprotein-containing immune complexes, and accumulation of cholesterol in the subendothelial cells of human aortic intima were all shown to decrease. Likewise, directly applying a soybean protein isolates 500 E water-alcohol extract into a culture of atherosclerotic plaque of human aortic intima decreased both the cholesterol content in the cells and cell proliferation (Tutel'ian et al. 1989).

In hamsters, a rice protein diet in comparison with a casein diet reduced early lesions of aortic atherosclerosis by approximately 80% (Tran and Nicolosi 1997). In *Macaca fascicularis* monkeys fed on a basal cholesterol-rich (0.014 mg/calorie) diet, aortic lesions declined from 86.25% to 53.38% when the diet was supplemented with soybean hull (Piliang et al. 1996).

New Zealand white rabbits fed on fish meal (130 g/kg) for a 1-year period developed extensive aortic atherosclerosis in comparison with rabbits fed on an isonitrogenous diet (30%) containing soybean protein or skimmed milk (Goulding et al. 1983).

4.1.4 AMINO ACIDS

4.1.4.1 Arginine

In hypercholesterolemic animals and humans with atherosclerosis, a high-cholesterol diet increased plasma cholesterol concentrations and promoted the development of xanthoma. Endothelium-dependent vasodilation was reduced and the intimal wall thickened (Cooke et al. 1991, 1992; Böger et al. 1995). The reduced endothelium-dependent vasodilator responses of coronary and peripheral vessels were probably due to impaired biological activity of nitric oxide (review in Böger et al. 1995, 1996a, 1996b; Garini et al. 1996; Aji et al. 1997). L-Arginine counteracts these effects (Böger et al. 1995; Davies et al. 1996) and prevents atherosclerosis (Aji et al. 1997; Thorne et al. 1988).

L-Arginine is the substrate for nitric oxide (NO) synthase, which catalyzes the production of NO in vascular endothelial cells (Palmer et al. 1987, 1988; Böger et al. 1995; Bode-Böger et al. 1996a, 1996b). It exerts an antihypertensive and antiproliferative effect on vascular smooth muscles and produces nitric oxide, a potent vasodilator (Nakaki and Kato 1994; Bode-Böger et al. 1996b; Ignarro et al. 1999). Plasma concentrations of asymmetrical dimethylarginine (ADMA), an endogenous inhibitor of NO synthesis (Vallance et al. 1992a), are elevated in hypercholesterolemic rabbits (Bode-Böger et al. 1996a), as are native and oxidized LDL levels, which influence the biological activity of NO *in vitro* (Jacobs et al. 1990; Liao et al. 1995; Mehta et al. 1995). The addition of L-arginine raises the plasma-L-arginine/ADMA ratio but does not modify plasma cholesterol levels. It does, however, increase NO formation and reduce endothelial superoxide radical release, which improves the endothelium-dependent vasodilator function and reduces the progression of atherosclerosis (Böger et al. 1997). Supplementation of a diet with L-arginine prevented xanthoma formation and reduced atherosclerosis in the LDL receptor of knockout mice, an animal model of familial hypercholesterolemia, whereas supplementation with L-arginine and N^ω-nitro-L-arginine (L-NA), an inhibitor of NO synthase, suppressed these beneficial effects (Aji et al. 1997).

L-Arginine may well prove to be a useful protector of vessel integrity. However, in male *New Zealand white* rabbits fed on a cholesterol diet, although plasma cholesterol levels were increased, no significant difference was found in plasma L-arginine levels between the cholesterol-fed and control animals. Impaired endothelial relaxation as described in this animal model of hypercholesterolemia would therefore not appear to result from a deficiency in plasma L-arginine (Williams et al. 1993).

Average atheromatous lesions (arch plus thoracic) are more extensive with casein and casein plus arginine than with soybean protein or soybean protein plus lysine. The benefit of adding arginine to casein remains unclear, whereas the addition of lysine to soybean protein increases the risk of atherogenesis (Czarnecki and Kritchevsky 1979). In the hypercholesterolemic rabbit model of atherosclerosis, oral administration of L-arginine increased NO activity, improved endothelial dysfunction and endothelium-dependent vasodilation in the thoracic aorta, reduced the formation of atheromatous plaque, and inhibited platelet aggregation and activation (Cooke et al. 1992; Tsao et al. 1994a). Monocyte adhesion to endothelial cells was reduced (Cooke et al. 1992; Tsao et al. 1994a, 1994b; Böger et al. 1995; Adams et al. 1997a, 1997b, 1997c). However, aortae excised from normal and cholesterol-fed (1% for 4 months) *New Zealand white* rabbits and incubated for 1 hour with 5 mM L-arginine showed no reaction to acetylcholine relaxation in contrast with the normal vessels. These results suggest that an L-arginine deficiency is unlikely to be the underlying cause of impaired endothelium-dependent relaxation in the aorta of cholesterol-fed rabbits (Mügge and Harrison 1991).

In rabbits subjected to an environment of tobacco smoke, chronic L-arginine supplementation (2.25% solution ad libitum) in the context of diet-induced hyper-cholesterolemia and atherosclerosis, had a preventive effect and compensated for the endothelial dysfunction generally associated with environmental tobacco smoke (Hutchinson et al. 1997).

In male *New Zealand white* rabbits, supplementation of a chow diet for 10 weeks, with cholesterol (1%) and L-arginine (2.25%) or L-methionine (0.9%) corresponding to a sixfold increase in daily L-arginine or L-methionine intake, respectively, produced different effects on atherogenesis. The L-methionine supplementation increased inti-mal accumulation of macrophages and the intima-media surface area of the left main coronary artery, whereas in L-arginine treated rabbits, adherent monocytes and tissue macrophages were absent. Intima-media thickness of the aorta and coronary arteries did not progress (Wang et al. 1994). When this species of rabbits was fed on a cholesterol-rich chow diet (1% cholesterol) for 10 weeks, endothelium-dependent relaxation in response to acetylcholine and calcium ionophore A 23187 was signif-icantly impaired. However, if the diet was supplemented with L-arginine (2.25%), the endothelium-dependent relaxation was significantly improved. Responses to norepinephrine or nitroglycerin were not modified by either diet. Arginine, the precursor of an endothelium-derived relaxing factor that is associated with a reduced lesion surface area and intimal thickening in these hypercholesterolemic animals, thus plays a role in the protection of arteries against atherogenesis (Cooke et al. 1992). The same results were observed in *New Zealand white* rabbits when L-arginine was added to a cholesterol-rich diet. The contrast between the potent effect of dietary arginine on vascular structure and its relatively weak influence on vascular reactivity suggests that the strong anti-atherogenic effects of the NO precursor may not be mediated entirely by its effect on the endothelium (Singer et al. 1995). L-Arginine supplementation decreased bradykinin hypersensitivity and improved and restored normal venous endothelial cell-dependent relaxation in adult male *New Zealand white* rabbits, but compared to control substances, it had no effect on norepinephrine, serotonin, or histamine responses (Davies et al. 1996).

In adult *New Zealand white* rabbits, a chow diet containing cholesterol (2%) and supplemented or not with L-arginine (2.25% solution) for 7 or 14 weeks, increased plasma arginine levels, reduced the development of atherosclerosis in the descending aorta and preserved endothelium-dependent vasodilation in resistance arteries. However, these effects were not sustained. Dietary L-arginine may therefore not be of long-term benefit in the prevention of atherosclerosis in humans (Jeremy et al. 1996). The addition of L-arginine (2.5%) to a cholesterol diet (1%) fed to female *New Zealand white* rabbits for 10 weeks reduced the intimal lesion surface area of the aorta (atherosclerotic plaques covering 60% of the surface) in comparison with the control subjects without L-arginine (95% surface area), even though the baseline hypercholesterolemia was similar. L-Arginine is associated with an increase in anti-oxidative reserves. The activities of aorta antioxidant enzymes, malondial-dehyde, catalase, and glutathione peroxidase, were decreased in rabbits fed on cholesterol plus L-arginine compared to rabbits fed on cholesterol without L-arginine (Mantha 1999). Although the plasma cholesterol levels of adult male *New Zealand white* rabbits fed on a diet containing 1% cholesterol were higher than those of control subjects on a standard diet, the plasma L-arginine levels were similar with both diets. The impaired endothelium-dependent relaxation described in the animal model of hypercholesterolemia would not appear to result from a deficiency in plasma L-arginine (Williams et al. 1993).

Intravenous administration of pharmacologic doses of L-arginine produced an acute improvement in endothelium-dependent vasodilation (Creager et al. 1990; Girerd et al. 1990; Cooke et al. 1991; Rossitch et al. 1991; Drexler et al. 1991b; Creager et al. 1992; Kuo et al. 1992). This effect is stereospecific since D-arginine does not mimic the action of its enantiomer in these experiments (Girerd et al. 1990; Cooke et al. 1991).

4.1.4.2 Lysine

Weigensberg et al. (1964) suggested that lysine may be a factor of atherogenicity. As previously mentioned, average atheromatous lesions (arch plus thoracic) are more extensive with casein and casein plus arginine than with soybean protein and soybean protein plus lysine. The benefit of adding arginine to casein remains unclear, whereas the addition of lysine to soybean protein increases atherogenicity (Czarnecki and Kritchevsky 1979).

4.1.4.3 Lysine/L-Arginine and L-Arginine/Aspartic Acid Ratios

The influence of the lysine/L-arginine ratio on the development of atherosclerosis was extensively studied by Kritchevsky et al. (1982a, 1982b). In rabbits fed with fish or casein or whole milk, which have lysine/L-arginine ratios of 1.44, 1.89, and 2.44, respectively, the average extent of atherosclerosis is positively correlated with the lysine/L-arginine ratio (Kritchevsky et al. 1982a).

Cholesterol content of the thoracic aorta of *Watanabe heritable hyperlipidemic (WHHL)* rabbits is higher than in the *New-Zealand white* rabbit aorta. The

L-arginine/lysine and L-arginine/aspartic ratios were lower in the thoracic aorta of *WHHL* rabbits than in that of *New-Zealand* rabbits. The difference is due to the reduced L-arginine content in the aorta since the lysine/aspartic ratio is not significantly different in these two species of rabbits. The reduction in the L-arginine content may well be responsible for the effect of the impaired metabolic status caused by lipid infiltration and also an expression of a genetically determined composition of the vascular tissue (Chinellato et al. 1992). In adult male *Sprague-Dawley* rats, although portal insulin concentrations were not correlated with the aortic levels of any amino acid, portal glucagonemia would appear to be weakly correlated with the aortic level of arginine (Jarrousse et al. 1980).

4.1.4.4 Methionine

The relationship between both sulfur amino acid metabolism and homocysteine metabolism, and arteriosclerotic lesions has been clearly demonstrated (McCully 1969). Animal proteins are rich in methionine, which is partly responsible for their atherogenic effect. Methionine increases plasma lipid levels and may contribute to endothelial cell injury or dysfunction. Indeed, endothelial cell metabolism is widely influenced by the protective or aggressive influences of nutrients (Hennig et al. 1994a, 1994b).

The histopathologic examination of male *New Zealand white* rabbits fed on a chow diet enriched with 0.3% methionine for 6 to 9 months showed typical atherosclerotic changes, such as intimal thickening, cholesterol deposits, and calcification. The stimulation of lipid peroxidation by methionine could be a possible mechanism influencing the atherogenic lesions (Toborek et al. 1995). In *New Zealand white* rabbits, a high level of methionine supplementation (3%) in a diet with or without cholesterol produced a greater increase in plasma triacylglycerol, cholesterol, homocysteine, cysteine, and lipid peroxide levels than in the group with the same cholesterol diet but without a methionine supplementation (Koyama 1995).

In *Stroke-Prone Spontanepously Hypertensive* rats (*SHR-SP*), a high-fat, cholesterol, low-protein diet containing 1% methionine had a marked preventive effect on atherogenesis in the cerebral and mesenteric arteries (Horie et al. 1987). A methionine-enriched diet may increase the serum triacylglycerol concentrations in rats (Yagasaki et al. 1986c). *In vitro*, the remnants resulting from the lipolysis of triacylglycerol-rich lipoproteins injured cultured endothelial cells and decreased the barrier function of the vascular endothelium (Hennig et al. 1992). Hydrolysis of these lipoproteins by lipoprotein lipase produced a high level of free fatty acids (Zilversmith 1973), and caused various types of damage, including oxidative stress and disruption of endothelial barriers (review in Hennig et al. 1992, 1994a, 1994b).

Despite the adaptability of sulfur-amino acid liver metabolism to high methionine supplies in rats (Finkelstein and Martin 1986), the same would not appear to apply in humans (Anderson et al. 1990). Plasma homocysteine levels were 70% higher in rats fed on a high rather than a moderate protein diet (60% versus 20%) for 1 week. However, the rise in homocysteine levels was suppressed by the addition of serine to the diet (Stead et al. 2000). This effect may well be explained by the role of dietary serine in homocysteine catabolism (Finkelstein et al. 1986; Gregory et al. 2000).

Increasing numbers of endothelial cells in the blood, which is a sign of endothelial damage, were observed in *Wistar* rats receiving an oral DL-methionine supplementation (100 mg/kg/day) for 20 weeks, and, after 10 weeks, a second supplementation with cholesterol and bile acids (50 mg cholesterol/kg/day) (Mhrova et al. 1988). Parenteral administration (or via a synthetic diet) of DL-methionine (80 mg/kg daily) or homocysteine thiolactone hydrochloride (80 mg/kg daily) to male *New Zealand white* rabbits resulted in the development of arteriosclerotic plaque in the aorta and arteries (McCully and Wilson 1975). L-Methionine supplementation (2%) of a cholesterol-free casein (10%) diet in male *Wistar* rats for 2 years, caused thickening of the intima-media resulting from hypertrophy of smooth muscular cells with collagen enrichment and diffuse fibrosis (Fau et al. 1988). Oral administration of high doses of methionine to normotensive and spontaneously hypertensive (*SHR*) rats produced an even greater increase in serum homocysteine and cystathion concentrations in arterial vessels. This methionine loading caused a more potent angiotoxic effect on the aorta with endothelial cell loss and degeneration. Serum homocysteine and cystathion concentrations were higher in *SHR* than in normotensive animals; endothelial lesions were also more extensive (Matthias et al. 1996). However, in stroke-prone spontaneously hypertensive rats (*SHR-SP*), a cholesterol diet with a high-fat and low-protein content and containing 1% methionine had a marked preventive effect on atherogenesis in the cerebral and mesenteric arteries (Horie et al. 1987). In *Macaca radiata* monkeys fed on a methionine-enriched and pyridoxine-deficient diet, in spite of a significant decrease in hepatic cystathionine synthase activity due to the pyridoxine deficiency, arterial wall morphology was not altered (Krishnaswamy and Rao 1977). In *Cebus* monkeys, a casein or soybean protein (10%) diet that is high in cholesterol and low in sulfur amino acids, administered over periods of 18 to 30 weeks, increased serum cholesterol levels within 2 to 8 weeks. After 18 or 23 weeks, vascular lesions were observed in the ascending aorta extending from the valves of the left ventricle to the proximal portions of the carotid and femoral arteries whereas in the coronary arteries the lesions were minimal. This hypercholesterolemia can, however, be prevented using 1 mg DL-methionine or L-cystine as dietary supplements. Supplementation by L-cystine is less effective (Mann et al. 1953).

Dietary methionine (20.0 g/kg) for a 7-week period caused a significant reduction in hepatic and erythrocyte copper-zinc superoxide dismutase activities in male *Wistar* rats. It increased catalase and glutathione peroxidase activities, and iron-level hepatic lipid peroxidation. A high-methionine diet may induce atherosclerosis in rats and in rabbits (Lynch and Strain 1989). Likewise, in male *New Zealand white* rabbits fed for 6 or 9 months on a chow diet supplemented with 0.3% methionine, compared to rabbits on a chow diet without methionine, plasma and aortic thiobarbituric acid reactive substances (TBARS) and aortic antioxidant enzyme activities were increased, whereas plasma antioxidant activity was decreased. Typical atherosclerotic changes with intimal thickening, cholesterol deposits, and calcification were observed in methionine-fed rabbits (Toborek et al. 1995). However, long-term consumption of excess methionine is hepatotoxic. Indeed, in male *Wistar* rats fed on either a methionine-supplemented (16.0 g/kg) or a control diet for 1, 3, 6, or 9 months, iron, ferritin, and TBARS levels in the liver were greater in those on the methionine-supplemented diet. The activities of hepatic glutathione peroxidase and catalase and total glutathione concentrations were higher in rats on a methionine-supplemented diet but only during the first 3 months and not at 6 and 9 months of the experiment (Mori and Hirayama 2000). Methionine may influence lipid composition and affect the integrity of endothelial cells directly or indirectly through homocysteine metabolism. Its ability to increase oxidative stress in vascular endothelial cells is one of its main mechanisms (review in Toborek et al. 1990; Toborek and Hennig 1996).

The role of homocysteine should also be considered. Methionine is the only dietary source of homocysteine. A methionine-rich diet increases the level of homocysteinemia. Homocysteine induces damage to the arterial connective tissue metabolism (McCully 1983) and increases thrombogenicity (Lenz and Sadler 1991). The enhanced plasma-tissue homocysteine concentrations, resulting from a methionine imbalance and possibly from B_6, B_{12}, riboflavin, and folic acid deficiencies, induces oxidative stress and endothelial cell injury (review in Toborek and Hennig 1996). The activities of the enzyme that regulates the transsulfuration pathway are modified in methionine-fed rabbits, promoting the accumulation of homocysteine. Homocysteine may therefore be partly responsible for the atherogenic effects of methionine (Starkebaum and Harlan 1986; Toborek et al. 1990; review in Kang et al. 1992 and Toborek and Hennig 1996).

4.1.4.5 Taurine

In pathogen-free-specific male and female cats fed for 6 weeks on diets containing either 25% or 50% casein and taurine (1 g/kg dry matter), plasma taurine concentrations were similar. However, if casein was replaced with soybean protein, a significant reduction in plasma taurine concentrations was observed in the soybean protein group at levels equivalent to 50% casein but not 25%. In another experiment, plasma taurine concentrations were lower in cats fed on diets containing 60% soybean protein or casein than when the diet contained 30% casein. In addition, fecal total bile acid and total taurine excretions were greater (Kim et al. 1995).

Taurine is responsible for numerous effects that have been reviewed by Schaffer et al. (2000). These effects include promotion of natriuresis and diuresis due to osmoregulatory activity in the kidney, modulation of atrial natriuretic factor secretion (Mozaffari et al. 1997), and possible regulation of vasopressin release (Dlouha and McBroom 1986; Miyata et al. 1997; Mozaffari et al. 1997); positive inotropic effect by regulating Na^+ and Na^+/Ca^{2+}; and reduction of the influence of angiotensin II on Ca^{2+} transport, protein synthesis, and angiotensin II signaling.

Taurine exhibits marked effects on calcium levels in a number of systems. Taurine supplementation (3% in tap water *ad libitum*) in the diet of mice with severe myocardial and aortic calcinosis due to the combined administration of vitamin D and nicotine, increased their survival rate and reduced the elevation of calcium content in both the aorta and the myocardium. The regulatory effect on calcium flux may well prevent the progression of arteriosclerosis (Yamauchi-Takihara et al. 1986).

Taurine deficiency induces cardiomyopathy (Azuma et al. 1984, 1985; Pion et al. 1987; Novotny et al. 1991; Fox and Sturman 1992; Elizarova et al. 1993). Taurine exerts a modest positive inotropic effect in the hemodynamically depressed heart (Schaffer and Azuma 1992); enhances renal sodium excretion (Mozaffari et al. 1997); improves cardiac contractile function (Takihara et al. 1986; Awata et al. 1987); and has been proposed as therapeutic agent in vascular pain (Sicuteri et al. 1970). Taurine also mimics certain actions of angiotensin-converting enzyme inhibitors. Despite species variations, taurine has an antagonistic action on angiotensin II (review in Schaffer et al. 2000). In comparison with *C57BL/6J* mice fed on a high-fat diet containing 15% fat and 1.25% cholesterol for 6 months, the surface area of aortic lipid accumulation was reduced by 20% in the group supplemented with taurine dissolved in the drinking water (1% w/v). In rats, oxygen consumption that is hampered by potassium cyanide (7.2 mg/kg) is improved by intraperitoneal injection of taurine (250 mg/kg) or cysteine (250 mg/kg) (Guidotti et al. 1967). Taurine also reduced oxygen saturation in patients with arterial disease (Becattini 1967) and increased intracellular calcium levels (Kato et al. 1951; Mori and Takeuchi 1955; Minami 1955; Baskin and Finney 1979).

4.1.4.6 Summary

The effects of the amount and nature of proteins or amino acids on the development of atherosclerosis are strongly influenced by the animal species, particularly with a high-protein diet. A moderately low-protein diet prevents the development of fatty streaks in pigeons and reduces the aortic cholesterol content in rats. However, in pigs and monkeys, this type of diet has no effect. The reduced sulfur-amino-acid content in a low-protein diet increases plasma cholesterol levels, although these may return to normal if methionine or cystine is added to the diet.

Most proteins, regardless of their nature, have similar effects in pigeons, whereas in the other animals, the prevalence of atherosclerosis is higher with casein or fish proteins than with soybean protein diets. The amino acids arginine, methionine, and taurine induce different effects on the development of atherosclerosis. Arginine increases nitric oxide synthesis since it is a substrate of nitric oxide synthase. It induces antihypertensive and antiproliferative effects, inhibits platelet aggregation, increases endothelium-dependent vasodilation, and reduces the development of atherosclerosis in cholesterol-fed rabbits. However, the addition of arginine to a casein diet produces equivocal results. Methionine increases lipid peroxidation, intimal thickening, and enhances cholesterol deposits, calcification, arteriosclerotic plaque formation, and endothelial cell numbers in the blood. It leads to the production of homocysteine and the subsequent angiotoxic effects. Taurine may prevent the development of atherosclerosis since it regulates osmolarity, reduces calcium levels in the aorta and myocardium, prevents the development of atheroma, improves cardiac contractile function, and mimics certain actions of angiotensin-converting enzyme inhibitors.

4.1.5 IMMUNOLOGIC EFFECTS OF PROTEINS

Scebat et al. (1980) have put forward the hypothesis of immune mechanisms being a possible cause of atherosclerosis in rabbits. Dietary proteins, especially animal proteins, are responsible for considerable immunologic reactions (Gallagher and Gibney 1983). Oligopeptides can be widely absorbed through the intestine, sometimes even faster than amino acids from equivalent mixtures (Silk et al. 1975; Adibi 1971). Thirty-six percent of a casein hydrolysate is absorbed as peptides rather than as free amino acids (Gardner 1975). Trace amounts of large polypeptides can also be absorbed through the intestine.

Hexapeptides and tripeptides have a number of immunologic properties (Jollès et al. 1982; Parker et al. 1984; Berthou et al. 1987; Gattegno et al. 1988), as demonstrated with soybean protein (Kishino and Moriguchi 1984; Moriguchi et al. 1985). Depending on their nature, proteins may modify the immunologic interactions between the host and intestinal microflora (Bounous et al. 1983). Enzymatic release of immunomodulating peptides may well occur during the digestive process (Jollès et al. 1982). Trypsin interaction with casein produces an immune activation of tri- and hexapeptides (Migliore-Samour et al. 1989). In *Fischer* rats, phagocytosis of opsonized sheep red-blood cells by alveolar macrophages and mitogenic activity are both greater if the diet contains peptides derived from soybean protein rather than from casein (Yamauchi and Suetsuna 1993).

Rabbits fed on a cholesterol-free diet develop serum antibodies to dietary protein and an anatomical form of atherosclerosis that is more typical of human atherosclerosis (Gallagher et al. 1978). Young animals fed with the same protein as their dams have lower amounts of food antigen-specific antibodies than rabbits fed on a novel protein during weaning; however, the extent of atherosclerosis is similar. Perinatal exposure of rabbits to dietary antigens may therefore modulate the systemic immune reaction to antigens (Gallagher et al. 1982).

The possible role of arginine immune effects on atherosclerosis is still unknown. This amino acid increases the total number of lymphocytes in the thymus (Rettura et al. 1979; Barbul et al. 1980a, 1980b; Barbul 1993). In *New Zealand white* rabbits fed for 90 days on a hyperenergetic diet (17 MJ/kg) containing soybean protein isolates or casein (308 g/kg), with (10 g/kg) or without cholesterol, both diets being supplemented by methionine, the serum cholesterol concentrations were significantly higher with the cholesterol-free casein diet and with the cholesterol enriched soybean-protein-isolates diet. With both diets, the changes in the cholesterol levels were mainly associated with LDL cholesterol. Serum antibody levels were higher in the soybean-fed animals than in those on casein. Marked atherosclerosis, typical of cholesterol-fed rabbits, was not significantly influenced by the nature of the protein source. With a cholesterol-free diet, only the casein diet induced small lesions of atherosclerosis. The level of antibodies in these food proteins therefore does not cause sufficiently strong immunologic injury to influence the induced atherosclerosis (Pathirana et al. 1979). Lastly, previously established atheroma in male *New Zealand white* rabbits did not regress when the atherogenic stimulus was removed. Male *New Zealand white* rabbits were fed an atherogenic diet (cholesterol 1% and corn oil 4%) mixed into a commercial ration for 2 months. The animals were then separated into four groups fed on (1) commercial ration, (2) commercial ration plus 4% corn oil, (3) semipurified diet containing 14% coconut oil and 25% soybean protein, and (4) semipurified diet containing 14% coconut oil and 25% casein. After 2 months, serum cholesterol levels had fallen by 91%, 80%, 81%, and 64%, respectively. Aortic sudanophilia had increased by 106%, 213%, 238%, and 25%, respectively (Kritchev-sky et al. 1988b). Nevertheless, despite the presence of many factors that may be involved in immunologically provoked lesions of the arterial tissues and despite potentially significant effects (Sugano 1983), their true role in atherogenesis has not as yet been confirmed (Redgrave 1984). Although ample experimental evidence is available to demonstrate the capacity of immune damage to promote atherogenesis in animals, the same cannot be said for human models (Constantinides 1980).

4.1.6 GLUTATHIONE

The nature and amount of protein and sulfur amino acid intake influence the synthesis of glutathione (Morand et al. 1997; Hunter et al. 1997; Griffith 1999; Lyons et al. 2000; Therond et al. 2000; Petzke et al. 2000). Glutathione, the major antioxidant, limits the formation of toxic oxygen radicals. The endogenous glutathione conjugates influence the action of nitric oxide on the endothelium (Wang and Ballatori 1998). Glutathione protects LDL and the arterial cells against oxidation and reduces the development of atherosclerotic plaques (Rosenfeld 1998; Cho et al. 1999).

4.1.7 INFLUENCE OF FOOD ENVIRONMENTS ON DIETS

The food environments of diets influence the effects of proteins as Kritchevsky and Tepper (1968) have shown in rabbits.

4.1.7.1 Copper and Zinc

Weanling rats developed cardiomyopathy when they were fed a copper-deficient purified diet; angiopathy was observed when the diet was low in zinc (Stemmer et al. 1985). The copper and zinc content in a diet may therefore modify the results of experiments investigating the effects of protein.

4.1.7.2 Choline and Lecithin

In rats fed on a choline-deficient diet, pathologic changes in heart and coronary arteries were observed (Wilgram and Hartroft 1955; Wilgram et al. 1955a, 1955b). In contrast, if these rats had been submitted to surgical bilateral renal decapsulation, the pathologic changes were very weak. These data support the view that cardio-vascular changes with choline deficiency are primarily due to severe bilateral haemorragic, renal cortical necrosis in the presence of increased intrarenal pressure (Wilgram and Blumenstein 1956).

The addition of 3.4% soy lecithin for 8 weeks to the American Heart Association (AHA) Step 1 diet in *Cynomolgus* monkeys produced a greater reduction in plasma cholesterol (−32%) and non HDL-cholesterol (−45%) concentrations, compared to the same diet without lecithin (Wilson et al. 1998b). In another experiment, male *F1B* hamsters were fed on three modified nonpurified diets for 8 weeks. With regard to the hypercholesterolemic diet (0.05% cholesterol), the hamsters fed on the same diet supplemented with 3.4% soybean lecithin had significantly lower plasma total cholesterol levels (−58%) and non-HDL cholesterol (−73%). They had also lower plasma total cholesterol (−33%) and non-HDL cholesterol (−50%) than the hamsters fed the hypercholesterolemic diet without lecithin but supplemented with linoleate and choline equivalent to lecithin. The aortic fatty streak area was significantly reduced (−90% and −79%, respectively) in hamsters fed lecithin compared with those fed the hypercholesterolemic diet without lecithin, and with hamsters fed on linoleate and choline (Wilson and Nicolosi 1997; Wilson et al. 1998b).

4.1.7.3   Dietary Fibers

Depending on their nature, dietary fibers may play a role in the prevention of atheroclerosis. Their effects on lipid metabolism in animals, and on lipoproteins in particular, have already been described in Section 2.4.6 on lipid metabolism, and are reviewed by Kritchevsky et al. (Kritchevsky and Story 1974; Kritchevsky et al. 1974; 1977; Kritchevsky 1978; Kritchevsky and Story 1978; Kritchevsky et al. 1982b, 1983; Smith and Pickney 1989; Kritchevsky 1999). On the basis of experimental results in male *New Zealand white* rabbits, Lo et al. (1987) have suggested that soybean fibers and soybean protein isolates may well have complementary roles. In male *New Zealand white* rabbits, fed for 36 weeks on either casein or soybean protein isolates with cellulose or soybean fibers, plasma cholesterol levels, cholesterol contents in the liver and heart, and incidence of atherosclerotic lesions in the aorta were lower in rabbits fed soybean protein isolates and soybean fibers than with casein (Lo et al. 1987). However, it is difficult to distinguish between the respective effects of food proteins, fats, and dietary fibers when assessing the correlations between a normal diet and autopsy observations (Moore et al. 1981).

4.1.7.4   Isoflavones

The consumption of soybean protein or of vegetable and fruit leads to considerable exposure to dietary phenolic antioxidants that can protect the LDL particle against oxidation (Wang et al. 1996). This antoxidative effect has previously been proven and is described in Section 2.7.4.4. Arterial lipid peroxidation levels of 46 ovariectomized *Cynomolgus* monkeys were lower (−17%) when they were fed on soybean protein isolates with isoflavones instead of casein/lactalbumin (Wagner et al. 1997). They significantly improve the metabolism of LDL cholesterol and HDL cholesterol (Anthony et al. 1998) and affect the apolipoprotein metabolism of HDL and LDL cholesterol (Deeley et al. 1985; Anthony and Clarkson 1997).

Genistein, the most abundant isoflavone in soybean protein, has been frequently shown to be a potent inhibitor of tyrosine kinase, angiogenesis, and oxidation of LDL. In atherosclerotic female macaques, after administration of acetylcholine, the arteries were seen to constrict or dilate according to whether the animals were fed on a low- or high-isoflavone diet. In addition intravenous injection of genistein in female macaques fed on a low-isoflavone diet, caused dilation of the constricted arteries (Honoré et al. 1997). Increased levels of isoflavonoids, in particular genistein, via consumption of a soybean protein diet, inhibited cell adhesion of monocytes and T-cells and also proliferation of cells involved in the formation of arterial lesions. Genistein inhibits the migration and proliferation of smooth muscle cells *in vitro* (Fujio et al. 1993; Shimokado et al. 1994, 1995; Mäkelä et al. 1999). The activities of growth factors, namely platelet-derived growth factor (PDGF), which modulate matrix synthesis and degradation, angiogenesis, cell–cell adhesion, and lipid cell uptake, are impaired in atherosclerotic plaque, and the increase of isoflavones, genistein in particular, inhibited cell adhesion, altered growth factor activity, and inhibited cell proliferation (Raines and Ross 1995).

In male *Sprague-Dawley* rats, genistein and daidzein have been shown to be capable of dilating the cerebral arteries by a direct action on these arteries. Moreover, they increased vascular diameter immediately after injection (Knutson et al. 1997). In *Stroke-Prone Spontaneously Hypertensive* rats (*SHR-SP*), soybean isoflavones inhibit the proliferation and DNA synthesis of aortic smooth muscle cells in a concentration-dependent manner; the function of the PDGF, which induces smooth muscle cell proliferation, is also impaired. These isoflavones therefore inhibit a basic mechanism of atherosclerotic vascular change (Pan et al. 2001). Aglycone-rich isoflavone extracts without soybean protein are capable of slowing down the development of atherosclerosis in cholesterol-fed rabbits. Indeed, in 12-week-old *New Zealand white* rabbits fed a cholesterol diet (1 g/100 g) for 8 weeks, the levels of plasma LDL cholesterol and cholesteryl ester hydroperoxide induced by $CuSO_4$ were significantly lower in the cholesterol-fed group with aglycone isoflavones than in the cholesterol-fed group without isoflavones. In the aortic arch, cholesterol concentrations and the extent of atherosclerotic lesions of the aortic arch were also lower. There were only a small number of oxidized LDL-positive, macrophage-derived foam cells in the atherosclerotic lesions in the aglycone isoflavone group. The antioxidative action of isoflavones can therefore be said to exert an antiatherosclerotic effect (Yamakoshi et al. 2000).

There is no difference in serum total cholesterol levels or thoracic aorta lesion surface areas between male *C57BL/6J* apo E-deficient mice fed on cholesterol-free diets containing ethanol-extracted soybean protein isolates or casein plus soybean protein ethanol extracts for 9 weeks (Ni et al. 1998). Likewise, in young male and female *Cynomolgus* monkeys fed on casein the degree of atherosclerosis was slightly greater than that observed when they were fed on soybean protein isolates from which the isoflavones had been alcohol extracted, and considerably greater than when they were fed on isoflavone-intact soybean protein (Anthony et al. 1998).

Intact soybean protein inhibited the constrictor response to intracoronary infusion of collagen or angiotensin II in monkeys, promoted adaptive arterial modeling delaying the development of atherosclerosis in surgically postmenopausal monkeys, and inhibited the development of restenosis after angioplasty in premenopausal monkeys. These effects are less marked with alcohol-extracted soybean protein since the active components have been removed by alcohol extraction (Williams et al. 1997).

Isoflavones probably act like estrogens, but whether they possess all of the following protective effects of estrogens has yet to be determined: reduced endothelin production; lower cytokine-induced endothelial-cell-adhesion molecule expression; reduced rate of cell proliferation and migration; decreased calcium influx into smooth muscle cells; and increased secretion of nitric oxide and production of prostaglandin I_2. Isoflavones also enhance macrophage phagocytosis, ester hydrolysis, and inhibit cytokine synthesis (review in St Clair 1997). The protective effect of isoflavones against atherosclerosis would appear to be due to the reduction in plasma lipids, antioxidant effects, and antiproliferative and antimigratory actions on smooth muscle cells. Moreover, they inhibit thrombus formation (Anthony et al. 1998). Lastly, via their effect on the estrogen receptor (ERβ), they may also exert a protective effect on the arterial wall. Indeed, when ERβ is overexpressed 7 days after arterial injury (endothelial denudation of rat arteries), treatment based on 0 to 2.5 mg/kg of genistein or 17β-estradiol ensures greater protection against neointima formation. On other hand, the same dose of genistein or 17β-estradiol has the same inhibitory effect on atherosclerosis (Mäkelä et al. 1999). However, the role of isoflavones in the prevention of cardiovascular disease has still not been demonstrated (Rossouw 1998).

4.1.8 Conclusion

The effects of the amount and nature of proteins and amino acids on the development of atherosclerosis depend on the animal species; this is even more significant with regard to high-protein diets. A moderately low-protein diet prevents the development of fatty streaks in pigeons and decreases the aortic cholesterol content in rats. However, in pigs and monkeys, it has no effects. A decrease in the sulfur amino acid content of a low-protein diet causes plasma cholesterol levels to rise, although they may return to normal levels if methionine or cystine is added to the diet. Although various types of proteins have similar effects in pigeons, in other animal species the prevalence of atherosclerosis is higher with casein or fish protein than with soybean protein diets.

Amino acids arginine, methionine, and taurine have been shown to induce different effects on the development of atherosclerosis. Arginine increases nitric oxide synthesis since it is a substrate of nitric oxide synthase. It induces antihypertensive and antiproliferative effects, inhibits platelet aggregation, increases endothelium-dependent vasodilatation, and reduces the development of atherosclerosis in cholesterol-fed rabbits. However, the addition of arginine to a casein diet produces equivocal results. Methionine increases lipid peroxidation, intimal thickening, and enhances cholesterol deposits, calcification, arteriosclerotic plaque formation, and endothelial cell numbers in the blood, and leads to the production of homocysteine and the subsequent angiotoxic effect.

Taurine may prevent the development of atherosclerosis since it regulates osmolarity, reduces calcium levels in the aorta and myocardium, improves cardiac contractile function, and mimics a number of the actions of angiotensin-converting enzyme inhibitors.

Despite the existence of numerous factors that may be involved in immunologically provoked lesions of the arterial tissues, and despite the potential significance of their effects, their true role in atherogenesis has not as yet been confirmed (Redgrave 1984). Although ample experimental evidence is available to demonstrate the capacity of immune damage to promote atherogenesis the same cannot be said for human models (Constantinides 1980).

Lecithin decreases serum cholesterol concentrations and reduces the extent of atheroclerotic lesions.

The effects of dietary fibers are more complex. The nature of the dietary fibers and the food environments in general are of particular importance.

Isoflavones reduce serum lipid concentrations, and have several protective effects, such as antioxidative, antiproliferative, and antimigratory actions. However, to date it is not yet clear whether they have all the protective effects of estrogens.

As the amounts of polyphenols, dietary fibers, and isoflavones vary from one experiment to another, depending on the composition of protein diet, their respective contribution to the prevention or reduction in cardiovascular risk cannot be evaluated accurately.

Most of the studies concerning the relationship between proteins and atherosclerosis have been carried out on growing animals consuming a single protein source. The results should therefore only be extrapolated to adult humans on a mixed diet with the greatest of caution (Finot 1992).

4.2 DATA ON HUMANS

4.2.1 EPIDEMIOLOGIC DATA

As in animals, it is difficult in humans to take into consideration the impact of inherited susceptibility to coronary heart disease (Tyroler 2000). Although a strong positive correlation has been observed in various countries between the amount of animal proteins in the diet and mortality from coronary heart disease (Carroll and Hamilton 1975; Carroll 1978a), a strong positive correlation is also observed with the consumption of fats. However, the correlation between mortality and coronary heart disease is stronger with dietary animal proteins than with dietary fat (Yerushalmy and Hilleboe 1957). Nevertheless, according to Yudkin (1957), the data available do not support any theory that supposes a single or major dietary cause of coronary thrombosis. In his report at the Conference on Atherosclerosis and Coronary Heart Disease, Hilleboe (1957) did not mention the effect of protein on atherosclerosis. In the Athens case-control study of diet and heart disease, there was no association between coronary heart disease and dietary protein, cholesterol, or vitamin C (Tzonou et al. 1993). In a general review of nutrient high-density lipoprotein relationships, Rifkind (1983), describing the results of the Lipid Research Clinic Prevalence Study, demonstrated the reality of the correlations with certain nutrients but not with the amount or nature of the proteins.

Consumption of a diet that is high in cereals, grains, legumes, and various vegetables is associated with a reduced incidence of cardiovascular disease (Brown and Karmally 1985). In the cohort of 80,082 women aged 34 to 59 years and enrolled in the Nurses' Health Study, 939 cases of ischemic heart disease were observed during the follow-up period of 14 years, although at baseline, no cases were reported. After elimination of confounding factors, a high animal or vegetable protein intake in low- or high-fat diets was shown to be associated with a low risk of ischemic heart disease. Thus, a high level of protein consumption, regardless of nature, does not enhance the risk for ischemic heart disease, and substituting carbohydrates with proteins is even associated with a decreased risk (Hu et al. 1999). In the Swedish male population, total apo A-I in plasma is a protective factor and a plasma lipoprotein(a) level above 200 mg/L is a risk factor for primary acute myocardial infarction (Dahlen et al. 1988). Casein lowers lipoprotein(a) serum levels by an average of 50% compared with soybean proteins (Nilausen and Meinertz 1999).

A correlation has been shown between the amount of dietary protein intake and fasting plasma total homocysteine levels. A long-term, high sulfur-amino-acids intake may enhance the activity of the enzymes that clear homocysteine, thus compensating or overcompensating for the higher amount of sulfur amino acids (Stolzenberg-Solomon et al. 1999).

4.2.1.1 Animal Proteins

Although a strong positive correlation between the amount of animal proteins in the diet and mortality from coronary heart disease has been observed in various countries (Carroll and Hamilton 1975; Carroll 1978a), a strong positive correlation is also observed with the consumption of fats. It is therefore impossible to determine from surveys if one or another or both factors are the real risk factors of atherosclerosis. Kritchevsky (1999) recently reviewed the relation between diet and atherosclerosis and concluded that there are many areas of diet and heart disease that still need to be assessed.

4.2.1.1.1 Fish and Meat Proteins

The possibility that coronary heart disease may be prevented by the consumption of fish is a particularly important field of research yet to be exploited. Interest has grown since the observation that in two populations with a high consumption of fish, Greenland Eskimos (Bang et al. 1971) and the Japanese (Keys 1980), the incidence of coronary heart disease is lower. Likewise, in the Netherlands, a negative correlation between the risk of coronary heart disease and the consumption of fish has been shown (Kromhout et al. 1985; Shekelle et al. 1985; Norrell et al. 1986; Kromhout et al. 1995), whereas Snowdon et al. (1984) established a positive correlation between meat consumption and fatal ischemic heart disease in the Seventh-Day Adventist population. Nevertheless, no relationship between fish intake and rates of total or fatal coronary heart disease has been demonstrated (Curb and Reed 1985; Vollset et al. 1985) and epidemiologic data in the United States have shown that increased consumption of fish (one to two servings/wk to five to six servings/wk) does not reduce the risk of coronary heart disease in healthy men (Ascherio et al. 1995). The data from a survey on fish consumption and coronary heart disease mortality in Finland, Italy, and the Netherlands clearly confirm the difficulties encountered in identifying the respective role of each food component. Indeed, in this survey, the pooled relative risk for the highest quartile of total fish compared with no fish consumption in the three countries was 1.08. Lean fish consumption is not associated with coronary heart disease mortality in any country and fatty fish consumption compared to non–fatty-fish is associated with lower mortality, the pooled risk for fatty-fish consumers being 0.66 (Oomen et al. 2000b).

Clearly, the respective roles of lipids and proteins warrant further investigation and evaluation (Kagawa et al. 1982).

4.2.1.1.2 Dairy Proteins

McLachlan (2001) has estimated the correlation (r^2 = 0.86) between dairy protein consumption (milk protein in cheese excluded) and mortality due to ischemic heart disease in several countries (Europe, United States, Australia, New Zealand, Israel, Japan). Although the populations of Toulouse and Belfast have almost identical collective "traditional" risk factors for heart disease, the mortality rate is three times higher in Northern Ireland where the consumption of β-casein A_1 is 3.23 times that in Toulouse. Although suspected, the possible atherogenic effect of β-casein A_1 has not been proven. To date, no experimental study has been undertaken to verify whether β-casein A_1 is really a risk factor for atherosclerotic disease (McLachlan et al. 2001).

In 1971, Oster suggested that consumption of homogeneized milk may well be a causal factor in the development of atherosclerosis. This suggestion has been supported by several subsequent articles (review in Deeth 1983). Indeed, xanthine oxydase, an enzyme in milk, could enter into the circulatory system and initiate atherosclerosis in arterial wall and heart tissue. However, according to the extensive reviews by Carr et al. (1975, quoted by Deeth 1983) and Deeth (1983), there is considerable doubt about the significance of milk xanthine oxidase as a causal factor of atherosclerosis. The action of the enzyme when absorbed would still appear to be highly speculative. Therefore, this hypothesis is unlikely to be generally accepted and additional research is still necessary.

4.2.1.2 Taurine

In the Cardiac Study, which has assessed 10,000 participants from 58 populations of 25 countries over the past 12 years, total coronary heart disease mortality is significantly positively correlated with serum cholesterol levels and significantly inversely related to urinary taurine excretion (Yamori et al. 1987; Yamori 1989; Yamori et al. 1992a, 1992b, 1994). The Japanese populations who regularly eat fish four to five times a week showed the highest taurine urinary excretion and the lowest incidence of coronary heart disease mortality. The lowest level of taurine urinary excretion and the highest level of severe hypertension were observed in Tibetans, who never eat fish for religious reasons. In contrast, the frequency of hypertension among the Japanese population of northeastern Japan who had a salt intake close to that of the Tibetans is half that of Tibetans (Yamori et al. 1996). The results of this survey confirm the previous data analyzed by Rifkind (1983).

4.2.1.3 Biological Parameters

4.2.1.3.1 Triacylglycerols

The relationships between plasma triacylglycerol levels and atherosclerosis are still under discussion. While Grundy (1998) considered that elevated plasma levels of triacylglycerol-rich lipoproteins, including very-low-density lipoproteins, and chylomicrons and their remnants, should be considered as risk factors for cardio-vascular disease, Sprecher (1998) regarded the same parameters as an independent factor. Triacylglycerol-rich lipoproteins have indeed been shown to interact with lipoprotein receptors on monocytes, macrophages, and endothelial cells. An abnormal ability to bind to low-density lipoprotein receptors via apo E is observed in hypertriglyceridemic subjects, whereas plasma chylomicrons bind to apo B-48 receptors of monocytes, macrophages, and endothelial cells. These interactions have a role in the formation of macrophage-derived "foam cells" of arteriosclerotic lesions and in endothelial dysfunction-derived defective fibrinolysis (Gianturco and Bradley 1999). The combined pooled data from 21 prospective studies in 46,413 men and 10,684 women confirm that independently of HDL-cholesterol levels, plasma triacylglycerol levels are indeed a risk factor for cardiovascular disease in the general population (Hokanson and Austin 1996). In univariate analyses, serum triacylglycerol levels are often more strongly correlated with the incidence of future coronary heart disease than serum cholesterol concentrations. However, in multiple logistic regression analyses, particularly when HDL cholesterol is included, the strength of the apparent independent relationship between triacylglycerol levels and the incidence of coronary heart disease is weakened (Durrington 1998). The development of severe and moderate lesions is associated with cholesterol- and triacylglycerol-rich lipoproteins (Hodis et al. 1994; Hodis and Mack 1995; Hodis et al. 1999), and a possible linking of atherogenesis to the interaction of endothelial lipoprotein lipase with triglyceride-rich lipoproteins had already been proposed by Zilversmith (1973). Data from prospective studies have shown that subjects with a high LDL-/HDL-cholesterol ratio and a high plasma triacylglycerol level have the highest risk for coronary artery disease (Ooi and Ooi 1998). Other epidemiologic surveys and meta-analyses are in favor of a relationship between the incidence of coronary artery diseases or mortality and plasma triacylgycerol levels (Austin et al. 1998; Gotto 1998a, 1998b; Jeppesen et al. 1998; Krauss 1998; Miller 1999). Later, however, Avins and Neuhaus (2000) carried out a secondary analysis of data from the Multiple Risk Factor Intervention Trial, the Lipid Research Clinics Coronary Primary Prevention Trial, and the Lipid Research Clinic Prevalence and Mortality Follow-up Study. They came to the conclusion that the level of serum triacylglycerols does not provide as much clinically meaningful information about the risk of coronary heart disease as that obtainable from the level of serum cholesterol subfractions.

Thus, although univariate analysis shows a positive correlation between plasma triacylglycerol levels and the risk for coronary heart disease, multivariate analysis does not confirm that a high plasma triacylglycerol level is an independent risk factor, except in women and diabetic individuals.

4.2.1.3.2 Homocysteine

Observations of premature vascular disease occuring in patients with homocysti-nuria, have lead to the role of homocytseine being investigated by a large numbers of review and epidemiological, clinical, or experimental studies (McCully 1969; McCully and Wilson 1975; McCully 1983; Starkebaum and Harlan 1986; Lentz and Sadler 1991; Kang et al. 1992; Nygärd et al. 1995; Bostom et al. 1995; Lentz et al. 1996; Stamler and Slivka 1996; McCully 1996, 1997; Nygard et al. 1997; Bates et al. 1997; Freyburger et al. 1997; Harpel 1997; Tawakol et al. 1997; McCully 1998; De Jong et al. 1998; Refsum and Ueland 1998; Stein and McBride 1998; Kuller and Evans 1998; Folsom et al. 1998; Nygärd 1999; Folsom 1999; Blacher et al. 1999; Bostom et al. 1999; Gherard and Duell 1999; Guthikonda and Haynes 1999; Hankey and Eikelbloom 1999; Eikelbloom et al. 1999; Lambert et al. 1999; Langman and Cole 1999; Jakubowski 1999; Meleady and Graham 1999; Perry 1999; Tyagi 1999; Tyagi et al. 1999; Nygärd et al. 1999; Selhub 1999; Voutilainen et al. 2000; Ueland et al. 2000; Thambyrajah and Townend 2000; Fukagawa et al. 2000; Brattström and Wilcken 2000; McKinley 2000; Scott 2000; Blacher and Safar 2001).

However, the data from prospective studies are sometimes conflicting or less conclusive, and although a relationship between hyperhomocysteinemia and cardiovascular diseases has been reported, no cause–effect relationship has been established (Eikelbloom et al. 1999; Perry 1999; Ueland et al. 2000; Scott 2000). Moreover, no randomized, controlled trials have been conducted to investigate whether lowering plasma homocysteine levels influences the incidence of atherosclerotic vascular events (Guthikonda and Haynes 1999; Blacher and Safar 2001). The differences in plasma homocysteine concentrations between men and women can be partially explained; indeed, women had significantly higher remethylation rates than did men and a tendency toward higher transmethylation (Fukagawa et al. 2000).

Several traditional risk factors are associated with homocysteinemia and may be confounding factors. Vitamin content in diet and vitamin status have to be taken into consideration since folate, vitamin B_6, and B_{12} levels play a key role in plasma homocysteine concentrations (Selhub 1999). Compared to omnivores, the fasting plasma homocysteine concentrations of Buddhist female lactovegetarians were significantly higher. In the vegetarian group, fasting plasma homocysteine levels correlated negatively with serum threonine, lysine, histidine, arginine, and cystine and these amino acids contributed to 38.7% of homocysteine variation. However, multiple regression analysis revealed that plasma folate, vitamin B_{12}, and creatinine were independent determinants of homocysteine variation and contributed to 38.6% of homocysteine variation in vegetarians (Hung et al. 2002).

For Ueland et al. (2000), only a placebo-controlled intervention study of total plasma homocysteine-low vitamin B levels and clinical endpoints can provide valid additional arguments on the potential role of homocysteinemia as a cardiovascular disease risk factor. As mildly elevated plasma homocysteine levels in atherosclerotic patients are frequently associated with impaired renal function, which alone causes elevated plasma homocysteine, a high plasma homocysteine level may well be an effect rather than a cause of atherosclerotic disease (Brattström and Wilcken 2000). Further studies are therefore still necessary to confirm the real influence of the amount and nature of dietary protein on plasma homocysteine levels, and whether elevated homocysteinemia is really a cause of atherosclerotic disease and an independent factor (Blacher et al. 1999; Nygärd et al. 1999; Gherard and Duell 1999).

The exact mechanism of the atherogenic and thrombogenic alterations that account for the vascular toxicity of elevated homocysteine levels is still unknown (McKinley 2000). However, the possible effect of homocysteine on the vessels and on endocardial endothelial function could be due to various mechanisms (Tyagi et al. 1999; Thambyrajah and Townend 2000). Some of these mechanisms follow.

- Homocysteine as a chelating agent for calcium. The uptake of calcium ions from cellular zonal adhesions induces their dissociation and promotes damage to vascular tissue through blood pressure, plasma cholesterol, and lipids, but also to the development of inflammatory processes (Wang 1999).
- Metabolic conversion of homocysteine to thiolactone (protein homocysteinylation), and resulting protein damage may be key factors of the involvement of homocysteine in atherosclerotic disease (Jakubowski 1999).
- Endothelial cellular and DNA damage.
- Reduced activity of glutathione peroxidase.
- Stimulation of procoagulant and impairment of anticoagulant and fibrinolytic pathways.
- Mitogenic effect on smooth muscle cell proliferation.
- Promotion of endothelial–leukocyte interactions.
- Alteration of the vascular and endocardium endothelium due to the inhibiting action of homocysteine on the vasodilatator effect of nitric oxide (NO) (Lentz et al. 1996; Tawakol et al. 1997; Tyagi et al. 1999).

4.2.2 EXPERIMENTAL DATA

4.2.2.1 Dairy Proteins

In 19 hypercholesterolemic adult men with a daily consumption for 8 weeks of either 750 ml of 2% cow's milk or a drink containing soybean protein isolates and 2% corn oil (in addition to their usual mixed diet, the average daily intake corresponding to dietary recommendations), the substitution of soybean beverages for 2% cow's milk significantly reduced serum cholesterol levels in hypercholesterolemic but not in healthy men. No change was observed with regard to zinc, copper, or iron status. This dietary modification could be a safe method of reducing the risk of coronary heart disease in hypercholesterolemic patients (Gibson et al. 1988).

4.2.2.2 Amino Acids

Amino acids have a very important function in the metabolism of vascular endothelium. The glutamine contained in glutamic acid is an energy source for endothelial cells (Hinshaw et al. 1990; Spolarics et al. 1991) and L-arginine, the nitric oxide (NO) synthase precursor in vascular endothelial cells (Palmer et al. 1987, 1988; Vallance et al. 1989; Moncada et al. 1991), influences vascular tone (Kuo et al. 1992; Cooke et al. 1992). In subjects with coronary heart disease, basal production of nitric oxide is reduced (Quyyumi et al. 1997; Sumino et al. 1998). In hypercholesterolemia, before the formation of atherosclerotic plaque, endothelial function is impaired and endothelial-dependent relaxation attenuated (Drexler et al. 1991a; Zeiher et al. 1991; Cohen et al. 1988).

The plasma free amino-acid pattern can be modified. This was demonstrated in 73 subjects fed on a balanced, predominantly plant protein diet for 4 weeks. Plasma levels of arginine, glycine, serine, and threonine were significantly increased, whereas those of histidine, leucine, tyrosine, and valine were decreased. The lysine/arginine ratio decreased from 3.46 to 2.72. This change in the amino acid pattern is more favorable to the prevention of atherosclerosis (Sanchez et al. 1983). The potential drawback of soybean protein, the insufficient supply of sulfur amino acids as postulated from data in rodents (Moundras et al. 1995), would not appear to be of any significance in humans (Sirtori et al. 1998).

4.2.2.2.1 Arginine

Following an arginine load, about 40% is degraded in the intestine, 50% enters the systemic circulation, and 15% of portal arginine is taken up by the liver (Wu and Morris 1998). Nutritional supplementation with L-arginine can increase nitric oxide production in humans (Girerd et al. 1990; Kharitonov et al. 1995), whereas a deficiency impairs nitric oxide synthesis in rats (Wu et al. 1999). High concentrations of L- and D-arginine have unspecific vasodilator effects in humans (Calver et al. 1991; MacAllister et al. 1995), and arginine has been shown to regulate blood pH and inhibit O_2 production by endothelial cells (Wascher et al. 1997).

Intravenous infusion of arginine reduced the plasma concentration of angiotensin II in humans. Indeed arginine is an inhibitor of the angiotensin-converting enzyme (Higashi et al. 1995). L-Arginine exerts antihypertensive and antiproliferative effects on vascular smooth muscle cells (Nakaki and Kato 1994; Ignarro et al. 1999). In 30 patients with diabetes mellitus, 1 gram of L-arginine twice a day for 3 months reduced lipid peroxidation as demonstrated by decreased urine malondialdehyde levels (Lubec et al. 1997).

As described in Section 4.1.4.1, arginine restores cholinergic relaxation in the thoracic aorta of hypercholesterolemic rabbits (Cooke et al. 1991). In hypercholesterolemic patients, a similar effect of L-arginine has been observed (Drexler et al. 1991b). L-Arginine plasma concentrations were significantly lower in hypercholesterolemic patients without lipid-lowering therapy than in age-matched normocholesterolemic patients. This reduction may well be one factor in the impairment of endothelium relaxation. The mechanism behind this plasma arginine reduction is still unknown (Jeserich et al. 1992). However, in 11 patients with type IIA hypercholesterolaemia and 11 age-matched patient controls with normal cholesterol concentrations, the serum L-arginine concentrations were similar. All 22 patients had serum triacylglycerol concentrations below 2.5 mmol/L and none had previously received lipid-lowering agents (Oleesky et al. 1982). L-Arginine enhances vasodilation in smokers (Thorne et al. 1988; Campisi et al. 1999) and in hypercholesterolemic humans (Clarkson et al. 1996). In subjects with coronary heart disease, the basal production of nitric oxide was reduced (Quyyumi et al. 1997; Sumino et al. 1998) and L-arginine decreased tobacco smoke–related infarct size (Zhu et al. 1996). *In vitro* L-arginine reduces human monocyte adhesion to vascular endothelium and endothelial expression of cell adhesion molecules (Adams et al. 1997b) and nitric oxide donors, which have the capacity to modulate surface expression of the vascular cell-adhesion molecules-1 (VCAM-1) and E-selectin (De Caterina et al. 1995; Adams et al. 1997b).

Arginine reverses the age-related decrease in vasodilatory capacity (Chauhan et al. 1996), reduces lipid peroxidation (Lubec et al. 1997), and cardiac hypertrophy has been seen to regress (Matsuoka et al. 1996). In healthy subjects, intravenous infusion of L-arginine induced NO-dependent peripheral vasodilation (Kanno et al. 1992; Bode-Böger et al. 1994; Böger et al. 1996b) via an NO-dependent mechanism that was observed in a randomized placebo-controlled study in patients with critical limb ischemia (Bode-Böger et al. 1996b). The treatment of 22 patients with peripheral arterial occlusive disease by intravenous infusion of L-arginine for 7 days suppressed platelet aggregation and shortened the euglobulin clot lysis time (Gryglewski et al. 1996). This treatment improves the response of endothelium-dependent coronary vasodilation following intracoronary injection of acetylcholine (Drexler et al. 1991b) and the clinical status of patients with peripheral arterial occlusive disease (Slawinski et al. 1996). Likewise, in patients with hypercholesterolemia and/or atherosclerosis, L-arginine induced vasodilation (Imaizumi et al. 1992) and enhanced the effects of endothelium-dependent vasodilatators (Creager et al. 1992; Casino et al. 1994). However, in hypercholesterolemic patients, infusion of L-arginine compared to a placebo did not improve the working capacity index of myocardial ischemia. This lack of effect could mean that in these patients, a deficiency of the precursor of nitric oxide formation did not seem to impair maximal exercise capacity, myocardial perfusion during maximal exercise, or maximal vasodilator capacity in skeletal muscle or skin (Wennmalm et al. 1995).

The effects of oral L-arginine and intravenous infusion of L-arginine have been studied in patients with coronary artery disease. Oral L-arginine improved endothelium-dependent dilation, inhibited platelet aggregation, and reduced monocyte adhesion to endothelial cells in young men with coronary artery disease (Adams et al. 1995, 1997a; Clarkson et al. 1996). In 21 patients with luminal reduction of the coronary arteries, L-arginine infusion was shown to reverse the vasoconstriction induced by intracoronary injection of acetylcholine but only in the early stages of atherosclerosis. In the more advanced stages, this infusion was without effect (Otsuji et al. 1995).

The effects of exogenous L-arginine are mediated by mechanisms that remain largely unknown (review in Böger et al. 1996a; Adams et al. 1997a). L-Arginine is a precursor of nitric oxide and competitively overcomes asymmetrical dimethylarginines, which are inhibitors of NO synthase (Vallance et al. 1992b). Plasma dimethylarginine concentrations are high in cholesterol-fed rabbits (Yu et al. 1994), although their levels are unknown in hypercholesterolemic subjects.

The action of L-arginine may be independent of hormonal influences (Bode-Böger et al. 1996b), but could also act by mediating the release of insulin, glucagon, and growth hormone (Pedrinelli et al. 1995). The metabolism of L-arginine into agmatine may also induce peripheral vasodilation since agmatine stimulates central α_2-adrenoreceptors (Sakuma et al. 1992; Li et al. 1994; Jun and Wennmalm 1994). Lastly, L-arginine may also have beneficial actions *in vivo* through its capacity to inhibit lipid peroxidation (Philis-Tsimikas and Witzum 1995; Engelman et al. 1995; Lubec et al. 1997) and the formation of lesions after balloon angioplasty (Schwarzacher et al. 1997).

Numerous authors have advocated the routine use of L-arginine in clinical practice (Cooke and Tsao 1997; Chowienczyk and Ritter 1997; Cooke 1998) for the prevention of atherosclerotic lesions. However, considering the large number of nutrients that are potentially useful supplements for the prevention of coronary heart disease, arginine supplementation would appear to be unrealistic (De Lorgeril 1998). Moreover, in the Zuphten Elderly Study of 806 men aged 64 to 84 years, the 10-year follow-up period failed to demonstrate any relationship between dietary arginine intake and the risk of coronary heart disease after adjustment for potential confounding factors (Oomen et al. 2000a).

4.2.2.2.2 Methionine

Depending on the dietary methionine/protein ratio, methionine-enriched diets can be hypercholesterolemic, hypocholesterolemic, or without any influence on plasma cholesterol levels (Yagasaki et al. 1986a, 1986b; Sugiyama et al. 1986c). Since methionine is hypercholesterolemic but its demythelated derivatives are hypocholesterolemic, the methyl group of methionine is responsible for its hypercholesterolemic effect. Glycine has been shown to lower plasma cholesterol levels in methionine-fed rats because it promotes the utilization of methionine via the trans-sulfuration pathway (Sugiyama et al. 1986c).

In 139 healthy male subjects (18 vegans, 43 ovolacto vegetarians, 60 moderate meat eaters, and 18 high meat eaters), although the meat eaters' group consumed significantly greater levels of methionine and had a significantly lower serum folate concentration relative to vegans, the plasma homocysteine concentrations were significantly higher in the vegans. The inverse relation between dietary protein intake and plasma homocysteine levels may well result from the relation between dietary protein and vitamin B_{12} intake. Indeed, the vitamin B_{12} content is relatively high in animal proteins that are consumed in large amounts by humans, and their vitamin B_{12} status is strongly related to methionine intake (Mann et al. 1999). In an older population (151 women and 109 men), an independent, negative dose–response relationship has been shown between dietary protein consumption and blood total homocysteine levels (Stolzenberg-Solomon et al. 1999).

Fasting homocysteine concentrations and response to a L-methionine load (100 mg/kg) were similar in healthy young men and premenopausal women. However, the remethylation rates were higher in women than in men (Fukagawa et al. 2000). In humans, the L-methionine-loading test is not affected by a low or normal previous protein intake (den Heijer et al. 1996). Moderate or relatively high dietary methionine intake does not affect fasting plasma total homocysteine levels in humans, unless this level reached four or six times the usual quantity (Verhoef et al. 1996; Ward et al. 2000, 2001).

In subjects with mild fasting hyperhomocysteinemia, the plasma homocysteine level increases strongly after a methionine-loading test (Bostom et al. 1995). A diet rich in methionine elevates the plasma homocysteine levels in both normo- and hyper-homocysteinemic subjects, thus modifying the markers of endothelial or platelet function (Bellamy et al. 1998; Constans et al. 1999). In 91 healthy children and adolescents, no significant relationship was observed between dietary methionine and plasma homocysteine levels (Divine et al. 1998).

A meal rich in animal proteins increased the total plasma homocysteine levels of volunteers by up to 14%, as compared to fasting values (Guttormsen et al. 1994). In elderly people, elevated homocysteinemia depressed endothelium-dependent vasodilation (Tawakol et al. 1997). This effect may be due to reduced nitric oxide (NO) production (Selhub 1999), as has been observed in cell cultures (Stamler et al. 1993).

In 16% of 99 patients with coronary artery disease, plasma homocysteine concentrations were higher 6 hours after an oral loading dose of L-methionine (0.1 g/kg) than in those of 39 subjects with normal coronary arteries, all possible confounding factors being taken into account. Thus, mild methionine intolerance is a risk factor for individuals exposed to the high methionine content of Western diets (Murphy-Chutorian et al. 1985). Mild fasting and post–methionine load hyperhomocysteinemia is associated with premature atherosclerosis. In 123 healthy first-degree relatives of patients with mild hyperhomocysteinemia and coronary, cerebral, or peripheral artery disease, the increase in homocysteine concentrations after a standard methionine load was a significant determinant of impaired flow-mediated vasodilatation of the brachial artery. In these subjects therefore, elevated homocysteine levels after a methionine load were an independent predictor of endothelial dysfunction (Lambert et al. 1999). The relationships between homocysteine and atherosclerosis have been extensively reviewed by Guthikonda and Haynes (1999).

4.2.2.2.3 Taurine

Serum taurine concentrations were increased in patients with ischemic coronary disease, whereas they were normal in those suffering from severe cardiac pain of various origins (tachycardia, acute pericarditis, etc.) (Lombardini 1975). The effects of adding taurine for a 4-week period to conventional treatment in 14 patients with congestive heart failure have been investigated in a double-blind, randomized, crossover, placebo-controlled study. No patient worsened during taurine administration, but four patients did during placebo administration. Before taurine treatment, the pre-ejection period (corrected for heart rate) is 148 ms, and it decreases to 137 ms after taurine treatment. The quotient pre-ejection period/left ventricular ejection time decreased from 47% to 42% (Azuma et al. 1985).

Intravenous injection of taurine (5 to 10 g/day) improved the electrocardiogram status in patients affected by coronary ischemia (De Rango and Del Corso 1974). Likewise, oral supplementation with 5 g/day of taurine or intramuscular (0.4 g/day) or intravenous injections of taurine (0.5 g/day [Sicuteri et al. 1970] or 1 g/day [Nigro et al. 1971]) have been shown to have a positive effect on clinical symptoms, muscular endurance, and the electrocardiogram status of patients. Cardiac pain was reported to disappear in 21 out of 30 patients following intravenous taurine injections of 5 g/day for 5 to 20 days (Cagliarducci 1974).

4.2.2.2.4 Tryptophan

Tryptophan, a precursor of serotonin, may play a role in atherosclerosis. Elevated cholesterol levels in the synaptic membranes of mouse brain enhanced the serotonin receptors (Heron et al. 1980). Serum cholesterol levels may therefore influence the function of serotonin in the central nervous system (Engelberg 1992). The presence of tryptophan was confirmed in atheromatous plaque of the carotid arteries of 16 patients subjected to surgical endoarteriectomy; it was shown to bind to LDL and HDL_2 lipoproteins. Tryptophan is chiefly transported by HDL_2 lipoproteins, as shown by the ratio between tryptophan and cholesterol bound to LDL and HDL_2. HDL_2 plays a role in the removal of tryptophan, thus reducing its availability for serotonin biosynthesis (Baldo-Enzi et al. 1996).

4.2.2.3 Immunologic Effects of Proteins

Mann et al. (1964) and Mann and Spoerri (1974) observed that the plasma cholesterol concentrations in Masaï people were very low in spite of high consumption of fermented milk. The low ischemic heart disease mortality rate observed in the Masaï population (Ho et al. 1971) may be due to their high, exclusive consumption of fermented milk, although according to Gibney and Burstyn (1980), this fact may also be due to a generally low energy intake with high energy expenditure, as well as to genetic factors. The effect of fermented milk has, however, been confirmed by Ritzel (1975), who observed a negative correlation in Basel between the consumption of yogurt and plasma lipid concentrations.

In his review of epidemiologic data on populations free of cardiovascular diseases, consuming no milk protein or fresh milk, lacto-vegetarians, not protected or only partially protected against cardiovascular diseases, and consuming boiled and/or pasteurized milk, as compared with populations with a high incidence of cardiovascular mortality and consuming milk treated by prolonged heat treatment, Annand (1967) suggested the possibility of a relationship between the effect of heat treatment on the milk protein and the pathogenesis of thrombosis. As antibodies to milk protein have frequently been found in healthy adults, a modified cell-mediated immune reaction might well be involved in the pathogenesis of atherosclerotic lesions. A heat-denaturated bovine immunoglobulin (BGG) may be a major risk factor in the pathogenesis of atherosclerosis. Indeed, Annand (1986) has established that not only the consumption of denatured BGG correlates at all three major epidemiologic levels — historical, international, and social class — but that this highly reactive and invasive molecule seems to possess the biological and/or pathologic properties that can be a factor for atherosclerosis (Annand 1986). When BGG was injected intravenously into guinea pigs, a cell-mediated tissue reaction developed 10 days later (Benacerraf and Cell 1961; Streilein and Hildreth 1966). Heating milk denatures its proteins by inducing the formation of antibodies (Annand 1986). Heat-dried milk powder has been used in various trials (Toivanen et al. 1975), but the antibodies can only be detected if the milk has been heated for 15 minutes from 40° to 70°C or for 3 to 4 hours at 90°C (Muscari et al. 1989). The cleavage of IgG molecules during acid fermentation (cheese, yogurt) suppresses their antigenic capacity (Butler 1983). This could explain why in 20 countries the correlation between ischemic cardiovascular mortality is better with the consumption of milk proteins (cheese excluded) (r = 0.93) than with that of all milk proteins (cheese included) (r = 0.91). The intestinal permeability of milk antigens may be selective but this mechanism is unknown (Marcon Genty et al. 1989).

The levels of antibodies to reconstituted dried cow's milk proteins, as measured by passive hemaglutination (Davies 1971; Davies et al. 1969, 1974), or of antibodies to bovine milk xanthine oxidase (Ross et al. 1975), were higher in myocardial infarction patients than in control subjects. However, the frequency and the quantity of IgM and IgG antibodies against milk proteins, as measured by radioimmunoassay, were comparable in controls and in myocardial infarction patients (Toivanen et al. 1975; Scott et al. 1976; Romano et al. 1984; Muscari et al. 1989). The levels of these immunoglobulins were also observed to be similar in 37 patients with three coronary vessel disease and in 37 patients with no evidence of occlusive coronary atheroma (Gibney et al. 1980). In 19 men with myocardial infarction, no correlation was found with anti-milk protein antibodies (Scott et al. 1976). Nevertheless, an association between anti-milk IgA antibodies and atherosclerosis has been observed for the following antigens: β-lactoglobulin, xanthine oxidase, and casein (Muscari et al. 1988, 1989).

High production of IgA immunoglobulins following normal consumption of milk protein could be due to a genetic factor (Muscari et al. 1989). The development of atherosclerosis may also be related to a genetic factor since the IgA plasma level, but not that of other immunoglobulins, was elevated in atheromatous monozygotic twins affected by ischemic heart disease (Björkholm et al. 1980). The comparative levels of IgA and of several antigens (β-lactoglobulin, casein, xanthine-oxidase) are strongly correlated with atherosclerosis (Muscari et al. 1992). Most correlations between IgA anti-apoproteins or anti-lipoproteins and IgA anti-milk-proteins were significantly positive in atherosclerotic patients in comparison with healthy subjects (Muscari et al. 1992). However, this association does not prove the existence of a cause–effect relationship. It may well be the consequence of impaired liver function due to atheroclerosis and of enhanced antigen intestinal permeability provoked by chronic hypoxia of mesenteric arteries.

Since milk immunoglobulins are known to fix to milk fat globules, eliminating them from skimmed milk may well explain a further effect on cardiovascular mortality of reduced fat consumption (Butler 1983; Romano et al. 1984). Food antigens/antibodies in immune complex form were observed in 7 of 14 patients with early myocardial infarction and persistently high circulating immune complex levels. As these patients have lower expression of conventional risk factors, the formation of these circulating immune complexes may well be a triggering factor for myocardial infarction (Mustafa et al. 2001). Finally casein, lactalbumin, and soybean protein do not have the same effects on immune responses to a T-dependent antigen; the dietary protein, lactalbumin, has the strongest enhancing effect on the immune response to sheep erythrocytes (Parker and Goodrun 1990). Further research is still required to confirm immunoglobulin atherogenicity, especially in milk consumers.

4.2.2.4 Dietary Fibers

According to Walker and Arvidson (1954), the absence of coronary heart disease in black African populations may be due to the high consumption of dietary fibers. In humans, soluble fibers (pectin, psyllium, guar gum) have certain hypocholesterolemic properties, whereas insoluble fibers such as wheat bran have no effects (Truswell and Beynen 1992). Humble (1997) and Kris-Etherton et al. (1988) reviewed the influence of dietary fibers on atherosclerosis in epidemiologic studies.

4.2.2.5 Isoflavones

The relationships reported between the intake of isoflavonoids and cardiovascular disease are somewhat contradictory. The Netherland Zuphten Elderly Study reported a negative correlation between the intake of the flavonol quercetin and coronary mortality (Hertog et al. 1993; Keli et al. 1996), but this result was not so apparent in the Finland Study (Knekt et al. 1996). The incidence of nonfatal coronary heart disease was not associated with the intake of isoflavonoids in the U.S. Health Professionals Study (Rimm et al. 1996) nor in men in the Great Britain Caerphilly Study (Hertog et al. 1997). Nevertheless, the existence of a possible protective effect of flavonoids during the development of coronary heart disease cannot be denied (Rimm et al. 1996). These differences may be due to the influence of confounding factors and further randomized clinical trials are necessary to improve our understanding of the real effect of the intake of isoflavonoids on cardiovascular mortality (Katan and Hollman 1998). Not all soybean products contain isoflavonoids. For example, unlike soybean flour, the textured soybean products used in several clinical studies (Anderson et al. 1995) are virtually free of isoflavones (Sirtori et al. 1997).

In postmenopausal women, the antioxidant capacity of isoflavones has been observed after 12 weeks of daily consumption of 40 g of soybean protein isolates (1.8 to 2.3 mg of total isoflavones/g of protein) (Chait 1996). Likewise, in 24 adult men and women, the consumption of diets enriched with soybean protein (high or low in isoflavones) in a crossover study, with each diet lasting 17 days and separated by a 25-day wash-out period, the plasma concentrations of 8-epi-PGF2α, a biomarker of *in vivo* lipid peroxidation, were significantly lower after the high-isoflavone diet than after the low-isoflavone dietary treatments. Soybean product containing naturally occurring amounts of isoflavone phytoestrogen reduced lipid peroxidation *in vivo* and increased LDL resistance to oxidation (Wiseman et al. 2000).

A significant improvement in systemic arterial elasticity was observed after administration of genistein (45 mg for 5 to 10 weeks) in perimenopausal women, even though plasma lipid concentrations were not affected by the consumption of isoflavones (Nestel et al. 1997). In healthy women, a treatment comprising 40 mg and then 80 mg daily of isoflavones from red clover in two successive 5-week periods raised arterial compliance of 23% only with 80 mg isoflavones. The 80 mg dose contained 8 mg of genistein and 7 mg of daidzein and their methylated precursors (49 mg of biochanin, 16 mg of formonetin) (Nestel et al. 1999).

According to recent reviews by Tikkanen et al. (1998), Meng et al. (1999), Tikkanen and Adlercreutz (2000), a diet containing soybean-derived isoflavones can result in various effects: reduced plasma cholesterol concentrations but only in subjects with initially elevated levels; antioxidation of LDL; improved vascular reactivity in nonhuman primates (Honoré et al. 1997) and in postmenopausal and perimenopausal women (Abebe and Agarwal 1995; Gould et al. 1995; Nestel et al. 1997; Dubroff and Decker 1999); and antiproliferative properties *in vitro* (Fotsis et al. 1995; Raines et al. 1995).

A beverage with 40 g of soybean protein containing 80 mg of isoflavones administered daily for 1 month was shown to improve flow-mediated dilation by 5.3% in

18 postmenopausal women with abnormal endothelium-dependent flow-mediated dilation. This effect persisted for 1 month after suppression of the beverage (Dubroff and Decker 1999). Likewise, a 5-week treatment with 80 mg/day of purified soybean isoflavones resulted in a 26% improvement in systemic arterial compliance (Nestel et al. 1997). This effect of purified isoflavones was, however, not observed by Simons et al. (2000) in postmenopausal women.

As discussed previously, the independent effects of isoflavonoids on serum cholesterol concentrations have been clearly demonstrated in rats, hamsters, and nonhuman primates (*Cynomolgus* monkeys), but also in humans (Cassidy et al. 1995; Balmir et al. 1996; Honoré et al. 1997; Clarkson et al. 1998; meta-analysis by Anderson et al. 1995). Nevertheless, apo A-1, apo B, and lipoprotein plasma concentrations remained unchanged in two studies (Anthony et al. 1996a; Honoré et al. 1997).

Many studies published between 1991 and 1993 that were reviewed by Raines and Ross (1995) showed that increased isoflavonoid concentrations in cultured vascular cells impair the cellular processes associated with lesion development. Genistein (100μmol/L) has been shown to inhibit PDGF-induced thymidine incorporation and receptor autophosphorylation, and to increase intracellular calcium (Hill et al. 1990). It is also a specific inhibitor for tyrosine kinases with little or no effect on serine and threonine kinases. Evidence obtained from observations of cultured vascular cells suggests that certain cellular processes involved in lesion formation are inhibited by genistein (Raines and Ross 1995).

Recently, Anthony et al. (1998) summarized the potential mechanisms of soybean isoflavones in the prevention of animal and human atheroclerosis. Soybean isoflavones reduce plasma lipid concentrations and have a potent antioxidant activity, thereby reducing LDL oxidation (Hodgson et al. 1996; Wagner et al. 1997; Tikkanen et al. 1998; Ni et al. 1998; Wiseman et al. 2000; Yamakoshi et al. 2000). They inhibit atherosclerosis through estrogen receptor–mediated effects on tyrosine kinase activity, macrophage cytokine expression, the migration or proliferation of arterial smooth muscle cells, endothelium-dependent arterial dilation, arterial elasticity, and platelet aggregation or activation (Anthony et al. 1998; Anthony 2000, 2001). The alcohol-extracted and intact soybean protein isolate effects on plasma lipoproteins and atherosclerosis are different. Indeed, in monkeys (Anthony et al. 1997) and in humans (Crouse et al. 1999), intact soybean protein isolates were more effective in lowering plasma LDL- plus VLDL-cholesterol concentrations, elevating HDL-cholesterol levels, and inhibiting the progression of coronary artery atherosclerosis than isoflavone-deficient soybean protein. In contrast, in other experiments administration of purified soybean protein isoflavone concentrates had no effect on plasma LDL or HDL cholesterol in human subjects (Nestel et al. 1997; Hodgson et al. 1998) or in monkeys (Anthony et al. 1996a, 1996b, 1997).

4.2.3 CONCLUSION

The effects of dietary protein level on the development of atherosclerosis are largely dependent on the animal species; in addition, genetic factors would appear to be of a great importance. In humans, a high vegetable-protein diet may well have a protective effect against atherosclerosis. The specific nature of the proteins seems to be particularly important. In both animals and humans, soybean protein and lean fish protein have a protective effect against atherosclerosis, whereas casein would appear to promote it. The protective effects of vegetable proteins, particularly soybean protein, are due to a reduction in LDL cholesterol (about −13%) and plasma triacylglycerols (about −10%) and an increase in HDL cholesterol (about 2%) (Anderson et al. 1995).

LDL peroxidation is enhanced by casein peptides. Arginine and taurine both exert beneficial effects; the former promotes nitric oxide synthesis and the latter enhances diuresis and natriuresis and reduces the calcium level of atheromatous lesions. In contrast, methionine and homocysteine are both responsible for harmful effects via several mechanisms. Antibodies against milk proteins, and perhaps against milk proteins that have been denatured by heat processing, promote the development of atherosclerosis, whereas the isoflavone content of soybean protein has a protective effect. Lastly, the antioxidative effect of isoflavones protects against atherosclerosis.

According to Anthony (2001), the results of numerous studies have confirmed the benefits of soybean protein consumption for the preservation of a healthy cardiovascular system. Dieticians, nutrition specialists, educators, and the media have an important role to play in educating people and suggesting simple recipes and tasty soybean foods.

5 Data on Hypertension

The effects of the amount and the nature of protein consumption on blood pressure are often neglected in reviews of the relationship between nutrition and blood pressure. Numerous studies have nevertheless been conducted in both animals and humans.

5.1 DATA ON ANIMALS

In 1963, Okamoto and Aoki isolated a new strain of genetically hypertensive rats (*SHR*). The characteristics of hypertension in these animals are extremely close to those of human hypertensive disease. A decade later, Okamoto et al. (1974) obtained a substrain of the *SHR* rats with a very high incidence of stroke during their first year of life (*SHR-SP* rats). Lovenberg and Yamori reviewed the data relating to these different strains (Lovenberg 1987, Lovenberg and Yamori 1990, 1995).

Yamori et al. (1976a) suggested that the incidence of cerebral lesions in spontaneous hypertensive stroke-prone rats (*SHR-SP*) may result from dietary factors. The preventive effect against stroke of a protein-rich diet associated with salt restriction in *SHR* rats, and the lower incidence of cerebral lesions with a high-protein rather than a low-protein diet have now been demonstrated in several studies. However, a high-protein diet induced hypertension in weanling *Sprague-Dawley* rats after 9 to 12 months of a normal purified diet providing 25% of casein as a source of protein; females were more susceptible than males. If the level of casein was reduced to 10%, the blood pressure returned to normal (Engen and Swenson 1969). Yamori et al. (1979b) were the first to show the harmful influence of proteins on hypertension; they were working on *SHR-Ss* rats, a genetically hypertensive strain. Between the ages of 10 weeks and 10 months the animals were fed two types of diet: a Japanese diet and a National Institutes of Health (NIH) open formula diet. The main difference between the two diets was their amino acid content of 17% and 24%, respectively. With the Japanese diet, 56% of the animals died or exhibited stroke symptoms, whereas with the NIH diet, none of the rats suffered from cerebral lesions (Yamori et al. 1979b). Detailed investigation of the nutritional composition of these diets led to the conclusion that the protective factor in the NIH diet was the higher protein content. The results of this study have been confirmed by other experiments (Yamori et al. 1984a, 1984b). In the NIH diet, methionine was the only predominant essential amino acid, and minor amino acids such as taurine, hydroxyproline, ornithine, and methylhistidine were also more abundant than in the Japanese diet. Supplementing a Japanese diet with additional protein results in a significant reduction in the incidence of stroke (Yamori et al. 1982).

A soybean protein diet has been shown to cause a light increase in blood pressure (Bursztyn and Vas Dias 1985) or to be without effect (Bursztyn and Firth 1975; Bursztyn and Husbands 1980). In spontaneously hypertensive (*SHR*) male and female rats, the incidence of hypertension was lower when they were fed on soybean protein than with casein although both casein and soybean protein diets induced renal hypertrophy when compared to a chow diet. These effects were independent of gender (Nevala et al. 2000). A high-protein diet has a beneficial effect on the development of hypertension and stroke incidence in *SHR* rats (Zicha and Kunes 1999). Likewise, in *SHR-SP* rats, a protein-rich diet reduced hypertension and the incidence of stroke, particularly if the hypertension was enhanced by excess dietary salt (Yamori 1981; Yamori et al. 1982, 1984b). In rats subjected to prenatal protein restriction, blood pressure is already high after weaning due to corticoid secretion, and adrenalectomy lowers the blood pressure (Gardner et al. 1997). When *SHR-SP* rats were fed high-fat cholesterol diets with or without 3%-taurine supplementation, taurine not only suppressed reactive hypercholesterolemia but also attenuated the hypertension (Yamori et al. 1981c). In hypertensive rats, elevated blood pressure levels also decline and the incidence of stroke was reduced by taurine dietary supplementation (Usui et al. 1983). On the whole, these data once again demonstrate the importance of genetic factors, not only with regard to the effects of a protein diet, but also for the effects of the salt content of a diet, which are also dependent upon genetic characteristics.

Arterial hypertension had already been observed in common weanling rats fed over a period of 4 to 12 months on a diet composed of rice, fish, soybean products, and vegetables. According to the authors, the salt content of this diet (4% dry NaCl) was not sufficient to account for the elevation in blood pressure (Hilker et al. 1965). Replacing all the fish and soybean products with isocaloric substitutions of casein, dried milk powder, cornstarch, corn oil, and appropriate amounts of NaCl (4%) completely cancels the effect of the diet on blood pressure and renal structure (Lichton and Wenkam 1967).

These results have been confirmed by other experiments. In weanling rats of a *Wistar*-derived strain that were fed for 3 months on a fresh diet of rice, skipjack tuna, soybean products, and vegetables simulating the Japanese diet (4% dry NaCl), blood pressure levels were increased, whereas no elevation occurred in similar animals fed on a control diet or a fresh diet without fish and soybean products as well as in pair-fed animals on a salt diet (4% NaCl) and 20% casein or 2.9% soybean proteins plus 17.1% casein. The consumption of fresh or defatted fish (skipjack tuna) is therefore clearly responsible for the hypertensive effect (Chakkaphak and Lichton 1970). However, the opposite effect was observed by Yamori et al. (1979a, 1979b, 1981a) since a diet supplemented with fish protein reduced both blood pressure levels and overall mortality in spontaneously hypertensive rats (*SHR*) and stroke-prone *SHR (SHR-SP)* rats. The data currently available concerning the possible effects of fish consumption on blood pressure levels are still contradictory. Moreover, with fish, other components such as dietary fats also have an influence on blood pressure.

The systolic blood pressure of normotensive *Wistar* rats was not influenced by various diets regardless of their content in casein, whey protein concentrates, skimmed milk protein concentrates, and dried yogurt; this contrasts with the effects of a chow diet or a soybean protein isolates diet (Yuan and Kitts 1993). However, the blood pressure levels of offspring were increased when normotensive mothers were fed on a low-protein diet (Langley and Jackson 1994; Petry et al. 1997).

Although intravenous infusion of 0.5 g/kg of arginine in children and 30 g in adult subjects resulted in decreased blood pressure levels in pulmonary and in salt-induced hypertension (Maxwell and Cooke 1998) in animal studies, the effect was not always significant, but this could possibly be explained by the anesthesia (Nakaki et al. 1990).

Making allowances for all dietary components is important. For example, the blood pressure of 10-week-old male *Sprague-Dawley* rats was 17% higher in rats fed on saturated fats (lard) and 8% higher in rats fed on polyunsaturated fats (corn oil) than in control rats (Kaufman et al. 1994). Moreover, dietary protein regulated the production of polyunsaturated fats, since in *SHR-SP* rats, casein, in comparison with soybean protein, stimulates linoleic acid and α-linolenic acid metabolism and the production of prostacyclin. The 20:3n-6 + 20:4n-6/18:n-6 ratio, the linoleic acid desaturation index of liver microsomes and in the aorta, was higher with casein (Ikeda et al. 1994). Likewise, the mineral content of diets (sodium, potassium, magnesium, calcium, and chloride) exerts a direct influence on blood pressure levels (Reusser et al. 1994).

5.1.1 SUMMARY

The effects of dietary protein have still not been clearly demonstrated in animal experiments. In rats that are genetically predisposed to hypertension, elevated protein levels would appear to reduce arterial hypertension. However, there are conflicting data concerning the influence of specific proteins (i.e., varied effects of diverse types of protein). In normotensive rats, blood pressure is not modified by either the quantity or the nature of proteins.

5.2 DATA ON HUMANS

5.2.1 EPIDEMIOLOGIC DATA

As in animal models, studies on human hypertension should take into account the influence of genetic factors (Yamori et al. 1981a; Cowley 1997; Rantala et al. 1997; Kurokawa and Okuda 1998; Luft 1998; Dominiczak et al. 1998; Gerber and Halberstein 1999; Gavras et al. 1999). The effect of diet on blood pressure in humans has been studied by several researchers (McDonald 1987).

Vegetarian populations have lower blood pressure than otherwise similar groups of omnivorous subjects (Malhotra 1970; Sacks et al. 1974; Armstrong et al. 1977; Rouse et al. 1983a, 1983b; Rouse and Beilin 1984). In addition, the blood pressure of vegetarians rises when they include meat in their diets for a period of time (Donaldson 1924; Sacks et al. 1981). However, in one study, this effect was not observed (White 1981). When omnivorous individuals consume a vegetarian diet, their blood pressure has been shown to decrease (Bursztyn 1982; Rouse et al. 1983a,

1983b). The effect of a vegetarian diet on blood pressure compared to an omnivorous diet is chiefly due to differences in fat and dietary fiber consumption rather than to the nature of proteins (Rouse and Beilin 1984; Bursztyn and Vas Dias 1985). In the dietary factors assessed in the Northern and Southern China Farmers Survey, the average daily intake of animal protein, including fish protein, was very low in the Yushien and Hanzhong groups, but relatively higher among Wuming farmers who have the lowest prevalence of hypertension (Tao et al. 1984). The relation between animal protein consumption and blood pressure is controversial (World Health Organization 1983; Burstyn 1982), in spite of the favorable effect of fish and animal protein observed in *SHR* rats (Yamori et al. 1981c; Yamori et al. 1984a, 1984b). Recently, Yamori et al. (1996) have again demonstrated epidemiologic evidence supporting the beneficial effect of fish protein intake on blood pressure in various populations worldwide. Nevertheless, the hypotensive effects of fish fats resulting from their ω-3 fatty-acid content must be considered (Beilin 1993). According to McCarron (1982), in human studies, it is difficult to alter one nutrient without changing the others. Although potassium, calcium, and protein are negatively correlated with blood pressure independently of several confounding variables, none of these are strongly related to blood pressure (Reed 1984).

A negative correlation has been shown between protein intake and systolic and diastolic blood pressures in several epidemiologic surveys analyzed by Obarzanek et al. (1996), in 12 cross-sectional studies, and in two longitudinal studies (Liu et al. 1992, 1993, 1996).

- The Japanese Rural Farming Men and Women Study. In this study of 1,120 men and women, the negative relationship between systolic blood pressure and the amount of animal protein consumed was only observed in men (Yamori et al. 1981b), thus confirming previous suspicions (Kimura 1977).
- In 61 young men and women, systolic blood pressure decreased as total protein consumption was increased (Pellum and Medeiros 1983).
- Japanese study. In the above study, a negative relationship between systolic blood pressure and the amount of animal protein consumed was only observed in men (Kihara et al. 1984). These data concord with the results of Yamori et al. (1981b).
- Honolulu Heart Study. This study of 6,496 Japanese-American men, a negative relationship was observed between systolic and diastolic blood pressures and the amount of total protein consumed (Reed et al. 1985).
- Chinese study. In this investigation of 2,672 adult men and women, a negative relationship was found between systolic blood pressure and the amount of animal protein consumed (Zhou et al. 1989).
- Study of 402 adult male twins. In this work, increased diastolic blood pressure levels were correlated with increasing total protein intake (Havlik et al. 1990).
- Intersalt Study. Based on 1,190 adult men and women, a negative relationship was observed between systolic blood pressure and the amount of total and animal protein consumed (Elliott et al. 1991).

- Intersalt Study. Based on 2,325 adult men and women, a negative relationship was found between systolic blood pressure and the amount of total protein consumed (Dyer et al. 1992).
- MRFIT Study. Based on 11,342 adult men, investigators observed a negative relationship between systolic blood pressure and the amount of total protein consumed (Stamler et al. 1992).
- British Nutritional Survey. In this study of 1,992 adult men and women, a negative relationship between diastolic blood pressure and the amount of protein consumed was observed in both men and women, and between systolic blood pressure and total protein consumed in women (Elliott et al. 1992).
- Chinese study. Based on 705 adult men and women, a negative relationship was found between systolic blood pressure and the amount of animal protein consumed (Zhou et al. 1994).
- CARDIA Study. In this study of 3,809 adult men and women, a negative relationship in black men and in white and black women was observed between diastolic blood pressure and obesity (Liu et al. 1992).
- Western Electric Study. Based on 1,804 adult men, a direct relationship was observed between diastolic blood pressure and vegetable protein consumption (Liu et al. 1993).

On the whole, these epidemiologic data confirm those observed in *SHR* rats (Zicha and Kunes 1999).

A loading dose of methionine increased the plasma homocysteine levels and in the Hordaland Study, a positive relationship was observed between methionine and hyperhomocysteinemia (Nygärd et al. 1995, 1999). Likewise, plasma homocysteine levels were higher in patients with peripheral arterial occlusive disease (Malinow et al. 1989), or hypertension with cerebral infarction, or cerebral infarction without hypertension (Araki 1989). This correlation existed only in younger men and women and not in older individuals (>65 years) of both sexes (Bates et al. 1997). However, in normotensive older adults, elevated homocysteine levels were independently correlated to isolated systolic hypertension in the study by Sutton-Tyrell et al. (1997) and would appear to be an independent risk factor for atherosclerosis. Nevertheless, in elderly subjects, no correlation was found between homocysteine levels and myocardial infarction (Dalery et al. 1995). A methionine-rich diet may well modify blood pressure levels (Perry 1999), but this hypothesis has yet to be confirmed by further studies.

5.2.2 EXPERIMENTAL DATA

5.2.2.1 Nature of Proteins

As was shown by the results of a study on experimental data on humans described in Section 3.2.1, no modification in blood pressure was observed after 2 years of either a casein- or a soybean-protein diet (Lembke et al. 1983). In vegetarians, daily dietary supplementation with 58 g of a mixture of soybean and wheat proteins and 7 g of rice protein had no effect on blood pressure levels (Sacks et al. 1984). Likewise, in groups of healthy young adults, soybean protein or casein dietary supplementation caused no variation in blood pressure levels (Brussard et al. 1981). In 32 young volunteers of both sexes, the introduction of textured vegetable proteins (TVP) into the diet did not affect blood pressure levels (Bursztyn and Vas Dias 1985); the dietary soybean protein level was, however, relatively weak. Soybean protein supplementation (20 g containing 34 mg of phytoestrogens) in the diet of 51 nonhypercholesterolemic, nonhypertensive perimenopausal women significantly reduced the diastolic blood pressure level (−5 mmHg) (Washburn et al. 1999). In a study of 22 healthy control subjects and 18 age-matched hypertensive patients, ingestion of 1 g/kg weight of tuna (40 g of protein) had no effect on systolic or diastolic blood pressure in controls but, in hypertensive subjects, resulted in significant reductions in both systolic and diastolic pressure levels over 2 hours, and reached lower levels than in the control period without protein and 3 hours after protein ingestion, but not lower than in control subjects. Hypertensive subjects have attenuated natriuretic and plasma free-dopamine responses and less free-epinephrine increase (Kuchel 1998).

The effects of meat and nonmeat protein sources on blood pressure were studied in a 12-week randomized study of 50 healthy men and women with normal blood pressure. No significant baseline or end-of-trial blood pressure differences were observed between the meat and nonmeat groups (Prescott et al. 1987, 1988).

In a placebo-controlled study conducted in 30 elderly hypertensive subjects, daily ingestion of 95 mL of sour milk for 8 weeks significantly decreased both systolic and diastolic blood pressures. Sour milk contains two kinds of tripeptides: Val-Pro-Pro (1.5 mg/100 g) and Ile-Pro-Pro (1.1mg/100 g), which inhibit the angiotensin I-converting enzyme (ACE) and have been shown to exert a hypertensive effect in *SHR* rats (Nakamura et al. 1995b). They have been isolated in the aorta of rats after oral administration of sour milk (Masuda et al. 1996).

With an elevated dietary salt level, the pathologic sequelae of hypertension may be reduced or increased, depending on the type of protein (Yamori et al. 1979a, 1979b).

Despite these studies, Bursztyn (1987) did not expand on the possible influence of the amount and/or nature of protein intake on the risk of high blood pressure in his book on the relationship between nutrition and blood pressure. Likewise, two recent reviews of nutritional factors failed to mention the effects of protein on blood pressure (McGregor 1999) and as a risk factor for stroke (Gariballa 2000). According to two recent general reviews on dietary protein and blood pressure published by Lovenberg and Yamori (1990, 1995) and Obarzanek et al. (1996), although a large amount of data from experiments and epidemiologic surveys would appear to support the effects of protein on blood pressure, they have not as yet been confirmed unequivocally. Further well-controlled studies and trials are still necessary to provide clear arguments for or against the protein–blood pressure hypothesis.

5.2.2.2 Amino Acids

5.2.2.2.1 Arginine

After an oral arginine load, 40% was degraded in the intestine, hepatic uptake accounted for 15%, and 45% was available in the systemic circulation (Wu and Morris 1998). In 40 healthy males, serum creatinine and urine L-arginine were shown to be negatively correlated to blood pressure levels (Penttinen et al. 2000). L-Arginine also reduced blood pressure in salt-sensitive subjects (Campese et al. 1997). Intravenous infusion of 0.5 g/kg of arginine in children and 30 g in adult subjects resulted in decreased blood pressure levels in pulmonary and in salt-induced hypertension (Maxwell and Cooke 1998). Local infusion of L-arginine increases the response to endothelium-dependent vasodilators in healthy subjects and patients with hypercholesterolemia (Imaizumi et al. 1992; Panza et al. 1993; Creager et al. 1992). The results of trials investigating the effects of local infusion of L-arginine on blood pressure are discordant: blood pressure was shown to decrease in normotensive (Hishikawa et al. 1992; Kanno et al. 1992; Bode-Böger et al. 1994) and hypertensive subjects (Ebel et al. 1993; Hishikawa et al. 1993), whereas it remained unaltered in hypercholesterolemic subjects (Creager et al. 1992; Baudoin et al. 1993). Infusion of L- or D-arginine in the forearm vascular bed of control subjects and patients with essential hypertension or insulin-dependent diabetes increased the local concentration of arginine, but was without effect on blood flow or the vasodilator response to acetylcholine (MacAllister et al. 1995).

Intravenous infusion of L-arginine (500 mg/kg over 30 minutes) caused rapid-onset reduction of systolic and diastolic blood pressure in five healthy males and five hypertensive patients. Twenty minutes after cessation of infusion, blood pressure returned to previous levels. Intravenous infusion of 0.5 g/kg of arginine in children and 30 g in adult subjects resulted in decreased blood pressure levels in pulmonary and in salt-induced hypertension (Maxwell and Cooke 1998). L-Arginine intravenous infusion (500 mg/kg over 30 minutes) reduced mean blood pressure (from 81.2 to 74.0 mmHg) and renal vascular resistance in ten healthy male volunteers but increased heart rate (from 60 to 69 beats/minute) and renal flow (from 616.6 to 701.0 mL/minute). Serum angiotensin-converting enzyme and plasma angiotensin II levels were reduced (Higashi et al. 1995). The reduction in blood pressure is probably due to release of endothelium-derived relaxing factor that regulates vascular tone. Thus, arginine induces relaxation of smooth muscle cells within vascular walls (Ignarro 1989a, 1989b).

5.2.2.2.2 Taurine

In patients with congenital heart disease, intravenous infusion of taurine significantly reduces both systolic and diastolic blood pressure levels in the aorta but not in the pulmonary artery where blood flow is diminished (Nishimoto et al. 1983). Dietary taurine supplementation (6 g/day for 6 months) in hypertensive patients on a low-salt diet reduced blood pressure, whereas urinary excretion of taurine and sodium increased significantly. The Na/K ratio and urinary volume are both enhanced (Kohashi et al. 1983). Likewise, dietary taurine supplementation (6 g/day for 16 months) in elderly hypertensive patients increased taurine serum concentrations, and produced a weak but nonsignificant reduction in blood pressure levels. Serum uric acid, phospholipid, β-lipoprotein and free fatty-acid concentrations were also reduced (Himeno et al. 1984). With the same protocol, blood pressure levels have been shown to decrease in four normotensive and five hypertensive elderly patients hospitalized for stroke (Usui et al. 1983). The lowest level of taurine urinary excretion and the highest level of severe hypertension were observed in Tibetans who never ate fish for religious reasons. In contrast, the frequency of hypertension among the Japanese population living in northeastern Japan, whose salt intake is close to that of Tibetans, is 50% less than that of Tibetans. In this latter population, a taurine supplement (3 g/day) for a 2-month period significantly decreased both systolic and diastolic blood pressure levels in 11 mild hypertensive and borderline hypertensive subjects who took taurine regularly (Yamori et al. 1996).

5.2.2.3 Isoflavones

Two crossover trials have demonstrated the hypotensive capacity of isoflavones. Diastolic blood pressure was significantly reduced (−5 mmHg) in 51 perimenopausal women consuming 20 grams of soybean protein isolates containing 34 mg of isoflavones (Washburn et al. 1999). Likewise, in 62 women receiving either 25 g of casein or 25 g of soybean protein isolates containing different concentrations of isoflavones (3 to 62 mg isoflavones per 25 g of proteins), the diastolic blood pressure decreased progressively as the isoflavone dose increased. However, in a similar experiment in 94 men, isoflavone supplements had no effect (Crouse et al. 1999).

5.3 MECHANISMS

The following mechanisms could explain the effects discussed above (Lovenberg 1984):

- Role of sympathetic nervous system in regulating protein synthesis in small vessels
- Effect of dietary protein on natriuresis
- Effects of casein peptides
- Effects of amino acids and amino acid metabolites that may serve as neurohumoral agents

5.3.1 EFFECTS OF SYMPATHETIC NERVOUS SYSTEM

Studies on the incorporation of amino acids into proteins in small resistance vessels in *SHR-SP* rats have shown an increase in vascular protein synthesis even before the animals become hypertensive (Yamabe and Lovenberg 1974). The increase in sympathetic nerve activity, which doubles the rate of amino acid incorporation into vascular noncollagen protein, is one of the early stages in the development of hypertension in the rat. This enhancement can be suppressed by pharmacologic (ganglionic blockade) or surgical (splanchnichotomy) interruption of sympathetic nerve traffic to the vessels. When hypertensive rats are treated with hydralazine — a potent antihypertensive drug — blood pressure levels decrease, the activity of the sympathetic nerve system increases, and the rate of amino acid incorporation is greater (Yamori et al. 1976b). The trophic effect of sympathetic nerves has also been demonstrated by the decreased rate of amino acid incorporation into proteins within the vessel of denervated rabbit ear arteries (Bevan 1975), and by the reduced wall-to-lumen ratio in cerebral blood vessels within the denervated hemispheres of hypertensive rats fed on low-protein Japanese diets (Sadoshima et al. 1981). Thus, the enhanced amino acid incorporation into the vascular proteins of hypertensive rats is due to a trophic effect of the sympathetic nerves rather than a consequence of hypertension (Lovenberg 1984). These effects have been observed in rats fed on a low-protein Japanese diet and in specific animal species. They may well differ in other animal species or with other protein sources.

5.3.2 Dietary Protein and Natriuresis

In both normotensive and hypertensive rats, increasing the dietary protein level enhances both urine volume and the amount of sodium excreted, although the mechanism behind these effects is unknown (Ikeda et al. 1989) and still speculative (Lovenberg and Yamori 1990). One study in human volunteers with a family history of hypertension has shown that a high-protein diet may counteract the adverse effects of excessive salt intake, although in rats it induces a diuretic and natriuretic effect (Nara et al. 1978). In the previously described study by Kuchel (1998), hypertensive subjects, compared to controls, were shown to have a significant increase in plasma 3,4-dihydroxyphenylalanine sulfate, epinephrine sulfate, dopamine sulfate/free dopamine ratio, and plasma free dopamine. The rise in plasma dopamine was due to the larger amount of tyrosine from dietary protein. The natriuretic and plasma free-dopamine responses and free-epinephrine increases were attenuated.

5.3.3 Effects of Amino Acids

Numerous hypotheses have been put forward to explain the possible effects of proteins on hypertension, including a potential role for certain amino acids and the impact on the onset of hypertension of different amino acid compositions.

5.3.3.1 Arginine

The mechanisms behind the effects of arginine on atherosclerosis in animals and in humans are extensively described in Section 4.1.4.1 and Section 4.2.2.2, respectively. The hemodynamic effects of arginine are dependent on the production of nitric oxide, which is derived from the terminal guanidino nitrogen of L-arginine (Ignarro 1989b). L-Arginine is also a precursor for the synthesis of endothelium-derived relaxing factor(s) (EDRF) from cultured endothelial cells *in vitro* (Palmer et al. 1988; Schmidt et al. 1988; Sakuma et al. 1988). A positive correlation has been observed between dietary protein levels and the production of nitric oxide in rats (Wu et al. 1999). Girerd et al. (1990) demonstrated that the vasodilation of hind-limb resistance vessels in cholesterol-fed rabbits is impaired, and that exogenous L-arginine normalizes the endothelium-dependent vasodilation of these vessels (Girerd et al. 1990). In normocholesterolemic rabbits subjected to environmental tobacco smoke, chronic administration of dietary L-arginine prevents endothelial dysfunction (Hutchinson et al. 1997). Because arginine inhibits the angiotensin-converting enzyme, the plasma concentrations of angiotensin II have been shown to be reduced in humans after intravenous infusion of arginine (Higashi et al. 1995). In animal studies, the effect of intravenous infusion of arginine was not always significant perhaps on account of the anesthesia (Nakaki et al. 1990).

5.3.3.2 Lysine

Lysine was more rapidly incorporated into the protein of small blood vessels in *SHR*s than in normotensive control animals (Yamabe and Lovenberg 1974); this incorporation is controlled by the sympathetic nervous system (Yamori et al. 1976b). Animal proteins rich in sulfur amino acids decreased blood pressure levels and the incidence of stroke; likewise in *SHR-SP* rats, the addition of lysine, methionine, and particularly taurine to the diet had the same effects. However, to date, none of these hypotheses have been clearly proven (Yamori et al. 1984b; review in Lovenberg and Yamori 1990). A negative correlation between the ratio of urinary sulfate to urea and blood pressure has been observed (Kihara et al. 1984; Zhou et al. 1994).

5.3.3.3 Methionine

Methionine supplementation reduced the incidence of cerebral lesions in stroke-prone rats on a Japanese diet (Yamori et al. 1981c).

5.3.3.4 Taurine

A diet supplemented with fish protein decreased blood pressure in *SHR* and *SHR-SP*; the mortality rate was also reduced (Yamori et al. 1979a, 1979b; Yamori 1981c). As fish protein is rich in taurine, the effect of taurine has been studied (Nara et al. 1978). Taurine supplementation of the diet of *SHR-SP* rats, in which the liver and plasma taurine levels are lower than those of *SHR* rats, induced a slight decrease in blood pressure (Nara et al. 1978; Zaki et al. 1980; Yamori et al. 1981c; Himeno et al. 1984), reduced the incidence of apoplexy or brain infarct, and lowered the triacyl-glycerol serum level. The serum free-cholesterol concentration was higher in taurine-supplemented *SHR-SP* rats than in *SHR-SP* control subjects (Himeno et al. 1984). In these rats, administration of taurine during pre- and postnatal periods produced a blood pressure reduction that persisted until 3 months of age (Horie et al. 1987). Dopa-decarboxylase activity in vessels and brain parenchyma that was decreased in *SHR-SP* and *SHR* rats (Himeno et al. 1984) may well be restored by dietary taurine supplementation.

The various mechanisms explaining the effects of taurine are complicated and as yet unidentified (Yamori et al. 1981c; Schaffer et al. 2000). However, dietary supplementation with taurine increased serotonergic nerve activity that was reduced in control *SHR-SP* rats (Himeno et al. 1984). Excessive urinary norepinephrine excretion in *SHR-SP* was significantly reduced by taurine-rich diets (Ikeda et al. 1989). Recently, Schaffer et al. (2000) reviewed the mechanism of the increasing effect of taurine on natriuresis and diuresis and also the reduced activity of angiotensin II.

5.3.3.5 Tyrosine and Tryptophan

Tyrosine and tryptophan hydroxylase are the limiting enzymes in the synthesis of the neurotransmitters, respectively catecholamines and serotonin. A high dose of L-tyrosine or L-tryptophan increased the turnover of catecholamines or serotonin in specific brain regions, and significantly reduced the blood pressure levels in adult *SHR* rats (Sved et al. 1979, 1982); central administration of tyrosine reduced blood pressure (Yamori et al. 1980). However, although L-tryptophan is the only form with a depressor effect, L- and D-tryptophan increased brain serotonin concentrations. Moreover, in both normotensive and hypertensive rats, small doses of L-tryptophan resulted in a mild increase in blood pressure levels, whereas large doses reduced these levels but only in hypertensive rats. Further studies are therefore still required to clarify this subject (Sved et al. 1982; Lovenberg 1984).

A diet supplemented with tryptophan provides partial protection against arterial hypertension, the development of cardiac hypertrophy in hypertensive and DOCA-salt rat models (Fregly and Fater 1986; Fregly et al. 1987), and against the hypertension caused by impaired renal function (Fregly et al. 1988). Chronic dietary intake of tryptophan (50 g/kg of food) also reduces the development of hypertension in inbred *Dahl salt-sensitive* (*DS/JR*) rats, but has no effect on the patterns of development of systolic hypertension in normotensive controls, inbred *DR/JR* rats, or outbred parental *Sprague-Dawley* rats. A high-tryptophan diet inhibits the cardiac hypertrophy generally associated with salt-induced hypertension. Although the hypotensive effect of tryptophan has been clearly demonstrated (Nakaki et al. 1990; Nakaki and Kato 1994) its mechanism is still unknown (Lark et al. 1990).

Five hours after a protein meal, natriuresis was increased and both systolic and diastolic blood pressure levels were reduced in hypertensive but not in normotensive subjects. This effect is related to an increase in plasma dopamine due to the larger amount of tyrosine from dietary protein. Dopamine may well inhibit the action of aldosterone and renin (Kuchel 1998).

5.4 EFFECTS OF CASEIN PEPTIDES

Some peptides of different forms of casein, α-lactalbumin bovine or β-lactoglobulin, have a hypertensive effect. Some are indicated by name and sequence but others only by sequence. The nature and the effects of the following peptides have been reviewed by Maubois and Leonil (1989), Shah (2000), and Leonil et al. (2001):

- From bovine casein α_{s1}: α_{s1}-casokinin 5 (23–27), α_{s1}-casokinin 12 (23–34), α_{s1}-casokinin 7 (28–34), α_{s1}-casokinin 2 (91–92), α_{s1}-casokinin 6 (194–199)
- From bovine casein α_{s2} bovine: peptides (189–192, 190–197, 198–202)

- From casein β: β-casokinin (43–69,; 158–175, 168–175); β-casokinin 7 (177–183); β-casokinin (191–209); human β-casokinin (39–52; 43–52)
- From bovine α-lactalbumin: α-lactokinin (50–51, 50–53, 50–52, 99–108, 104–108, 105–110)
- From β-lactoglobulin: lactokinin (78–80, 142–148), β-lactorphin (102–105, 102–103, 104–105); lactotensin (146–149)

Certain experiments have proven the antihypertensive effects of these casein peptides.

The 177–183 sequence of bovine casein β inhibits the angiotensin-converting enzyme of angiotensin (Maruyama et al. 1985). Angiotensin may therefore not be converted into angiotensin II, a potent vasoconstrictor. Hydrolysis of bovine casein by a protease of *Lactobacillus helveticus* releases numerous peptides that have an antihypertensive effect in *SHR* rats (Yamamoto et al. 1994) and perhaps in humans (Hata et al. 1996). The efficacy of antihypertensive peptides from the B variant of casein α_{s1} is situated in position 23–27; 23–34; 194–199 and has been demonstrated in spontaneously hypertensive rats (*SHR*) (Maruyama et al. 1987). Likewise, the peptides of casein α_{s2} (189–192, 190–197, 198–202) have been shown to exert antihypertensive effects (Maeno et al. 1996).

A large number of sequences of bovine β-lactoglobulin — such as in bovine α-lactalbumin, and principally dipeptides, tripeptides, and one hexapeptide, called lactokinins — also have antihypertensive effects (Mullaly et al. 1996, 1997).

L-Valyl-L-propyl-L-proline (Val-Pro-Pro) and L-isoleucyl-L-prolyl-L-proline (Ile-Pro-Pro) two angiotensin I-converting enzyme (ACE) inhibitory tripeptides isolated from sour milk, prepared by fermenting milk with *Lactobacillus helveticus* and *Saccharomyces cerevisiae*, are responsible for the majority of the ACE inhibitory activity of sour milk (Nakamura 1995a). Six hours after the absorption of these tripeptides, systolic blood pressure levels of spontaneously hypertensive rats (*SHR*) have been observed to decrease. The activity of the angiotensin I-converting enzyme was significantly reduced and the presence of these tripeptides was detected in abdominal aorta (Masuda et al. 1996).

However, the effects of these peptides are less potent than the pharmacologic products currently in use.

5.5 CONCLUSION

Epidemiologic studies have shown that blood pressure levels are lower in vegetarian than in omnivorous individuals. The data relating to the effects of protein level intake or the nature of protein consumed on blood pressure levels are conflicting. The roles of the food environment and a potential genetic predisposition must be taken into consideration. Various mechanisms have been suggested to explain the effects of proteins: the increased natridiuresis following high protein intake, a very probable role of certain peptides (particularly casein), on the conversion of angiotensin I to angiotensin II, the increase in sympathetic nervous system activity such as the effects of various amino acids. Arginine, an inhibitor of the angiotensin-converting enzyme, increases vasodilation and lysine, taurine, tryptophan and tyrosine may well have hypotensive effects. Blood pressure levels are decreased by increasing the production of nitric oxide; arginine reduces blood pressure levels. Sulfur amino acids such as methionine and taurine decrease blood pressure levels. Taurine, tryptophan, and tyrosine modify blood pressure levels by enhancing the neurotransmitters, particularly serotonin, and also interacting with catecholamines. Nevertheless, further studies are still required to clearly define the respective importance of each of these mechanisms.

6 Data on Thrombosis in Animals and Humans

6.1 EFFECTS OF PROTEINS

Based on similarities between milk and blood coagulation (Jollès 1975, Jollès et al. 1978, Jollès and Henschen 1982) and the functional similarities between the fibrinogen γ-chain and κ-casein or its glycomacropeptide segment, the effects of proteins on coagulation factors have been widely investigated (Mazoyer et al. 1992; review by Rutherfurd and Gill 2000). The level of dietary protein modifies platelet aggregation, which is increased in rats consuming a low-protein diet (10% casein) in comparison to a control group (20% casein) and a group on a high-protein diet (60% casein). The production of thromboxane A_2 is lower and prostaglandins I_2 higher in the low-protein group (Morita et al. 1985).

In female *New Zealand white* rabbits, the addition of walnut meal or soybean protein to a cholesterol-free diet reduced platelet aggregation, whereas it was enhanced by casein. Walnut meal lowered platelet aggregation induced by adenosine diphosphate (ADP) and collagen, whereas a soybean meal diet modified only the washed platelet aggregation. The relative effects of casein, soybean, and walnut protein were strongly correlated with the lysine/arginine ratio of the protein and with the HDL/LDL ratio. None of the three diets had any effect on coagulation tests (Ravel et al. 1988).

6.1.1 MILK PEPTIDES FROM CASEIN, SOYBEAN PROTEIN, LACTALBUMIN, LACTOTRANSFERRIN, AND OTHER PROTEINS

Some milk peptides have antithrombotic effects, which have been reviewed by Maubois and Leonil (1989), Shah (2000), and Leonil et al. (et al.2001). Bleeding and coagulation times were diminished in adult rats fed for 2 weeks on a semi-purified diet containing 18 g or 50 g or 100 g/day of casein and lactalbumin. This effect was more significant in those consuming the largest amount of proteins. Platelet aggregation was not modified, nor were prothrombin, thromboplastin, or thrombin times. It would therefore appear that these proteins act on other factors of coagulation (Chan et al. 1993). The relative effects of casein, soybean, and walnut proteins on platelet aggregation in rabbits were strongly correlated with the lysine/arginine ratio of the proteins and the HDL/LDL ratio. The addition of walnut meal to the diet decreased platelet aggregation and total serum cholesterol levels (Ravel et al. 1988).

A peptide composed of six kinds of amino acids (Asp-Glu-Gly-Leu-Phe-Arg) prepared from soybean protein inhibits platelet aggregation (Kanazawa 1996). The bovine caseinoglycopeptide (residues 106-169), the C-terminal part of κ-casein, inhibited the von Willebrand factor-dependent platelet aggregation in a dose-dependent manner. This caseinoglycopeptide selectively binds the platelet membrane glycoprotein GPIb alpha, which contains the von Willebrand factor–binding site (Chabance et al. 1997).

Several similarities have been observed between the clotting process of blood and milk and between fibrinogen and κ-casein. There are a number of matching characteristics between the sequence of cow κ-casein, the substrate of chymosin (milk-clotting process), and the γ-chain of human fibrinogen (Jollès 1975; Jollès and Henschen 1982; Jollès et al. 1986; Jollès and Caen 1991; Caen et al. 1991, 1992; Fiat et al. 1993). To date the activities of other caseins on thrombosis and aggregation have not been elucidated.

Several peptides of bovine κ-casein have been shown to have antithrombotic effects. The undecapeptide of sequence 106 to 116 inhibits fibrinogen binding to the platelet receptors and ADP-induced aggregation. Several caseinglycomacropeptides (bovine κ-casein residues 106 to 169) have demonstrated either antithrombotic or antiaggregant activities or both. In the guinea pig, numerous peptides of ovine and human κ-casein have been shown to possess these properties, the human peptides being the most potent (Bal dit Sollier et al. 1996). These κ-casein peptides follow:

- One decapeptide, Met-Ala-Ile-Pro-Pro-Lys-Lys-Asn-Gln-Asp-Lys (residues 106 to 116 of cow-milk κ-casein). This peptide, originating from chymosin, acts on caseinoglycomacropeptide, residues 106 to 169 of cow-milk κ-casein or casein. *In vitro*, it inhibits ADP-dependent human platelet aggregation and platelet binding with fibrinogen (Jollès et al. 1986, 1993; Maubois et al. 1991; Caen et al. 1992). This effect is maintained if the peptide is reduced to a pentapeptide, KNQDK[+] (Caen et al. 1992), and in rat experiments, intravenous injection of residues 106 to 116 reduces thrombogenesis by 65% (Drouet et al. 1990).
- One pentapeptide residue 112 to 116 (Caen et al. 1992) or 113 to 116 (Jollès et al. 1986), which inhibits platelet aggregation less strongly *in vitro* than the decapeptide.

The inhibition of platelet aggregation is greater when a lysine residue is included in the peptide. For example, the sequence 112 to 116, which possesses a lysine residue, is 222 times more active than peptide 113 to 116 (Maubois et al. 1991). The C-terminal caseinoglycopeptides (residues 106 to 171) of ovine κ-casein, inhibit thrombin and collagen-induced platelet aggregation in a dose-dependent manner (Qian et al 1995b).

Human lactotransferrin is antithrombotic, and sheep and human lactotransferrin inhibit platelet aggregation. Peptides situated at the N-terminal extremities of these lactotransferrin also exert antiaggregation activities: sheep lactotransferrin (sequences 27 to 33), human lactoferrin (octapeptide 30 to 37) (Leveugle et al. 1993), and residues 28 to 34 (Qian et al. 1995a).

One tetrapeptide (39 to 42, KRDS residues) inhibits fibrinogen binding to platelets and platelet aggregation *in vitro*; this effect is ADP dependent (Mazoyer et al.

1990, 1992). This tetrapeptide also inhibits thromboxane synthesis. These effects have been observed in models of experimental thrombosis in various animal species, including rats, guinea pigs, and dogs, and with caseinoglycopeptides of three species (cow, ewe, and human), which are antithrombotic, the most potent being the human form (Drouet et al. 1990; Wu et al. 1992; Caen et al. 1992; Bal dit Sollier et al. 1990, 1996). The longevity of the antithrombotic effect (80 m) is greater than that of the small peptides (100 to 200 seconds) (Bal dit Sollier et al. 1990).

In vivo, these peptides have also been shown to exert significant antithrombotic activities in guinea pigs with arterial lesions (Caen et al. 1992). They may have a potential preventive effect by inhibiting fibrinogen binding to the platelets. Ewe caseinoglycopeptides are also antithrombotic although the human form remains the most potent (Bal dit Sollier et al. 1996).

In 15 middle-aged women with mild hypercholesterolemia, daily intake of soybean protein (12 g) or low-fat milk protein (14 g) for 1 month each did not change the serum total cholesterol, HDL-cholesterol, apo A-I, A-II, B, C-II, C-III, E, and triacylglycerol levels or platelet aggregation induced by ATP and hemostatic markers, with the exception of plasminogen activator inhibitor I and D-dimer. With soybean protein intake, D-dimer is significantly lower than with milk intake. Soybean proteins may therefore have a favorable effect on the hemostatic system (Waki et al. 1996).

Soy cream suppresses platelet aggregation in heavy smokers and patients with myocardial infarction. A peptide of six amino acids with antiplatelet aggregation capacities has been isolated (Kanazawa and Osanai (1998).

Although the data from experimental studies support the hypothesis of a correlation between food components and thrombosis, in contrast, no association between these components and hemostatic factors, with the exception of fibrinogen, has been established in epidemiologic studies (Pearson et al. 1997). The individual variations observed in animals and humans are due to the modulation of coagulation factors by genetic factors, lipids, and proteins (Bernardi et al. 1997).

6.1.2 IMMUNOGLOBULINS

Anti–milk protein immunoglobulins show a strong binding affinity to platelets and promote thrombosis, especially in arterioles (Davis and Holtz 1969; Henson 1973). Elevated production of immunoglobulins IgA in response to a normal consumption of milk proteins could be due to a genetic factor (Muscari et al. 1989).

6.1.3 AMINO ACIDS

6.1.3.1 Arginine

L-Arginine is the substrate for nitric oxide synthesis. Nitric oxide (NO) is a potent platelet inhibitor and it improves endothelium-dependent vasodilation (Ignarro 1989a, 1989b; Kugiyama et al. 1990; Chin et al. 1992; Adams et al. 1995). Platelet adhesion to collagen fibrils and endothelial cell matrix is completely inhibited by NO (Radomski et al. 1987). Oxidized LDL impairs the release of NO and predisposes to vasoconstriction, leukocyte deposit, platelet-adhesion, and aggregation (Moncada et al. 1991; review in Chen et al. 1996). Deposition of T-lymphocytes and macrophages provokes various inflammatory and immunologic reactions, which in turn promotes the process of atherogenesis (Russel 1990). The stimulation of platelet activity is due mainly to inhibition of NO-synthase activity (Chen et al. 1996).

The L-arginine-nitric oxide pathway is involved in the effects of oxidized LDL, which stimulates platelets function primarily by diminishing NO-synthase expression as well as decreasing the uptake of arginine. Oxidized LDL promotes vasoconstriction and platelet aggregation (Chen et al. 1996). These effects of L-arginine have been clearly demonstrated by experiments in rabbits. Male *New Zealand white* rabbits were fed for 10 weeks a chow diet enriched with 1% cholesterol supplemented or not with either L-arginine (inducing a twofold increase in plasma arginine), or L-methionine (0.9%, a six-fold enrichment compared to the normal diet). Cholesterol levels were equally increased in the cholesterol- and arginine-fed animals. Plasma arginine concentrations doubled in the arginine group. Maximum platelet aggregation initiated by ADP in controls and methionine- and cholesterol-fed animals was similar, whereas that of arginine-fed rabbits was significantly reduced. This effect would appear to be due to the metabolization of L-arginine to nitrite oxide (Tsao et al. 1994a). In the same species of adult rabbits, supplementation or not of a chow cholesterol (2%) diet with L-arginine (2.25% solution) for 7 or 14 weeks increased plasma arginine levels, reduced the development of atherosclerosis in the descending aorta, and preserved endothelium-dependent vasodilation in the resistance arteries. These effects were all reported in both male and female subjects with the exception of vascular reactivity preservation, which was observed in male but not in female subjects. However, these treatment effects were not sustained (Jeremy et al. 1996).

In healthy (Bode-Böger et al. 1994) and hypercholesterolemic humans (Clarkson et al. 1996; Wolf et al. 1997), L-arginine reduces platelet aggregation. Likewise, in 12 healthy young men receiving 7 g of arginine three times daily for 3 days, inhibition of platelet aggregation was correlated with plasma levels of L-arginine. The higher level of platelet cyclic guanosine monophosphate following an oral dose of L-arginine was due to activation of guanylate cyclase (Adams et al. 1995).

6.1.3.2 Methionine and Homocysteine

Methionine, which is the only dietary source of homocysteine, increases thrombogenicity by enhancing the activities of platelets and coagulation factors (Lentz and Sadler 1991; Harpel 1997; De Jong et al. 1998), as well as factors V and XII (Loscalzo 1996) and factors VIIc and vWf (Freyburger et al. 1997). Hyperhomocysteinemia inhibits the function of thrombomodulin, which is the cofactor for activation of protein C by thrombin (Lentz and Sadler 1991; Lentz et al. 1996, Loscalzo 1996).

6.1.3.3 Taurine

In rats, taurine inhibits the platelet aggregation induced by ADP, collagen, or thrombin. This reduction is probably due to reduced formation of thromboxane A_2

(Huang and Rao 1995). The same observations have been made with platelets from normotensive and hypertensive humans (Kohashi et al. 1983).

In vivo platelet taurine concentrations were weaker and platelet aggregation induced by ADP was higher in hypertensive than in normotensive patients (Kohashi et al. 1983).

6.1.3.4 Tryptophan

A diet enriched with tryptophan (4 and 10 g/kg) enhances ADP-induced platelet aggregation in *Charles River CD* strain rats. *In vitro*, tryptophan has no effect on ADP platelet aggregation, whereas its metabolite, serotonin, enhances this effect in a dose-dependent pattern.

The possible involvement of serotonin in enhancing platelet aggregation has been demonstrated by the increased urinary excretion of 5-hydroxyindole acetic acid, a catabolite of serotonin (Mokady et al. 1990).

6.2 EFFECTS OF ISOFLAVONES

Diets that are rich in soybean protein may affect the development of atherosclerosis because they increase the plasma concentrations of genistein (Adlercreutz et al. 1993), which intervenes in several stages of the process of thrombogenesis (review in Wilcox and Blumenthal 1995).

Genistein is a potent inhibitor of growth factors that enhance the formation of tyrosine kinase. Thus, decreasing activity of protein tyrosine kinase slightly blocks platelet aggregation, the release of serotonin induced by thrombin, and the intracellular Ca^{2+} concentration induced by thrombin. It also inhibits the formation of reactive oxygen species (ROS) during activation of rat platelets in whole blood (Akiyama et al. 1987; Asahi et al. 1992; Sargeant et al. 1993a, 1993b; Schoene and Guidry 1996). However, as the protein tyrosine phosphorylation induced by thrombin is not affected by genistein, the inhibitory effect of genistein on polyphosphoinositides is unrelated to tyrosine kinase inhibition (Ozaki et al. 1993).

In vitro, genistein inhibits activation of thromboxane A_2 collagen–induced platelets (Nakashima et al. 1991), the ADP-induced activation of platelets (Sargeant et al. 1993b), and serotonin uptake in platelets (Helmeste and Tang 1995). Thrombin-induced platelet activation (Ozaki et al. 1993; Sargeant et al. 1993a) and aggregation are blocked by the action of genistein on tyrosine kinase (Asahi et al. 1992). Likewise, platelet aggregation *in vitro* is reduced in animals fed on intact soybean protein isolates (with isoflavones) due to activation by thrombin or serotonin. This contrasts with the platelet aggregation of animals fed on alcohol-washed soybean protein isolates (Williams and Clarkson 1998). The volume of platelets was significantly lower in rats fed on soybean protein isolates with intact isoflavones than in rats on soybean protein isolates without isoflavones (Schoene and Guidry 1996).

However, the effects of genistein have been observed *in vitro* and further investigation is still necessary to ascertain whether they are also present *in vivo*. Indeed, in 20 male normocholesterolemic subjects in two groups consuming either a soybean-protein-isolate beverage powder (60 g/day for 28 days) or a casein supplement, a dramatic rise in plasma isoflavone concentrations was observed in the soybean protein group, but this increase was not sufficient to significantly inhibit platelet aggregation (Gooderham et al. 1996). However, Williams and Clarkson (1998) have shown that in 12 female non-human primates, the reduction in blood flow is greater (−26%) after collagen-induced platelet activation in the group fed on soybean protein isolates without isoflavones than in the group on soybean-protein isolates with isoflavones.

6.3 CONCLUSION

In animal experiments, platelet aggregation is increased by protein deficiency and suppressed by several peptides from casein, lactalbumin, lactotransferrin, and soybean protein, in a dose-dependent manner in some cases. Amino acids have different effects on platelet aggregation. L-Arginine decreases platelet aggregation in animals and in normocholesterolemic and hypercholesterolemic humans, whereas it is inhibited by taurine *in vitro*. In contrast, tryptophan enhances platelet aggregation due to serotonin and its metabolites. Methionine, the only dietary source of homocysteine, increases thrombogenicity by enhancing platelet and coagulation factor activities. Finally, genistein inhibition of tyrosine kinase depresses platelet aggregation.

7 General Conclusions

It is clear that our knowledge regarding the effects of low-protein and high-protein diets for each species is influenced by the number of studies and experimental conditions. It is therefore quite impossible to attempt to suggest an accurate general conclusion. Moreover, as the effects of low- and high-protein diets differ according to species, any extrapolation of the data to human use must take into consideration the species investigated. When the level of proteins in the diet decreases or increases, the serum cholesterol concentrations are enhanced in birds, rabbits, and rodents (rats, mice, hamsters). Chickens, however, react differently from other species. In calves and monkeys, reactions vary according to subspecies. In pigs, serum cholesterol would appear to be particularly sensitive to varying levels of dietary proteins. In dogs, too few experiments have been conducted for any conclusion to be proposed. Of all the proteins investigated, casein produces the greatest increase in serum cholesterol concentrations. In monkeys, a protein intake in conformity with protein requirements can maintain normal lipid, lipoprotein, and cholesterol serum levels. A low-protein diet increases VLDL and HDL particle levels, whereas a high-protein diet increases serum cholesterol, lipid, and lipoprotein concentrations.

Differences in experimental protocols, particularly the nature and quantity of dietary components, may well explain most of the conflicting results. The lipid and cholesterol contents of a diet modulate effects of protein and sulfur amino acids. The food environment is therefore an important parameter to be taken into account. On the whole, the data concerning the effects of protein levels on serum cholesterol concentrations clearly show that only an adequate coverage of protein requirements will ensure normal levels of serum cholesterol concentrations.

When experiments are performed, the nutritional value of the proteins chosen for the diet is another essential factor, as is the use of protein levels that are similar to protein requirements. The widely varying reactions observed in different animal species underline the importance, before any extrapolation can be made to humans, of conducting experiments in monkeys and pigs since their metabolic reactions are the closest to those of humans.

Although, in the majority of cases, a casein diet is hypercholesterolemic whereas a soybean protein diet is hypocholesterolemic, their effects can vary not only according to the animal species and genetic factors but also to the age and sex of the animals. The effects of proteins also depend on the proportion included in the diet and on the amount of cholesterol. In comparison with soybean protein, casein increases VLDL-, LDL-, and HDL-cholesterol levels, and reduces their turnover because of the reduction in LDL-apo B receptor affinities. Casein also decreases cholesterol turnover and down-regulates the enzymatic activities of LCAT and lipoprotein lipase. Depending on the species, these effects can vary. Sirtori et al. (1995)

suggested that soybean protein up-regulates LDL receptors that are depressed by hypercholesterolemia or by dietary cholesterol administration.

Several soybean and casein products processed by various technologies are utilized for animals and humans. They are more or less hypocholesterolemic or hypercholesterolemic according to the products and the animal species. Germinated products and ethanol extracts are less hypocholesterolemic because the partial or total loss of isoflavones.

Soybean protein and casein are the most extensively studied but investigations have also focused on several other vegetable and animal proteins. Although it is widely accepted that vegetable proteins are hypocholesterolemic, it is still difficult to rank animal proteins according to the extent of their effects on cholesterol and lipid metabolisms. Several factors — animal species; age of animals; amount of proteins; diet composition, particularly the nature of fats and amount of fats and cholesterol; and study duration — are known to modify the results of experiments. There have also been too few studies in animal models, such as pigs or monkeys, for any valid extrapolation of the results to human use. Existing results have, however, given several interesting indications. It is obvious that the different effects of various food proteins are related to their amino acid composition.

The data concerning the influence of amino acids on cholesterol and lipid metabolisms are often inconsistent since they too are modified by the same factors as those described for proteins. Moreover, most experiments have been carried out on rats and too few on other animals. Sulfur amino acids have the most potent effects. On the whole, arginine, cystine, glycine, leucine, methionine, and taurine are hypocholesterolemic, whereas histidine, lysine, and tyrosine are hypercholesterolemic. Methionine may be hyper- or hypocholesterolemic according to species and composition of diet, particularly the methionine proportion. The effects of glutamic acid differ according to species, and tyrosine-induced hypercholesterolemia varies according to the nature of proteins in the diet. Tryptophan enhances lipid peroxidation in chickens. The cystine-induced increase in liver lipids can be prevented by methionine and also by taurine, depending on the endogenous synthesis of taurine that is specific to the animal species studied. HMG-CoA reductase activity is increased by cystine and methionine.

Amino acid mixtures simulating the composition of casein, soybean protein, or wheat gluten have respectively the same effects as casein, soybean protein, or wheat gluten. When all the essential amino acids, except arginine, are included in the diet, the reduction in serum cholesterol levels is greater and the LDL receptors are down-regulated. Effects of amino acid mixtures vary according to their composition. A mixture of lysine, leucine, methionine, isoleucine, and valine results in the same type of hypercholesterolemia as a mixture of lysine, leucine, and methionine, whereas one containing histidine, phenylalanine, tryptophan, and glycine has only a moderate effect. Partial hydrolysates of casein or soybean protein have similar effects to those of casein or soybean protein.

The effects of various proteins on lipid metabolism have chiefly been investigated with soybean protein or casein diets and somewhat less with fish proteins. In the majority of cases, although not systematically, animal proteins are hypercholesterolemic in comparison with soybean protein. These effects have still not been clearly understood despite numerous studies. They have been well described particularly by Sugano (1983), Pfeuffer and Barth (1990), West et al. (1990), and Lovati et al. (1991b). It is, however, difficult to propose a schematic summary of these effects because they vary according to animal species, genetic factors, age, sex, amount of proteins in the diet, food environments, particularly cholesterol and fats, and study duration. Consequently, it is impossible to generalize any of these effects and further investigation into these mechanisms is still necessary. This brief summary focuses exclusively on the differences between soybean protein and casein.

The following factors must be considered.

- Amino acid composition of proteins
  - Arginine, cystine, leucine, methionine, and taurine are hypocholesterolemic, whereas histidine, lysine and tyrosine are hypercholesterolemic. The differences in the amino acid composition of soybean protein and casein account for their contrasting effects on plasma cholesterol.
  - The 7S and 11S globulins of soybean protein have a hypocholesterolemic effect that up-regulates LDL receptors and increases the resistance of LDL to oxidation.
- The endocrine response to the proteins in diets
  - The response to insulin, glucagon, thyroid hormones, corticosterone, cortisol, and growth hormone secretion varies — thus modifying the activities of several enzymes — according to amino acid composition and protein quantity.
  - Flavonoids may also displace thyroid hormones from their serum transport proteins, increase serum concentrations, and decrease serum cholesterol concentrations.
- Changes in enzyme activities
  - Of interest are changes in HMG-CoA reductase, β-hydroxy-β-methylglutaryl coenzyme A reductase, cholesterol 7-α-monooxygenase, lipoprotein lipase, hepatic lipase, $\Delta 5$- and $\Delta 6$-desaturases, and also the induction of hepatic apo B and apo E receptor activities.
- Nonprotein components
  - Saponins increase the fecal excretion of endogenous and exogenous neutral steroids and bile acids, which counteracts the effects of hypercholesterolemia-inducing diets.
  - Isoflavones reduce serum lipid concentrations, and have several protective effects such as antioxidative, antiproliferative, and antimigratory actions. However, to date it is not yet clear whether they have all the protective effects of estrogens.
- Food environments modify the effects of soybean protein and casein but also those of other dietary proteins
  - The amount of cholesterol in a diet increases the hypocholesterolemic effect of soybean protein compared to casein.
  - Choline or soybean lecithin in a diet alleviates hypercholesterolemia.

- The nature and amount of minerals (calcium, zinc, and copper) modulate the hypocholesterolemic effect of proteins in the absence of phytate in the diet. However, the data observed in a number of animal species are not systematically comparable.
- The nature of fats (saturated or polyunsaturated) and the amount of fats can influence the effects of proteins; these are greater when the dietary level is either too high or too low.
- The role of carbohydrates and dietary fibers may be important. Depending on the animal species, sucrose but not starch in a diet may or may not increase the hypercholesterolemic effect of casein.

The effects of the nature and amount of dietary fibers are more complex to evaluate. Differences in the water-holding capacity of dietary fibers may account for the various effects of dietary fibers on minerals, bile acids, digestive enzymes, and the absorption time of different components of the intestinal chyme (Kay 1982; Schneeman and Gallaher 1980; Dutta and Hlasko 1985). Dietary fibers reduce intestinal transit time and intestinal reabsorption due to the binding of bile acids; cause damage to the bacterial flora; and enhance bacterial conversion of cholesterol and production of short-chain fatty acids, including propionate, by fermentation of dietary fibers. Supplementing diets with propionate decreases the plasma cholesterol concentrations in pigs, and intracaecal infusion of propionic acid in ileally fistulated rats limits the plasma cholesterol increase caused by a casein diet, without any alteration of total liver lipids or cholesterol. Moreover, according to Pfeuffer and Barth (1990), the morphologic changes in intestinal mucosa caused by dietary fibers (Jacobs 1983) or soybean protein (Seegraber and Morril 1982) could be implicated in the effects of dietary fibers and soybean protein fibers.

These various mechanisms all induce the following changes when soybean protein is substituted for casein.

- Reduced intestinal absorption of cholesterol and/or bile acids and their influx into the liver
- Increased fecal excretion of cholesterol and bile acids
- Stimulation of metabolic turnover of cholesterol in the body
- Decreased hepatic intracellular cholesterol concentrations
- Reduced hepatic production of lipoproteins and increased number of LDL receptors

The mechanism behind the effects of fish proteins is not the same as those of casein and soybean protein. There are probably less changes in hepatic cholesterol metabolism than with casein or soybean protein. Moreover, with fish proteins, the lipoprotein pattern is different: LDL and HDL concentrations rise with fish proteins and VLDL levels are increased with casein. Nevertheless, this field still requires further research (West et al. 1990).

Numerous mechanisms have been put forward in an attempt to explain the various effects of food proteins on lipid metabolism in humans, and cholesterol metabolism in particular; no single theory would appear to apply. Further studies are necessary because of the numerous factors presumed to be involved and also because the effect of each would appear to vary according to genetic factors and the food environment. However, the hypocholesterolemic action of soybean protein and the absence of side effects have been sufficiently clearly demonstrated to justify recommending this protein as a drug in the treatment for type II hyperlipoproteinemia (Beynen et al. 1987b).

The effects of the amount and nature of proteins or amino acids on the development of atherosclerosis are strongly influenced by the animal species, particularly with a high-protein diet. A moderately low-protein diet prevents the development of fatty streaks in pigeons and reduces the aortic cholesterol content in rats. However in pigs and monkeys it is without effect. The reduced sulfur amino acid content in a low-protein diet increases plasma cholesterol levels although these may return to normal if methionine or cystine is added to the diet.

Although most proteins, regardless of their nature, have similar effects in pigeons, in other animals the prevalence of atherosclerosis is higher with casein or fish protein than with soybean protein diets.

Three amino acids have been shown to induce different effects on the development of atherosclerosis. Arginine increases nitric oxide synthesis since it is a substrate of nitric oxide synthase. It induces antihypertensive and antiproliferative effects, inhibits platelet aggregation, increases endothelium-dependent vasodilation, and reduces the development of atherosclerosis in cholesterol-fed rabbits. However, the addition of arginine to a casein diet produces equivocal effects.

Methionine increases lipid peroxidation and intimal thickening, and enhances cholesterol deposits, calcification, arteriosclerotic plaque formation, and endothelial cell numbers in the blood. It leads to the production of homocysteine and the subsequent angiotoxic effects.

Taurine may prevent the development of atherosclerosis since it regulates osmolarity, reduces calcium levels in the aorta and myocardium, prevents the development of atheroma, improves cardiac contractile function, and mimics certain actions of angiotensin-converting enzyme inhibitors.

Despite the presence of numerous factors that may be involved in immunologically provoked lesions of the arterial tissues, and despite the potential significance of their effects, their true role in atherogenesis has not as yet been confirmed (Redgrave 1984). Although ample experimental evidence is available to demonstrate the capacity of immune damage to promote atherogenesis in experimental animals, the same cannot be said for human models (Constantinides 1980).

Lecithin decreases serum cholesterol concentrations and reduces the extent of atherosclerotic lesions.

The effects of the protein level of a diet on the development of atherosclerosis are largely dependent on the animal species; in addition, genetic factors would appear to be of great importance. In humans, a high vegetable-protein diet may well have a protective effect against atherosclerosis and the specific nature of the proteins would appear to be particularly important. In both animals and humans, soybean protein and lean fish protein have a protective effect against atherosclerosis, whereas casein would appear to promote it. The protective effects of vegetable proteins, particularly soybean protein, are due to a reduction in LDL cholesterol (about 13%), and plasma triacylglycerols (about 10%), and to an increase in HDL cholesterol (about 2%) (Anderson et al. 1995).

LDL peroxidation is increased by casein peptides. Arginine and taurine both have beneficial effects: arginine promotes nitric oxide synthesis and taurine enhances diuresis and natriuresis and reduces the calcium level in atheromatous lesions. In contrast, methionine and homocysteine are both harmful via several mechanisms. Antibodies against milk proteins, and perhaps against milk, that result from denatured proteins by heat processing, increase the development of atherosclerosis, whereas the isoflavone content of soybean protein has a protective action. The hypocholesterolemic action of soybean protein and the absence of side effects have been sufficiently well demonstrated to justify recommending this protein as a therapy in the treatment of type II hyperlipoproteinemia (Beynen et al. 1987b). According to Anthony (2001), the benefits of soybean protein consumption for the preservation of a healthy cardiovascular system are widely supported by numerous scientific studies. Dieticians, nutrition specialists, and the media have an important role to play in educating people by suggesting simple recipes and tasty soybean foods.

In epidemiologic studies, blood pressure levels have been shown to be lower in vegetarian than in omnivorous individuals. The data relating to the effects on blood pressure of protein intake or the nature of the protein consumed are conflicting. The role of the food environment and genetic predisposition must be taken into consideration. Several mechanisms have been suggested to explain the effects of proteins, including enhanced sodium excretion due to the consumption of proteins; and a very probable role for certain peptides, particularly casein, in the conversion of angiotensin I to angiotensin II, as well as various amino acids. By increasing the production of nitric oxide, arginine reduces blood pressure levels. Sulfur amino acids such as methionine and taurine tend to reduce blood pressure. Taurine, tryptophan, and tyrosine modify blood pressure levels by enhancing neurotransmitters, particularly serotonin, and also by acting on catecholamines. Nevertheless, further research is still necessary to provide a clear explanation of the importance of each of these mechanisms.

In animal experiments, platelet aggregation is increased by protein deficiency and suppressed by several peptides from casein, lactalbumin, lactotransferrin, and soybean protein, in a dose-dependent manner. Amino acids have diverse effects on platelet aggregation. L-Arginine decreases platelet aggregation in animals as in normocholesterolemic and hypercholesterolemic humans, whereas taurine inhibits this process *in vitro*. In contrast, the serotonin content of tryptophan (and that of its metabolites) enhances platelet aggregation. Methionine, the only dietary source of homocysteine, increases thrombogenicity by enhancing platelet and coagulation factor activities. Lastly, inhibition of tyrosine kinase by genistein suppresses platelet aggregation.

Despite numerous studies that have investigated the relationships between food proteins, plasma lipids, and cholesterol on the one hand, and atherosclerosis, hypertension, and thrombosis on the other, it is still too early to precisely define these relationships. However, the compelling data thus far obtained clearly confirm the necessity of continuing these investigations.

References

Abebe W and Agarwal DK. 1995. Role of tyrosine kinases in norepinephrine-induced contraction of vascular smooth muscle. *J. Cardiovasc. Pharmacol.* 26: 153–159.

Abreu de J and Millan N. 1994. Effect of addition of brewer's yeast to soy protein and casein on plasma cholesterol levels of rabbits. *Archiv. LatinoAmer. Nutr.* 44: 18–22.

Adams CWM, Abdulla YH, Bayliss OB and Morgan RS. 1967. Modification of aortic atheroma and fatty liver in cholesterol-fed rabbits by intravenous injection of saturated and polyunsaturated lecithins. *J. Pathol. Bacteriol.* 94: 77–87.

Adams MR, Forsythe CJ, Jessup W, Robinson J and Celermajer DS. 1995. Oral L-arginine inhibits platelet aggregation but does not enhance endothelium-dependent dilatation in healthy young adults. *J. Am. Coll. Cardiol.* 26: 1054–1061.

Adams MR, McCredie R, Jessup W, Robinson J, Sullivan D and Celermajer DS. 1997a. Oral L-arginine improves endothelium-dependent vasodilatation and reduces monocyte adhesion to endothelial cells in young men with coronary artery disease. *Atherosclerosis* 129: 261–269.

Adams MR, Jessup W, Hailstones D and Celermajer DS. 1997b. L-arginine reduces human monocyte adhesion to vascular endothelium and endothelial expression of cell adhesion molecules. *Circulation* 95: 662–668.

Adams MR, Jessup W and Celermajer DS. 1997c. Cigarette smoking is associated with increased human monocyte adhesion to endothelial cells: Reversibility with oral L-arginine but not vitamin C. *J. Am. Coll. Cardiol.* 29: 491–497.

Adams MR, Golden DL, Anthony MS, Register TC and Williams JK. 2002. Inhibitory effect of soy protein isolate on atherosclerosis in mice does not require the presence of LDL receptors or alteration of plasma lipoproteins. *J. Nutr.* 132: 43–49.

Adeyeye SO, Oyenuga VA and Fetuga BL. 1989. Serum cholesterol and triacylglycerol in rats fed different protein sources. *Nutr. Rep. Int.* 40: 323–334.

Adibi SA. 1971. Intestinal absorption of dipeptides in man. Relative importance of hydrolysis and intact absorption. *J. Clin. Invest.* 50: 2266–2275.

Adibi SA. 1980. Roles of branch chain amino acids in the metabolic regulation. *J. Lab. Clin. Med.* 95: 475–484.

Adibi SA, Gray SJ and Menden E. 1967. The kinetics of amino acid absorption and alteration of plasma composition of free amino acids after intestinal perfusion of amino acid mixtures. *Am. J. Clin. Nutr.* 20: 24–33.

Adler AJ and Holub BJ. 1997. Effect of garlic and fish-oil supplementation on serum lipid and lipoprotein concentrations in hypercholesterolemic men. *Am. J. Clin. Nutr.* 65: 445–450.

Adlercreutz H. 1990. Western diet and Western diseases: Some hormonal and biochemical mechanisms and associations. *Scand. J. Clin. Lab. Invest.* 201 (Suppl.): 3–23.

Adlercreutz H, Hoeckerstedt K, Bannwart C, Bloigu S, Hamalainen E, Fotsis T and Ollus A. 1987. Effect of dietary components, including lignans and phytoestrogens, on enterohepatic circulation and liver metabolism of estrogens and on sex hormone binding globulin (SHBG). *J. Steroid Biochem.* 27: 1135–1144.

Adlercreutz H, Markkanen H and Watanabe S. 1993. Plasma concentrations of phytooestrogens in Japanese men. *Lancet* 342: 1209–1210.

Agbedana EO. 1980. Changes in serum postheparin and tissue lipoprotein lipase activities in protein malnourished rats. *Nutr. Rep. Int.* 32: 157–165.

Agbedana EO, Johnson AO and Oladunni Taylor G. 1979a. Studies on hepatic and extrahepatic lipoprotein lipases in protein-calorie malnutrition. *Am. J. Clin. Nutr.* 32: 292–298.

Agbedana EO, Johnson AO and Oladunni Taylor G. 1979b. Selective deficiency of hepatic triglyceride lipase and hypertriglyceridemia in kwashiorkor. *Br. J. Nutr.* 42: 351–356.

Aji W, Ravalli S, Szaboles M, Jiang XC, Sciacca RR, Michler RE and Cannon PJ. 1997. L-arginine prevents xanthoma development and inhibits atherosclerosis in LDL receptor knockout mice. *Circulation* 95: 430–437.

Akiba Y, Jensen LS, Barb CR and Kraeling R. 1982. Plasma estradiol, thyroid hormones, and liver lipid content in laying hens fed different isocaloric diets. *J. Nutr.* 112: 299–308.

Akiba Y and Jensen LS. 1983. Temporal effect of change in diet composition on plasma estradiol and thyroxine concentrations and hepatic lipogenesis in laying hens. *J. Nutr.* 113: 2078–2084.

Akiyama T, Ishida J, Nagakawa S, Ogawara H, Watanabe S, Itch N, Shibuya M and Fuani Y. 1987. Genistein a specific inhibitor of tyrosine-specific protein kinase. *J. Biol. Chem.* 262: 5592–5595.

Albanese AA, Higgons RA, Lorenze EJ and Orto LA. 1959. Effect of dietary protein on blood cholesterol of adults. *Geriatrics* 14: 237–243.

Aljawad NS, Fryer EB and Fryer HC. 1991. Effects of casein, soy and the whey proteins and amino acid supplementation on cholesterol metabolism in rats. *J. Nutr. Biochem.* 2: 150–155.

Alladi S, Gilbert R and Shanmugasundaram KR. 1989a. Lipids, lipoproteins and lipolytic activity in plasma with dietary protein changes. *Nutr. Rep. Int.* 40: 653–661.

Alladi S and Shanmugasundaram KR. 1989b. Induction of hypercholesterolemia by supplementing soy protein with acetate generating amino acids. *Nutr. Rep. Int.* 40: 893–900.

Allotta EC, Samman S and Roberts DCK. 1985. The importance of the non-protein components of the diet in the plasma cholesterol response of rabbits to casein. *Br. J. Nutr.* 54: 87–94.

Anderson A, Hoiriis-Nielsen J and Borg LAH. 1977. Effects of L-leucine on the insulin production, oxidative metabolism and mitochondrial ultrastructure of isolated mouse pancreatic islets in tissue culture. *Diabetologia* 13: 59–68.

Anderson A, Brattström L, Israelsson B, Isaksson A and Hultherg B. 1990. The effect of excess daily methionine on plasma homocysteine after a methionine loading test in humans. *Clin. Chim. Acta* 192: 69–76.

Anderson JT, Grande F and Keys A. 1971. Effect of man's serum lipids of two proteins with different amino acid composition. *Am. J. Clin. Nutr.* 24: 524–530.

Anderson JW and Chen WJL. 1979. Plant fiber. Carbohydrate and lipid metabolism. *Am. J. Clin. Nutr.* 32: 346–363.

Anderson JW, Story L, Sieling B, Lin Chen WJ, Petro MS and Story J. 1984. Hypercholesterolemic effect of oat-bran or bean intake for hypercholesterolemic men. *Am. J. Clin. Nutr.* 40: 1146–1155.

Anderson JW and Tietyen-Clark J. 1986. Dietary fiber: Hyperlipidemia, hypertension and coronary heart disease. *Am. J. Gastroenterol.* 81: 907–919.

Anderson RL and Wolf WJ. 1995. Compositional changes in trypsin inhibitors, phytic acid, saponins and isoflavones related to soybean processing. *J. Nutr.* 125 (Suppl.): 581S–588S.

Anderson RL, Johnstone BM and Cook-Newell ME. 1995. Meta-analysis of the effects of soy protein intake on serum lipids. *N. Engl. J. Med.* 333: 276–282.

Anitschkow N and Chalatow S. 1913. Über experimentelle Cholesterin-Steatose und ihre Bedeutung für die Entstehung einiger pathologischer Prozesse. *Zentralbl. Allg. Pathol. Pathol. Anat.* 24: 1–9.

Annand JC. 1967. Hypothesis: Heated milk protein and thrombosis. *J. Atheroscl. Res.* 7: 797–801.

Annand JC. 1986. Denaturated bovine immunoglobulin pathogenic in atherosclerosis. *Atherosclerosis* 59: 347–351.

Anonymous. 1991. Casein versus soy protein: Further elucidation of their differential effect on serum cholesterol in rabbits. *Nutr. Rev.* 49: 121–123.

Anthony MS. 2000. Soy and cardiovascular disease: Cholesterol lowering and beyond. *J. Nutr.* 130 (Suppl.): 662S–663S.

Anthony MS. 2001. Soy protein and heart disease. In Descheemaeker K and Debruyne I., Eds., *Soy and Health 2000: Clinical Evidence, Dietetic Applications*, Garant, Leuven, pp. 11–16.

Anthony MS, Clarkson TB and Hughes CL Jr. 1994. Plant and mammalian estrogens effects on plasma lipids of female monkeys. *Circulation* 90: I-235, Abstract 1261.

Anthony MS, Clarkson TB, Hughes CL Jr, Lorgan TM and Burke GL. 1996a. Soybean isoflavones improve cardiovascular risk factors without affecting the reproductive system of peripubertal *Rhesus* monkeys. *J. Nutr.* 126: 43–50.

Anthony MS, Clarkson TB and Williams JK. 1996b. Effects of soy isoflavones on atherosclerosis: Potential mechanisms. Second International Symposium on the Role of Soy in Preventing and Treating Chronic Disease, Brussels, Sept. 15–18, 1996, Abstract, p. 26.

Anthony MS and Clarkson TB. 1997. Association between plasma isoflavone and plasma lipoprotein concentrations. Symposium on Phytoestrogen Research Methods: Chemistry, Analysis, and Biological Properties, Tucson, AZ, Sept. 21–24, 1997, Abstract.

Anthony MS, Clarkson TB, Bullock BC and Wagner JD. 1997. Soy protein versus soy phytoestrogens in the prevention of diet-induced coronary artery atherosclerosis of male *Cynomolgus* monkeys. *Arterioscl. Thromb. Vasc. Biol.* 17: 2524–2531.

Anthony MS, Clarkson TB and Williams JK. 1998. Effects of soy isoflavones on atherosclerosis: Potential mechanisms. *Am. J. Clin. Nutr.* 68 (Suppl.): 1390S–1393S.

Aoyama Y and Ashida K. 1972. Effect of excess and deficiency of individual essential amino acids in diet on the liver lipid content of growing rats. *J. Nutr.* 102: 1025–1032.

Aoyama Y, Nakanishi M and Ashida K. 1973. Effect of methionine on liver lipid content and lipid metabolism of rats fed a protein-free diet. *J. Nutr.* 103: 54–60.

Aoyama Y, Ohmura E and Yoshida A. 1977. Effect of dietary composition on lipids in serum and in liver of rats fed a cystine-excess diet. *Agric. Biol. Chem.* 51: 3125–3131.

Aoyama Y and Ashida K. 1979. Prevention by urea cycle intermediates and adenine on the lipid accumulation in the liver induced by refeeding an arginine-devoid diet. *Nutr. Rep. Int.* 20: 483–490.

Aoyama Y, Yoshida A and Ashida K. 1981. Effects of some dietary additions to either an arginine-devoid diet or a diet supplemented with orotic acid refed after starvation on liver lipid content during essential fatty acid deficiency in rats. *J. Nutr.* 111: 895–906.

Aoyama Y, Yoshida A and Ashida K. 1983a. Changes in lipids in liver and serum of rats fed a histidine-excess diet. *Nutr. Rep. Int.* 28: 643–651.

Aoyama Y, Sakaida K, Yoshida A and Ashida K. 1983b. Effects on liver and serum lipids of dietary supplements of methionine and excess lysine given to previously-starved rats. *Br. J. Nutr.* 50: 627–636.

Aoyama Y, Matsumoto H, Tsuda T, Ohmura E and Yoshida A. 1988. Effect on liver and serum lipids in rats of dietary additions of fibers and cholestyramine a cystine-excess diet. *Agric. Biol. Chem.* 52: 2811–2816.

Aoyama Y, Hitomi-Ohmura E and Yoshida A. 1991. Effect of a dietary excess of histidine and subsequent starvation on serum lipids in rats. *Agric. Biol. Chem.* 55: 1161–1162.

Aoyama Y, Matsumoto H, Hitomi-Ohmura E and Yoshida A. 1992a. Fatty liver induced by the addition of excess cystine to a soya-bean protein diet in rats. *Comp. Biochem. Physiol.* 102A: 185–189.

Aoyama Y, Ishikawa T, Amano N and Yoshida A. 1992b. Lipid accumulation in the liver of rats fed a soy protein isolate diet with excess cystine, and its prevention by methionine or choline. *Biosci. Biotechnol. Biochem.* 56: 656–659.

Aoyama Y, Inaba T and Yoshida A. 1998. Dietary cystine and liver triacylglycerol in rats: Effects of dietary lysine and threonine. *Comp. Biochem. Physiol.* 119A: 543–546.

Araki A, Sako Y and Fukushima Y. 1989. Plasma sulfhydryl-containing amino acids in patients with cerebral infarction and in hypertensive subjects. *Atherosclerosis* 79: 139–146.

Arbeeny CM and Rifici BA. 1984. The uptake of chylomicron remnant and very low-density lipoprotein remnants by the perfused rat liver. *J. Biol. Chem.* 1984: 9662–9666.

Aritsuka T, Tanaka K and Kiriyama S. 1989. Effect of beet dietary fiber on lipid metabolism in rats fed a cholesterol-free diet in comparison with pectin and cellulose. *J. Jpn. Soc. Nutr. Food Sci.* 42: 295–304.

Aritsuka T, Tanaka K and Kiriyama S. 1992. Long-term effects on serum cholesterol concentrations of beet dietary fiber in normal and cecectomized rats fed a cholesterol-free diet casein diet. *J. Agr. Chem. Soc. Jpn.* 66: 881–889.

Arjmandi BH, Khan DA, Juma SS and Svanborg A. 1997. The ovarian hormone deficiency induced hypercholesterolemia is reversed by soy protein and the synthetic isoflavone, ipriflavones. *Nutr. Res.* 17: 885–894.

Armstrong B, van Merwyk AJ and Coates H. 1977. Blood pressures in Seventh-Day Adventist vegetarians. *Am. J. Epidemiol.* 105: 444–459.

Armstrong BK, Mann JI, Adelstein AM and Eskin F. 1975. Commodity consumption and ischemic heart disease mortality, with special reference to dietary practices. *J. Chronic Dis.* 28: 455–469.

Asahi M, Yanagi S, Ohta S, Inazu T, Sakai K, Takeuchi F, Taniguchi T and Yamamura H. 1992. Thrombin-induced human platelet aggregation is inhibited by protein-kinase inhibitors, ST638 and genistein. *F.E.B.S. Lett.* 309: 10–14.

Asato L, Kina T, Sugiyama BS, Shimabukuro T and Yamamoto S. 1994. Effect of dietary peptides on plasma lipids and its mechanism studied in rats and mice. *Nutr. Res.* 14: 1661–1669.

Asato L, Wang MF, Chan YC, Yeh SH, Chung HM, Chida S, Uezato T, Suzuki I, Yamagata N, Kokubu T and Yamamoto S. 1996. Effect of egg white on serum cholesterol concentration in young women. *J. Nutr. Sci. Vitaminol.* 42: 87–96.

Asayama K, Amemiya S, Kusano S and Kato K. 1984. Growth-hormone-induced changes in postheparin plasma lipoprotein lipase and hepatic triglyceride lipase activities. *Metabolism* 31: 129–131.

Ascherio A, Rimm EB, Stampfer MJ, Giovannucci EL and Willet WC. 1995. Dietary intake of marine n-3 fatty acids, fish intake, and the risk of coronary disease among men. *N. Engl. J. Med.* 332: 977–982.

Aschkenazy A, Nataf B and Sfez M. 1961. Iodide concentrating ability of the rat thyroid gland as affected by the dietary content of proteins and certain amino acids. *Compt. Rend. Soc. Biol.* 155: 986–990.

Ashton E and Ball M. 2000. Effects of soy as tofu vs. meat on lipoprotein concentrations. *Eur. J. Clin. Nutr.* 54: 14–19.

Asp NG, Schweizer TF, Southgate DAT and Theander O. 1992. Dietary fiber analysis. In Schweizer TF and Edwards CA, Eds., *Dietary Fibre — A Component of Food: Nutritional Function in Health and Disease*, Springer-Verlag, London, pp. 57–101.

Assmann G, Schmitz G, Menzel HJ and Schulte H. 1984. Apolipoprotein E polymorphism and hyperlipidemia. *Clin. Chem.* 30: 641–643.

Astuti M. 1996. The role of tempe on lipid profile and lipid peroxidation. In Second International Symposium on the Role of Soy in Preventing and Treating Chronic Disease, Brussels, Sept. 15–18, 1996, Abstract, pp. 27–28.

Atinmo T , Baldijao C, Pond WG and Barnes RH. 1978. The effect of dietary protein restriction on serum thyroxine levels of pregnant or growing swine. *J. Nutr.* 108: 1546–1553.

Atwal AS, Kubow S and Wolynetz MS. 1997. Effects of protein source and amino acid supplementation on plasma cholesterol in guinea pigs. *Int. J. Vitam. Nutr. Res.* 67: 192–195.

Aubert R and Flament C. 1991. Changes in rat plasma apolipoproteins and lipoproteins during moderate protein deficiency: Potential use in the assessment of nutritional status. *J. Nutr.* 121: 653–662.

Auboiron S, Durand D, Robert JC, Chapman MJ and Bauchart D. 1995. Effects of dietary fat and L-methionine on the hepatic metabolism of very low density lipoproteins in the preruminant calf, *Bos* spp. *Reprod. Nutr. Dev.* 35: 167–178.

Auboiron S, Catala I, Juste C, Bornet FRJ, Corring T and Guy-Grand B. 1996. Effects of soy protein on plasma lipoproteins in healthy men. Second International Symposium on the Role of Soy in Preventing and Treating Chronic Disease, Brussels, Sept. 15–18, 1996, Abstract, p. 23.

Auboiron S, Catala I, Juste C, Bornet FRJ, Corring T and Guy-Grand B. 1997. Effet des proteines de soja sur les lipoprotéines plasmatiques chez l'homme sain. *Cah. Nutr. Diet.* 32: 189.

Auboiron S, Catala I. Juste C, Bornet FRJ, Corring T and Guy-Grand B. 1998. Effects of soy protein on plasma lipoproteins in healthy men. *Am. J. Clin. Nutr.* 68 (Suppl.): 1519S.

Aust L, Poledne R, Elhahet A and Noack R. 1980. The hypolipaemic action of a glycine rich diet in rats. *Nahrung* 24: 663–671.

Austin MA, Hokanson JE and Edwards KL. 1998. Hypertriglyceridemia as a cardiovascular risk factor. *Am. J. Cardiol.* 81: 7B–12B.

Avins AL and Neuhaus JM. 2000. Do triglycerides provide meaningful information about heart disease risk. *Arch. Intern. Med.* 160: 1937–1944.

Aviram M, Cogan U and Mokady S. 1991. Excessive dietary tryptophan enhances plasma lipid peroxidation in rats. *Atherosclerosis* 88: 29–34.

Awata N, Azuma J, Hamaguchi T, Tanaka Y, Ohta H, Takihara K, Harada H, Sawamura A and Kishimoto S. 1987. Acute haemodynamic effect of taurine on hearts *in vivo* with normal and depressed function. *Cardiovasc. Res.* 21: 241–247.

Azuma J, Takihara K, Awata N, Ohta M, Sawanaura A, Hamada H and Kishimoto S. 1984. Beneficial effect of taurine on congestive heart failure induced by chronic aortic regurgitation in rabbits. *Res. Commn. Chem. Pathol. Pharmacol.* 45: 261–270.

Azuma J, Sawamura A, Awata N, Ohta H, Hamaguchi T, Harada H, Takihara K, Hasegawa H, Yamagami T, Ishiyama T, Iwata H and Kishimoto S. 1985. Therapeutic effect of taurine in congestive heart failure; a double blind cross-over trial. *Clin. Cardiol.* 8: 276–282.

Baba N, Radwan H and Van Itallie T. 1992. Effects of casein versus soy protein diets on body composition and serum lipid levels in adult rats. *Nutr. Res.* 12: 279–288.

Bagchi K, Ray R and Datta T. 1963. The influence of dietary protein and methionine on serum cholesterol level. *Am. J. Clin. Nutr.* 13: 232–237.

Bakhit RM, Potter SM, Essex-Sorlie D, Ham JO and Erdman JW Jr. 1993. Hypolipidemic response to soy protein and fiber in mildly hypercholesterolemic men. *F.A.S.E.B. J.* 7: Part II, A802, Abstract 4635.

Bakhit RM, Klein BP, Essex-Sorlie D, Ham JO, Erdman JW and Potter SM. 1994. Intake of 25 g of soybean protein with or without soybean fiber alters plasma lipids in men with elevated cholesterol concentrations. *J. Nutr.* 124: 213–222.

Bakhit RM, Adams VL and Chen C. 1999. The effect of soy protein intake on plasma lipid profiles and plasma TBARS in male college subjects. *F.A.S.E.B. J.* 13: A904, Abstract 676.4.

Bal dit Sollier C, Drouet L, Fiat AM, Jollès P and Caen JP. 1990. The antithrombotic effect of the peptides of lactotransferrin. *Compt. Rend. Soc. Biol.* 184: 201–210.

Bal dit Sollier C, Drouet L, Pignaud G, Chevallier C, Caen J, Fiat AM, Izquierdo C and Jollès P. 1996. Effect of κ-casein split peptides on platelet aggregation and on thrombus formation in the guinea-pig. *Thromb. Res.* 81: 427–437.

Baldner GL, Beitz DC and Jacobson NL. 1985. Effect of animal and vegetable fats and proteins on cholesterol concentration in plasma and tissue of pigs. *Fed. Proc.* 44: 1497, Abstract 6355.

Baldo-Enzi G, Baiocchi MR, Bertazo A, Costa CVL and Allegri G. 1996. Tryptophan and atherosclerosis. In GA Filipinn, CVL Costa and A Bertazzo, Eds., *Recent Advances in Tryptophan Research: Tryptophan and Serotonin Pathways, Adv. Exp. Biol. Med.* 398: 429–432.

Balmir F, Potter SM, Essex-Sorlie D, Bakhit RM, Ham JO and Erdman JW Jr. 1993. Endocrinological reponses to soy protein and fiber in mildly hypercholesterolemic men. *F.A.S.E.B. J.* 7: Part II, A802, Abstract 4634.

Balmir F, Staack R, Jeffrey E, Jimenez MDB, Wand L and Potter SM. 1996. An extract of soy flour influences serum cholesterol and thyroid hormones in rats and hamster. *J. Nutr.* 126: 3046–3053.

Balogun EA, Balogun OO and Odutuga AA. 1982. Arginine: Lysine ratio as a contributory factor to the hypercholesterolemic effect of plant protein sources. *IRCS Med. Sci.* 10: 643–644.

Banerjee U and Chakrabarti CH. 1973. Effect of supplementation of some essential amino acids on tissue levels of cholesterol and phospholipid of *albino* rats fed different pulse proteins. *Ind. J. Nutr. Diet.* 10: 68–74.

Bang HO, Dyerberg J and Nielsen AB. 1971. Plasma lipids and lipoprotein pattern in Greenlandic West-coast Eskimos. *Lancet* 1: 1143–1146.

Barbul A. 1993. The role of arginine as an immune modulator. In Cunningham-Rundles S, Ed., *Nutrient Modulation of the Immune Response.* Marcel Dekker, New York, 1993, pp. 47–61.

Barbul A, Wasserkrug HL, Seifter E, Rettura G, Levenson SH and Efron G. 1980a. Immunostimulatory effects of arginine in normal and injured rats. *J. Surg. Res.* 29: 228–235.

Barbul A, Wasserkrug HL, Sisto DA, Seifter E, Rettura G, Levenson SH and Efron G. 1980b. Thymic and immune stimulatory actions of arginine. *J. Parentol. Enterol. Nutr.* 4: 446–449.

Barichello AW and Fedoroff S. 1971. Effect of ileal bypass and alfalfa on hypercholesterolaemia. *Br. J. Exp. Pathol.* 52: 81–87.

Barnes RH, Kwong E, Fiala G, Rechcigl M, Lutz RN and Loosli JK. 1959a. Dietary fat and protein and serum cholesterol. I. Adult swine. *J. Nutr.* 69: 261–268.

Barnes RH, Kwong E, Pond W, Lowry R and Loosli JK. 1959b. Dietary fat and protein and serum cholesterol. II. Young swine. *J. Nutr.* 69: 269–273.

Barth CA, Pfeuffer M and Hahn G. 1984. Influence of dietary casein or soy protein on serum lipids and lipoproteins of monkeys. (*Macaca fascicularis*). *Ann. Nutr. Metab.* 28: 137–143.

Barth CA and Pfeuffer M. 1988. Dietary protein and atherogenesis. *Klin. Wochenschr.* 66: 135–143.

Barth CA, Scholz-Ahrens KE, Pfeuffer M and de Vrese M. 1989. Endocrine response to animal and vegetable protein. In Barth CA and Schlimme E, Eds., *Milk Proteins*, Steinkopff-Verlag, Darmstadt, pp. 62–67.

Barth CA, Pfeuffer M and Scholtissek J. 1990a. Animal models for the study of lipid metabolism, with particular reference to the *Göttingen minipig*. In Kirchgessner M., Ed., *Advances in Animal Physiology and Animal Nutrition*. Paul Parey, Hamburg, pp. 39–49.

Barth CA, Scholz-Ahrens KE, Pfeuffer M and Hotze A. 1990b. Response of hormones and lipid metabolism to different dietary proteins. In Beynen AC, Kritchevsky D and Pollack OJ, Eds., *Dietary Proteins, Cholesterol Metabolism and Atherosclerosis*, Monographs on Atherosclerosis, Vol. 16, S. Karger, Basel, pp. 110–125.

Barth CA, Scholtz-Ahrens KE, de Vrese M and Hotze A. 1990c. Difference of plasma amino acids following casein or soy protein intake: Significance for differences of serum lipid concentrations. *J. Nutr. Sci. Vitaminol.* 36 (Suppl.): 111S–117S.

Baskin SI and Finney CM. 1979. Effects of taurine and taurine analogues on the cardiovascular system. *Sulfur-Containing Amino Acids* 2: 1–18.

Bassat M and Mokady S. 1985. The effect of amino-acid-supplemented wheat gluten on cholesterol metabolism in the rat. *Br. J. Nutr.* 53: 25–30.

Bates CJ, Mansoor A, van der Pols J, Prentice A, Cole TJ and Finch S. 1997. Plasma total homocysteine in a representative sample of 972 British men and women aged 65 and over. *Eur. J. Clin. Nutr.* 51: 691–697.

Batta AK, Salen G, Shefer S, Tint GS and Dayal B. 1982. The effect of tauroursodeoxycholic acid and taurine supplementation on biliary bile acid composition. *Hepatology* 2: 811–816.

Bau HM. 1987. Les constituants biochimiques de quelques graines d'oléagineux et de légumineuses, PhD diss., Université de Nancy I.

Bau HM, Poullain B, Beaufrand MJ and Debry G. 1978a. Comparison of cold acid and salt precipitated soy proteins. *J. Food Sci.* 43: 106–111.

Bau HM, Poullain B, Sere Y and Debry G. 1978b. Etude de l'activité trypsique et des propriétés physico-chimiques de diverses fractions protéiques de soja. *Can. Invest. Food Sci. Technol. J.* 11: 7–11.

Bau HM and Debry G. 1979. Germinated soybean products: Chemical and nutritional evaluations. *J. Am. Oil Chem.* 56: 160–162.

Bau HM, Mohtadi-Nia D, Mejean L and Debry G. 1983. Preparation of colorless sunflower protein products: Effects of processing in physicochemical and nutritional properties. *J. Am. Oil Chem. Soc.* 60: 1141–1148.

Bau HM, Mothadi-Nia DJ, Gianangelli F and Debry G. 1987. Isolement des protéines de colza en milieu acide. (pH 4,5): Effets des traitements sur le rendement et les qualités physico-chimiques et nutritionnelles. Etude de faisabilité. *Sci. Aliment.* 7: 337–359.

Baudoin SV, Bath P, Martin JF, Du Bois R and Evans TW. 1993. L-arginine infusion has no effect on systemic haemodynamics in normal volunteers, or systemic and pulmonary haemodynamics in patients with elevated pulmonary vascular resistance. *Br. J. Pharmacol.* 36: 45–49.

Bauer JE. 1987. Serum lipoprotein of rabbits fed semi-purified diets varying in protein and carbohydrate source. *J. Am. Oil Chem. Soc.* 64: 1183–1192.

Bauer JE. 1990. Increased serum and liver lipid mass and hepatic 3–hydroxy-3–methylglu-taryl-CoA reductase activities in rabbits fed soy protein saturated fat diets. *Artery* 17: 176–188.

Bauer JE. 1991. Serum lipoprotein alterations of rabbits fed high fat soy protein-dextrose diets. *Nutr. Res.* 11: 771–782.

Bauer JE and Covert SJ. 1984. The influence of protein and carbohydrate type on serum and liver lipids and lipoprotein cholesterol in rabbits. *Lipids* 19: 844–850.

Baum JA, Teng H, Erdman JW, Weigel RM, Klein BP, Perksy VW, Freels S, Surya P, Bakhit RM, Ramos E, Shay NF and Potter SM. 1998. Long-term intake of soy protein improves blood lipid levels and increases mononuclear cell low-density-lipoprotein receptor messenger RNA in hypercholesterolemic postmenopausal women. *Am. J. Clin. Nutr.* 68 (Suppl.): 545S–551S.

Bauman JW, Hill R, Nejad NS and Chaikoff IL. 1959. Effect of bovine pituitary growth hormone on hepatic cholesterogenesis of hypophysectomized rats. *Endocrinology* 65: 73–79.

Bazzano G. 1969. Hypocholesterolemic effect of glutamic acid in the *Mongolian* gerbil. *Proc. Soc. Exp. Biol. Med.* 131: 1463–1465.

Bazzano G, d'Elia JA and Olson RE. 1970. Monosodium glutamate: Feeding of large amount in man and gerbils. *Science* 169: 1208–1209.

Bazzano G, Williams CA and Bazzano GS. 1972. The hypocholesterolemic effect of a-ketoglutarate in the *Mongolian* gerbil. *Fed. Proc.* 31: 727, Abstract.

Becattini U. 1967. Prospettive di un nuovo farmaco nella terapia delle vasculopati. *Sett. Med.* 55: 1355–1361.

Beilin LJ. 1993. Dietary fats, fish, and blood pressure. *Ann. N. Y. Acad. Sci.* 683: 35–45.

Bellamy MF, McDowell IF, Ramsey MW, Brownlee RGN, Bones C, Newcombe RG and Lewis MJ. 1998. Hyperhomocysteinemia after an oral methionine load acutely impairs endothelial function in healthy adults. *Circulation* 98: 1848–1852.

Bellentani S, Pecorari M, Cordoma M, Marchegiano P, Manenti F, Bosisio E, De Fabiani E and Galli G. 1987a. Taurine increases bile acid pool size and reduces bile saturation index in the hamster. *J. Lip. Res.* 28: 1021–1027.

Bellentani S, Bosisio E, Pecorari M, de Fabiani E, Cordoma P, Crestani M and Manenti F. 1987b. Effect of tauroursodeoxycholate feeding, with or without taurine supplementation on hepatic bile acids and cholesterol metabolism in the hamster. *Pharmacol. Res. Commn.* 19: 327–339.

Benacerraf B and Cell PG. 1961. Delayed hypersensitivity to homologous γ-globulin in the guinea pig. *Nature* 189: 586–587.

Benevenga NJ and Harper AE. 1970. Effect of glycine and serine on methionine metabolism in the rat and rabbit. *J. Nutr.* 100: 1205–1214.

Berg K. 1992. Lp(a) lipoprotein: An important genetic risk factor for atherosclerosis. In Lusis AJ, Rotter JI and Sparkes RS, Eds., *Molecular Genetics of Coronary Artery Disease: Candidate Genes and Processes in Atherosclerosis,* Monographs in Human Genetics, Vol. 14, Sparkes RS, Ed., S. Karger, Basel, pp. 189–207.

Bergeron N and Jacques H. 1989. Influence of fish protein as compared to casein and soy protein on serum and liver lipids, and serum lipoprotein cholesterol levels in the rabbit. *Atherosclerosis* 78: 113–121.

Bergeron N and Jacques H. 1990. Influence of dietary carbohydrates on cholesterol metabolism in casein-fed rabbits. *Nutr. Res.* 10: 1455–1462.

Bergeron N, Deshaies Y, Lavigne C and Jacques H. 1991. Interaction between dietary proteins and lipids in the regulation of serum and liver lipids in the rabbit. Effect of fish protein. *Lipids* 26: 759–764.

Bergeron N, Deshaies Y and Jacques H. 1992a. Factorial experiment to determine influence of fish protein and fish oil on serum and liver lipids in rabbits. *Nutrition* 8: 354–358.

Bergeron N, Deshaies Y and Jacques H. 1992b. Dietary fish protein modulates high density lipoprotein choleterol and lipoprotein lipase activity in rabbits. *J. Nutr.* 122: 1731–1737.

Bergeron N, Deshaies Y and Jacques H. 1992c. Modulation of high density lipoprotein cholesterol and lipoprotein lipase activity by dietary fish protein in the rabbit. *F.A.S.E.B. J.* 6: Part I, A1107, Abstract 991.

Bernardi F, Arcieri P, Bertina RM, Chiarotti F, Corral J, Pinotti M, Prydz H, Samama M, Sandset PM, Strom R, Garcia VV and Mariani G. 1997. Contribution of factor VII genotype to activated FVII levels. Differences in genotype frequencies between Northern and Southern European populations. *Arterioscler. Thromb. Vasc. Biol.* 17: 2548–2553.

Berthou J, Migliore-Samour D, Lifshitz A, Delettre J, Floc'h F and Jollés P. 1987. Immuno-modulating properties and three-dimensional structure of two tripeptides from human and cow caseins. *F.E.B.S. Lett.* 218: 55–58.

Bevan RD. 1975. Effect of sympathetic denervation on smooth muscle cell proliferation in the growing ear artery. *Circ. Res.* 37: 14–19.

Beveridge JMR, Connel WF and Robinson C. 1963. Effect of the level of dietary protein with and without added cholesterol on plasma cholesterol levels in man. *J. Nutr.* 79: 289–295.

Beynen AC. 1990a. Dietary proteins, cholesterol metabolism and atherosclerosis. In Sing RB, Lochan R, Rastogi SS and Mori H, Eds., *Nutrition and Cardiovascular Disease: Recent Advances in Nutriology*, Vol. 2, Shyam Printing Press, Moradabad, India, pp. 21–24.

Beynen AC. 1990b. Mode of cholesterolemic action of dietary proteins. In Beynen AC, Kritchevsky D and Pollak OJ, Eds., *Dietary Proteins, Cholesterol Metabolism and Atherosclerosis*, Monographs on Atherosclerosis, Vol. 16, S. Karger, Basel, pp. 153–159.

Beynen AC. 1990c. Comparison of the mechanism proposed to explain the hypocholester-olemic effect of soybean protein versus casein in experimental animals. *J. Nutr. Sci. Vitaminol.* 36 (Suppl.): S87–S93.

Beynen AC and Schouten JA. 1983. Influence of dietary soybean protein and casein on the level of plasma cholesterol in hamsters. *Nutr. Rep. Int.* 28: 835–841.

Beynen AC, den Engelsman G, Scholz KE and West CE. 1983a. Casein-induced hypercho-lesterolemia in rabbits: Distribution of cholesterol, triglycerides and phospholipids between serum and liver. *Ann. Nutr. Metab.* 27: 117–124.

Beynen AC, Terpstra AHM, West CE and van Tintelen G. 1983b. The concentration of serum cholesterol in rats fed cholesterol-free, low-fat semipurified diets containing either casein or soybean protein. *Nutr. Rep. Int.* 28: 363–374.

Beynen AC, Winnubst ENW and West CE. 1983c. The effect of replacement of dietary soybean protein by casein on the fecal excretion of neutral steroids in rabbits. *Z. Tierphys. Tierern. Futtermittelkunde* 49: 43–49.

Beynen AC, West CE, van Raaij JMA and Katan MB. 1983d. Dietary casein, soybean protein and serum cholesterol in experimental animals and man. In Hollo J, Ed., *Fat Science 1983: Proceedings of the ISF Congress, Budapest, 4–7 October 1983*, Elsevier, Amsterdam, pp. 1079–1088.

Beynen AC, van Gils LGM, Scholz KE and West CE. 1983e. Serum cholesterol levels of calves and rabbits fed milk replacers containing skim milk powder or soybean protein concentrate. *Nutr. Rep. Int.* 27: 757–764.

Beynen AC, Boogaard A, van Laack HLJM and Katan MB. 1984. Cholesterol metabolism in two strains of rats with high or low response of serum cholesterol to a cholesterol-rich diet. *J. Nutr.* 114: 1640–1645.

Beynen AC, West CE and Huisman J. 1985a. Differential cholesterolemic effects of dietary casein and soy protein in pigs: Role of protein digestibility. In Beynen AC, Geelen MJA, Katan MB and Schouten JA, Eds., *Cholesterol Metabolism in Health and Disease: Studies in the Netherlands.* Ponsen and Lojen, Wageningen, pp. 145–150.

Beynen AC, West CE, van Tintelen G, van Gils LGM and van der Meer R. 1985b. Effect of formaldehyde treatment of dietary casein on serum cholesterol levels in rats. *Nutr. Rep. Int.* 32: 325–335.

Beynen AC and Katan MB. 1986. Hypo and hyperresponders to dietary cholesterol. *Am. J. Clin. Nutr.* 43: 974–987.

Beynen AC, West CE, Katan MB and van Zuphten LFM. 1986a. Hyperresponsiveness of plasma cholesterol to dietary cholesterol saturated fatty acid and casein in inbred rabbits. *Nutr. Rep. Int.* 33: 65–70.

Beynen AC, van der Meer R and West CE. 1986b. Mechanisms of casein induced hypercholesterolemia: Primary and secondary features. *Atherosclerosis* 60: 291–293 (Letter).

Beynen AC, West CE, van Zuphten LFM and Katan MB. 1986c. Relation between the response of serum cholesterol to dietary cholesterol and to the type of dietary fat in random-bred rabbits. *Nutr. Rep. Int.* 33: 71–78.

Beynen AC and Lemmens AG. 1987. Dietary glycine and cholesterol metabolism in rats. *Z. Ernährungswiss.* 26: 161–164.

Beynen AC and Liepa GU. 1987. Dietary cottonseed protein and cholesterol metabolism. *Z. Ernährungswiss.* 26: 219–225.

Beynen AC and West CE. 1987. Cholesterol metabolism in swine fed diets containing either casein or soybean protein. *J. Am. Oil Chem. Soc.* 64: 1178–1182.

Beynen AC, Katan MB and van Zuphten LF. 1987a. Hypo- and hyperresponders: Individual difference in the response of serum cholesterol concentration to changes in diet. *Adv. Lipid Res.* 22: 115–171.

Beynen AC, Sirtori CR and West CE. 1987b. Vegetable protein as drugs. *Pharmacol. Res. Commn.* 19: 387–394.

Beynen AC and Sugano M. 1990. Dietary protein as a regulator of lipid metabolism: State of the art and new perspectives. *J. Nutr. Sci. Vitaminol.* 36 (Suppl.) 2: 185S–188S.

Beynen AC, West CE, Spaaij CJK, Huisman J, van Leeuwen P, Schutte JB and Hackeng WHK. 1990. Cholesterol metabolism, digestion rates and posprandial changes in serum of swine fed purified diets containing either casein or soybean protein. *J. Nutr.* 120: 422–430.

Bierman EL and Glomset JA. 1995. Disorders of lipid metabolism. In Wilson J and Foster DW, Eds., *Williams Textbook of Clinical Endocrinology,* W.B. Saunders, Philadelphia, pp. 1108–1136.

Björkholm M, de Faire U and Golm G. 1980. Immunologic evaluation of patients with ischemic heart disease. Genetic determination and relation to disease. *Atherosclerosis* 36: 195–200.

Blacher J, Ducimetiere P and Safar M. 1999. Homocysteine et pathologies cardiovasculaires: quel lien? *Presse Med.* 28: 1717–1722.

Blacher J and Safar M. 2001. Homocysteine, acide folique, vitamines du groupe B et risque cardiovasculaire. *Age Nutr.* 12: 158–162.

Blacher J and Safar ME. 2001. Homocysteine, folic acid, B vitamins and cardiovascular risk. *J. Nutr. Health Aging* 5: 196–199.

Blackett PR, Weech PK, McConathy WJ and Fesmire JD. 1982. Growth hormone in the regulation of hyperlipidemia. *Metabolism* 31: 117–120.

Blumenschein S, Torres E, Kushmaul E, Crawford J and Fixler D. 1991. Effect of oat bran/soy protein in hypercholesterolemic children. *Ann. N. Y. Acad. Sci.* 623: 413–415.

Bode-Böger SM, Böger RH, Creutzig A, Tsikas D, Gutzki FM, Alexander K and Fröhlich JC. 1994. L-arginine infusion decreases peripheral arterial resistance and inhibits platelet aggregation in healthy subjects. *Clin. Sci.* 87: 303–310.

Bode-Böger SM, Böger RH, Kienke S, Junker W and Fröhlich JC. 1996a. Elevated L-arginine/dimethyl arginine ratio contributes to enhanced systemic NO production by dietary L-arginine in hypercholesterolemic rabbits. *Biochem. Biophys. Res. Commn.* 19: 598–603.

Bode-Böger SM, Böger RH, Alfke H, Heinzel D, Tsikas D, Creutzig A, Alexander K and Fröhlich JC. 1996b. L-arginine induces nitric oxide-dependent vasodilatation in patients with critical limb ischemia. A randomized controlled study. *Circulation* 93: 85–90.

Bodwell CE, Schuster EM and Steele PS. 1980. Effects of dietary protein on plasma lipid profiles of adult men. *Fed. Proc.* 39: 1113.

Boerwinckle E, Brown SA, Rohrbach K, Gotto AM Jr and Patsch W. 1991. Role of apolipoprotein E and B gene variation in determining response of lipid, lipoprotein and apolipoprotein levels to increased dietary cholesterol. *Am. J. Hum. Genet.* 49: 1145–1154.

Böger RH, Bode-Böger SM, Mügge AV, Kienke S, Brandes R, Dwenger A and Fröhlich JC. 1995. Supplementation of hypercholesterolaemic rabbits with L-arginine reduces the vascular release of superoxide anions and restores NO production. *Atherosclerosis* 117: 273–284.

Böger RH, Bode-Böger SM and Fröhlich JC. 1996a. The L-arginine-nitric-oxide pathway: Role in atherosclerosis and therapeutic implications. *Atherosclerosis* 127: 1–11.

Böger RH, Bode-Böger SM and Fröhlich JC. 1996b. Pathogenetische Bedeutung des L-Arginin-NO-Stoffwechselwegs bei Arteriosklerose und mögliche therapeutische Aspekte. *Vasa* 25: 305–316.

Böger RH, Bode-Böger SM, Brandes RP, Phivthong-ngam L, Böhme M, Nafe R, Mügge A and Fröhlich JC. 1997. Dietary L-arginine reduces the progression of atherosclerosis in cholesterol-fed rabbits. Comparison with lovastatin. *Circulation* 96: 1282–1290.

Bohman VR, Wade MA and Torell CR. 1962. Effect of dietary fat and graded levels of alfalfa on growth and tissue lipids of the bovine. *J. Anim. Sci.* 21: 241–247.

Borradaile NM, Carroll KK and Kurowska EM. 1999. Regulation of HepG$_2$ cells apolipoprotein B metabolism by the citrus flavanones hesperetin and naringenin. *Lipids* 34: 591–598.

Bosaeus I, Sandstrom B and Anderson H. 1988. Bile acid and cholesterol excretion in human beings given soya-bean and meat-protein-based diets: A study in ileostomy subjects. *Br. J. Nutr.* 59: 215–221.

Bosello O, Cominacini L, Zocca I, Garbin U, Compri R, Davoli A and Brunetti L. 1988. Short- and long-term effects of hypocaloric diets containing proteins of different sources on plasma lipids and apoproteins of obese subjects. *Ann. Nutr. Metab.* 32: 206–214.

Bosisio E, Ghiselli GC, Kienle GM, Galli G and Sirtori CR. 1980. Experimental studies on the mechanism of the hypocholesterolemic effect of soy protein. *Proceedings of the VII International Symposium on Drugs Affecting Lipid Metabolism*, Fumagalli R, Kritchevsky D and Paoletti R. Eds., Milan, May 1980, Elsevier, Amsterdam, p. 274.

Bosisio E, Ghiselli GC, Kienle GM, Galli G and Sirtori CR. 1981. Effects of dietary soy protein on liver catabolism and plasma transport of cholesterol in hypercholesterolemic rats. *J. Steroid Biochem.* 14: 1201–1207.

Bostom AG, Jacques PF, Nadeau MR, William RR, Ellison RC and Selhub J. 1995. Postmethionine load hyperhomocysteinemia in persons with normal fasting total plasma homocysteine: Initial results from the NHLBI Family Heart Study. *Atherosclerosis* 116: 147–151.

Bostom AG, Silbershatz H, Rosenberg IH, Selhub J, D'Agostino RB, Wolf PA, Jacques PF and Wilson PW. 1999. Nonfasting plasma total homocysteine levels and all-cause and cardiovascular disease mortality in elderly Framingham men and women. *Arch. Intern. Med.* 159: 1077–1080.

Boualga A, Bouchenak M and Belleville J. 2000. Low-protein diet prevents tissue lipoprotein lipase activity increase in growing rats. *Br. J. Nutr.* 84: 663–671.

Bounous G, Letourneau L and Kongshavn PAL. 1983. Influence of dietary protein type on immune system of mice. *J. Nutr.* 113: 1415–1421.

Bouziane M, Prost J and Belleville J. 1992. Changes in serum and lipoprotein fatty acids of growing rats fed protein-deficient diets with low or adequate linolenic acid concentrations. *J. Nutr.* 122: 2037–2046.

Bouziane M, Prost J and Belleville J. 1994a. Changes in fatty acid compositions of total serum and lipoprotein particles, in growing rats given protein-deficiency diets with either hydrogenated coconut or salmon oils as fat sources. *Br. J. Nutr.* 71: 375–387.

Bouziane M, Prost J and Belleville J. 1994b. Dietary protein affects n-3 and n-6 polyunsaturated fatty acids hepatic storage and very low density lipoprotein transport in rats on different diets. *Lipids* 29: 265–272.

Boyd EM. 1942. Species variation in normal plasma lipids estimated by oxidative micromethods. *J. Biol. Chem.* 143: 131–132.

Bragdon JH and Mikelsen O. 1955. Experimental atherosclerosis in the rat. *Am. J. Pathol.* 31: 965–973.

Brattsand R. 1976. Distribution of cholesterol and triglycerides among lipoproteins fractions in fat-fed rabbits at different levels of serum cholesterol. *Atherosclerosis* 23: 97–110.

Brattström L and Wilcken DEL. 2000. Homocysteine and cardiovascular disease: Cause or effect? *Am. J. Clin. Nutr.* 72: 315–323.

Bremer J. 1955. The conjugation of glycine with cholic acid and benzoic acid in rat liver homogenates. Bile acids and steroids. *Acta Chem. Scand.* 9: 268–271.

Bremer J. 1956. Species differences in the conjugation of free bile acids with taurine and glycine. *Biochem. J.* 63: 507–513.

Bremer J. 1983. Carnitine — Metabolism and function. *Physiol. Rev.* 63: 1420–1480.

Brink EJ, Dekker PR, Beresteijn van ECH and Beynen AC. 1991. Inhibitory effect of dietary soybean protein vs. casein on magnesium absorption in rats. *J. Nutr.* 121: 1374–1381.

Bronte-Stewart B, Antonis A, Eales L and Brock JF. 1956. Effects of feeding different fats on the serum cholesterol level. *Lancet* 1: 525–526.

Brooks YR and Morr CV. 1992. Current aspects of soy protein fractionation and nomenclature. *J. Am. Oil Chem. Soc.* 62: 1347–1354.

Brown MS, Kovanen PT and Goldstein JL. 1981. Regulation of plasma cholesterol by lipoprotein receptors. *Science* 212: 628–635.

Brown WV and Karmally W. 1985. Coronary heart disease and the consumption of diets high in wheat and other grains. *Am. J. Clin. Nutr.* 41: 1163–1171.

Brussard JH, van Raaij JMA, Stasse-Wolthuis M, Katan MB and Hautvast JAGJ. 1981. Blood pressure and diet in normotensive volunteers: Absence of an effect of dietary fibre, protein or fat. *Am. J. Clin. Nutr.* 34: 2023–2029.

Bulpitt CJ. 1985. Epidemiology of hypertension. In Kirkehäger WH and Reid JL, Eds., *Handbook of Hypertension*, Elsevier, Amsterdam, p. 6.

Burns MJ and Self KS. 1969. Effects of cystine, niacine and taurine on cholesterol and bile acid metabolism in rabbits. *Metabolism* 18: 427–432.

Burslem J, Schonfeld G, Howald MA, Weidman SW and Miller JP. 1978. Plasma apoprotein and lipoprotein lipid levels in vegetarians. *Metabolism* 27: 711–719.

Burston D, Addison JM and Matthews DM. 1972. Uptake of dipeptides containing basic and acidic amino acids by rat small intestine *in vitro*. *Clin. Sci.* 43: 823–837.

Bursztyn PG. 1982. Effect of meat on blood pressure. *J.A.M.A.* 248: 29–30.

Bursztyn PG. 1987. *Nutrition and Blood Pressure*. John Libbey, London.

Bursztyn PG and Firth WR. 1975. Effect of three fat-enriched diets on the arterial pressure of rabbits. *Cardiovasc. Res.* 9: 807–810.

Bursztyn PG and Husbands DR. 1980. Fat induced hypertension in rabbits. Effects of dietary fibre on blood pressure and blood lipid concentration. *Cardiovasc. Res.* 14: 185–191.

Bursztyn PG and Vas Dias FW. 1985. Dietary protein and blood pressure. *Clin. Exp. Hypertens.* 7: 1553–1562.

Butler JE. 1983. Bovine immunoglobulins: An augmented review. *Vet. Immunol. Immunopathol.* 4: 43–152.

Bydlowski SP, Stivaletti VLG and Douglas CR. 1984. Biochemical observations on rat aortas: Effect of protein refeeding after a protein depletion period. *Ann. Nutr. Metab.* 28: 85–91.

Bydlowski SP, Stivaletti VLG and Douglas CR. 1986. Biochemical observations on rat aortas: Interaction of dietary protein and cholesterol. *Br. J. Nutr.* 55: 295–304.

Caen JP, Bal dit Sollier C, Mazoyer E, Drouet L, Jollés P and Fiat AM. 1991. Des peptides à activité antithrombotique dans les protéines du lait: Un lien entre thérapeutique et diététique. *Med. Sci.* 7: 500–501.

Caen JP, Jollés P, Bal dit Sollier C, Fiat AM, Mazoyer E and Drouet L. 1992. Activité antithrombotique de séquences peptidiques de protéines de lait. *Cah. Nutr. Diet.* 27: 33–35.

Cagliarducci U. 1974. Sul trattamento delle cardiopatie ischemiche acute con taurina. *Clin. Ther.* 68: 261–270.

Calver A, Collier J and Vallance P. 1991. Dilator actions of arginine in human peripheral vasculature. *Clin. Sci.* 81: 695–700.

Calvert GD, Blight L, Illman RJ, Topping DL and Potter JD. 1981. A trial of the effects of soya bean flour and soya bean saponins on plasma lipids, faecal bile acids and neutral sterols in hypercholesterolemic men. *Br. J. Nutr.* 45: 277–281.

Campbell AM, Swendseid ME, Griffith WH and Tuttle SG. 1965. Serum lipids of men fed diets differing in protein quality and linoleic acid content. *Am. J. Clin. Nutr.* 17: 83–87.

Campbell KL, Czarnecki-Maulden GL and Schaeffer JD. 1995. Effects of animal and soy fats and proteins in the diet on fatty acid concentrations in the serum and skin in dogs. *Am. J. Vet. Res.* 56: 1465–1469.

Campbell M, Rhodes GL and Levinson JP. 1952. The effects of α-tocopherol on experimental atherosclerosis. *Angiology* 3: 397–403.

Campese VM, Amar M, Anjali C, Medhat T and Wurgaft A. 1997. Effect of L-arginine on systemic and renal haemodynamics in salt-sensitive patients with essential hypertension. *J. Hum. Hypertens.* 11: 527–532.

Campisi R, Czernin J, Schröder H, Sayre JW and Schelbert HR. 1999. L-arginine normalizes coronary vasomotion in long term smokers. *Circulation* 99: 491–497.

Cantafora A, Mantovani A, Masella R, Mechelli L and Alvaro D. 1986. Effect of taurine administration on liver lipids in guinea pig. *Experientia* 42: 407–408.

Cantafora A, Blotta I, Ross SS, Hofmann AF and Sturman JA. 1991. Dietary taurine content changes liver lipids in cats. *J. Nutr.* 121: 1522–1528.

Cantafora A, Yan CC, Sun Y and Masella R. 1994. Effects of taurine on microsomal enzyme activities involved in liver lipid metabolism of *Wistar* rats. In Huxtable R and Michalk DV, Eds., *Taurine in Health and Disease*, Plenum Press, New York, pp. 99–110.

Carlile SI and Lacko AG. 1981. Strain differences in the age related changes of rat lipoprotein metabolism. *Comp. Biochem. Physiol. B. Biochem. Mol. Biol.* 70: 753–758.

Carlile SI, Kudchodkar BJ, Wang CS and Lacko AG. 1986. Age-related changes in the rate of esterification of plasma cholesterol in *Fischer-344* rats. *Mech. Ageing Dev.* 33: 211–220.

Carr CJJ, Talboot M, Fischer KD. 1975. A review of the significance of bovine milk xanthine oxidase in the etiology of atherosclerosis. (Contract FDA 223–75–2090.) F.A.S.E.B. Life Sciences Research Office, Division of Nutrition, Bureau of Foods, Bethesda MD.

Carroll KK. 1967. Diet, cholesterol metabolism and atherosclerosis. *J. Am. Oil Chem. Soc.* 44: 607–614.

Carroll KK. 1971. Plasma cholesterol levels and liver cholesterol biosynthesis in rabbits fed commercial or semi-synthetic diets with and without added fats or oils. *Atherosclerosis* 13: 67–76.

Carroll KK. 1978a. Dietary protein in relation to plasma cholesterol levels and atherosclerosis. *Nutr. Rev.* 36: 1–5.

Carroll KK. 1978b. The role of dietary protein in hypercholesterolemia and atherosclerosis. *Lipids* 13: 360–365.

Carroll KK. 1981a. Soy protein and atherosclerosis. *J. Am. Oil Chem. Soc.* 58: 416–419.

Carroll KK. 1981b. Dietary protein and cardiovascular disease. In New Trends in Nutrition, Lipid Research and Cardiovascular Disease. In Bazan NG, Paoletti R and Iacono JM, Eds., *Current Topics in Nutrition and Disease*, Vol. 5, Alan R. Liss, New York, pp. 167–177.

Carroll KK. 1982. Hypercholesterolemia and atherosclerosis: Effect of dietary protein. *Fed. Proc.* 41: 2792–2796.

Carroll KK. 1983. Dietary proteins and amino acids: Their effects on cholesterol metabolism. In Gibney MJ and Kritchevsky D, Eds., *Animal and Vegetable Proteins in Lipid Metabolism and Atherosclerosis*, Alan R. Liss, New York, pp. 9–17.

Carroll KK. 1991a. Review of clinical studies on cholesterol-lowering response to soy protein. *J. Am. Diet. Assoc.* 91: 820–827.

Carroll KK. 1991b. Vegetable proteins: Potential lipid-lowering effects. *Med. North Am. 4th Ser.* 17: 2279–2282.

Carroll KK. 1992. Dietary protein, cholesterolemia and atherosclerosis. *Can. Med. Assoc. J.* 147: 900.

Carroll KK and Hamilton RMG. 1975. Effects of dietary protein and carbohydrate on plasma cholesterol levels in relation to atherosclerosis. *J. Food Sci.* 40: 18–23.

Carroll KK, Giovanetti PM, Huff MW, Moase O, Roberts DCK and Wolfe BM. 1978. Hypocholesterolemic effect of substituting soybean protein for animal protein in the diet of healthy young women. *Am. J. Clin. Nutr.* 31: 1312–1321.

Carroll KK, Huff MW and Roberts DCK. 1979. Vegetable protein and lipid metabolism. In Wilcke HL, Hopkins DT and Waggle DH, Eds., *Soy Protein and Human Nutrition*, Academic Press, New York, pp. 261–280.

Carroll KK, Hrabek-Smith JM and Kurowska EM. 1989. Effects of dietary protein on serum total and lipoprotein cholesterol levels. In Grepaldi G, Gotto AM, Manzato E and Baggio G, Eds., *Atherosclerosis VIII*, Elsevier, Amsterdam, pp. 693–696.

Carroll KK and Kurowska EM. 1995. Soy consumption and cholesterol reduction: Review of animal and human studies. *J. Nutr.* 125: 594S–597S.

Casino PR, Kilcoyne CM, Quyyumi AA, Hoeg JM and Panza JA. 1994. Investigation of decreased availability of nitric oxide precursor as the mechanism responsible for impaired endothelium-dependent vasodilatation in hypercholesterolemic patients. *J. Am. Coll. Cardiol.* 23: 844–850.

Cassidy A, Bingham S and Setchell K. 1995. Biological effects of isoflavonoids in young women: Importance of the chemical composition of soyabean products. *Br. J. Nutr.* 74: 587–601.

Caterina de R, Libby P, Peng HB, Thannical VJ, Rajavashist TB, Gimbrone MA, Shin WS and Liao JK. 1995. Nitric oxide decreases cytokine-induced endothelial activation. Nitric oxide selectively reduces endothelial expression of adhesion molecules and proinflammatory cytokines *J. Clin. Invest.* 96: 60–68.

Chabance B, Quian ZY, Migliore Samour D, Jollès P and Fiat AM. 1997. Binding of the bovine caseinoglycopeptide to the platelet membrane glycoprotein GPIb alpha. *Biochem. Mol. Biol. Int.* 42: 77–84.

Chait A. 1996. Effects of isoflavones on LDL-cholesterol *in vitro* but not *in vivo*. Second International Symposium on the Role of Soy in Preventing and Treating Chronic Diseases, Brussels, Sept. 15–18, 1996, Abstract, p. 28.

Chait A. 1998. Effects of isoflavones on LDL-cholesterol *in vitro* but not *in vivo*. *Am. J. Clin. Nutr.* 68 (Suppl.): 1523S.

Chait A, Bierman EL and Albers JJ. 1979. Regulatory role of triiodothyronine in the degradation of low density lipoprotein by cultured human skin fibroblast. *J. Clin. Endocrinol. Metab.* 48: 887–889.

Chakkaphak MS and Lichton IJ. 1970. Elevation of systolic blood pressure in rats fed diets containing fish and soybean proteins. *J. Nutr.* 100: 1081–1088.

Chalatow S. 1912. Über das Verhalten der Leber gegenüber den verschiedenen Arten von Speisefett. *Virchows Arch. Pathol. Anat. Physiol. Klin. Med.* 207: 452–469.

Chan KC, Lou PP and Hargrove JL. 1993. High casein-lactalbumin diet accelerates blood coagulation in rats. *J. Nutr.* 123: 1010–1016.

Chandler PT, McCarthy RD and Kesler EM. 1968. Effect of dietary lipids and protein on serum proteins, lipids and glucose in the blood of dairy calves. *J. Nutr.* 95: 461–468.

Chandrasiri V, Bau HM, Villaume C, Gianangeli F, Lorient D and Méjean L. 1987. Effet de la germination de la graine de soja sur la composition et la valeur nutritionnelle de sa farine. *Sci. Alim.* 7: 139–150.

Chandrasiri V, Bau HM, Villaume C, Gianangeli F and Méjean L. 1990. Effect of germinated and heated soybean meals on plasma cholesterol and triglycerides in rats. *Reprod. Nutr. Dev.* 30: 611–618.

Chandrasiri V, Villaume C, Bau HM and Méjean L. 1991. Effects of the nature of dietary proteins, lecithin and methionine on rat plasma lipids. *Arch. Int. Physiol. Biochim. Biophys.* 99: 291–295.

Chang MLW and Johnson MA. 1980. Effect of pectin and protein levels on cholesterol-4-^{14}C metabolism in rats. *Nutr. Rep. Int.* 22: 91–99.

Chango A, Villaume C, Bau HM, Schwertz A, Nicolas JP and Méjean L. 1998. Effects of casein, sweet white lupin and sweet yellow lupin diet on cholesterol metabolism in rats. J. *Sci. Food Agric.* 76: 303–309.

Chanussot F, Polichetti E, Luna A and La Droitte P. 1996. La lécithine de soja en alimentation humaine. *Cah. Nutr. Diet.* 31: 305–311.

Chanusssot F, Polichetti E, Domingo N, Janissson A, Lechene De la Porte P, Lafont H, Luna A and La Droitte P. 1998. Stimulation by soybean lecithin of cholesterol transfer from plasma to biliary compartment: Mechanisms of cholesterol- and triglyceride-lowering effects in liver. *Am. J. Clin. Nutr.* 68 (Suppl.): 1520S.

Chao YS, Yamin TT and Alberts AW. 1982. Effects of cholestyramine on low density lipo-protein binding sites on liver membranes from rabbits with endogenous hypercho-lesterolemia induced by a wheat starch-casein diet. *J. Biol. Chem.* 257: 3623–3627.

Chao YS, Kroon PA, Yamin TT, Thompson GM and Alberts AW. 1983. Regulation of hepatic receptor-dependent degradation of LDL by mevinolin in rabbits. *Biochim. Biophys. Acta* 754: 134–141.

Chao YS, Yamin TT, Seidenberg J and Kroon PA. 1986. Secretion of cholesterol-ester rich lipoproteins by the perfused livers of rabbits fed a wheat starch-casein diet. *Biochem. Biophys. Acta* 876: 392–398.

Chapman MJ. 1980. Animal lipoproteins: Chemistry, structure and comparative aspects. *J. Lipid Res.* 21: 789–853.

Chauhan A, More RS, Mullins PA, Taylor G, Petch MC and Schofield PM. 1996. Aging-associated endothelial dysfunction in humans is reversed by L-arginine. *J. Am. Coll. Cardiol.* 28: 1796–1804.

Cheeke PR. 1976. Nutritional and physiological properties of saponins. *Nutr. Rep. Int.* 13: 315–324.

Chen C and Bakhit RM. 1999. The effect of genistein on antioxidative defense systems and plasma lipid profiles in aged rats. *F.A.S.E.B. J.* 13: A904, Abstract 676.5.

Chen LH, Liao S and Packett LV. 1972. Interaction of dietary vitamin E and protein level or lipid source with serum cholesterol level in rats. *J. Nutr.* 102: 729–732.

Chen LY, Mehta P and Mehta JL. 1996. Oxidized LDL decreases L-arginine uptake and nitric oxide synthase protein expression in human platelets. Relevance of the effect of oxidized LDL on platelet functions. *Circulation* 93: 1740–1746.

Chen WJL, Anderson JW and Jennings D. 1984. Propionate may mediate the hypocholester-olemic effects of certain soluble plant fibers in cholesterol-fed rats. *Proc. Soc. Exp. Biol. Med.* 175: 215–218.

Cheraskin E and Ringsdorf WM. 1970. Daily vitamin E consumption and reported cardio-vacular findings. *Nutr. Rep. Int.* 2: 107–111.

Chervan J. 1980. Phytic acid interactions in food systems. *Crit. Rev. Food Sci. Nutr.* 13: 297–335.

Chiji H, Harayama K and Kiriyama S. 1990. Effects of feeding rats low protein diets containing casein or soy protein isolate supplemented with methionine or oligo-methionine. *J. Nutr.* 120: 166–171.

Chin JH, Azhar S and Hoffman BB. 1992. Inactivation of endothelial derived relaxing factor by oxidized lipoproteins. *J. Clin. Invest.* 89: 10–18.

Chinellato A, Ragazzi E, Polverino de Laureto P and Fassina G. 1992. Reduced L-argin-ine/lysine and L-arginine/aspartic acid ratios in aorta from *Watanabe heritable hyper-lipidemic (WHHL)* rabbit. *Pharmacol. Res.* 25: 255–258.

Cho BH, Egwin PO and Fahey GC Jr. 1985. Plasma lipid and lipoprotein cholesterol levels in swine. Modification of protein-induced responses by added cholesterol and soy fiber. *Atherosclerosis* 56: 39–49.

Cho ES, Johnson N and Snider BCF. 1984. Tissue glutathione as a cyst(e)ine reservoir during cystine depletion in growing rats. *J. Nutr.* 114: 1853–1862.

Cho S, Hazama M, Urata Y, Goto S, Horiuchi S, Sumikawa K and Kondo T. 1999. Protective role of glutathione synthesis in response to oxidized low density lipoprotein in humans vascular endothelial cells. *Free Radical Biol. Med.* 26: 589–602.

Choi IS and Chee KM. 1995a. Effect of paired-fed diets containing soy protein, casein and fish oil on cholesterol levels in plasma and liver of young chicks. *Korean J. Anim. Sci.* 37: 117–126.

Choi IS and Chee KM. 1995b. Effects of dietary casein and fish oil on plasma cholesterol levels in young chicks. *Korean J. Anim. Sci.* 37: 127–135.

Choi YS and Sugano M. 1988. Effects of dietary alpha- and gamma-linolenic acid on lipid metabolism in young and adult rats. *Ann. Nutr. Metab.* 32: 169–176.

Choi YS, Horigome T, Sakaguchi E and Uchida S. 1988. Effects of feeding of leaf proteins on serum cholesterol concentrations in rats. *Nippon Eyyō Shokuryō Gakkaishi* 41: 127–132 (in Japanese).

Choi YS, Goto S, Ikeda I and Sugano M. 1989a. Interaction of dietary protein, cholesterol and age on lipid metabolism of the rat. *Br. J. Nutr.* 61: 531–543.

Choi YS, Ikeda I and Sugano M. 1989b. The combined effect of dietary proteins and fish oil on cholesterol metabolism in rats of different ages. *Lipids* 24: 506–510.

Choi YS, Ikeda I and Sugano M. 1990. Dietary fats modulate age-dependent effects of dietary proteins on cholesterol metabolism of rats. *J. Nutr. Sci. Vitaminol.* 36 (Suppl.): 181S–184S.

Chopra IJ, Chopra U, Smith SR, Reza M and Solomon DH. 1975. Reciprocal changes in serum concentrations of 3, 3', 5–triiodothyronine (T3) in systemic illness. *J. Clin. Endocrinol. Metab.* 41: 1043–1049.

Chowienczyk P and Ritter J. 1997. Arginine: NO more than a simple amino acid? *Lancet* 150: 901.

Chu EL and Kies C. 1993. Protein and lipid status in human fed diets containing pork, beef, fish, soy and poultry. *F.A.S.E.B. J.* 7: A179, Abstract 1035.

Clarkson P, Adams MR, Powe AJ, Donald E, McCredie R, Robinson J, McCarty SN, Keech A, Celermajer DS and Deanfield E. 1996. Oral L-arginine improves endothelium-dependent dilatation in hypercholesterolemic young adults. *J. Clin. Invest.* 97: 1989–1994.

Clarkson S and Newburgh LH. 1926. The relation between atherosclerosis and ingested cholesterol in the rabbit. *J. Exp. Med.* 43: 595–612.

Clarkson TB, Prichard RW, Lofland HB and Goodman HO. 1962. Interactions among dietary fat, protein, and cholesterol in atherosclerosis-susceptible pigeons. *Circ. Res.* 11: 400–404.

Clarkson TB, Anthony MS, Williams JK, Honore EK and Cline JM. 1998. The potential of soybean phytoestrogens for postmenopausal hormone replacement therapy. *Proc. Soc. Exp. Biol. Med.* 217: 365–368.

Clifton PM and Abbey M. 1997. Genetic control of response to dietary fats and cholesterol. *World Rev. Nutr. Diet.* S. Karger, Basel, 80: 1–14.

Cobb MM, Teitelbaum H, Risch N, Jekel J and Ostfeld A. 1992. Influence of dietary fat, apolipoprotein E phenotype, and sex on plasma lipoprotein levels. *Circulation* 86: 849–857.

Cobb MM and Risch N. 1993. Low-density lipoprotein cholesterol responsiveness to diet in normolipemic subjects. *Metabolism* 42: 7–13.

Coccodrilli GD, Chandler PT and Polan CE. 1970. Effects of dietary protein on blood lipids of the calf with special reference to cholesterol. *J. Dairy Sci.* 53: 1627–1631.

Coggins CH, Dwyer JT, Greene T, Petot G, Snetselaar LG and Van Lente F. 1994. Serum lipid changes associated with modified protein diets: Results from the feasibility phase of the Modification of Diet in Renal Disease Study. *Am. J. Kidney Dis.* 23: 514–523.

Cohen JC. 1989. Protein ingestion does not affect postprandial lipaemia or chylomicron-triglyceride clearance. *Eur. J. Clin. Nutr.* 43: 497–499.

Cohen RA, Zitnay KM, Haudenschild CC and Cunningham LD. 1988. Loss of selective endothelial cell vasoactive function caused by hypercholesterolemia in pig coronary arteries. *Circ. Res.* 63: 903–910.

Cohn JS, Kimpton WG and Nestel PJ. 1984. The effect of dietary casein and soy protein on cholesterol and very low density lipoprotein metabolism in the rat. *Atherosclerosis* 52: 219–231.

Cohn JS and Nestel PJ. 1985. Hepatic lipoprotein receptor activity in rats fed casein and soy protein. *Atherosclerosis* 56: 247–250.

Connor WE and Connor SL. 1972. The key role of nutritional factors in the prevention of coronary heart disease. *Prev. Med.* 1: 49–83.

Constans J, Blann AD, Resplandy F, Parrot F, Seigneur M, Renard M, Amiral J, Guerin V, Boisseau MR and Couri CL. 1999. Endothelial dysfunction during acute methionine load in hyperhomocysteinamic patients. *Atherosclerosis* 147: 411–413.

Constantinides P. 1980. Present evidence for the role of immune factors in atherogenesis. In Constantinides P, Pratesi F, Cavallero C and di Perri T, *Immunity and Atherosclerosis*, Academic Press, London, pp. 23–30.

Cooke J. 1998. Is atherosclerosis an arginine deficiency disease? *J. Invest. Med.* 46: 377–380.

Cooke JP, Andon NA, Girerd XJ, Hirsch AT and Creager MA. 1991. Arginine restores cholinergic relaxation of hypercholesterolemic rabbits thoracic aorta. *Circulation* 83: 1057–1062.

Cooke JP, Singer AH, Tsao P, Zera P, Rowan RA and Billingham ME. 1992. Antiatherogenic effects of L-arginine in the hypercholesterolemic rabbit. *J. Clin. Invest.* 90: 1168–1172.

Cooke JP and Tsao PS. 1997. Arginine: A new therapy for atherosclerosis? *Circulation* 95: 311–312.

Cookson FB, Alstchul R and Fedoroff S. 1967. The effects of alfalfa on serum cholesterol and in modifying or preventing cholesterol induced atherosclerosis in rabbits. *J. Atheroscler. Res.* 7: 69–81.

Cookson FB and Fedoroff S. 1968. Quantitative relationship between administered cholesterol and alfalfa required to prevent hypercholesterolemia in rabbits. *Br. J. Exp. Pathol.* 49: 348–355.

Coulson CB and Evans RA. 1960. The effects of saponin and linoleic acid on the weight increase of growing rats. *Br. J. Nutr.* 14: 121–134.

Cowan JW and Margossian S. 1966. Thyroid function in female rat severely depleted of body protein. *Endocrinology* 79: 1023–1026.

Cowley AW. 1997. Genetic and non genetic determinants of salt sensitivity and blood pressure. *Am. J. Clin. Nutr.* 65 (Suppl.): 587S–593S.

Cranwell K and Liebman M. 1989. Effect of soybean fiber and phytate on serum zinc response. *Nutr. Res.* 9: 127–132.

Creager MA, Gallagher SJ, Girerd XJ, Dzau VJ and Cooke JP. 1990. L-arginine normalizes endothelial response in the forearm circulation of hypercholesterolemic human. *Circulation* 82 (Suppl. 3): III-346, Abstract.

Creager MA, Gallagher S, Girerd XJ, Coleman SM, Dzau VJ and Cooke JP. 1992. L-arginine improves endothelium-vasodilatation in hypercholesterolemic humans. *J. Clin. Invest.* 90: 1248–1253.

Cree TC and Schalch DS. 1985. Protein utilization in growth: Effect of lysine deficiency on serum growth hormone, somatomedins, insulin, total thyroxine (T_4) and triiodothyronine, free T_4 index, and total corticosterone. *Endocrinology* 117: 667–673.

Critchfield JW, Ney D, Schneeman B and Rucker R. 1990. Protein quality: Plasma cholesterol and apolipoprotein levels in the rats. *Nutr. Res.* 10: 655–662.

Crouse JR III, Morgan T, Terry JG, Ellis J, Vitlins M and Burke GL. 1999. A randomized trial comparing the effect of casein with that of soy protein containing varying amounts of isoflavones on plasma concentrations of lipids and lipoproteins. *Arch. Intern. Med.* 159: 2070–2076.

Cryer A and Jones HM. 1978. Changes in the lipoprotein lipase (clearing-factor lipase) activity of white adipose tissue during development of the rat. *Biochem. J.* 172: 319–325.

Curb JD and Reed DM. 1985. Fish consumption and mortality from coronary heart disease. *N. Engl. J. Med.* 313: 821–822.

Czarnecki SK and Kritchevsky D. 1979. The effects of dietary proteins on lipoprotein metabolism and atherosclerosis in rabbits. *J. Am. Oil Chem. Soc.* 56: 388A.

Dahlen GH, Weinehall L, Stenlund H, Jansson JH, Hallmans G, Huhtasaari F and Wall S. 1988. Lipoprotein(a) and cholesterol levels act synergistically and apolipoprotein A-I is protective for the incidence of primay acute myocardial infarction in middle-aged males. An incident case-control from Sweden. *J. Intern. Med.* 244: 425–430.

Dalery K, Lusier-Cacan S, Selhub J, Davignon J, Latour Y and Genest J Jr. 1995. Homocysteine and coronary artery disease in French Canadian subjects: Relation with vitamin B_{12}, B_6, pyridoxal phosphate and folate. *Am. J. Cardiol.* 75: 1107–1111.

Daley SJ, Herderick EDE, Cornhill JF and Rogers KA. 1994a. Cholesterol-fed and casein-fed rabbit models of atherosclerosis. Part 1: Differing lesion area and volume despite equal plasma cholesterol levels. *Arterioscler. Thromb. Vasc. Biol.* 14: 95–104.

Daley SJ, Klemp KF, Guyton JR and Rogers KA. 1994b. Cholesterol-fed and casein-fed rabbit models of atherosclerosis. Part 2: Differing morphological severity of atherogenesis despite matched plasma cholesterol levels. *Arterioscler. Thromb. Vasc. Biol.* 14: 105–114.

Damasceno NRT, Gidlund MA, Goto H, Dias CTS, Okawabata FS and Abdalla DSP. 2000. Casein and soy protein isolate in experimental atherosclerosis: Influence on hyperlipidemia and lipoprotein oxidation. *Ann. Nutr. Metab.* 45: 38–46.

D'Amato L. 1908. Neue Untersuchungen über die Experimentelle Pathologie der Blutgefässe. *Virchows Arch. Pathol. Anat. Physiol. Klin. Med.* 192: 86–112.

D'Amico G, Gentile MG, Manna G, Fellin G, Ciceri R, Cofano F, Petrini C, Lavarda F, Perolini S and Porrini M. 1992. Effect of vegetarian soy diet on hyperlipidaemia in nephrotic syndrome. *Lancet* 339: 1131–1134.

Darley-Usmar VM, Crawford J, Patel R, Moellering D and Barnes S. 1997. Effects of phytosterols on lipid peroxidation. Symposium on Phytoestrogen Research Methods: Chemistry, Analysis, and Biological Properties, Tucson, AZ, Sept. 21–24, 1997, Abstract.

Davies DF. 1971. Hypothesis: An immunological view of atherogenesis. *J. Atheroscler. Res.* 10: 253–256.

Davies DF, Davies JR and Richards MA. 1969. Antibodies to reconstituted dried cow's milk protein in coronary heart disease. *J. Atheroscler. Res.* 9: 103–107.

Davies DF, Johnson AP, Rees BWG, Elwood PC and Abernethy M. 1974. Food antibodies and myocardial infarction. *Lancet* 1: 1012–1017.

Davies MG, Barber E, Dalen H and Hagen PO. 1996. L-arginine supplementation improves venous endothelial cell but not smooth muscle cell dysfunction induced by prolonged diet-induced hypercholesterolemia. *J. Invest. Surg.* 9: 415–422.

Davignon J, Gregg RE and Singh CF. 1988. Apolipoprotein E polymorphism and atherosclerosis. *Atherosclerosis* 8: 1–21.

Davis R, Boogaerts JR, Borchardt RA, Malone-McNeal M and Archambault-Schexnayder J. 1985. Intrahepatic assembly of very-low density lipoproteins. *J. Biol. Chem.* 260: 14137–14144.

Davis RB and Holtz GC. 1969. Clumping of blood platelets by heat aggregated gamma globulin. *Thromb. Diath. Haemorrhage* 21: 65–75.

Davis SR, Murkies AL and Wilcox G. 1998. Phytoestrogens in clinical practice. *Integrative Med.* 1: 27–34.

Dawber TR. 1980. *The Framingham Study: The Epidemiology of Atherosclerotic Disease.* Harvard University Press, Cambridge, MA.

Day CE, Phillips WA and Schurr PE. 1979. Animal models for an integrated approach to the pharmacologic control of atherosclerosis. *Artery* 5: 90–99.

Deb C, Mallick N and Goswami U. 1973. Effect of different percentages of protein intake on thyroid activity, protein bound iodine, total thyroxine and free thyroxine level of blood of rats. *Endokrinologie* 62: 321–326.

Debry G. 1976. Comportement alimentaire et maladies cardiovasculaires. *Ann. Nutr. Aliment.* 30: 219–233.

Debry G. 1987a. Food proteins and atherosclerosis. In Schlierf G and Mörl H, Eds., *Expanding Horizons in Atherosclerosis Research.* Springer-Verlag, Berlin, pp. 309–316.

Debry G. 1987b. Nutrition and heart disease in the aging. In Watson RR, Ed., *Nutrition and Heart Disease*, Vol. 2. CRC. Press, Boca Raton, FL, pp. 119–140.

Debry G. 2001a. Lait et athérosclérose. In Debry G, Ed., *Lait, Nutrition et Santé*, Editions Tec et Doc Lavoisier, Paris, pp. 395–433.

Debry G. 2001b. Lait, thrombose, hypertension artérielle et accidents vasculaires cérébraux. In Debry G, Ed., *Lait, Nutrition et Santé*, Editions Tec et Doc Lavoisier, Paris, pp. 435–465.

Debry G, Drouin P, Pointel JP, Louis J and Gross P. 1984. Alimentation et athérosclérose. *J. Annu. Diabetol.* 223–234.

Deeley RG, Tam SP and Archer TK. 1985. The effects of estrogen on apolipoprotein synthesis (review). *Can. J. Biochem. Cell Biol.* 63: 882–889.

Deeth HC. 1983. Homogenized milk and atherosclerotic disease: A review. *J. Dairy Sci.* 66: 1419–1435.

Delgado M, Gutiérrez A, Cano MD and Castillo MJ. 1996. Elimination of meat, fish, and derived products from the Spanish-Mediterranean diet: Effects on the plasma lipid profile. *Ann. Nutr. Metab.* 40: 202–211.

Delhumeau G, Pratt GV and Gitler C. 1962. The absorption of amino acid mixtures from the small intestine of the rat. I. Equimolar mixtures and those simulating egg albumen, casein and zein. *J. Nutr.* 77: 52–60.

Demigne C, Fafournoux P and Remesy C. 1985. Enhanced uptake of insulin and glucagon by liver in rats adapted to a high protein diet. *J. Nutr.* 115: 1065–1072.

Demonty I, Deshaies Y and Jacques H. 1998. Dietary proteins modulate the effects of fish oil on triglyceridemia in the rat. *Lipids* 33: 913–921.

Deo MG, Sood SK and Ramalingaswani V. 1965. Experimental protein deficiency. Pathologic features in the *Rhesus* monkey. *Arch. Pathol.* 80: 14–23.

Dermers JM and Alary JG. 1966. Effect of different dietary carbohydrates on the lipid metabolism in the duckling. Proceedings of Seventh International Congress on Nutrition, Vol. 5, p. 381 (Abstract).

Descovich GC, Gaddi A, Mannino G, Cattin L, Senin U, Caruzzo C, Fragiacomo C, Sirtori M, Ceredi C, Benassi MS, Colombo L, Fontana G, Mannarino E, Bertelli E, Noseda G and Sirtori CR. 1980. Multicentre study of soybean protein diet for outpatient hypercholesterolemic patients. *Lancet* 2: 709–712.

Després JP, Moorjani S, Tremblay A, Lupien PJ, Nadeau A, Thériault G and Bouchard C. 1990. Genotype-associated changes in plasma lipoprotein levels following long-term overfeeding in men. *F.A.S.E.B. J.* 4: A367, Abstract 587.

Diecke O. 1926. Beobachtungen an Kaninchen mitkunstlicher Cholesterinzufuhr. *Krankheitsforschung* 3: 399–418.

Diersen-Schade DA, Richard MJ, Beitz DC and Jacobson NL. 1985. Effects of beef, soy and conventional diets on body composition and plasma lipids of young pigs fed restricted or liberal amounts of diet. *J. Nutr.* 115: 1016–1024.

Diersen-Schade DA, Richard MJ, Beitz DC and Jacobson NL. 1986. Plasma tissue and fecal cholesterol of young pigs fed restricted or liberal amounts of beef, soy or conventional diets. *J. Nutr.* 116: 2086–2095.

Dietschy JM and Wilson JD. 1970a. Regulation of cholesterol metabolism (first of three part). *N. Engl. J. Med.* 282: 1128–1138.

Dietschy JM and Wilson JD. 1970b. Regulation of cholesterol metabolism (second of three part). *N. Engl. J. Med.* 282: 1179–1183.

Dietschy JM and Wilson JD. 1970c. Regulation of cholesterol metabolism (third of three part). *N. Engl. J. Med.* 282: 1241–1249.

DiFrancesco I, Allen OB and Mercer NH. 1990. Long-term feeding of casein or soy protein with or without cholesterol in *Mongolian* gerbils. II. Plasma lipids and liver cholesterol responses. *Acta Cardiol.* 45: 273–290.

Divine JK, Hine RJ, Hakkak R and Demenci L. 1998. Dietary methionine and its relationship to plasma homocysteine levels in children and adolescents. *F.A.S.E.B. J.* 12: Part I, A228, Abstract 1334.

Dlouha H and McBroom MJ. 1986. Atrial natriuretic factor in taurine-treated normal and cardiomyopathic hamsters. *Proc. Soc. Exp. Biol. Med.* 181: 411–415.

Dodge JA, Glasebrook AL, Magee DE, Philips DL, Sato M, Short LL and Bryant HU. 1996. Environmental estrogens: Effects on cholesterol lowering and bone in the ovariectomized rat. *J. Steroid Biochem. Mol. Biol.* 59: 155–161.

Dominiczak AF, Jeffs B and McConnell JMC. 1998. New genetic concepts in hypertensive cardiovascular disease. *Curr. Opin. Cardiol.* 13: 304–311.

Donaldson AN. 1924. The relation of protein foods to hypertension. *Calif. West. Med.* 26: 328–331.

Doucet C, Flament C, Sautier C and Lemonnier D. 1987. Effect of an hypercholesterolemic diet on the level of several serum lipids and apolipoproteins in nine rat strains. *Reprod. Nutr. Dev.* 27: 897–906.

Dreon DM and Krauss RM. 1992. Gene-diet interactions in lipoprotein metabolism. In Lusis AJ, Rotter JI and Sparkes RS, Eds., *Molecular Genetics of Coronary Artery Disease: Candidate Genes and Processes in Atherosclerosis*, Monographs on Human Genetics, Vol. 14, S. Karger, Basel, 14, 325–349.

Drexler H and Zeiher AM. 1991a. Endothelial function in human coronary arteries *in vivo*. Focus on hypercholesterolemia. *Hypertension* 18 (Suppl. 2): 1–10.

Drexler H, Zeiher AM, Meinzer K and Just H. 1991b. Correction of endothelial dysfunction in coronary microcirculation of hypercholesterolaemic patients by L-arginine. *Lancet* 338: 1546–1560.

Drouet L, Bal dit Sollier C, Cisse M, Pignaud G, Fiat AM, Jollès P and Caen JP. 1990. The antithrombic effect of KDRS a lactotransferrin peptide, compared with RGDS. *Nouv. Rev. Fr. Hematol.* 32: 59–62.

Duane WC. 1999. Effects of soybean protein and very low dietary cholesterol on serum lipids, biliary lipids, and fecal sterols in humans. *Metabolism* 48: 489–494.

Dubroff R and Decker P. 1999. Soy phytoestrogens improve endothelial dysfunction in postmenopausal women. North American Menopause Society Meeting Abstracts, Abstract 99085, p. 53.

Dunn C and Liebman M. 1986. Plasma lipid alterations in vegetarian males resulting from the substitution of tofu for cheese. *Nutr. Res.* 6: 1343–1352.

Durrington PN. 1998. Triglycerides are more important in atherosclerosis than epidemiology has suggested. *Atherosclerosis* 141 (Suppl.): 57S–62S.

Dutta SK and Hlasko MS. 1985. Dietary fiber in pancreatic disease: Effect of high fiber diet on fat malabsorption in pancreatic insufficiency and *in vitro* study of the interaction of dietary fiber with pancreatic enzymes. *Am. J. Clin. Nutr.* 112: 158–166.

Duvillard von SP, Stucchi AF, Terpstra AHM and Nicolosi RJ. 1992. The effect of dietary casein and soybean protein on plasma lipids in *Cebus* monkeys fed cholesterol-free or cholesterol-enriched semipurified diets. *J. Nutr. Biochem.* 3: 71–74.

Dwyer JY, Goldin BR, Saul N, Gualtieri L, Barakat S and Adlercreutz H. 1994. Tofu and soy drinks contain phytoestrogens. *J. Am. Diet. Assoc.* 94:749–743.

Dyer A, Elliott P, Kesteloot H, Stamler J, Stamler R, Freeman J, Shipley M, Marmot M and Rose G. 1992. Urinary nitrogen excretion and blood pressure in INTERSALT. *J. Hypertens.* 10 (Suppl. 4): S122, Abstract P95.

Ebel M, Catapano M, Colombo G, Clerico A, Giannesi D, del Chicca M, Lupetti S, Materazzi F and Pedrinelli R. 1993. The humoral, renal and pressor effects of systemic L-arginine infusion in hypertensive patients. *J. Hypertens.* 11 (Suppl. 5): 140S–141S.

Ebihara K, Miyada T and Nakajima A. 1993. Hypocholesterolemic effect of cecally infused propionic acid in rats fed a cholesterol-free casein diet. *Nutr. Res.* 13: 209–217.

Edgwin PO. 1985. Plasma and lipoprotein cholesterol in weanling and postweanling rats fed casein and soya protein diets. *Nutr. Res.* 5: 1237–1245.

Eikelboom JW, Lonn E, Genest J, Hankey G and Salim Y. 1999. Homocyst(e)ine and cardiovascular disease: A critical review of the epidemiologic evidence. *Ann. Intern. Med.* 131: 363–375.

Eklund A and Sjöblom L. 1980. Effects of the source of dietary protein on serum lower density lipoprotein (VLDL + LDL) and tocopherol levels in female rats. *J. Nutr.* 110: 2321–2335.

Eklund A and Sjöblom L. 1986. Effects of dietary proteins on hepatic and plasma lipids, and some properties of major plasma lipoprotein fractions during dietary-induced hypercholesterolemia in male rats. *Biochim. Biophys. Acta* 877: 127–134.

Elizarova EP, Orlova TR and Medvedeva NV. 1993. Effects on heart membranes after taurine treatment in rabbits with congestive heart failure. *Artzneimittelforschung* 43: 308–312.

Elkind RG, Featherston WR and Rogler JC. 1980. Dietary phenylalanine and trypsine on thyroid hormones levels and growth in the chick. *J. Nutr.* 110: 130–138.

Elliott P, Kesteloot H, Dyer A, Freeman J, Shipley M, Stamler J, Rose G, Marmot M and Stamler R. 1991. 24–hour urinary nitrogen excretion and blood pressure: INTERSALT findings. *Circulation* 84 (Suppl. 2): 698, Abstract 2774.

Elliott P, Kesteloot H, Stamler J, Stamler R, Freeman J, Shipley M, Marmot M and Rose G. 1992. Urinary nitrogen excretion and blood pressure in Intersalt. *J. Hypertens.* 10 (Suppl. 4): S122, Abstract P95.

Elson CE, Humleker E and Pascal L. 1971. Dietary protein level and serum and erythrocytes lipids in young adult males. *Am. J. Clin. Nutr.* 24: 194–199.

Engelberg H. 1992. Low serum cholesterol and suicide. *Lancet* 339: 727–729.

Engelman DT, Watanabe M, Maulik N, Cordis GA, Engelman RM, Ronson JA, Flack JE 3rd, Deaton DW and Dask DK. 1995. L-arginine reduces endothelial inflammation and myocardial stunning during ischemia/reperfusion. *Ann. Thorac. Surg.* 60: 1275–1281.

Engen RL and Swenson MJ. 1969. Influence of diet on indirect systolic blood pressure of rats. *J. Nutr.* 97: 19–24.

Englyst HN and Cummings JH. 1990. Non-starch polysaccharides (dietary fiber) and resistant starch. In Furda I and Brine CJ, Eds., *New Developments in Dietary Fiber*, Plenum Press, New York, pp. 205–225.

Enle FR, Robertson JB and van Soest PJ. 1982. Influence of dietary fibers on fermentation in the human large intestine. *J. Nutr.* 112: 2158–2166.

Enselme J, Cottet J and Fray G. 1962. Action d'un pool d'acides aminés sur l'athérosclérose expérimentale du lapin. *Arch. Mal. du Coeur, Rev. Atheroscl.* 4 (Suppl.) 2: 15–20.

Enselme J, Cottet J and Fray G. 1963. Etude de diverses influences alimentaires sur l'athérosclérose provoquée par une alimentation privée de cholestérol. *Rev. de l'Athéroscl.* 5: 52–59.

Erdman JW Jr. 1995. Control of serum lipids with soy protein. *N. Engl. J. Med.* 333: 313–315.

Erdman JW and Forbes. 1981. Effect of soya protein on mineral availability. *J. Am. Oil Chem. Soc.* 58: 489–493.

Erdman JW Jr, Forbes RM and Kondo H. 1983. Zinc bioavailability from processed soybean products. In Inglett GE, Ed., *Nutritional Bioavailability of Zinc*, American Chemical Society, Washington, DC, pp. 173–183 (ACS Symposium series 210).

Erdman JW Jr and Fordyce EJ. 1989. Soy products and the human diet. *Am. J. Clin. Nutr.* 49: 725–737.

Fache W. 1997. Effects of soy protein and isoflavones on plasma lipid profiles in patients with cardiovascular disease. Symposium on Phytoestrogen Research Methods: Chemistry, Analysis, and Biological Properties, Tucson, AZ, Sept. 21–24, 1997, Abstract.

Fahr T. 1912. Beitrage zur experimentellen Atherosklerose unter besonderer Berücksichtung der Frage nach dem Zusammenhang zwischen Nebenierenveranderungen und Atherosklerose. *Verh. Dtsch. Ges. Pathol.* 15: 234–249.

Fajans SS, Floyd JC, Knopf RF and Conn JW. 1967. Effects of amino acids and proteins on insulin secretion in man. *Recent Prog. Horm. Res.* 23: 617–662.

Farber E, Simpson MV and Tarver H. 1950. Studies on ethionine. II. The interference with lipid metabolism. *J. Biol. Chem.* 182: 91–99.

Fau D, Peret J and Hadjiisky P. 1988. Effects of ingestion of high protein or excess methionine diets by rats for two years. *J. Nutr.* 118: 128–133.

Feinberg H, Rubin L, Hill R, Entenman C, Chaikoff IL. 1954. Reduction of serum lipids and lipoproteins by ethionine feeding in the dog. *Science* 120: 317–318.

Feland B, Fuqua EG and Smith JT. 1973. Effect of dietary sulfur on serum cholesterol and the glycocholic: Taurocholic acid ratio of the rat. *J. Nutr.* 103: 1561–1565.

Fernandez ML, and McNamara DJ. 1991. Regulation of cholesterol and lipoprotein metabolism in guinea pigs mediated by dietary fat quality and quantity. *J. Nutr.* 121: 924–943.

Fernandez ML, Wilson TA, Conde K, Vergara-Jimenez M and Nicolosi RJ. 1999a. Hamsters and guinea pigs differ in their plasma lipoprotein cholesterol distribution when fed diets varying in animal protein, soluble fiber, or cholesterol content. *J. Nutr.* 129: 1323–1332.

Fernandez ML, Wilson TA and Conde K. 1999b. Hamsters and guinea pigs have similar response to dietary cholesterol. *F.A.S.E.B. J.* 13: Part II, A1026, Abstract 759.4.

Fernandez Ortega MF. 1989. Effect of dietary lysine level and protein restriction on the lipids and carnitine levels in the liver of pregnant rats. *Ann. Nutr. Metab.* 33:162–169.

Ferns GAA and Lamb DJ. 2001. Coronary heart disease: Pathophysiological events and risk factors. *Nutr. Bull.* 26: 213–218.

Fiat AM, Migliore Samour D, Jollès P, Drouet L, Bal dit Sollier C and Caen J. 1993. Biologically active peptides from milk proteins with emphasis on two examples concerning antithrombotic and immunomodulating activities. *J. Dairy Sci.* 76: 301–310.

Fillios LC and Mann GV. 1954. Influence of sulfur amino-acid deficiency on cholesterol metabolism. *Metabolism* 3: 16–26.

Fillios LC, Andrus SB, Mann GV and Stare FJ. 1956. Experimental production of gross atherosclerosis in the rat. *J. Exp. Med.* 104: 539–554.

Fillios LC, Naito C, Andrus SB, Portman OW and Martin RS. 1958. Variations in cardiovascular sudanophilia with changes in the dietary level of protein. *Am. J. Physiol.* 194: 275–279.

Finkelstein JD and Martin JJ. 1986. Methionine metabolism in mammals. Adaptation to methionine excess. *J. Biol. Chem.* 261: 1582–1587.

Finking G and Hanke H. 1997. Nikolaj Nikolajewitsch Anitschkow (1885–1964) established the cholesterol-fed rabbit as a model for atherosclerosis research. *Atherosclerosis* 135: 1–7.

Finnigan TJA. 1983. The effect of whole and air-classified legumes on serum lipids in hypercholesterolaemic rabbits. J. *Sci. Food Agric.* 34: 275–276.

Finot PA. 1992. Proteins and cardiovascular problems. In Somogyi JC, Gy B and Hötzel D, Eds., *Nutrition and Cardiovascular Risks*, Bibliography, Nutrition Dieta, Vol. 49, S. Karger, Basel, pp. 83–92.

Fisher H, Feigenbaum A, Leveille GA, Weiss HS and Griminger P. 1959. Biochemical observations on aortas of chickens. Effect of different fats and varying levels of protein, fat and cholesterol. *J. Nutr.* 69: 163–171.

Fleury Y, Welti DH, Philipossian G and Magnoloto D. 1992. Soybean (malonyl) isoflavones: Characterization and antioxidant properties. In Huang MT, Lee CY and Ho CT, Eds., *Phenolic Compounds in Food and their Effects on Health. II: Antioxidants and Cancer Prevention*, American Chemical Society, Washington DC, pp. 99–113.

Flores H, Sierralta W and Monckeberg F. 1970a. Triglyceride transport in protein-depleted rat. *J. Nutr.* 100: 375–379.

Flores H, Pak N, Macioni A and Monckenberg F. 1970b. Lipid transport in kwashiorkor. *Br. J. Nutr.* 24: 1005–1011.

Floyd JC Jr, Fajans SS, Conn JW, Knopf RF and Rull J. 1966. Stimulation of insulin secretion by amino acids. *J. Clin. Invest.* 45: 1487–1502.

Floyd JC, Fajans SS, Pek S, Thiffault CA, Knoph RF and Conn JW. 1970a. Synergistic effects of essential amino acids pairs upon insulin secretion in man. *Diabetes* 19: 102–108.

Floyd JC, Fajans SS, Pek S, Thiffault CA, Knoph RF and Conn JW. 1970b. Synergistic effects of certain amino acids and glucose upon insulin secretion in man. *Diabetes* 19: 109–115.

Foley MK, Beitz DC and Young JW. 1988. Dietary protein: Does type influence cholesterolemia? *J. Am. Oil Chem. Soc.* 65: 173–178.

Folsom AR. 1999. "New" risk factors for atherosclerotic diseases. *Exp. Gerontol.* 34: 483–490.

Folsom AR, Nieto J, McGovern PG, Tsai MY, Malinow MR, Eckfeldt JH, Hess DL and Davis CE. 1998. Prospective study of coronary heart disease incidence in relation to fasting total homocysteine, related genetic polymorphisms, and B vitamins. The Atherosclerosis Risk in Communities (ARIC) Study. *Circulation* 98: 204–210.

Food and Agriculture Organization (F.A.O.). 1970. *Amino Acid Content of Foods and Biological Data on Proteins*, F.A.O. Report 24, F.A.O., Rome.

Food and Agriculture Organization, World Health Organization, and United Nations University. 1985. *Energy and Protein Requirements. Report of a Joint FAO/WHO/UNU Expert Consultation*, Technical Report Series 724, World Health Organization, Geneva.

Forbes RM, Parker HM and Erdman WJ Jr. 1984. Effect of dietary phytate calcium and magnesium levels of zinc bioavailability to rats. *J. Nutr.* 114: 1421–1425.

Fordyce EJ, Forbes RM, Robbins KR and Erdman JW Jr. 1987. Phytate X calcium/zinc molar ratios are they predictive of zinc bioavailability? *J. Food Sci.* 52: 440–444.

Forsythe III WA. 1986. Comparison of dietary casein or soy protein effects on plasma lipids and hormone concentration in the gerbil (*Meriones ungiculatus*). *J. Nutr.* 116: 1165–1171.

Forsythe III WA. 1990. Dietary proteins, cholesterol and thyroxine: A proposed mechanism. *J. Nutr. Sci. Vitaminol.* 36 (Suppl.): 101S–104S.

Forsythe III WA. 1995. Soy protein, thyroid regulation and cholesterol. *J. Nutr.* 125 (Suppl.) 619S–623S.

Forsythe III WA, Miller ER, Hill GM, Romsos DR and Simpson RC. 1980. Effects of dietary protein and fat sources on plasma cholesterol parameters, LCAT activity and amino acid levels and on tissue lipid content of growing pigs. *J. Nutr.* 110: 2467–2479.

Forsythe III WA, Green MS and Anderson JJB. 1986. Dietary protein effects on cholesterol and lipoprotein concentrations: A review. *J. Am. Coll. Nutr.* 5: 533–549.

Fotsis T, Pepper M, Adlercreutz H, Hase T, Montesano R and Schweigerer L. 1995. Genistein, a dietary ingested isoflavonoid, inhibit cell proliferation *in vitro* angiogenesis. *J. Nutr.* 125: 790S–797S.

Fox PF and Flynn A. 1997. Biological properties of milk proteins. In Fox PF, Ed., *Advanced Dairy Chemistry*, Vol. 1, *Proteins*, Blackie Academic and Professional, London, pp. 255–284.

Fox PR and Sturman JA. 1992. Myocardial taurine concentrations in cats with cardiac disease and in healthy cats fed taurine-modified diets. *Am. J. Vet. Res.* 53: 237–241.

Fregly MJ and Fater DC. 1986. Prevention of DOCA-induced hypertension in rats by chronic treatment with tryptophan. *Clin. Exp. Pharmacol. Physiol.* 13: 767–776.

Fregly MJ, Lockley OE, van der Voort J, Sumers C and Henley WN. 1987. Chronic dietary administration of tryptophan prevent the development of deoxycorticosterone acetate salt induced hypertension in rats. *Can. J. Physiol. Pharmacol.* 65: 753–764.

Fregly MJ, Lockley OE and Cade JR. 1988. Effect of chronic dietary treatment with L-tryptophan on the development of renal hypertension in rats. *Pharmacology* 36: 91–100.

Freyberg RH. 1937. Relation of experimental atherosclerosis to diets rich in vegetable proteins. *Arch. Intern. Med.* 59: 660–666.

Freyburger G, Labrouche S, Sassoust G, Rouanet F, Javorschl S and Parrot T. 1997. Mild hyperhomocysteinemia and hemostatic factors in patients with arterial vascular diseases. *Thromb. Haemostas.* 77: 466–471.

Friedlander Y, Leitersdorf E, Vecsler R, Funke H and Kark J. 2000. The contribution of candidate genes to the response of plasma lipids and lipoproteins to dietary challenge. *Atherosclerosis* 152: 239–248.

Friedman M, Byers SO and Elek SR. 1970. Pituitary growth hormone essential for regulation of serum cholesterol. *Nature* 225: 464–467.

Friedman M, Byers SO, Rosenman RH, Li CH and Neuman R. 1974. Effect of subacute administration of human growth hormone on various serum lipid and hormone levels of hypercholesterolemic and normocholesterolemic subjects. *Metabolism* 23: 905–912.

Friedman M, Gumbmann MR and Grosjean OKK. 1984. Nutritional improvement of soy flour. *J. Nutr.* 114: 2241–2246.

Fujio Y, Fumiko Y, Takahashi K and Shibata N. 1993. Responses of smooth muscle cells to platelet-derived growth factor are inhibited by herbimycin-A tyrosine kinase inhibitor. *Biochem. Biophys. Res. Commn.* 195: 79–83.

Fujisawa K, Yagasaki K and Funabiki R. 1994. Reduction of hyperlipidemia and proteinuria without growth retardation in nephritic rats by amino acids-fortified low casein diets. *J. Nutr. Biochem.* 5: 21–27.

Fujisawa K, Yagasaki K and Funabiki R. 1995. Reduction of hyperlipidemia and proteinuria without growth retardation in nephritic rats by amino acids-fortified low casein diets. *Am. J. Nutr. Biochem.* 61: 603–606.

Fujiwara M, Itokawa Y, Uchino H and Inoue K. 1972. Anti-hypercholesterolemic effect of sulfur containing amino acids *S*-methyl-L-cysteine sulfoxide isolated from cabbage. *Experientia* 28: 254–255.

Fukagawa NK, Martin JM, Wurthmann A, Prue AH, Ebenstein D and O'Rourke B. 2000. Sex-related differences in methionine metabolism and plasma homocysteine concentrations. *Am. J. Clin. Nutr.* 72: 22–29.

Fukuda H and Iritani N. 1984. Effect of aging on changes in substrate and effector levels of rat-liver glycolytic and lipogenic enzymes during induction. *Biochim. Biophys. Acta* 795: 79–84.

Fukuda N, Hidaka T, Toda T and Sugano M. 1990. Altered hepatic metabolism of free fatty acid in rats fed a threonine-imbalanced diet. *J. Nutr. Sci. Vitaminol.* 36: 467–474.

Fumagalli R, Paoletti R and Howard AN. 1978. Hypocholesterolaemic effect of soya. *Life Sci.* 22: 947–952.

Fumagalli R, Soleri L, Farina R, Musanti R, Mantero O, Noseda G, Gatti E and Sirtori CR. 1982. Fecal cholesterol excretion studies in type II hypercholesterolemic patients treated with the soybean protein diet. *Atherosclerosis* 43: 341–353.

Furman RH, Norcia LN, Robinson CW and Gonzalez IE. 1957. Influence of testosterone, methyltestosterone and *dl*-ethionine on canine liver lipids, serum lipids and lipoproteins. *Am. J. Physiol.* 191: 561–572.

Furman RH, Howard RP and Norcia LN. 1958. Effects of isocaloric substitution of carbohydrate for dietary protein on serum lipids and lipoproteins and their response to gonadal steroid administration. *Circulation* 18: 492.

Gaddi A, Descovich GC, Noseda G, Fragiocomo C, Nicolini A, Montanari G, Vanetti G, Sirtori M, Gatti E and Sirtori CR. 1987. Hypercholesterolaemia treated with soybean protein diet. *Arch. Dis. Child.* 62: 274–278.

Gaddi A, Ciarrocchi A, Matteucci A, Rimondi S, Ravaglia G, Descovich GC and Sirtori CR. 1991. Dietary treatment for familial hypercholesterolemia — differential effects of dietary soy protein according to the apolipoprotein E phenotypes. *Am. J. Clin. Nutr.* 53: 1191–1196.

Galibois I, Jacques H, Montminy C, Bergeron N and Lavigne C. 1992. Independent effects of protein and fibre sources on glucose and cholesterol metabolism in the rat. *Nutr. Res.* 12: 643–655.

Gallagher PJ, Muir CA and Taylor TG. 1978. Immunological aspects of arterial disease. *Atherosclerosis* 30: 361–363.

Gallagher PJ, Goulding NJ, Pathirana C, Gibney MJ, Jones DB and Taylor TG. 1982. Immune tolerance and atherosclerosis in rabbits. *Atherosclerosis* 45: 115–127.

Gallagher PJ and Gibney MJ. 1983. Immunological aspects of atherosclerosis. The role of dietary proteins. In Gibney MLG and Kritchevsky D, Eds., *Animal and Vegetable Protein in Lipid Metabolism and Atherosclerosis*, Current Topics in Nutrition and Disease, Vol. 8, Alan R. Liss, New York, pp. 149–168.

Gandhi VM, Cherian KM and Mulky MJ. 1992. Hypolipidemic action of taurine in rats. *Ind. J. Exp. Biol.* 30: 413–417.

Gardner CD, Newell KA, Cherin R and Haskell WL. 2001. The effect of soy protein with or without isoflavones relative to milk protein on plasma lipids in hypercholesterolemic postmenopausal women. *Am. J. Clin. Nutr.* 73: 728–735.

Gardner DS, Jackson AA and Langley-Evans SC. 1997. Maintenance of maternal diet-induced hypertension in the rat is dependent on glucocorticoids. *Hypertension* 30: 1525–1530.

Gardner MLG. 1975. Absorption of amino acids and peptides from a complex mixture in the isolated small intestine in the rat. *J. Physiol.* 253: 233–256.

Gariballa SE. 2000. Nutritional factors in stroke. *Br. J. Nutr.* 84: 5–17.

Garini G, Savazzi G and Borghetti A. 1996. The L-arginine nitric oxide system: Physiology, physiopathology and clinical relevance. *Rec. Prog. Med.* 88: 90–99.

Garlich JD, Bazzano G and Olson RE. 1970. Changes in plasma free amino acid concentrations in human subjects on hypocholesterolemic diets. *Am. J. Clin. Nutr.* 23: 1626–1638.

Garnier M and Simon LG. 1907. De l'état du foie chez les lapins soumis au régime carné. *C. R. Hebdom. Sci. Mém. Soc. Biol.* 63: 250–252.

Garrel DR, Verdy M, PetitClerc C, Martin C, Brulé D and Hamet P. 1991. Milk- and soy protein ingestion: Acute effect on serum uric acid concentration. *Am. J. Clin. Nutr.* 53: 665–669.

Gascon A, Jacques H, Moorjani S, Deshaies Y, Brun LD and Julien P. 1996. Plasma lipoprotein profile and lipolytic activities in response to the substitution of lean white fish for other animal protein sources in premenopausal women. *Am. J. Clin. Nutr.* 63: 315–321.

Gatchalian-Yee M, Imamura M, Nonaka M, Gu JY and Sugano M. 1994. Effect of dietary fats on cholesterol metabolism protein and eicosanoid production in hamsters fed undigested fraction of soybean protein. *J. Nutr. Sci. Vitaminol.* 40: 499–504.

Gatchalian-Yee M, Imamura M, Nonaka M, Gu JY and Sugano M. 1995. Effects of different dietary fats and proteins on cholesterol metabolism and eicosanoid production in hamsters. *Nutr. Res.* 15: 1149–1158.

Gatchalian-Yee M, Arimura Y, Ochiai E, Yamada K and Sugano M. 1997. Soyabean protein lowers serum cholesterol levels in hamsters: Effect of debittered undigested fraction. *Nutrition* 13: 633–639.

Gattegno L, Migliore-Samour D, Saffar L and Jollès P. 1988. Enhancement of phagocytic activity of human monocytic macrophagic cells by immunostimulating peptides from human casein. *Immunol. Lett.* 18: 27–32.

Gaul GEH, Pesantes Morales H and Charles E. 1985. Taurine in human nutrition; overview. *Prog. Clin. Biol. Res.* 179: 3–21.

Gavras I, Manolis A and Gavras H. 1999. Genetic epidemiology of essential hypertension. *J. Hum. Hypertens.* 13: 225–230.

Geison RL and Waisman HA. 1970. Plasma and tissue cholesterol and lipid levels in rabbits on L-histidine-supplemented diets. *Proc. Soc. Exp. Biol. Med.* 133: 234–237.

Gerber DA, Sklar JE and Niedwiadowiez. 1971. Lack of an effect of oral-L-histidine on the serum cholesterol in human subjects. *Am. J. Clin. Nutr.* 24: 1382–1383.

Gerber LM and Halberstein RA. 1999. Blood pressure: Genetic and environmental influences. *Hum. Biol.* 71: 467–473.

Gestetner G, Assa Y, Henis Y, Tencer Y, Rotman M, Birk Y and Bondi A. 1972. Interaction of lucerne saponins with steroids. *Biochim. Biophys. Acta* 270: 181–185.

Gherard GT and Duell PB. 1999. Homocysteine and atherosclerosis *Curr. Opin. Lipidol.* 10: 417–428.

Ghosh P and Misra UK. 1987. Rice deficient in lysine and threonine alters normal cholesterol metabolism of rat hepatic Golgi apparatus. *Nutr. Res.* 7: 637–643.

Gianturco SH and Bradley WA. 1999. Pathophysiology of triglyceride-rich lipoproteins in atherothrombosis: Cellular aspects. *Clin. Cardiol.* 22 (Suppl. 2): 7–24.

Gibney MJ. 1982. Hypocholesterolemic effect of soya-bean proteins. *Proc. Nutr. Soc.* 41: 19–26.

Gibney MJ. 1983. The effect of dietary lysine to arginine ratio on cholesterol kinetics in rabbits. *Atherosclerosis* 47: 263–270.

Gibney MJ and Burstyn PG. 1980. Milk, serum cholesterol, and the Maasai. A hypothesis. *Atherosclerosis* 35: 339–343.

Gibney MJ, Gallagher PJ, Sharratt GP, Benning HS, Taylor G and Pitts JM. 1980. Antibodies to heated milk protein in coronary heart disease. *Atherosclerosis* 37: 151–155.

Gibson RS, Laidlaw M, MacDonald AC, Mercer NJH. 1988. Effect of substitution of a soy beverage for 2% cow's milk on the iron, zinc and copper status of hypercholesterolemic men. *Trace Elements Med.* 5: 16–21.

Giovanetti PM, Carroll KK and Wolfe BM. 1986. Constancy of fasting serum cholesterol of healthy young women upon substitution of soy protein isolate for meat and dairy protein in medium and low fat diets. *Nutr. Res.* 6: 609–618.

Girerd XJ, Hirsch AT, Cooke JP, Dzau VJ and Creager MA. 1990. L-arginine augments endothelium-dependent vasodilatation in cholesterol-fed rabbit. *Circ. Res.* 67: 1301–1308.

Giroux I, Lavigne C, Moorjani S and Jacques H. 1997. Simvastatin further enhances the hypocholesterolemic effect of soy protein in rabbits. *J. Am. Coll. Nutr.* 16: 166–174.

Giroux I, Kurowska EM and Carroll KK. 1998. Effects of dietary lysine, methionine, arginine and glycine on cholesterolemia and liver lipids in rats. *F.A.S.E.B. J.* 12: Part I, A238, Abstract 1389.

Giroux I, Kurowska EM, Freeman DJ and Carroll KK. 1999a. Addition of arginine but not glycine to lysine plus methionine-enriched diets modulates serum cholesterol and liver phospholipids in rabbits. *J. Nutr.* 129: 1807–1813.

Giroux I, Kurowska EM, Carroll KK. 1999b. Role of dietary lysine, methionine, and arginine in the regulation of hypercholesterolemia in rabbits. *J. Nutr. Biochem.* 10: 166–171.

Glatz JFC, Demacker PNM, Turner PR and Katan MB. 1991. Response of serum cholesterol to dietary cholesterol in relation to apolipoprotein E phenotype. *Nutr. Metab. Cardiovasc. Dis.* 1: 13–7.

Glickman RM. 1980. Intestinal lipoprotein formation. *Nutr. Metab.* 24 (Suppl. 1): 3–11.

Glickman RM and Kirsch K. 1973. Lymph chylomicrons formation during inhibition of protein synthesis, studies of chylomicron apoproteins. *J. Clin. Invest.* 52: 2910–2920.

Golay A, Ferrara JM, Felber JP and Schneider H. 1990. Cholesterol lowering effect of skim milk from immunized cows in hypercholesterolemic patients. *Am. J. Clin. Nutr.* 52: 1014–1019.

Goldberg AC. 1995. Perspectives on soy protein as a nonpharmacological approach for lowering cholesterol. *J. Nutr.* 125 (Suppl. 3): 675S–678S.

Goldberg AC and Schonfeld G. 1985. Effect of diet on lipoprotein metabolism. *Annu. Rev. Nutr.* 5: 195–212.

Goldberg AP, Lim A, Kolar JB, Grundhauser JJ, Steinke FH and Schonfeld G. 1982. Soybean protein independently lowers plasma cholesterol levels in primary hypercholesterolemia. *Atherosclerosis* 43: 355–368.

Goldner MG, Loewe L, Lasser R and Stern I. 1954. Effect of caloric restriction on cholesterol atherogenesis in the rabbit. *Proc. Soc. Exp. Biol. Med.* 87: 105–108.

Gooderham MJ, Adlercreutz H, Ojala ST, Wahala K and Holub BJ. 1996. A soy protein isolate rich in genistein and diadzein and its effects on plasma isoflavone concentrations, platelet aggregation, blood lipids, and fatty acid composition of plasma phospholipid in normal men. *J. Nutr.* 126: 2000–2006.

Goodman HO and Shihabi ZK. 1990. Supplemental taurine in diabetics rats: Effects on plasma glucose and triglycerides. *Biochem. Med. Metab. Biol.* 43: 1–9.

Gordon T, Castelli WP, Hjortland MC, Kannel WB and Dawber TR. 1977. High density lipoprotein as a protective factor against coronary heart disease. The Framingham Study. *Am. J. Med.* 62: 707–714.

Gottfries A, Schersten T and Ekdahl PH. 1966. The capacity of human liver homogenates to synthezise taurocholic and glycocholic acid *in vitro. Scand. J. Clin. Lab. Invest.* 18: 643–653.

Gotto AM. 1998a. Triglyceride. The forgotten risk factor. *Circulation* 97: 1027–1028.

Gotto AM. 1998b. Triglyceride as a risk factor for coronary heart disease. *Am. J. Cardiol.* 82: 22Q–25Q.

Gouache P, Le Moullac B, Bleiberg-Daniel F, Aubert R and Flament C. 1991. Changes in rat plasma apolipoproteins and lipoproteins during moderate protein deficiency: Potential use. *J. Nutr.* 121: 653–662.

Gould EM, Rembold CM and Murphy RA. 1995. Genistein, a tyrosine kinase inhibitor, reduces Ca^{2+} mobilization in swine carotid media. *Am. J. Physiol.* 268: C1425–C1429.

Goulding NJ, Gibney M, Taylor TG and PJ Gallagher. 1983. Reversible hypercholesterolemia produced by cholesterol-free fish meal protein diets. *Atherosclerosis* 439: 127–137.

Graf E. 1983. Application of phytic acid determination in soybean. *J. Am. Oil Chem. Soc.* 60: 1861–1867.

Greaves KA, Parks JS, Williams JK and Wagner JD. 1999. Intact dietary soy protein, but not adding an isoflavones-rich soy extract to casein, improves plasma lipids in ovariectomized *Cynomolgus* monkeys. *J. Nutr.* 129: 1585–1592.

Greaves KA, Wilson MD, Rudel LL, Williams JK and Wagner JD. 2000. Consumption of soy protein reduces cholesterol absorption compared to casein protein alone or supplemented with an isoflavone extract or conjugated equine estrogen in ovariectomized *Cynomolgus* monkeys. *J. Nutr.* 130: 820–826.

Greer SAN, Hays VW, Speer VC and McCall JT. 1966. Effect of dietary fat, protein and cholesterol on atherosclerosis in swine. *J. Nutr.* 90: 183–190.

Gregory JF III, Cuskelly GJ, Shane B, Toth JP, Baumgartner TG and Stacpoole PW. 2000. Primed, constant infusion with [2H3] serine allows *in vivo* kinetic measurement of serine turnover, homocysteine remethylation, and transsulfuration processes in human one-carbon metabolism. *Am. J. Clin. Nutr.* 72: 1535–1541.

Griffin BA. 1999. Cholesterol-lowering effects of high-protein soya milk. *Br. J. Nutr.* 82: 79–80.

Griffith OW. 1999. Biology and pharmacologic regulation of mammalian glutathione synthesis and delivery by the liver. *Free Radical Biol. Med.* 27: 922–935.

Griminger P and Fisher H. 1958. Dietary saponin and plasma cholesterol in the chicken. *Proc. Soc. Exp. Biol. Med.* 99: 424–426.

Groot de AP. 1958. The influence of dietary protein on the serum cholesterol levels in rats. *Voeding* 19: 715–718.

Groot de AP. 1959. Dietary protein and serum cholesterol in rats. *Nature* 184: 903–904.

Groot de AP. 1960. De invloed van eiwitten en andere nutriënten op de cholesterolspiegel van het bloed. *Voeding* 21: 374–386.

Grove RI, Mazucco CE, Radka SF, Shoyab H and Kiener PA. 1991. Oncostatin M up-regulates low-density lipoprotein receptors in HepG2 cells by a novel mechanism. *J. Biol. Chem.* 266: 18194–18199.

Grundy SM. 1998. Hypertriglyceridemia, atherogenic dyslipemic and the metabolic syndrome. *Am. J. Cardiol.* 81: 18B–25B.

Grundy SM and Abrams JJ. 1983. Comparison of action of soy protein and casein on metabolism of plasma lipoproteins and cholesterol in humans. *Am. J. Clin. Nutr.* 38: 245–252.

Gryglewski RJ, Grodzinska L, Kostka-Trabka E, Korbut R, Bieron K, Goszcz A and Slawinski M. 1996. Treatment with L-arginine is likely to stimulate generation of nitric oxide in patients with peripheral arterial obstructive disease. *Wien. Klin. Woschenschr.* 108: 111–116.

Grynspan F and Cheryan M. 1989. Phytate-calcium interactions with soy protein. *J. Am. Oil Chem. Soc.* 66: 93–97.

Guder W, Nolte I and Wieland O. 1968. The influence of thyroid hormones β-hydroxy-β-methylglutaryl coenzyme A reductase of rat liver. *Eur. J. Biochem.* 4: 273–278.

Gueguen L. 2001. Minéraux et oligoéléments. In Debry G, Ed., *Lait, Nutrition et Santé*, Editions Tec et Doc Lavoisier, Paris, pp. 125–149.

Guermani L, Villaume Ch, Bau HW, Méjean L and Nicolas JP. 1992. Effect of different kinds of dietary casein on blood cholesterol and triglycerides in pair fed rats. *Nutrition* 8: 101–104.

Guermani L, Villaume C, Bau HM, Nicolas JP and Méjean L. 1993. Modification de l'effet hypocholestérolémiant des protéines de soja après fermentation par *Rhizopus oligosporus* spT3. *Sci. Aliments* 13: 317–324.

Guidotti A, Buffoni F and Giotti A. 1967. Azione della taurina e di alcuni suoi derivati sulla riduzione del consumo di ossigeno prodotta dal cianuro nel ratio. *Bull. Soc. Ital. Biol. Sper.* 43: 1390–1395.

Guigoz Y, Stasse-Wolthuis M and Hermus RJJ. 1979. Sources de protéines, taux de cholestérol et composition des lipoprotéines du rat, normal et obèse. *Int. J. Vitam. Nutr. Res.* 20: 32–42.

Guillaume M, Lapidus L and Lambert A. 2000. Differences in associations of familial and nutritional factors with serum lipids between boys and girls: The Luxembourg Child Study. *Am. J. Clin. Nutr.* 72: 384–388.

Gupta PP, Tandon HD, Karmakar HD and Ramalingaswami V. 1974. Experimental atherosclerosis in swine: Effect of dietary protein and high fat. *Exp. Mol. Pathol.* 20: 115–131.

Guthikonda S and Haynes WG. 1999. Homocysteine as a novel risk factor for atherosclerosis. *Curr. Opin. Cardiol.* 14: 283–291.

Guttormsen AB, Schneede J, Fiskerstrand T, Leland PM and Refsum HM. 1994. Plasma concentration of homocysteine and other aminothiol compounds and related to food intake in healthy human subjects. *J. Nutr.* 124: 1934–1941.

Guzman MA and Strong JP. 1987. Nutritional and pathological aspects of atherosclerosis in aging adults. In Watson RR, Ed., *Nutrition and Heart Disease*, Vol. 1, CRC Press, Boca Raton, FL, pp. 117–137.

Gylling H and Miettinen T. 1992. Cholesterol absorption and synthesis related to low density lipoprotein metabolism during varying cholesterol intake in men with different apo E phenotypes. *J. Lipid Res.* 33: 361–371.

Haban P and Stanova E. 1989. Effect of dietary proteins on Nile red fluorescence from the arch of aorta in guinea pigs. *Bratisl. Lek. Listy* 90: 120–124.

Hafez YS, Mohamed AI, Hewedi FM and Singh G. 1985. Effects of microwave heating on solubility, digestibility and metabolism of soy protein. *J. Food Sci.* 50: 415–417.

Hagemeister H, Scholz-Ahrens KE, Schulte-Koerne H and Barth CA. 1990. Plasma amino acids and cholesterol following dietary casein or soy protein in minipigs. *J. Nutr.* 120: 1305–1311.

Ham JO, Karen MS, Chapman KM, Essex-Sorlie D, Bakhit RM, Prabhudesai M, Winter L, Erdman JW and Potter SM. 1993. Endocrinological response to soy protein and fiber in mildly hypercholesterolemic men. *Nutr. Res.* 13: 873–884.

Hamaguchi E and Aoyagi K. 1974. Clinical study of taurine on the secretion of bile. *Kiso to Rinsho* 8: 128–138.

Hambraeus L. 1997. Nutritional aspects of milk proteins. In Fox PF, Ed., *Advanced Dairy Chemistry*, Vol. 1: *Proteins*, Blackie Academic & Professional, London, pp. 457–490.

Hamilton RMG and Carroll KK. 1974. Effect of dietary protein on plasma cholesterol levels in rabbits fed cholesterol-free semi-synthetic diets. In Schletter G and Weizel A, Eds., *Atherosclerosis*, Proceedings of 3rd International Symposium 1973, Springer Verlag, Berlin, pp. 406–409.

Hamilton RMG and Carroll KK. 1976. Plasma cholesterol levels in rabbits fed low fat, low cholesterol diets. Effect of dietary proteins, carbohydrates and fiber from different sources. *Atherosclerosis* 24: 47–62.

Hankey GH and Eikelbloom JW. 1999. Homocysteine and vascular disease. *Lancet* 354: 407–413.

Hardinge MG and Stare FJ. 1954. Nutritional studies of vegetarians. II. Dietary and serum levels of cholesterol. *Am. J. Clin. Nutr.* 2: 83–88.

Hardinge MG, Crooks H and Stare FJ. 1962. Nutritional studies on vegetarians. IV. Dietary fatty acids and serum cholesterol levels. *Am. J. Clin. Nutr.* 10: 516–524.

Hardison WGM and Grundy SM. 1983. Effect of bile acid conjugation pattern on bile acid metabolism in normal humans. *Gastroenterology* 84: 617–620.

Harman D. 1960. Vitamin E effect of serum cholesterol and lipoproteins. *Circulation* 22: 151–153.

Harpel PC. 1997. Homocysteine, atherogenesis and thrombosis. *Fibrinol. Proteol.* 11 (Suppl.): 77–80.

Harper AE. 1958. Nutritional fatty livers in rats. *Am. J. Clin. Nutr.* 6: 242–253.

Harper AE. 1964. Amino acids toxicities and imbalances. In Munro HN and Allison JB, Eds., *Mammalian Protein Metabolism*, Vol. 2, Academic Press, New York, pp. 87–134.

Harper AE, Benevenga NJ and Wohlhueter RM. 1970. Effects of ingestion of disproportionate amounts of amino acids. *Physiol. Rev.* 50: 428–558.

Harrill I, Minarik G and Gifford ED. 1965. Effects of vitamin A and E on lipids in selected rat tissues. *J. Nutr.* 87: 424–428.

Harris WS. 1997. *n*–3 fatty acids and serum lipoproteins: Animal studies. *Am. J. Clin. Nutr.* 65 (Suppl.): 1611S–1616S.

Harvey PW and Allen KG. 1981. Decreased plasma lecithin: Cholesterol acyl transferase activity in copper-deficient rats. *J. Nutr.* 11: 1855–1858.

Harvey PW, Hunsaker HA and Allen KGD. 1981. Dietary L-histidine-induced hypercholesterolemia and hypercupremia in the rat. *J. Nutr.* 111: 639–647.

Hassan AS. 1986. Role of hepatic glutathione and glucocorticoids in the regulation of hepatic 7 α-hydroxylase. *Biochem. Pharmacol.* 35: 4592–4594.

Hassan AS. 1989. Effect of chronic inhibition of glutathione biosynthesis on cholesterol and bile acid metabolism in rats. *Biochim. Biophys. Acta* 963: 131–138.

Hassan AS, Hackley JJ and Jeffery EH. 1984. Role of glutathione in the regulation of hepatic cholesterol 7 α-hydroxylase, the rate limiting enzyme of bile acid biosynthesis. *Steroids* 44: 373–380.

Hassan AS, Logas LL and Hackley JJ. 1985. Dietary protein and atherosclerosis: Effect of exposure to dietary casein in early life on cholesterol and bile acid metabolism in the adult rabbit. *Fed. Proc.* 44: 1856, Abstract 8441.

Hata Y, Yamamoto M, Ohni M, Nakajima K and Nakamura Y. 1996. A placebo controlled study of the effect of sour milk on blood pressure in hypertensive subjects. *Am. J. Clin. Nutr.* 64: 767–771.

Havel RJ. 1986. Functional activities of hepatic lipoprotein receptors. *Annu. Rev. Physiol.* 48: 119–134.

Havlik RJ, Fabsitz RR, Kalousdian S, Borhani NO and Christian JC. 1990. Dietary protein and blood pressure in monozygotic twins. *Prev. Med.* 19: 31–39.

Hayashi S, Miyazaki Y, Yamashita J, Nakagawa M and Takiawa H. 1994. Soy protein has no hypocholesterolemic action in mice because it does not stimulate fecal steroid excretion in that species. *Cell. Mol. Biol.* 40: 1021–1028.

Heaney RP, Weaver CM and Fitzsimmons ML. 1991. Soybean phytate content: Effect on calcium absorption. *Am. J. Clin. Nutr.* 53: 745–747.

Heijer den M, Bos GM, Brouwer IA, Gerrits WB and Blom HJ. 1996. Variability of the loading test: No effect of a low protein diet. *Ann. Clin. Biochem.* 33: 551–554.

Hellstrom K and Sjövall J. 1961. Conjugation of bile acids in patients with hypothyroidism. *J. Atheroscler. Res.* 1: 205–209.

Helmeste DM and Tang SW. 1995. Tyrosine kinase inhibitors regulate serotonin uptake in platelets. *Eur. J. Pharmacol.* 280: R5–R7.

Hennig B and Chow CK. 1988. Lipid peroxidation and endothelial cell injury: Implications in atherosclerosis. *Free Radical Biol. Med.* 4: 99–106.

Hennig B, Chung BH, Watkins BA and Alvarado A. 1992. Disruption of endothelial barrier function by lipolytic remnants of triglyceride-rich lipoproteins. *Atherosclerosis* 95: 235–247.

Hennig B, Toborek M, Alvarado Cader A and Decker E. 1994a. Nutrition, endothelial cell metabolism, and atherosclerosis. *Crit. Rev. Food Sci. Nutr.* 34: 253–282.

Hennig B, Diana JN, Toborek M and McClain CJ. 1994b. Influence of nutrients and cytokines on endothelial cell metabolism. *J. Am. Coll. Nutr.* 13: 224–231.

Henson PM. 1973. Release of serotonin from human platelets induced by aggregated immunoglobulins of different classes and subclasses. *J. Clin. Invest.* 52: 1282–1288.

Hermus RJJ. 1975. Experimental atherosclerosis in rabbits on diets with milk fat and different proteins. Thesis, Centre Agricultural Publishing and Documentation, Wageningen.

Hermus RJJ and Stasse-Wolthuis M. 1978. Lipids and lipoproteins in rabbits fed semisynthetic diets containing different proteins. In Peeters PH, Ed., *Protides of the Biological Fluids*, Pergamon Press, Oxford, pp. 457–460.

Hermus RJ and Dallinga-Thie GM. 1979. Soya saponins and plasma cholesterol. *Lancet* 2: 48.

Hermus RJJ, Terpstra AHM and Dallinga-Thie GM. 1979. Aanwijzingen voor een rol van voedingseiwitten bij, de beïnvloeding van het serum cholesterolgehalte. *Voeding* 40: 95–99.

Hermus RJJ, West CE and van Weerden EJ. 1983. Failure of dietary-casein-induced acidosis to explain the hypercholesterolemia of casein-fed rabbits. *J. Nutr.* 113: 618–629.

Heron DS, Shinitzky M, Herrshkowitz M and Samuel D. 1980. Lipid fluidity markedly modulates the binding of serotonin to mouse brain membranes. *Proc. Natl. Acad. Sci. U. S. A.* 77: 7463–7467.

Herrmann RG. 1959. Effect of taurine, glycine and β-sitosterols on serum and tissue cholesterol in the rat and rabbit. *Circ. Res.* 7: 224–227.

Hertog MGL, Feskens EJM, Hollman PCH, Katan MB and Kromhout D. 1993. Dietary antioxidant flavonoids and risk of coronary heart disease. The Zuphten Elderly Study. *Lancet* 342: 1007–1011.

Hertog MGL, Sweetnam PM, Fehily AM, Eldwood PC and Kromhout D. 1997. Antioxidants flavonols and ischemic heart disease in a Welsh population of men. The Caerphilly Study. *Ann. Intern. Med.* 125: 384–389.

Herzberg GR and Rogerson M. 1981. The role of dietary protein in hepatic lipogenesis in the young rat. *Br. J. Nutr.* 45: 529–538.

Herzberg GR and Rogerson M. 1984. Hepatic lipogenesis in rats given proteins of different quality. *Br. J. Nutr.* 52: 131–137.

Heubi JE, Burstein S, Sperling MA, Gregg D, Subbiah MTR and Matthews DE. 1983. The role of human growth hormone in the regulation of cholesterol and bile acid metabolism. *J. Clin. Endocrinol. Metab.* 57: 885–891.

Hevia P and Visek WJ. 1979a. Dietary protein and plasma cholesterol in chickens. *J. Nutr.* 109: 32–38.

Hevia P and Visek WJ. 1979b. Serum and liver lipids in rats fed casein or soybean protein with sucrose or dextrin or sucrose and cholesterol. *Nutr. Rep. Int.* 20: 539–548.

Hevia P and Visek WJ. 1980. Liver and serum lipids and lipoproteins of rats fed 5% L-lysine. *Lipids* 15: 95–99.

Hevia P, Kari FW, Ulman EA and Visek WJ. 1980a. Serum and liver lipids in growing rats fed casein with L-lysine. *J. Nutr.* 110: 1224–1230.

Hevia P, Ulman EA, Kari FW and Visek WJ. 1980b. Serum lipids of rats fed excess L-Lysine and different carbohydrates. *J. Nutr.* 110: 1231–1239.

Higashi Y, Oshima T, Ono N, Hiraga H, Yoshimura M, Watanabe M, Matsuura H, Kambe M and Kajiyama G. 1995. Intravenous administration of L-arginine inhibits angiotensine-converting enzyme in humans. *J. Clin. Endocrinol. Metab.* 80: 2198–2202.

Hilker DM, Wenkam NS and Lichton. 1965. Blood pressure elevation and renal pathology in rats fed simulated Japanese diets. *J. Nutr.* 87: 371–384.

Hill EG. 1966. Effects of methionine menhaden oil and ethoxyquin on serum cholesterol of chicks. *J. Nutr.* 89: 143–148.

Hill TD, Dean NM, Mordan LJ, Lau AF, Kanemitsu MY and Boynton AL. 1990. PDGF-induced activation of phospholipase C is not required for induction of DNA synthesis. *Science* 248: 1660–1663.

Hilleboe HE. 1957. Some epidemiologic aspects of coronary artery disease. *J. Chronic Dis.* 6: 210–228.

Himeno A, Kunisada K, Niwa M, Ozaki M, Tsuchiyama H and Kurihara M. 1984. Taurine and experimental hypertension. In Lovenberg W and Yamori Y, Eds., *Nutritional Prevention of Cardiovascular Disease*, Academic Press, Orlando, FL, pp. 53–58.

Hinshaw DB, Burger JM, Delius RE and Hyslop PA. 1990. Mechanism of protection of oxidant-injured endothelial cells by glutamine. *Surgery* 108: 298–304.

Hishikawa K, Nakaki T, Tsuda M, Esumi H, Ohshima H, Suzuki H, Saruta T and Kato R. 1992. Effect of systemic L-arginine administration on hemodynamics and nitric oxide release in man. *Jpn. Heart J.* 33: 41–48.

Hishikawa K, Nagaki T, Suzuki H, Kato R, Saruta T. 1993. Role of L-arginine-nitric oxide pathway in hypertension. *J. Hypertens.* 11: 639–645.

Hitomi Y and Yoshida A. 1989. Effect of methionine and threonine on the hypercholesterolemia induced by polychlorinated biphenyls in rats fed a nonprotein diet. *J. Nutr. Sci. Vitaminol.* 35: 589–596.

Ho HT, Kim DN and Lee KT. 1989. Intestinal apolipoprotein B-48 synthesis and lymphatic cholesterol transport are lower in swine fed high fat, high cholesterol diet with soy protein than with casein. *Atherosclerosis* 77: 15–23.

Ho K, Biss K, Mikkelson B and Lewis LA. 1971. The Masaï of East Africa: Some unique biological characteristics. *Arch. Pathol.* 91: 387–410.

Hodges RE, Krehl WA, Stone DB and Lopez A. 1967. Dietary carbohydrates and low cholesterol diets: Effects on serum lipids in man. *Am. J. Clin. Nutr.* 20: 198–208.

Hodgson JM, Croft KD, Puddey IB, Mori TA and Beilin LJ. 1996. Soybean isoflavonoids and their metabolic products inhibit *in vitro* lipoprotein oxidation in serum. *J. Nutr. Biochem.* 7: 664–669.

Hodgson JM, Puddey IB, Beilin LJ, Mori TA and Croft KD. 1998. Supplementation with isoflavonoid phytoestrogens does not alter serum lipid concentrations: A randomized controlled trial in humans. *J. Nutr.* 128: 728–732.

Hodis HN, Mack WJ, Azen SP, Alaupovic P, Pogoda JM, LaBree L, Hemphill LC, Kramsch DM and Blankenhorn DH. 1994. Triglyceride- and cholesterol-rich lipoproteins have a differential effect on mild, moderate and severe lesion progression as assessed by quantitative coronary angiography in a controlled trial of lovastatin. *Circulation* 90: 42–49.

Hodis HN and Mack WJ. 1995. Triglyceride-rich lipoproteins and the progression of coronary artery disease. *Curr. Opin. Lipidol.* 6: 209–214.

Hodis HN, Mack WJ, Krauss RM and Alaupovic P. 1999. Pathophysiology of triglyceride-rich lipoproteins in atherothrombosis: Clinical aspects. *Clin. Cardiol.* 22 (Suppl. 2): 1115–1120.

Hokanson JE and Austin A. 1996. Plasma triglyceride level is a risk factor for cardiovascular disease independent of high-density lipoprotein cholesterol level: A meta-analysis of population-based prospective studies. *J. Cardiovasc. Risk* 3: 213–219.

Holmes WL, Rubel GB and Hood SS. 1980. Comparison of the effect of dietary meat versus dietary soybean protein on plasma lipid of hyperlipidemic individuals. *Atherosclerosis* 36: 379–387.

Holt LE Jr, Sorydeman SE, Norton PM, Roitman E and Finch J. 1963. The plasma aminogram in kwashiorkor. *Lancet* 2: 1343–1348.

Honoré EK, Williams JK, Anthony MS and Clarkson TB. 1997. Soy isoflavones enhance coronary vascular reactivity in atherosclerosis female macaques. *Fertil. Steril.* 67: 148–154.

Horie R, Yamori Y, Nara Y, Sawamura M and Mano M. 1987. Effects of sulfur amino acids on the development of hypertension and atherosclerosis in stroke-prone spontaneously hypertensive rats. *J. Hypertens.* 5 (Suppl.): 223–225.

Horigome T and Cho YS. 1992. Dietary casein and soybean protein affect the concentrations of serum cholesterol, triglyceride and free amino acids in rats. *J. Nutr.* 122: 2273–2282.

Horton JD, Cuthbert JA and Spady DK. 1993. Dietary fatty acids regulate hepatic low density lipoprotein (LDL) transport by altering LDL receptor protein and mRNA levels. *J. Clin. Invest.* 92: 743–749.

Howard AN, Gresham GA, Jones D and Jennings IW. 1965. The prevention of rabbit athero-sclerosis by soya bean meal. *J. Atheroscler. Res.* 5: 330–337.

Howard AN and Gresham GA. 1968. Dietary aspects of atherosclerosis and thrombosis. *Int. J. Vitam. Nutr. Res.* 38: 545–559.

Howes JB, Sullivan D, Lai N, Nestel P, Pomeroy S, West L, Eden JA and Howes LG. 2000. The effects of dietary supplementation with isoflavones from red clover on the lipoprotein profiles of post menopausal women with mild to moderate hypercholester-olemia. *Atherosclerosis* 152: 143–147.

Hrabek-Smith J and Carroll KK. 1987. A comparative study of serum lipoproteins in rabbits fed a natural ingredient diet or low-fat, cholesterol-free, semipurified diets containing casein or isolated soy protein. *Biochem. Cell Biol.* 65: 610–616.

Hrabek-Smith JM, Kurowska E and Carroll KK. 1989. Effects of cholesterol-free, semipurified diets containing different levels of casein or soy protein on distribution of cholesterol and protein among serum lipoproteins of rabbits. *Atherosclerosis* 76: 125–130.

Hu FB, Stampfer MJ, Manson JAE, Rimm E, Colditz GA, Speizer FE, Hennekens CH and Willett WC. 1999. Dietary protein and risk of ischemic heart disease in women. *Am. J. Clin. Nutr.* 70: 221–227.

Huang HL and Rao MR. 1995. Effect of neferine and its combination with taurine on platelet aggregation and experimental thrombosis in rats. *Yao Hsueh Hsueh Pao* (China) 30: 486–490.

Huang YS. 1990a. Effects of dietary protein levels and cholesterol on tissue lipids of rats. *J. Nutr. Sci. Vitaminol.* 36 (Suppl.): 151S–156S.

Huang YS. 1990b. Regulation of cholesterol metabolism by dietary protein and n-6 poly-unsaturated fatty acids. *J. Nutr. Sci. Vitaminol.* 36 (Suppl.): S169–S172.

Huang YS, Cunane SC and Horrobin DF. 1986. Effect of different dietary proteins on plasma and liver fatty acid compositions in growing rats. *Proc. Soc. Exp. Biol. Med.* 181: 399–403.

Huang YS, Watanabe Y, Horrobin DF and Simmons SV. 1990. The effects of dietary protein and cholesterol on tissue cholesterol contents and n-6 fatty acid composition in rats and mice fed a gamma-linoleate-rich diet. In Beynen AC, Kritchevsky D and Pollak OJ, Eds., *Dietary Proteins, Cholesterol Metabolism and Atherosclerosis*, Monographs on Atherosclerosis, Vol. 16, S. Karger, Basel, pp. 11–25.

Huang YS, Koba K, Horrobin DF and Sugano M. 1993. Interrelationship between dietary protein, cholesterol and n-6 polyunsaturated fatty acid metabolism. *Prog. Lipid Res.* 32: 123–137.

Hubbard R, Kosch CL, Sanchez A, Sabate J, Berk L and Shavlik G. 1989. Effect of dietary protein on serum insulin and glucagon levels in hyper- and normocholesterolemic men. *Atherosclerosis* 76: 55–61.

Hubbard RW, Sanchez A. 1990. Dietary protein control of serum cholesterol by insulin and glucagon. In Beynen AC, Kritchevsky D and Pollak OJ, Eds., *Dietary Proteins, Cholesterol Metabolism and Atherosclerosis*, Monographs on Atherosclerosis, Vol. 16, S. Karger, Basel, pp. 139–147.

Huff MW, Hamilton RMG and Carroll KK. 1977. Plasma cholesterol levels in rabbits fed low fat, low cholesterol semi-purified diets. Effect of dietary proteins, protein hydroly-sates and amino acid mixtures. *Atherosclerosis* 28: 187–195.

Huff MW and Carroll KK. 1980a. Effect of dietary proteins and aminoacid mixtures on plasma cholesterol level in rabbits. *J. Nutr.* 110: 1676–1685.

Huff MW and Carroll KK. 1980b. Effects of dietary protein on turnover, oxidation, and absorption of cholesterol, and on steroid excretion in rabbits. *J. Lipid Res.* 21: 546–558.

Huff MW, Roberts DCK and Carroll KK. 1982. Long-term effects of semipurified diets containing casein and soy protein isolate on atherosclerosis and plasma lipoproteins in rabbits. *Atherosclerosis* 41: 327–336.

Huff MW, Giovanetti PM and Wolfe BM. 1984. Turnover of very low density lipoprotein-apoprotein B is increased by substitution of soybean protein for meat and dairy protein in the diets of hypercholesterolemic men. *Am. J. Clin. Nutr.* 39: 888–897.

Human Nutrition Information Service, U.S. Department of Agriculture. 1993. USDA Nutrient Data Base for Standard Reference, release 10, National Technical Information Service, Springfield, VA.

Humble C. 1997. The evolving epidemiology of fiber and heart disease. In Kritchevsky D and Bonfield C, Eds., *Dietary Fiber in Health and Disease*, Plenum Press, New York, pp. 15–26.

Hung CJ, Huang PC, Lu SC, Li YH, Huang HB, Lin BF, Chang SJ and Chou HF. 2002. Plasma homocysteine levels in Taiwanese vegetarians are higher than those of omnivores. *J. Nutr.* 132: 152–158.

Hunninghake DB, Miller VT, LaRosa JC, Kinosian B, Jacobson T, Brown V, Howard WM, Edezlman DA and O'Connor RR. 1984. Long-term treatment of hypercholesterolemia with dietary fiber. *Am. J. Med.* 97: 504–508.

Hunter EA and Grimble RF. 1997. Dietary sulfur amino acid adequacy influences glutathione synthesis and glutathione-dependent enzymes during the inflammatory response to endotoxin and tumor necrosis factor-alpha in rats. *Clin. Sci. (Colch.)* 92: 297–305.

Hurley C, Galibois I and Jacques H. 1995. Fasting and postprandial lipid and glucose metabolism are modulated by dietary proteins and carbohydrates: Role of plasma insulin concentrations. *J. Nutr. Biochem.* 6: 540–546.

Hutchins AM, Slavin JL and Lampe JW. 1995. Urinary isoflavonoid phytoestrogen and lignan excretion after consumption of fermented and unfermented soy products. *J. Am. Diet. Assoc.* 95: 545–551.

Hutchinson SJ, Reitz MS, Sudhir K, Sievers RE, Zhu BQ, Sun YP, Chou TM, Deedwania PC, Chatterjee K, Glantz A and Parmley WW. 1997. Chronic dietary L-arginine prevents endothelial dysfunction secondary to environmental tobacco smoke in normocholesterolemic rabbits. *Hypertension* 29: 1186–1191.

Ide T, Murata M and Sunada Y. 1992. Soybean protein dependent changes in triacylglycerol synthesis and concentration of diacylglycerol in the liver microsomes of fasted-refed rats. *Ann. Nutr. Metab.* 36: 87–96.

Ignarro LJ. 1989a. Endothelium-derived nitric oxide: Actions and properties. *Circulation* 3: 31–36.

Ignarro LJ. 1989b. Biological actions and properties of endothelium-derived nitric oxide formed and released from artery and vein. *Circ. Res.* 65: 1–21.

Ignarro LJ, Cirino G, Casini A and Napoli C. 1999. Nitric oxide as a signaling molecule in the vascular system. An overview. *J. Cardiovasc. Pharmacol.* 34: 879–886.

Ignatowski A. 1908a. Changes in parenchymatous organs and in the aorta of rabbits under the influence of animal protein. *Izvestizy Imperatorskoi Voyenno-Meditsinskoi Akademii* (St Petersburg) 18: 231–244.

Ignatowski A. 1908b. Influence de la nourriture animale sur l'organisme des lapins. *Arch. Med. Exp. Anat. Pathol.* 20: 1–20.

Ignatowski A. 1909. Uber die Wirkung des tierischen Eiweisses auf die Aorta und die parenchymatosen Organe der Kaninchen. *Virchow Arch. Pathol. Anat. Physiol. Klin. Med.* 198: 248–270.

Ikeda A, Imaizumi K and Sugano M. 1993. Interaction of dietary protein and fat on plasma cholesterol and amino acid levels, fatty acid desaturation, and prostacyclin production in exogenous hypercholesterolemic rats. *Biosci. Biotechnol. Biochem.* 11: 1867–1872.

Ikeda A, Wakamatsu K, Umeda T, Shikada S, Ikeda I, Imaizumi K and Sugano M. 1994. Effects of dietary protein and fat on linoleic and α-linolenic acid metabolism and prostacyclin production in *Stroke-Prone Spontaneous Hypertensive* rats. *J. Nutr. Biochem.* 5: 248–255.

Ikeda K, Nara Y, Horie R and Yamori Y. 1989. Diets modify pressor and catecholamines response to stress in *Stroke-Prone Spontaneously Hypertensive Rats (SHRSP)*. In Yamori Y and Strasser T, Eds., *New Horizons in Prevention of Cardiovascular Diseases*, Elsevier, Amsterdam, pp. 23–25.

Imaizumi T, Hirooka Y, Masaki H, Harada S, Momohara M, Tagawa T and Takeshita A. 1992. Effects of L-arginine on forearm vessels and responses to acetylcholine. *Hypertension* 20: 511–517.

Iritani N, Narita R, Fujita T and Tanaka T. 1985. Effects of dietary fish protein, soybean protein and casein on cholesterol turnover in rats. *J. Nutr. Sci. Vitaminol.* 31: 385–392.

Iritani N, Nagashima K, Fukuda H, Katsurada A and Tanaka T. 1986. Effects of dietary proteins on lipogenic enzymes in rat liver. *J. Nutr.* 116: 190–197.

Iritani N, Suga A, Fukuda H, Katsurada A and Tanaka T. 1988. Effects of dietary casein and soybean protein on triglyceride turnover in rat liver. *J. Nutr. Sci. Vitaminol.* 34: 309–315.

Iritani N, Hosomi H, Fukuda H, Tada K and Ikeda H. 1996. Soybean protein suppresses hepatic lipogenic enzyme gene expression in *Wistar* fatty rats. *J. Nutr.* 126: 380–388.

Ishibashi S, Brown MS, Goldstein JL, Gerard RD, Hammer RE and Herz J. 1993. Hypercholesterolemia in low density lipoprotein receptor knockout mice and its reversal by adenovirus-mediated gene delivery. *J. Clin. Invest.* 92: 883–893.

Ishinaga M, Hamada M, Ohnaka K, Fukunaga K and Minato Y. 1993. Effects of casein and soy protein on accumulation of cholesterol and dolichol in rat liver. *Proc. Soc. Exp. Biol. Med.* 203: 74–77.

Itokawa Y, Inoue K, Sasagawa S and Fujiwara M. 1973. Effect of *S*-methylcysteine sulfoxide and related sulfur-containing amino acids on lipid metabolism of experimental hypercholesterolemic rats. *J. Nutr.* 103: 88–92.

Iwami K, Kitagawa M, Nagasaki T and Ibuki F. 1987. Comparison on intestinal taurocholate uptake in rats given soy protein- or casein based-diet. *Nutr. Res.* 10: 547–554.

Iwami K, Kitigawa M and Ibuki F. 1990. Effect of dietary proteins and/or their digestive products on intestinal taurocholate absorption. *J. Nutr. Sci. Vitaminol.* 36 (Suppl.): 141S–146S.

Jackson JA and Burns MJ. 1974. Effects of cystine, niacin and taurine on cholesterol concentration in the *Japanese* quail with comments on bile acid metabolism. *Comp. Biochem. Physiol.* 48A: 61–68.

Jackson RL, Taunton OD, Morrisett JD and Gotto AM. 1978. The role of dietary polyunsaturated fat in lowering blood cholesterol in man. *Circ. Res.* 42: 447–453.

Jacobs LR. 1983. Effects of dietary fiber on mucosal growth and cell proliferation in small intestine of the rat: A comparison of oat bran, pectin and guar with total deprivation. *Am. J. Clin. Nutr.* 37: 954–960.

Jacobs M, Plane F and Brückdorfer NR. 1990. Native and oxidized low-density lipoproteins have different inhibitor effects on endothelium-derived relaxing factor in the rabbit aorta. *Br. J. Pharmacol.* 100: 21–26.

Jacobsen JG and Smith LH Jr. 1968. Biochemistry and physiology of taurine and taurine derivatives. *Physiol. Rev.* 48: 425–511.

Jacobsson L and Lindholm L. 1982. Experimental atherosclerosis in hypercholesterolemic minipigs. *Atherosclerosis* 45: 129–148.

Jacques H. 1990. Effects of dietary fish protein on plasma cholesterol and lipoproteins in animal models and in humans. In Beynen AC, Kritchevsky D and Pollack OJ, Eds., *Dietary Proteins, Cholesterol Metabolism and Atherosclerosis*, Monographs on Atherosclerosis, Vol. 16, S. Karger, Basel, 59–70.

Jacques H, Deshaies Y and Savoie L. 1986. Relationship between dietary proteins, their *in vitro* digestion products, and serum cholesterol in rats. *Atherosclerosis* 61: 89–98.

Jacques H, Deshaies Y and Savoie L. 1988a. Relationship between dietary tyrosine and plasma cholesterol in the rat. *Can. J. Physiol. Pharmacol.* 66: 1023–1027.

Jacques H, Deshaies Y, Carroll KK, Hrabek-Smith JM and Savoie L. 1988b. Effects of dietary proteins on the cholesterol and soluble apolipoprotein composition of plasma lipoproteins in the rat. *Nutrition* 4: 439–445.

Jacques H, Deshaies Y and Savoie L. 1990. Relationship between protein digestion products and plasma cholesterol in the rat. *J. Nutr. Sci. Vitaminol.* 36 (Suppl. 2): 133S–136S.

Jacques H, Noreau L and Moorjani S. 1992a. Effects on plasma lipoproteins and endogenous sex hormones of substituting lean white fish for other animal-protein sources in diets of postmenopausal women. *Am. J. Clin. Nutr.* 55: 896–901.

Jacques H, Laurin D, Moorjani S, Steinke FH, Gagne C, Brun D and Lupien PJ. 1992b. Influence of diets containing cow's milk or soy protein beverage on plasma lipids in children with familial hypercholesterolemia. *J. Am. Coll. Nutr.* 11 (Suppl.): 69S–73S.

Jacques H, Chaumette P and Lavigne C. 1993a. Further investigation on the hypocholesterolemic effect of vegetable protein in the rabbits. *F.A.S.E.B. J.* 7: Part II, A 802, Abstract 4636.

Jacques H, Chaumette P and Lavigne C. 1993b. Further investigation on the hypocholesterolemic effect of vegetable protein in the rabbits. *Nutr. Res.* 13: 969–977.

Jacques H, Gascon A, Bergeron N, Lavigne C, Hurley C, Deshaies Y, Moorjani S and Julien P. 1995. Role of dietary fish protein in the regulation of plasma lipids. *Can. J. Cardiol.* 11 (Suppl. G): 63G–71G.

Jakubowski H. 1999. Protein homocysteinylation: Possible mechanims underlying pathological consequences of elevated homocysteine levels. *F.A.S.E.B. J.* 13: 2277–2283.

James L, Bhuiyan AKMJ, Foster D and Seccombe D. 1995. Effect of L-carnitine treatment on very low density lipoprotein kinetics in the hyperlipidemic rabbit. *Clin. Biochem.* 28: 451–458.

Jarowski CI and Pytelewski R. 1975. Utility of fasting essential amino acids plasma levels in formulation of nutritionally adequate diets. III. Lowering of rat serum cholesterol levels by lysine supplementation. *J. Pharm. Sci.* 64: 690–691.

Jarrousse C, Lardeux B, Bourdel G, Girard-Globa A and Rosselin G. 1980. Portal insulin and glucagon in rats fed proteins as a meal: Immediate variations and circadian modulations. *J. Nutr.* 110: 1764–1773.

Jenkins DJA, Wolever TMS, Spiller G, Buckley G, Lam Y, Jenkins AL and Josse RG. 1989. Hypocholesterolemic effect of vegetable protein in a hypocaloric diet. *Atherosclerosis* 78: 99–107.

Jenkins DJA, Kendall CWC, Rosenberg-Zand RS, Jackson CJ, Agarwal S, Rao AV, Diamandis EP, Parker T, Faulkner D, Vuksan V and Vidgen E. 2000. Effects of soy protein foods on low-density lipoprotein oxidation and ex-vivo sex hormone receptor activity: A controlled cross over study. *Metabolism* 49: 537–543.

Jenkins DJA, Kendall WC, Vidgen E, Augustin LSA, van Erk M, Geelen A, Parker T, Faulkner D, Vuksan V, Josse RG, Leiter LA and Connelly PW. 2001. High-protein diets in hyperlipidemia: Effect of wheat gluten on serum lipids, uric acid, and renal function. *Am. J. Clin. Nutr.* 74: 57–63.

Jenkins MY, Mitchell GV and Vanderveen JE. 1983. Effects of dietary protein and lecithin on plasma and liver lipids and plasma lipoproteins in rats. *Nutr. Rep. Int.* 28: 621–634.

Jeppesen J, Hein HO, Suadicani P and Gyntelberg F. 1998. Triglyceride concentration and ischemic heart disease. An eight-year follow-up in the Copenhagen male study. *Circulation* 97: 1029–1036.

Jeremy RW, McCarron H and Sullivan D. 1996. Effects of dietary L-arginine on atherosclerosis and endothelium-dependent vasodilatation in the hypercholesterolemic rabbit. Response according to the treatment duration, anatomic site and sex. *Circulation* 94: 498–506.

Jeserich M, Münzel T, Just H and Drexler H. 1992. Reduced plasma L-arginine in hypercholesterolemia. *Lancet* 339: 561.

Johnson D, Léveillé GA and Fisher H. 1958. Influences of amino-acid deficiencies and protein level on the plasma cholesterol of the chick. *J. Nutr.* 66: 367–376.

Johnson FL, St Clair RW and Rudel LL. 1983. Studies on the production of low density lipoproteins by perfused livers from non human primates. Effects of dietary cholesterol. *J. Clin. Invest.* 72: 221–226.

Johnson JA, Beitz DC and Jacobson NL. 1987. Effect of animal and vegetable proteins on plasma cholesterol homeostasis. *Fed. Proc.* 46: 1473, Abstract 6748.

Johnson JA, Beitz DC and Jacobson NL. 1989. Effects of dietary beef and soy protein on tissue composition and low density lipoprotein uptake in young pigs. *J. Nutr.* 119: 696–705.

Jollès P. 1975. Structural aspects of the milk clotting process. Comparative features with the blood clotting process. *Mol. Cell Biochem.* 7: 73–85.

Jollès P, Loucheux-Lefebvre MH and Henschen A. 1978. Structural relatedness of κ-casein and fibrinogen γ-chain. *J. Mol. Evol.* 11: 271–278.

Jollès P and Henschen A. 1982. Comparison between the clotting of blood and milk. *Trends Biochem. Sci.* 7: 325–328.

Jollès P, Levy-Toledano S, Fiat AM, Soria C, Gillessen D, Thomaidis A, Dunn FW and Caen JP. 1986. Analogy between fibrinogen and casein. Effect of an undecapeptide isolated from κ-casein on platelet function. *Eur. J. Biochem.* 158: 379–382.

Jollès P and Caen JP. 1991. Parallels between milk clotting and blood clotting: Opportunities for milk-derived products. *Trends Food Sci. Technol.* 2: 42–43.

Jollès P, Fiat AM, Migliore-Samour D, Drouet L and Caen JP. 1993. Peptides from milk proteins implicated in antithrombosis and immunomodulation. In Renner B and Sawatzki G, Eds., *New Perspectives in Infant Nutrition*, Symposium Antwerp, Thieme Medical Publishers, New York, pp. 160–172.

Jones JD. 1964. Lysine-arginine antagonism in the chick. *J. Nutr.* 84: 313–321.

Jones JD, Wolters R and Burnett PC. 1966. Lysine-arginine electrolyte relationships in the rat. *J. Nutr.* 89: 171–188.

Jones PJH, Main BF and Frohlich JJ. 1993. Response of cholesterol synthesis to cholesterol feeding in men with different apolipoprotein E genotype. *Metabolism* 42: 1065–1071.

Jones RJR and Huffman S. 1956a. Chronic effect of dietary protein on hypercholesterolemia in the rat. *J. Nutr.* 66: 367–376.

Jones RJR and Huffman S. 1956b. Chronic effect of dietary protein on hypercholesterolemia in the rat. *Proc. Soc. Exp. Biol. Med.* 93: 519–522.

Jones RJR, Wisler RW and Huffman S. 1957. Certain dietary effects on the serum cholesterol and atherogenesis in the rat. *Arch. Pathol.* 63: 593–601.

Jong de SC and Schreiber G. 1987. Messenger RNA levels of plasma proteins in rat liver during protein depletion and refeeding. *J. Nutr.* 117: 1798–1800.

Jong de SC, van den Berg M, Rauwerda JA and Stehouver CD. 1998. Hyperhomocysteinemia and atherothrombotic disease. *Semin. Thromb. Hemost.* 24: 381–385.

Jonnalagadda SS, Angert RM and Hayes KC. 1993. Soy protein enhances bile excretion and reduces cholesterol gallstones in hamsters. *F.A.S.E.B. J.* 7: Part II, A802, Abstract 4633.

Joshida K, Masatoshi Y and Ahiko K. 1988. Effects of addition of arginine, cystine, and glycine to the bovine milk-simulated amino acid mixture on the level of plasma and liver cholesterol in rats. *J. Nutr. Sci. Vitaminol.* 34: 567–576.

Julius AD and Wiggers KD. 1979. Effect of infant formulas and source of fat and protein on blood and tissue cholesterol in weanling pigs. *Fed. Proc.* 38: 744, Abstract.

Julius CA and Richard JW. 1982. Studies on the mechanism by which tyrosine raises urinary catecholamines. *Biochem. Pharmacol.* 31: 3577–3581.

Jun T and Wennmalm A. 1996. L-arginine-induced hypotension in the rat: Evidence that NO synthesis is not involved. *Acta Physiol. Scand.* 152: 386–390.

Kabir Y and Ide T. 1995. Effect of dietary soybean phospholipid and fats differing in the degree of unsaturation on fatty acid synthesis and oxidation in rat liver. *J. Nutr. Sci. Vitaminol.* 41: 635–645.

Kagawa Y, Nishizawa M, Suzuki M, Miyatake T, Hamamoto T, Goto K, Motonage E, Izumikawa H, Hirata B and Ebihara E. 1982. Eicosapolyenoic acid of serum lipid of Japanese islanders with low incidence of cardiovascular diseases. *J. Nutr. Sci. Vitaminol.* 28: 441–453.

Kajikawa M, Ohta T, Takase M, Kawase K and Shimumura S. 1994. Lactoferrin inhibits accumulation in macrophages mediated by acetylated or oxidized low-density-lipoproteins. *Biochim. Biophys. Acta* 1213: 82–90.

Kanazawa T. 1996. Anti-atherogenic effects of soybean protein. Viewpoints from peroxidizability and molecular size of LDL and from antiplatelet aggregation. Second Symposium on the Role of Soy in Preventing and Treating Chronic Disease, Brussels, Sept. 15–18, 1996, Abstract, p. 27.

Kanazawa T, Tanaka M, Tsugumichi U, Osanai T, Onodera K, Okubo K, Metoki H and Oike Y. 1993. Antiatherogenicity of soybean protein. In Lee KT, Oike Y and Kanazawa T, Eds., Third International Conference on Nutrition in Cardio-Cerebrovascular Diseases. *Ann. N. Y. Acad. Sci.* 676: 202–214.

Kanazawa T, Osanai T, Zhang XS, Uemura T, Yin XZ, Onodera K, Oike Y and Ohkubo K. 1995. Protective effect of soy protein on the peroxidizability of lipoproteins in cerebrovascular disease. *J. Nutr.* 125: 639S–648S.

Kanazawa T and Osanai T. 1998. Effects of soy protein on peroxidizability, antiplatelet aggregability and enlargement of molecular size of low-density lipoprotein. *Am. J. Clin. Nutr.* 68 (Suppl.): 1523S.

Kang SS, Wong PWK and Malinow MR. 1992. Hypermocyst(e)inemia a a risk factor for occlusive vascular disease. *Annu. Rev. Nutr.* 12: 279–298.

Kanno K, Hirata Y, Emori T, Ohta K, Eguchi S, Imai T and Marumo F. 1992. L-arginine infusion induces hypotension and diuresis/natriuresis concomitant with increased urinary excretion of nitrite/nitrate and cyclic GMP in humans. *Clin. Exp. Pharmacol. Physiol.* 19: 619–625.

Kapiotis S, Hermann M, Held I, Seelos C, Ehringer H and Gmeiner BMK. 1997. Genistein, the dietary-derived angiogenesis inhibitor, prevents LDL oxidation and protects endothelial cells from damage by atherogenic LDL. *Arterioscler. Thromb. Vasc. Biol.* 17: 2868–2874.

Karpatti G, Carpenter S, Engel AW, Watters G, Allen J, Rothman S, Klassen G and Mamer OA. 1975. The syndrome of systemic carnitine deficiency. Clinical, morphologic, biochemical, and pathophysiologic features. *Neurology* 25: 16–24.

Karr SC, Lampe J, Hutchins AM and Slavin JL. 1997. Urinary isoflavonoid excretion in human is dose-dependent at low to moderate levels of soy-protein consumption. *Am. J. Clin. Nutr.* 66: 46–51.

Kassim PAK, Howe JC and Beecher GR. 1984. Effects of dietary protein level on lipid and glycogen metabolism in the rat. *Nutr. Rep. Int.* 30: 529–535.

Katan MB, Vroomen LHM and Hermus RJJ. 1982. Reduction of casein-induced hypercholesterolaemia and atherosclerosis in rabbits and rats by dietary glycine, arginine and alanine. *Atherosclerosis* 43: 381–391.

Katan MB, Beynen AC, DeVries JH, Nobles AA. 1986. Existence of consistent hypo and hyperresponders to dietary cholesterol in man. *Am. J. Epidemiol.* 123: 221–234.

Katan MB, Berns MA, Glatz JF, Knuiman JT, Nobels A and de Vries JH. 1988a. Congruence of individual responsiveness to dietary cholesterol and to saturated fat in humans. *J. Lipid Res.* 29: 883–892.

Katan MB, van Gastel AC, de Rover CM, van Montfort MAJ and Knuiman JT. 1988b. Differences in individual responsiveness of serum cholesterol to fat-modified diets in man. *Eur. J. Clin. Invest.* 18: 644–647.

Katan MB and Hollman PCH. 1998. Dietary flavonoids and cardiovascular disease. *Nutr. Metab. Cardiovasc. Dis.* 8: 1–4.

Kato M. 1951. Study of the perfusion of the intestine: The effects of sugar, protein and amino acids on the absorption of calcium to the intestine. *Showa Med. Univ. J.* 11: 216–225.

Kato N, Tani T and Yoshida A. 1980. Effect of dietary level of protein on liver microsomal drug-metabolizing enzymes, urinary ascorbic acid and lipid metabolism in rats fed PCB-containing diets. *J. Nutr.* 110: 1686–1694.

Kato N, Mochizuki S, Kawai K and Yoshida A. 1982. Effect of dietary level of sulfur-containing amino acids on liver drug metabolizing enzymes, serum cholesterol and urinary ascorbic acid in rats fed PCB. *J. Nutr.* 112: 848–854.

Kaufman LN, Peterson MM and Smith SM. 1994. Hypertensive effect of polyunsaturated dietary fat. *Metab. Clin. Exp.* 43: 1–3.

Kay R. 1982. Dietary fiber. *J. Lipid Res.* 23: 221–242.

Kay RM and Truswell AS. 1980. Dietary fibers: Effects on plasma and biliary lipids in man. In Spiller GA and Kay RM, Eds., *Medical Aspects of Dietary Fiber*, Plenum Press, New York, pp. 153–173.

Kayashita J, Shimaoka I and Nakajoh M. 1995. Hypocholesterolemic effect of buckwheat protein extract in rats fed cholesterol enriched diets. *Nutr. Res.* 15: 691–698.

Kayashita J, Shimaoka I, Nakajoh M and Kato N. 1996. Feeding of buckwheat protein extract reduces hepatic triglyceride concentration, adipose tissue weight and hepatic lipogenesis in rats. *J. Nutr. Biochem.* 7: 555–559.

Kayashita J, Shimaoka I, Nakajoh M, Yamazaki M and Kato N. 1997. Consumption of buckwheat protein lowers plasma cholesterol and raises fecal neutral sterols in cholesterol-fed rats because of its low digestibility. *J. Nutr.* 127: 1395–1400.

Keli SO, Hertog MGL, Feskens EJM and Kromhouth D. 1996. Dietary flavonoids, antioxidant vitamins, and incidence of stroke: The Zuphten Study. *Arch. Intern. Med.* 156: 637–642.

Kempner W. 1948. Treatment of hypertensive vascular disease with rice diet. *Am. J. Med.* 4: 545–577.

Kenney JJ and Fisher H. 1973. Effect of medium chain triglyceride and dietary protein on cholesterol absorption and deposition in the chicken. *J. Nutr.* 103: 923–928.

Kerr GR, Wolf RC and Waisman HA. 1965. Hyperlipemia in infant monkeys fed excess L-histidine. *Proc. Soc. Exp. Biol. Med.* 119: 561–562.

Kerr GR, Wolf RC and Waisman HA. 1966. A disorder of lipid metabolism associated with experimental hyperhistidinemia in *Macaca mulatta*. In *Some Recent Developments in Comparative Medicine*, Academic Press, New York, pp. 371–392.

Kerr SJ. 1972. Competing methyltransferases systems. *J. Biol. Chem.* 247: 4248–4252.

Kesaniemi YA and Grundy SM. 1986. Effects of dietary polyenylphosphatidylcholine on metabolism of cholesterol and triglycerides in hypertriglyceridemic patients. *Am. J. Clin. Nutr.* 43: 98–107.

Kestin M, Rouse IL, Correll RA and Nestel PJ. 1989. Cardiovascular disease risk factors in free-living men: Comparison of two prudent diets, one based on lacto-ovovegeterianism and the other allowing lean meat. *Am. J. Clin. Nutr.* 50: 280–287.

Keys A. 1980. *Seven Countries: A Multivariate Analysis of Death and Coronary Heart Disease.* Harvard University Press, Cambridge, MA.

Keys A and Anderson JT. 1957. Dietary protein and the serum cholesterol level in man. *Am. J. Clin. Nutr.* 5: 29–34.

Keys A and Hodges RE. 1967. Effects on serum lipids of different dietary proteins and carbohydrates *Am. J. Clin. Nutr.* 20: 1249–1251.

Khan A and Weaver CM. 1989. Bioavailability of zinc to rats from soybean and casein as affected by protein source and length of adaptation. *Nutr. Res.* 9: 327–336.

Kharitonov SA, Lubec G, Lubec B, Hjelm M and Barnes PJ. 1995. L-arginine increases exhaled nitric oxide in human subjects. *Clin. Sci.* 88: 135–139.

Khosla P, Samman S, Carroll KK and Huff MW. 1989. Turnover of ^{125}I-VLDL and ^{131}I-IDL apolipoprotein B in rabbits fed diets containing casein or soy protein. *Biochem. Biophys. Acta* 1002: 157–163.

Khosla P, Samman S and Carroll KK. 1991. Decreased receptor-mediated LDL catabolism in casein-fed rabbits precedes the increase in plasma cholesterol levels. *J. Nutr. Biochem.* 2: 203–209.

Kibe C, Wake C, Kuramoto T and Hoshita T. 1980. Effect of dietary taurine on bile acids metabolism in guinea pigs. *Lipids* 15: 224–229.

Kihara M, Fujikawa J, Ohtaka M, Mano M, Nara Y, Horie R, Tsunematsu T, Nota S, Fukase H and Yamori Y. 1984. Interrelationships between blood pressure, sodium, potassium, serum cholesterol, and protein intake in Japanese. *Hypertension* 6: 736–742.

Kim DN, Lee KT, Reiner JM and Thomas WA. 1978. Effects of soy protein product on serum and tissue cholesterol concentrations in swine fed high-fat, high-cholesterol diets. *Exp. Mol. Pathol.* 29: 385–399.

Kim DN, Lee KT, Reiner JM and Thomas WA. 1980a. Increased steroid excretion in swine fed high-fat, high-cholesterol diet with soy protein. *Exp. Mol. Pathol.* 33: 25–35.

Kim DN, Lee KT, Reiner JM and Thomas WA. 1980b. Studies of hypocholesterolemic effect of soy protein in swine. *Proceedings of the VII International Symposium on Drugs Affecting Lipid Metabolism*, Fumagalli R, Kritchevsky D and Paoletti R, Eds., Elsevier, Amsterdam, pp. 347–353.

Kim DN, Lee KT, Reiner J. M. and Thomas WA. 1981. Lack of beneficial effects of wheat bran cereals on cholesterol balance in swine. *Exp. Mol. Pathol.* 35: 301–313.

Kim DN, Lee KT, Reiner JM and Thomas WA. 1982. Hypolipidemic action of soy protein in swine. In Noseda G, Fragiacomo C, Fumagalli R and Paoletti R, Eds., *Lipoproteins and Coronary Atherosclerosis*, Elsevier, Amsterdam, pp. 265–270.

Kim DN, Lee KT, Reiner JM and Thomas WA. 1983. Effects of soy protein on cholesterol metabolism in swine. In Gibney MJ and Kritchevsky D, Eds., *Animal and Vegetable Proteins in Lipid Metabolism and Atherosclerosis*, Current Topics in Nutrition and Disease, Vol. 8, pp. 101–110.

Kim S, Chao PY and Allen KG. 1992. Inhibition of elevated hepatic gluthatione abolishes copper deficiency cholesterolemia. *F.A.S.E.B. J.* 6: 2467–2471.

Kim SW, Morris JG and Rogers QR. 1995. Dietary soybean protein decreases plasma taurine in cats. *J. Nutr.* 125: 2831–2837.

Kimura S. 1977. Atherosclerosis in Japan: Epidemiology. *Atheroscler. Rev.* 2: 209–221.

Kimura S, Chiang MT and Fujimoto H. 1990. Effects of eicosapentanoic acid and soybean protein on plasma cholesterol, blood pressure and platelet aggregation in *Stroke-Prone Spontaneously Hypertensive* rats. In Beynen AC, Kritchevsky D and Pollak OJ, Eds., *Dietary Proteins, Cholesterol Metabolism and Atherosclerosis*, Monographs on Atherosclerosis, Vol. 16, S. Karger, Basel, pp. 26–35.

Kirk EA, Sutherland P, Wang SA, Chait A and LeBoeuf RC. 1998. Dietary isoflavones reduce plasma cholesterol and atherosclerosis in *C57BL/6* mice but not LDL receptor deficient-mice. *J. Nutr.* 128: 954–959.

Kishino Y and Moriguchi S. 1984. The effects of soy protein on cellular immunologic response. *Nutr. Sci. Soy Protein Jpn.* 5: 67–70.

Kita T, Brown MS, Watanabe Y and Goldstein JL. 1981. Deficiency of LDL receptor in liver and adrenal gland of the *WHHl* rabbit, an animal model of familial hypercholesterolemia. *Proc. Natl. Acad. Sci. U.S.A.* 78: 2268–2272.

Kito M, Moriyama T, Kimura Y and Kambara H. 1993. Changes in plasma lipid levels in young healthy volunteers by adding an extruder-cooked soy protein to conventional meals. *Biosci. Biotechnol. Biochem.* 57: 354–355.

Klavins JV, Kinney TD and Kaufman N. 1963. Histopathologic changes in methionine excess. *Arch. Pathol.* 75: 661–673.

Klein M, Schadereit R and Kuchemmeister V. 2000. Energy metabolism and thyroid hormone levels of growing rats in response to different dietary proteins — soy protein or casein. *Arch. Tierernähr.* 53: 99–125.

Klevay LM. 1994. Soy protein may affect plasma cholesterol through copper. *Am. J. Clin. Nutr.* 60: 300–301.

Klevay LM, Sandstead HH, Jacob RA and Johnson L. 1979. The hypocholesterolemic effect of dietary calcium in normal men. *Fed. Proc.* 38: 551, Abstract 1705.

Knack AV. 1915. Uber Cholesterinsklerose. *Virchows Arch. Pathol. Anat. Physiol. Klin. Med.* 220: 36–52.

Knekt P, Järvinen R, Reunanen A and Maatela J. 1996. Flavonoid intake and coronary mortality in Finland: A cohort study. *B.M.J.* 312: 478–481.

Knuiman JT, Beynen AC and Katan MB. 1989. Lecithin intake and serum cholesterol. *Am. J. Clin. Nutr.* 49: 266–268.

Knutson MR, Hansen AJ, Martin DS, Eyster KM and Williams JL. 1997. Acute dilatory effects of estrogen and soy isoflavones on cerebral arteries in rats. Symposium on Phytoestrogen Research Methods: Chemistry, Analysis, and Biological Properties, Tucson, AZ, Sept. 21–24, 1997, Abstract.

Koba K and Sugano M. 1989. Protein-fat interaction on the cholesterol level and fatty acid desaturation in rats consuming alcohol. *Agric. Biol. Chem.* 53: 2769–2776.

Koba K and Sugano M. 1990. Dietary protein influences polyunsaturated fatty acid patterns of rat tissue lipids. *J. Nutr. Sci. Vitaminol.* 36 (Suppl.): 173S–176S.

Koba K, Abe K and Sugano M. 1990. Effects of amino acid composition of dietary protein on linoleic acid desaturation in rats. *Agric. Biol. Chem.* 54: 2711–2717.

Koba K, Abe K, Wakamatsu K and Sugano M. 1991. Effect of overnight fasting on the fatty acid composition of tissue lipids in rats fed with different proteins. *Agric. Biol. Chem.* 55: 1367–1373.

Koba K, Wakamatsu K, Obata K and Sugano M. 1993. Effects of dietary proteins on linoleic acid desaturation and membrane fluidity in rat liver microsomes. *Lipids* 28: 457–464.

Koba K, Rozee LA, Horrobin DF and Huang YS. 1994. Effects of dietary protein and cholesterol on phosphatidylcholine and phosphatidylethanolamine molecular species in mouse liver. *Lipids* 29: 33–39.

Kohashi N, Obayashi T, Hama J, Yagi T, Katori R, Morishima Y and Ohba Y. 1983. The relationship between taurine and platelet aggregation in normal and essential hypertension. *Sulfur-Containing Amino Acids* 6: 89–95.

Kohls KJ, Kies C and Fox HM. 1985. Blood serum lipid levels of humans: Effect of arginine, lysine and tryptophan supplements. *Fed. Proc.* 44: 1498, Abstract 6362.

Kohls KJ, Kies C and Fox HM. 1987. Blood serum lipid levels of humans given arginine, lysine and tryptophan supplements without food. *Nutr. Rep. Int.* 35: 5–13.

Köhrle J, Fang SL, Irmscher K, Esch RD, Pino S, Alex S and Braverman LE. 1989. Rapid effects of the flavonoid EMD 21388 on serum thyroid hormone binding and thyrotropin regulation in the rat. *Endocrinology* 125: 532–537.

Kokatnur MG, Rand NT, Kummerow FA and Scott HM. 1956. Dietary protein: A factor which may reduce serum cholesterol levels. *Circulation* 14: 962.

Kokatnur MG, Rand NT and Kummerow FA. 1958a. Effect of the energy to protein ratio on serum and carcass cholesterol levels in chicks. *Circ. Res.* 6: 424–431.

Kokatnur MG, Rand NT, Kummerow FA and Scott HM. 1958b. Effect of dietary protein and fat on changes in serum cholesterol in mature birds. *J. Nutr.* 64: 177–184.

Kokatnur MG, Klain G, Snetsinger D, Kummerow FA and Scott HM. 1959. Effect of various amino acids on serum cholesterol levels in chicks. *Fed. Proc.* 18: 532.

Kokatnur MG and Kummerow FA. 1961. Amino acid imbalance and cholesterol levels in chicks *J. Nutr.* 75: 319–329.

Kolb S and Sailer D. 1984. Soybean protein crispbread as additional dietetic measure in hypercholesterolemia. *Nutr. Rep. Int.* 30: 719–724.

Komatsu T, Komatsu K, Yamamoto T, Wang MF, Chung HM, Kohrin T, Kakinohana S and Yamamoto S. 1998. Soybean protein hydrolysates reduce serum cholesterol concentration and induce thermogenesis. *Am. J. Clin. Nutr.* 68 (Suppl.): 1520S–1521S.

Kon Y. 1913. Referat über Arteriosklerose. *Trans. Jpn. Pathol. Soc.* 3: 8–19.

Kon Y. 1914. Futterungsversuche an Saugetieren mit Leberpulver und eigelb. *Trans. Jpn. Pathol. Soc.* 4: 105–112.

Koo SI and Williams DA. 1981. Relationship between the nutritional status of zinc and cholesterol concentration of serum lipoproteins in adult male rats. *Am. J. Clin. Nutr.* 34: 2376–2381.

Kovanen PT, Brown MS, Basu SK, Bilheimer DW and Goldstein JL. 1981. Saturation and suppression of hepatic lipoprotein receptors: A mechanism for the hypercholesterolemia of cholesterol-fed rabbits. *Proc. Natl. Acad. Sci. U.S.A.* 78: 1396–1400.

Koyama J. 1995. The influence of methionine and its metabolites on the progression of atherosclerosis in rabbits. *Nippon Ika Daigaku Zasshi* 62: 596–604.

Koyanagi T, Wada S, Murashami M and Minura T. 1966. Effects of vitamins A and E on serum cholesterol and atherosclerosis in the hen. *Eiyo Shokuryo* 19: 81–86.

Kratky RG, Ivey J, Rogers KA, Daley S and Roach MR. 1993. The distribution of fibro-fatty atherosclerotic lesions in the aortae of casein- and cholesterol-fed rabbits. *Atherosclerosis* 99: 121–131.

Krauss RM. 1997. Genetic, metabolic, and dietary influences on the atherogenic lipoprotein phenotype. *World Rev. Nutr. Diet.* 80: 22–43.

Krauss RM. 1998. Atherogenicity of triglycerides-rich lipoproteins. *Am. J. Cardiol.* 81: 13B–17B.

Kris-Etherton PM, Krummel D, Russel ME, Dreon D, Mackey S, Borcher J and Wood PD. 1988. The effect of diet on plasma lipids, lipoproteins, and coronary heart disease. *J. Am. Diet. Assoc.* 88: 1373–1400.

Kris-Etherton PM and Dietschy J. 1997. Design criteria for studies examining individual fatty acid effects on cardiovascular risk factors: Human and animal studies. *Am. J. Clin. Nutr.* 65 (Suppl.): 1590S–1596S.

Krishnaswamy K and Rao SB. 1977. Failure to produce atherosclerosis in *Macaca radiata* on high-methionine, high-fat, pyridoxine-deficient diet. *Atherosclerosis* 27: 253–258.

Kritchevsky D. 1976. Diet and atherosclerosis. *Am. J. Pathol.* 84: 615–632.

Kritchevsky D. 1978. Fiber, lipids and atherosclerosis. *Am. J. Clin. Nutr.* 31: 565–574.

Kritchevsky D. 1979. Vegetable protein and atherosclerosis. *J. Am. Oil Chem. Soc.* 56: 135–140.

Kritchevsky D. 1980a. Age-related changes in lipid metabolism. *Proc. Soc. Exp. Biol. Med.* 165: 193–199.

Kritchevsky D. 1980b. Dietary protein in atherosclerosis. In Noseda G, Lewis B and Paoletti R, Eds., *Diet and Drug in Atherosclerosis*, Raven Press, New York, pp. 9–14.

Kritchevsky D. 1981. Experimental atherosclerosis in rabbits fed cholesterol-free diets. *Atherosclerosis* 39: 169–175.

Kritchevsky D. 1983a. Influence of animal and vegetable protein atherosclerosis and lipid metabolism. In Kaufmann W, Ed., *Role of Milk Proteins in Human Nutrition*, Verlag Th Mann KG, Geisenkirchen-Buer, pp. 389–396.

Kritchevsky D. 1983b. Nutritional theories of atherogenesis. *Contemp. Issues Clin. Nutr.* 6: 29–44.

Kritchevsky D. 1987. Animal and vegetable protein effects in experimental atherosclerosis. In Schlierf G and Mörl H, Eds., *Expanding Horizons in Atherosclerosis Research.* Springer-Verlag, Berlin, pp. 304–308.

Kritchevsky D. 1990. Protein and atherosclerosis. *J. Nutr. Sci. Vitaminol.* 36 (Suppl. 2): S81–S86.

Kritchevsky D. 1993. Dietary protein and experimental atherosclerosis. *Ann. N. Y. Acad. Sci.,* 676: 180–187.

Kritchevsky D. 1995. Dietary protein, cholesterol and atherosclerosis: A review of the early history. *J. Nutr.* 125 (Suppl. 3): 589S–593S.

Kritchevsky D. 1999. Diet and atherosclerosis. *Am. Heart J.* 138: 5426–5430.

Kritchevsky D, Kolman RR, Guttmacher RM and Forbes M. 1959. Influence of dietary carbohydrate and protein on serum and liver cholesterol in germ-free chickens. *Arch. Biochem. Biophys.* 85: 444–451.

Kritchevsky D and Tepper SA. 1968. Experimental atherosclerosis in rabbits fed cholesterol-free diets: Influence of chow components. *J. Atheroscler. Res.* 8: 357–369.

Kritchevsky D and Story JA. 1974. Binding of bile salts *in vitro* by non nutritive fiber. *J. Nutr.* 104: 458–462.

Kritchevsky D, Tepper SA, Story JA. 1974. Isocaloric, isogravic diet in rats. III. Effect of non-nutritive fiber (alfalfa and cellulose) on cholesterol metabolism. *Nutr. Rep. Int.* 9: 301–308.

Kritchevsky D, Tepper SA, Williams DE and Story WA. 1977. Experimental atherosclerosis in rabbits fed cholesterol-free diets. 7. Interaction of animal or vegetable protein with fiber. *Atherosclerosis* 26: 397–403.

Kritchevsky D and Story JA. 1978. Fiber, hypercholesterolemia and atherosclerosis. *Lipids* 13: 366–369.

Kritchevsky D, Tepper SA and Story JA. 1978. Influence of soy protein and casein on atherosclerosis in rabbits. *Fed. Proc.* 3: 747, Abstract 2801.

Kritchevsky D, Tepper SA, Czarnecki SK, Klurfeld DM, Story JA. 1981. Experimental atherosclerosis in rabbits fed cholesterol-free diets. Part 9. Beef protein and textured vegetable protein. *Atherosclerosis* 39: 169–175.

Kritchevsky D and Czarnecki SK. 1982. Dietary protein and atherosclerosis. In Descovich GC and Lenzi S, Eds., *Soy Protein in the Prevention of Atherosclerosis*, MTP Press Limited, Lancaster, England, pp. 1–11.

Kritchevsky D, Tepper SA, Czarnecki SK and Klurfeld DM. 1982a. Atherogenicity of animal and vegetable protein. Influence of the lysine to arginine ratio. *Atherosclerosis* 41: 429–431.

Kritchevsky D, Tepper SA, Czarnecki SK, Story JA and Marsh JB. 1982b. Experimental atherosclerosis in rabbits fed cholesterol-free diets. 11. Corn protein, wheat gluten and lactalbumin. *Nutr. Rep. Int.* 26: 931–936.

Kritchevsky D and Czarnecki SK. 1983. Dietary protein and experimental atherosclerosis: Early history. In Gibney MJ and Kritchevsky D, Eds., *Animal and Vegetable Proteins in Lipid Metabolism and Atherosclerosis*, Vol. 5, Alan R. Liss, New York, pp. 1–7.

Kritchevsky D, Tepper SA, Czarnecki SK, Klurfeld DM and Story JA. 1983. Effect of animal and vegetable protein in experimental atherosclerosis. In Gibney MG and Kritchevsky D, Eds., *Animal and Vegetable Protein in Lipid Metabolism and Atherosclerosis*, Current Topics in Nutrition and Disease, Vol. 8, Alan R. Liss, New York, pp. 85–100.

Kritchevsky D, Tepper SA, Czarnecki SK, Mueller MA, Klurfeld DM and Story JA. 1984. Effects of dietary protein on lipid metabolism in rats. *J. Natl. Acad. Sci.* (Washington) 74: 1–8.

Kritchevsky D and Klurfeld K. 1987. Protein and carbohydrate. Effects in atherosclerosis. In Gallo LL, Ed., *Cardiovascular Disease: Molecular Mechanisms, Prevention and Treatment*, Plenum Press, New York, pp. 521–531.

Kritchevsky D, Tepper SA and Klurfeld DM. 1987. Dietary protein and atherosclerosis. *J. Am. Oil Chem. Soc.* 64: 1167–1171.

Kritchevsky D, Davidson LM and Mendelsohn D. 1988a. Influence of increasing levels of dietary casein on serum lipids and atherosclerosis in *Vervet* monkeys. *Nutr. Rep. Int.* 38: 307–311.

Kritchevsky D, Tepper SA, Weber MM and Klurfeld DM. 1988b. Influence of soy protein or casein on pre-established atherosclerosis in rabbits. *Artery* 15: 163–169.

Kritchevsky D, Tepper SA, Davidson LM, Fisher EA and Klurfeld DM. 1989. Experimental atherosclerosis in rabbits fed cholesterol-free diets. 13. Interaction of proteins and fat. *Atherosclerosis* 75: 123–127.

Kromhout D, Bosschieter EB and Cor de Lezenne Coulander CL. 1985. The inverse relation between fish consumption and 20-year mortality from coronary heart disease. *N. Engl. J. Med.* 312: 1205–1209.

Kromhout D, Feskens JM and Bowled CH. 1995. The protective effect of a small amount of fish on coronary heart disease mortality in an elderly population. *Int. J. Epidemiol.* 24: 340–345.

Kroon PA, Hand UM, Huff JW and Alberts AW. 1982. The effect of mevinolin on serum cholesterol levels of rabbits with endogenous hypercholesterolemia. *Atherosclerosis* 44: 41–48.

Kroon PA, Thompson GM and Chao YS. 1985. β-very low density lipoproteins in cholesterol-fed rabbits are of hepatic origin. *Atherosclerosis* 56: 323–329.

Krul ES and Dolphin PJ. 1982. Secretion of nascent lipoproteins by isolated hepatocytes from hypothyroid and hypothyroid hypercholesterolemic rats. *Biochim. Biophys. Acta* 13: 609–621.

Kubow S, Goyette N, Noski KG. 1997. Tissue lipid peroxidation and serum lipoproteins in hamsters are affected by dietary protein composition. *Nutr. Res.* 17: 271–281.

Kuchel O. 1998. Differential catecholamine responses to protein intake in healthy and hypertensive subjects. *Am. J. Physiol.* 275: R1164–R1173.

Kudchodkar BJ, Lee MJ, Lee SM, DiMarco NM and Lacko AG. 1988. Effect of dietary protein on cholesterol homeostasis in diabetic rats. *J. Lipid Res.* 29: 1272–1287.

Kugiyama K, Kern SA, Morrisett JD, Roberts R and Henry PD. 1990. Impairment of endothelium-dependent arterial relaxation by lysolecithin in modified low-density lipoproteins. *Nature* 344: 160–162.

Kuiper GGJM, Carlsson B, Grandien K, Enmark E, Haggblad J, Nilsson E and Gustafsson JA. 1997. Comparison of the ligand binding specificity and transcript tissue distribution of estrogen receptor alpha and beta. *Endocrinology* 138: 863–870.

Kuiper GGJM, Lemmen JG, Carlsson B, Corton JC, Safe SH, van der Saag PT, van der Burg B and Gustafsson JA. 1998. Interaction of estrogenic chemicals and phytoestrogens with estrogen receptors β. *Endocrinology* 139: 4252–4263.

Kuller LH and Evans RW. 1998. Homocysteine, vitamins, and cardiovascular disease. *Circulation* 98: 196–199.

Kuo L, Davis MJ, Cannon MS and Chilian WM. 1992. Pathophysiological consequences of atherosclerosis extend into the coronary microcirculation: Restoration of endothelium-dependent response by L-arginine. *Circ. Res.* 70: 456–476.

Kurokawa K and Okuda T. 1998. Genetic and non genetic basis of essential hypertension: Maladaptation of human civilization to high salt intake. *Hypertens. Res.* 21: 67–71.

Kurowska EM. 2001. Soy protein in the regulation of apo B secretion. In Descheemaeker K and Debruyne I, Eds., *Soy and Health 2000: Clinical Evidence, Dietetic Applications*, Garant, Leuven/Apeldoorn, pp. 21–28.

Kurowska EM, Hrabek-Smith JM and Carroll KK. 1989. Compositional changes in serum lipoproteins during developing hypercholesterolemia induced in rabbits by cholesterol-free, semipurified diets. *Atherosclerosis* 78: 159–165.

Kurowska EM and Carroll KK. 1990. Essential amino acids in relation to hypercholesterolemia induced in rabbits by dietary casein. *J. Nutr.* 120: 831–836.

Kurowska EM and Carroll KK. 1991. Studies on the mechanism of induction of hypercholesterolemia in rabbits by high dietary levels of amino acids. *J. Nutr. Biochem.* 2: 656–662.

Kurowska EM and Carroll KK. 1992. Effects of high levels of selected dietary essential amino acids on hypercholesterolemia and down-regulation of hepatic LDL receptors in rabbits. *Biochim. Biophys. Acta* 1126: 185–191.

Kurowska EM and Carroll KK. 1993. Metabolic changes during hypercholesterolemia induced in rabbits by high levels of dietary amino acids. *F.A.S.E.B. J.* 7: Part 2, A803, Abstract 4639.

Kurowska EM and Carroll KK. 1994. Hypercholesterolemic responses in rabbits to selected groups of dietary essential amino acids. *J. Nutr.* 124: 364–370.

Kurowska EM, Moffart M and Carroll KK. 1994. Dietary soybean isoflurones counteract the elevation of VLDL but not LDL cholesterol produced in rabbits by feeding a cholesterol-free casein diet. *Proc. Can. Fed. Biol. Soc.* 37: 126, Abstract 365.

Kurowska EM and Carroll KK. 1996. LDL versus apolipoprotein B responses to variable proportions of selected amino acids in semipurified diets fed to rabbits and in the media of HepG$_2$ cells. *J. Nutr. Biochem.* 7: 418–424.

Kurowska EM, Jordan J, Spence JD, Wetmore S, Piché LA, Radzikowski M and Carroll KK. 1996. Role of the main components of whole soybean products, soy protein and soy oil, in reducing hypercholesterolemia. Second Symposium on the Role of Soy in Preventing and Treating Chronic Disease, Brussels, Sept. 15–18, 1996, Abstract, pp. 22–23.

Kurowska EM, Jordan J, Spence JD, Wetmore S, Piché LA, Radzikowski M, Dandona P and Carroll KK. 1997a. Effects of substituting dietary soybean protein and oil for milk protein and fat in subjects with hypercholesterolemia. *Clin. Invest. Med.* 20: 162–170.

Kurowska EM, Giroux I and Carroll KK. 1997b. Regulation of hypercholesterolemia by dietary proteins and certain amino acids. *Atherosclerosis* 134: 330, P163.

Kurowska EM, Jordan J, Spence JD, Wetmore S, Piché LA, Radzikowski M and Carroll KK. 1998. Role of the main components of whole soybean products, soy protein and soy oil, in reducing hypercholesterolemia. *Am. J. Clin. Nutr.* 68 (Suppl.): 1519S.

Kurowska EM, Manthey JA and Hasegawa S. 2000. Regulatory effects of tangeretin, a flavonoid from tengarines, and limonin, a limonoid from citrus, on apo B metabolism in HepG2 cells. *F.A.S.E.B. J.* 14: A298, Abstract 231.2.

Kurup GM, Leelamma S and Kurup PA. 1983. Effect of lysine and methionine on lipid metabolism in rats. *Ind. J. Biochem. Biophys.* 19: 347–351.

Kurzer MS and Xu X. 1997. Dietary phytoestrogens. *Annu. Rev. Nutr.* 17: 353–381.

Kushawaha RS and Hazzard WR. 1978. Catabolism of very low density lipoproteins in the rabbit: Effect of changing composition and pool size. *Biochim. Biophys. Acta* 528: 176–181.

Kushawaha RS, McGill HC. 1997. Mechanisms controlling lipemic reponses to dietary lipids. *World Rev. Nutr. Diet.* 80: 82–125.

Kuyvenhoven MW, West CE, van der Meer R and Beynen AC. 1986. Fecal steroid excretion in relation to the development of casein-induced hypercholesterolemia in rabbits. *J. Nutr.* 116: 1395–1404.

Kuyvenhoven MW, West CE, Hakkert BC, Mensink GBM and Beynen AC. 1987. Digestibility of dietary proteins and serum cholesterol in rats. *Nutr. Rep. Int.* 36: 537–549.

Kuyvenhoven MW, Roszkowski WF, West CE, Hogenboom RL, Vos RM, Beynen AC and Van der Meer R. 1989. Digestibility of casein, formaldehyde-treated casein and soyabean protein in relation to their effects on serum cholesterol in rabbits. *Br. J. Nutr.* 62: 331–342.

Laakso S. 1984. Inhibition of lipid peroxidation by casein. Evidence of molecular encapsulation of 1,4-pentadiene fatty acids. *Biochim. Biophys. Acta* 792: 11–15.

Lacaille B, Julien P, Deshaies Y, Lavigne C, Brun LD and Jacques H. 2000. Response of plasma lipoproteins and sex hormones to the consumption of lean fish incorporated in a prudent diet in normolipidemic men. *J. Am. Coll. Nutr.* 19: 745–753.

Lacombe C and Nibbelink M. 1980. Lipoprotein modifications with changing dietary proteins in rabbits on a high fat diet. *Artery* 6: 280–289.

Laidlaw M and Mercer NH. 1985. Serum cholesterol, triglycerides and lipoprotein response in hypercholesterolemic males to replacement of cow's milk with a soy beverage. *Fed. Proc.* 44: 1498, Abstract 6360.

Lakshmanan MR, Neprokoeff CM, Ness GC, Dugan RE, Porter JW. 1973. Stimulation by insulin of rat liver β-hydroxy-β-methylglutaryl coenzyme A reductase and cholesterol synthesising activities. *Biochem. Biophys. Res. Commn.* 50: 704–710.

Lambert GF, Miller JP, Olson RT and Frost DV. 1958. Hypercholesterolemia and atherosclerosis induced in rabbits by purified high fat rations devoid of cholesterol. *Proc. Soc. Exp. Biol. Med.* 97: 544–549.

Lambert J, van den Berg M, Steyn M, Rauwerda JA, Donker ABJM and Stehouver CDA. 1999. Familial hyperhomocysteinemia and endothelium-dependent vasodilatation and arterial distensibility of large arteries. *Cardiovasc. Res.* 42: 743–751.

Lampe JW, Karr SC, Hutchins AM and Slavin JL. 1998. Urinary equol excretion wih a soy challenge: Influence of habitual diet. *Proc. Soc. Exp. Biol. Med.* 217: 335–339.

Lamry MY, Meghelli-Bouchenak M, Boualga A, Belleville J and Prost J. 1995. Rat plasma VLDL composition and concentration and hepatic lipase and lipoprotein lipase activities are impaired during two types of protein malnutrition and unaffected by balanced refeeding. *J. Nutr.* 125: 2425–2434.

Langley SC and Jackson AA. 1994. Increased systolic pressure in adult rats induced by fetal exposure to maternal low-protein diets. *Clin. Sci. (Colch.)* 86: 217–222 (Discussion 121).

Langman LJ and Cole DEC. 1999. Homocysteine. *Crit. Rev. Clin. Lab. Sci.* 36: 345–406.

Lapré JA, West CE, Lovati MR, Sirtori CR and Beynen CA. 1989. Dietary animal proteins and cholesterol metabolism in rats. *Int. J. Vitam. Nutr. Res.* 59: 93–100.

Lark LA, Witt PA, Becker KB, Studzinski WM and Weyhenmeyer JA. 1990. Effect of dietary tryptophan on the development of hypertension in the Dahl salt-sensitive rat. *Clin. Exp. Hypertens.* 12: 1–13.

Larson M, Wilson C, Hassan A and Potter SM. 1992. Effects of dietary casein: Whey ratios on plasma lipids and lesion development in rabbits. *F.A.S.E.B. J.* 6: Part I, A1107, Abstract 992.

Larson MR, Wilson C and Potter SM. 1994. The role of dietary protein source in the development of cholesterol metabolism in rabbits. *J. Nutr. Biochem.* 5: 232–237.

Larson MR, Donovan SM and Potter SM. 1996. Effects of dietary protein source on cholesterol metabolism in neonatal pigs. *Nutr. Res.* 16: 1563–1574.

Lasekan JB, Guezth L and Sukur K. 1995. Influence of dietary golden pea proteins versus casein on plasma and hepatic lipids in rats. *Nutr. Res.* 15: 71–84.

Lau BW and Klevay LM. 1981. Plasma lecithin: Cholesterol acyltransferase in copper-deficient rats. *J. Nutr.* 111: 1698–1703.

Lau BW, Klevay LM. 1982. Postheparin plasma lipoprotein lipase in copper deficient rats. *J. Nutr.* 112: 928–933.

Laurent G. 1983. Contribution à l'étude du rôle des protéines alimentaires dans l'athérogenèse. Etude chez le lapin *Fauve de Bourgogne, Oryctolagus cuniculus Dom. L.* Ph.D. diss., Université de Nancy 1.

Laurin D, Jacques H, Moorjani S, Steinke FH, Gagné C, Brun D and Lupien PJ. 1991. Effects of a soybean beverage on plasma lipoproteins in children with familial hypercholesterolemia. *Am. J. Clin. Nutr.* 61: 98–103.

LeBlanc MJ, Gavino V, Pérea A, Yousef IM, Lévy E and Tuchweber B. 1998. The role of dietary choline in beneficial effects of lecithin on the secretion of biliary lipids in rats. *Biochim. Biophys. Acta* 1393: 223–234.

Leclerc J, Miller ML and Septier C. 1985. Comparative effects of carbohydrate content (fructose or glucose) and methionine supplement in the diet of lactating rat. Lipid concentrations in the plasma and liver of the dam. *Nutr. Rep. Int.* 32: 1003–1008.

Leclerc J, Chanussot B, Miller ML, Poisson JP and Belleville J. 1989. Effects of protein level, methionine supplementation and carbohydrate type of the diet on liver lipid and plasma free threonine contents in the lactating rat. *Reprod. Nutr. Dev.* 29: 269–276.

Lee HS, O'Donnell JAO and Hurt HD. 1981. Influence of various dietary protein sources on plasma and liver lipids in gerbils. *Fed. Proc.* 40: Part 1, 353, Abstract 685.

Lee KT, Onodera K and Tanaka K, Eds. 1990. Atherosclerosis III. Recent progress in atherosclerosis research. The Second Saratoga International Conference on Atherosclerosis in Towada. *Ann. N. Y. Acad. Sci.* 558.

Leelamma S, Menon PVG and Kump PA. 1978. Nature and quantity of dietary protein and metabolism of lipids in rats fed normal and atherogenic diet. *Ind. J. Exp. Biol. Med.* 16: 29–35.

Lefevre M and Schneeman BO. 1983. Relationship between plasma cholesterol and protein quality in weanling rats. *Nutr. Rep. Int.* 28: 1369–1374.

Lefevre M and Schneeman BO. 1984. High density lipoprotein composition in rats fed casein or soy protein isolate. *J. Nutr.* 114: 768–777.

Lehtimäki T, Moilanen T, Solakivi T, Laippala P and Enholm C. 1992. Cholesterol-rich diet induced changes in plasma lipids in relation to apolipoprotein E phenotype in healthy students. *Ann. Med.* 24: 61–66.

Lembke A, Greggersen H, Kay HW, Rathjen G and Steinicke F. 1981. Zur Frage der atherogenen Wirkung von Casein. *Milchwissenschaft* 36: 557–561.

Lembke A, Greggersen H, Kay HW, Rathjen G and Steinicke F. 1983. Comparative studies on atherogenic effects of soy protein and casein. *Milchwissenschaft* 38: 538–541.

Lentz SR and Sadler JE. 1991. Inhibition of thrombomodulin surface expression and protein C activation by the thrombogenic agent homocysteine. *J. Clin. Invest.* 88: 1906–1914.

Lentz SR, Sobey CG, Piegors DJ, Bhopatkar MY, Faraci M, Malinow MR and Heistad DD. 1996. Vascular dysfunction in monkeys with diet-induced hyperhomocysteinemia. *J. Clin. Invest.* 98: 24–29.

Leonil J, Bos C, Maubois JL and Tomé D. 2001. Protéines. In Debry G, Ed., *Lait, Nutrition et Santé*, Editions Tec et Doc Lavoisier, Paris, pp. 45–83.

Léveillé GA and Fisher H. 1958. Plasma cholesterol in growing chicken as influenced by dietary protein and fat. *Proc. Soc. Exp. Biol. Med.* 98: 630–632.

Léveillé GA, Feigenbaum AS and Fisher H. 1960. The effect of dietary protein, fat and cholesterol on plasma cholesterol and serum protein components of the growing chick. *Arch. Biochem. Biophys.* 86: 67–70.

Léveillé GA and Sauberlich HE. 1961. The influence of dietary protein level on serum protein components and cholesterol in the growing chick. *J. Nutr.* 74: 500–504.

Léveillé GA, Shockley JW and Sauberlich HE. 1961. Influence of dietary factors on plasma lipids relationships in the growing chick. *Proc. Soc. Exp. Biol. Med.* 108: 313–315.

Léveillé GA, Shockley JW and Sauberlich HE. 1962a. Influence of dietary protein level and amino acids on plasma cholesterol of the growing chick. *J. Nutr.* 76: 321–324.

Léveillé GA and Sauberlich HE, Powell RC and Nunes WT. 1962b. The influences of dietary protein on plasma lipids in human subjects. *J. Clin. Invest.* 41: 1007–1012.

Léveillé GA and Sauberlich HE and Schockley JW. 1962c. Protein value and the amino acid deficiencies of various algae for growth of rats and chicks. *J. Nutr.* 76: 423–428.

Léveillé GA and Sauberlich HE. 1964. Plasma and liver lipids of mice as influenced by dietary protein and sulfur-containing acid. *J. Nutr.* 84: 10–14.

Leveugle B, Mazurier J, Legrand D, Mazurier C, Montreuil J and Spik G. 1993. Lactotransferrin binding to its platelets receptor inhibits platelets aggregation. *Eur. J. Biochem.* 213: 1205–1211.

Lewis B, Hansen JDL, Witttman W, Krutm LH and Stewart F. 1964. Plasma free fatty acids in kwashiorkor and the pathogenesis of the fatty liver. *Am. J. Clin. Nutr.* 15: 161–168.

Lewis LA, Green AA and Page IH. 1952. Ultracentrifugal lipoprotein pattern of serum of normal, hypertensive, and hypothyroid animals. *Am. J. Physiol.* 171: 391–400.

Li G, Regunathan S, Barrow CJ, Eshragi J, Cooper R and Reis DJ. 1994. Agmatine: An endogenous clonidine-displacing substance in the brain. *Science* 263: 966–969.

Li TW and Freeman S. 1946. Experimental lipaemia and hypercholesterolemia in protein depletion and by cholesterol feeding in dogs. *Am. J. Physiol.* 145: 660–666.

Liao JK, Shin WS, Lee WY and Clark SL. 1995. Oxidized low-density lipoprotein decreases the expression of endothelial nitric oxide synthase. *J. Biol. Chem.* 270: 319–324.

Lichtenstein AH. 1998. Soy protein, isoflavones and cardiovascular disease risk. *J. Nutr.* 128: 1589–1592.

Lichton IJ and Wenkam NS. 1967. Renal disease in rats fed Japanese-type diets: Ameliorating effects of protein substitution and restriction of food intake. *Fed. Proc.* 26: 517, Abstract.

Lin ECK, Fernandez ML and McNamara DJ. 1992. Dietary fat type and cholesterol quantity interact to affect cholesterol metabolism in guinea pigs. *J. Nutr.* 122: 2019–2029.

Lin ECK, Fernandez ML, Tosca MA and McNamara DJ. 1994. Regulation of hepatic LDL metabolism in the guinea pig by dietary fat and cholesterol. *J. Lipid Res.* 35: 446–457.

Linassier C, Pierre M, LePecq JB and Pierre J. 1990. Mechanism of action in NIH–3T3 cells of genistein an inhibitor of EGF receptor tyrosine kinase activity. *Biochem. Pharmacol.* 39:187–193.

Lindholm M and Eklund A. 1991. The effects of dietary protein on the fatty acid composition and Δ6 desaturase activity of rat hepatic microsomes. *Lipids* 26: 107–110.

Lindholm M, Sjoblom L, Nordborg C, Ostlund-Lindqvist AM and Reklunf A. 1993. Comparison of dietary casein and soybean protein effects on plasma lipid and gastrin levels, hepatic delta-6-desaturase activity and coronary arteriosclerosis in male *Sprague-Dawley* rats. A 9 month study. *Ann. Nutr. Metab.* 37: 302–310.

Linton MF, Farese RV Jr, Chiesa G, Grass DS, Chin P, Hammer RE, Hobbs HH and Young SG. 1993. Transgenic mice expressing high plasma concentration s of human apolipoprotein B100 and lipoprotein(a). *J. Clin. Invest.* 92: 3029–3037.

Little JM and Angell EA. 1977. Dietary protein level and experimental aortic atherosclerosis. *Atherosclerosis* 26: 173–179.

Liu K, Ruth KJ, Flack J, Burke G, Savage P, Liang KY, Hardin M and Hulley S. 1992. Ethnic differences in 5-year blood pressure change in young adults: The CARDIA Study. *Circulation* 85: 867, Abstract 22.

Liu K, Ruth KJ, Shekelle RB and Stamler J. 1993. Macronutrients and long-term change in systolic blood pressure. *Circulation* 87: 679, Abstract 7.

Liu K et al. 1996. Personal written communication on Cardia Study, quoted by Obarzaneck et al., *J.A.M.A.* 275: 1598–1603.

Lo GS. 1990. Physiological effects and physico-chemical properties of soy cotyledon fiber. In Furda I and Brine CJ, Eds., *New Developments in Dietary Fiber*, Plenum Press, New York, pp. 49–66.

Lo GS, Goldberg AP, Lim A, Grundhauser JJ, Anderson C and Schonfeld G. 1986. Soy fiber improves lipid and carbohydrate metabolism in primary hyperlipidemic subjects. *Atherosclerosis* 62: 239–248.

Lo GS, Evans RH, Phillips KS, Dahlgren RR and Steinke FH. 1987. Effect of soy fiber and soy protein on cholesterol metabolism and atherosclerosis in rabbits. *Atherosclerosis* 64: 47–54.

Loewe L, Goldner MG, Rapoport SM and Stern I. 1954. Failure of protein to protect against cholesterol atherogenesis in underfed rabbits. *Proc. Soc. Exp. Biol.* 87: 360–362.

Lofland HB, Clarkson TB and Goodman HO. 1961. Interactions among dietary fat, protein and cholesterol in atherosclerosis-susceptible pigeons. Effect on serum cholesterol and aortic atherosclerosis. *Circ. Res.* 9: 919–924.

Lofland HB, Clarkson TB, Rhyne L and Goodman HO. 1966. Interrelated effects of dietary fats and proteins on atherosclerosis in the pigeon. *J. Atheroscler. Res.* 6: 395–403.

Lombardini JB. 1975. An enzymatic derivative double isotope assay for measuring tissue levels of taurine. *J. Pharmacol. Exp. Ther.* 193: 301–308.

Lönnerdal B, Cederblad A, Davidsson L and Sandström B. 1984. The effects of individual components of soy formula and cow's milk formula on zinc bioavailability. *Am. J. Clin. Nutr.* 40: 1064–1070.

Lopez-Miranda J, Ordovas JM, Mata P, Lichtenstein AH,Clevidence B, Judd JT, Schaefer EJ. 1994. Effect of apolipoprotein E phenotype on diet-induced lowering of plasma low density lipoprotein cholesterol. *J. Lipid Res.* 35: 1965–1975.

LoPresto L and Wada L. 1988. Effect of level and type of dietary protein on carbohydrate metabolism and serum lipids in rats. *F.A.S.E.B. J.* 5: Part 2, A1213, Abstract 5332.

Lorgeril de M. 1998. Dietary arginine and the prevention of cardiovascular disease. *Cardiovasc. Res.* 37: 560–563.

Loscalzo J. 1996. The oxidant stress of hyperhomocyst(e)inemia. *J. Clin. Invest.* 98: 5–7.

Loschiavo C, Ferrari S, Panebianco R, Bedogna V, Oldrizzi L, Bonazzi L and Maschio G. 1988. Effect of protein-restricted diet on serum lipids and atherosclerosis risk factors in patients with chronic renal failure. *Clin. Nephrol.* 29: 113–118.

Lovati MR. 2001. Soy proteins and regulation of LDL receptors. In Deescheemaeker K and Debruyne I, Eds., *Soy and Health 2000: Clinical Evidence, Dietetic Applications*, Garant, Leuven, pp. 17–20.

Lovati MR, Allievi L and Sirtori CR. 1985. Accelerated early catabolism of very low density lipoproteins in rats after dietary soy proteins. *Atherosclerosis* 56: 243–246.

Lovati MR, Manzoni C, Canavesi A, Sirtori M, Vaccarino V, Marchi M, Gaddi G and Sirtori CR. 1987. Soybean protein diet increases low density lipoprotein receptor activity in mononuclear cells from hypercholesterolemic patients. *J. Clin. Invest.* 80: 125–130.

Lovati MR, West CE, Sirtori CR and Beynen AC. 1990. Dietary animal proteins and cholesterol metabolism in rabbits. *Br. J. Nutr.* 64: 473–485.

Lovati MR, Manzoni C, Agostinelle P, Ciappellano S, Mannuccil and Sirtori CR. 1991a. Studies on the mechanism of the cholesterol lowering activity of soy proteins. Soy protein extract reduces plasma cholesterol and increases liver β-VLDL receptors in mice. *Nutr. Metab. Cardiovasc. Dis.* 1: 18–24.

Lovati MR, Manzoni C and Sirtori CR. 1991b. Animal versus vegetable proteins as a risk factors for atherosclerotic disease. *Cardiovasc. Risk Factors* 1: 300–305.

Lovati MR, Manzoni C, Corsini A, Granata A, Frattini R, Fumagalli R and Sirtori CR. 1992. Low-density lipoprotein receptor activity is modulated by soybean globulins in cell culture. *J. Nutr.* 122: 1971–1978.

Lovati MR, Manzoni C, Corsini A, Granata A, Fumagalli R and Sirtori CR. 1996. 7S globulin from soybean is metabolized in human cell cultures by a specific uptake and degradation system. *J. Nutr.* 126: 2831–2842.

Lovati MR, Manzoni C, Gianazza C, Sirtori CR. 1998. Soybean protein product as a regulator of liver low-density lipoprotein receptors, I - Identification of active-β-conglycinin subunits. *J. Agric. Food Chem.* 46: 2474–2480.

Lovati MR, Manzoni C, Gianazza E, Arnoldi A, Kurowska M, Carroll KK and Sirtori R. 2000. Soy protein peptides regulate cholesterol homeostasis in HepG2 cells. *J. Nutr.* 130: 2543–2549.

Lovenberg W. 1984. Possible relationship between nutrition and cardiovascular disease in experimental animals. In Lovenberg W and Yamori Y, Eds., *Nutritional Prevention of Cardiovascular Disease*, Academic Press, Orlando, FL, pp. 21–26.

Lovenberg W. 1987. Animal models for hypertension research. *Prog. Clin. Biol. Res.* 229: 225–240.

Lovenberg W and Yamori Y. 1990. The role of dietary protein in hypertensive disease. In Laragh JH and Brener BM, Eds., *Hypertension, Physiology, Diagnosis and Management*, Raven Press, New York, pp. 295–301.

Lovenberg W and Yamori Y. 1995. The role of dietary protein in hypertensive disease. In Laragh JH and Brenner BM, Eds., *Hypertension, Pathophysiology, Diagnosis and Management*, 2nd ed., Raven Press, New York, pp. 313–320.

Lu YF and Tang CY. 1996. Effects of protein sources and levels on fatty acid composition in rat tissues. *Nutr. Sci. J.* 21: 279–288.

Lu YF and Jian MR. 1997. Effects of soy protein and casein on lipid metabolism in mature and suckling rats. *Nutr. Res.* 17: 1341–1350.

Lubarsch O. 1909. Zur Pathogenese der Atherosklerose der Arterien. *Muench. Med. Wochenschr.* 56: 1819–1820.

Lubarsch O. 1910. Über alimentare Schlagaderverbolkung. *Muench. Med. Wochenschr.* 57: 1577–1580.

Lubec B, Hayn M, Kitzmüller E, Vierhapper H and Lubec G. 1997. L-Arginine reduces lipid peroxidation in patient with diabetes mellitus. *Free Radical Biol. Med.* 22: 355–357.

Lucas EA, Khalil DA, Daggy BP and Arjmandi BH. 2001. Ethanol extracted soy protein isolates does not modulate serum cholesterol in *Golden Syrian* hamsters: a model of postmenopausal hypercholesterolemia. *J. Nutr.* 131: 211–214.

Lueprasitsakul W, Alex S, Fang SL, Pino S, Irmscher K, Köhrle J and Braverman LE. 1990. Flavonoid administration immediately displaces thyroxine (T4) from serum trans-thyretin, increases serum free T4, and decreases serum thyrotropin in the rat. *Endocrinology* 126: 2890–2895.

Luft FC. 1998. Molecular genetics of human hypertension. *J. Hypertens.* 16: 1971–1878.

Lusas EW and Riaz MN. 1995. Soy protein products: Processing and use. *J. Nutr.* 125: 573S–580S.

Lusis A and Sparkes RS, Eds. 1989. *Genetic Factors in Atherosclerosis: Approaches and Model Systems*, Monographs on Human Genetics, Vol. 12, S. Karger, Basel.

Lutz RN, Barnes RH, Kwong E and Williams HH. 1959. Effect of dietary protein on blood serum cholesterol in men consuming mixed diets. *Fed. Proc.* 18: 534, Abstract.

Lynch SR. 1984. Iron. In Solomon NW and Rosenberg IH, Eds., *Absorption and Malabsorption of Mineral Nutrients*, Alan R. Liss, New York, pp. 89–124.

Lynch SM and Strain JJ. 1989. Increased hepatic lipid peroxidation with methionine toxicity in the rat. *Free Radical Res. Commn. Med.* 5: 221–226.

Lyons J, Rauch-Pfeiffer A, Yu YM, Lu XM, Zurakowski D, Tomkins RG Ajami AM, Young VR and Castillo L. 2000. Blood glutathione synthesis rates in healthy adults receiving a sulfur amino acid-free diet. *Proc. Natl. Acad. Sci. U. S. A.* 97: 5071–5076.

MacAllister RJ, Calver AL, Collier J, Edwards CMB, Herreros B, Nussey SS and Vallance P. 1995. Vascular and hormonal responses to arginine: Provision of substrate for nitric oxide or non-specific effect? *Clin. Sci.* 89: 183–190.

MacKinnon AM, Savage J, Gibson RA and Barter PJ. 1985. Secretion of cholesteryl ester-enriched very low density lipoproteins by the liver of cholesterol-fed rabbits. *Atherosclerosis* 54: 145–148.

Madani S, Lopez S, Blong JP, Prost J and Belleville J. 1998. Highly purified soybean protein is not hypocholesterolemic in rats but stimulates cholesterol synthesis and excretion and reduces polyunsaturated fatty acid biosynthesis. *J. Nutr.* 128: 1084–1091.

Madani S, Prost J and Belleville J. 2000. Dietary protein level and origin (casein and highly purified soybean protein) affect hepatic storage, plasma lipid transport and antioxidative defense status in the rat. *Nutrition* 16: 368–375.

Maeno M, Yamamoto N and Takano T. 1996. Isolation of an antihypertensive peptide from casein hydrolysate produced by a proteinase from *Lactobacillus helveticus* CP 790. *J. Dairy Sci.* 79: 1316–1321.

Mahalko JR, Sanstead HH, Johnson LK, Inman LF, Milne DB, Warner RC and Haunz EA. 1984. Effect of consuming fiber from corn bran, soy hulls, or apple powder on glucose tolerance and plasma lipids in type II diabetics. *Am. J. Clin. Nutr.* 39: 25–34.

Mahfouz-Cercone S, Johnson JE and Liepa GU. 1984. Effect of dietary animal and vegetable protein on gallstone formation and biliary constituents in the hamster. *Lipids* 19: 5–10.

Mahgoub A and Abu-Jayyab A. 1984. The cholesterolemic and triglyceridemic effects of some essential amino acids in rabbits. *IRCS Med. Sci.* 12: 431–432.

Mahgoub A and Abu-Jayyab A. 1987. Effect of some essential amino acids on serum lipids in the rabbit. *Nutr. Res.* 7: 771–778.

Mäkelä S, Savolainen H, Aavik E, Myllärniemi M, Strauss L, Taskinen E, Gustafsson JA and Hävry P. 1999. Differentiation between vasculoprotective and uterotrophic effects of ligands with different binding affinities to estrogens receptors α and β. *Proc. Natl. Acad. Sci.* 96: 7077–7082.

Malhotra SL. 1970. Dietary factors causing hypertension in India. *Am. J. Clin. Nutr.* 23: 1353–1363.

Malhotra S and Kritchevsky D. 1978. The distribution and lipid composition of ultra-centrifugally separated lipoproteins of young and old rat plasma. *Mech. Ageing Dev.* 8: 445–452.

Malinow MR. 1984. Saponins and cholesterol metabolism. *Atherosclerosis* 50: 117–119 (Letter).

Malinow MR, McLaughlin P, Papworth L, Naito HK, Lewis L, McNulty WP. 1976. A model for therapeutic intervention on established coronary atherosclerosis in a non human primate. *Adv. Exp. Med. Biol.* 76: 3–31.

Malinow MR, McLaughlin P, Kohler GO and Livingston AL. 1977a. Prevention of elevated cholesterolemia in monkeys by alfalfa saponins. *Steroids* 29: 105–109.

Malinow MR, Connor WE, McLaughlin P, Papworth L, Stafford C, Kohler GO, Livingston AL and Cheeke PR. 1977b. Effect of alfalfa saponins on intestinal cholesterol absorption in rats. *Am. J. Clin. Nutr.* 30: 2061–2067.

Malinow MR, McLaughlin P, Kohler GO and Livingston AL. 1977c. Alteration of alfalfa saponins and intestinal cholesterol absorption. *Fed. Proc.* 36: 1104, Abstract.

Malinow MR, McLaughlin P, Naito KK, Lewis LA and McNulty WP. 1978a. Effect of alfalfa meal on shrink-age regression of atherosclerotic plaques during cholesterol feeding in monkeys. *Atherosclerosis* 30: 27–43.

Malinow MR, McLaughlin P and Stafford C. 1978b. Prevention of hypercholesterolemia in monkeys *Macaca fascicularis* by digitonin. *Am. J. Clin. Nutr.* 31: 814–818.

Malinow MR, McLaughlin P, Stafford C, Livingston AL, Kohler GO and Cheeke PR. 1979. Comparative effects of alfalfa saponins and alfalfa fiber on cholesterol absorption in rats. *Am. J. Clin. Nutr.* 32: 1810–1812.

Malinow MR, Connor WE, McLaughlin P, Stafford C, Lin DS, Livingston AL, Kohler GO and Mc Nulty WP. 1981. Cholesterol and bile acid balance in *Macaca fascicularis*. Effects of alfalfa saponins. *J. Clin. Invest.* 67: 156–162.

Malinow MR, Kang SS, Taylor LM, Wong PW, Coull B, Inahara T, Mukerjee D, Sexton G and Upson B. 1989. Prevalence of hyperhomocyst(e)inemia in patients with peripheral arterial occlusive disease. *Circ. Res.* 79: 1180–1188.

Mann GV. 1960. Experimental atherosclerosis. Effects of sulfur compounds on hypercho-lesterolemia and growth in cysteine deficient monkeys. *Am. J. Clin. Nutr.* 8: 491–498.

Mann GV. 1977. A factor in yoghurt which lowers cholesterolemia in man. *Atherosclerosis* 26: 335–340.

Mann GV, Andrus SB, McNally A and Stare F. 1953. Experimental atherosclerosis in *Cebus* monkeys. *J. Exp. Med.* 98: 195–218.

Mann GV, McNally A and Prudhomme C. 1960. Experimental atherosclerosis. Effects of sulfur compounds on hypercholesterolemia and growth in cysteine-deficient monkeys. *Am. J. Clin. Nutr.* 8: 491–498.

Mann GV, Shaffer RD, Anderson RS and Sandstead HH. 1964. Cardiovascular disease in the Maasai. *J. Atheroscler. Res.* 4: 289–312.

Mann GV and Spoerri A. 1974. Studies of a surfactant and cholesterolemia in Maasai. *Am. J. Clin. Nutr.* 27: 464–469.

Mann NJ, Li D, Sinclair AJ, Dudman NPB, Guo XW, Elsworth GR, Wilson AK and Kelly FD. 1999. The effect of diet on plasma homocysteine concentration in healthy male subjects. *Eur. J. Clin. Nutr.* 53: 895–899.

Mänttäri M, Koskinen P and Enholm C, Huttunen JK and Manninen V. 1991. Apolipoprotein E polymorphism influences the serum cholesterol response to dietary intervention. *Metabolism* 40: 217–221.

Mantha SV. 1999. Mediation of L-arginine-induced retardation of hypercholesterolemic atherosclerosis in rabbits by antioxidant mechanisms. *Nutr. Res.* 19: 1529–1539.

Manzoni C, Lovati MR, Gianazza E, Morita Y and Sirtori CR. 1998. Soybean products as regulators of liver low-density lipoprotein receptors. II. α - α' rich commercial soy concentrate and α' deficient mutant differently affect low-density lipoprotein receptor activation. *J. Agric. Food Chem.* 46: 2481–2484.

March BE, Beily J, Tothill J and Haqq SA. 1959. Dietary modification of serum cholesterol in the chick. *J. Nutr.* 69: 105–110.

Marcon Genty D, Tomé D, Dumontier AM, Kheroua O and Desjeux FJ. 1989. Permeability of milk protein antigens across the intestinal epithelium *in vitro*. *Reprod. Nutr. Dev.* 29: 717–723.

Marenberg ME, Risch N, Berkman LF, Floderus B and de Faire U. 1994. Genetic susceptibility to death from coronary heart disease in a study of twins. *N. Engl. J. Med.* 330: 1041–1046.

Marion JE, Edwards HM and Driggers HM. 1961. Influence of diet on serum cholesterol in chick. *J. Nutr.* 74: 171–175.

Mariotti F, Huneau JF and Tomé D. 2001. Dietary protein and cardiovascular risk. *J. Nutr. Health Aging* 5: 200–204.

Marquez-Ruiz G, Richter BD and Schneeman BO. 1992. Modification of triacylglycerides and apolipoprotein B in rats fed diets containing whole milk, skim milk and milk proteins. *J. Nutr.* 122: 1840–1846.

Martin LJ, Connelly PW, Nancoo D, Wood N, Zhang ZJ, Maguire G, Quidet E, Tall R, Marcel YL and McPherson R. 1993. Cholesteryl ester transfer protein and high density lipoprotein responses to cholesterol feeding in men: Relationship to apolipoprotein E genotype. *J. Lipid Res.* 34: 437–446.

Maruyama S, Nakagomi K, Tomizuka N and Suzuki H. 1985. Angiotensin-converting enzyme inhibitor derived from an enzymatic hydrolase of casein. Isolation and bradykinin-potentiating activity on the uterus and the ileum of rats. *Agric. Biol. Chem.* 49: 1405–1409.

Maruyama S, Mitachi H, Awaya J, Kurono M, Tomizuka N and Suzuki H. 1987. Angiotensin I-converting enzyme inhibitory activity of the C-terminal hexapeptide of α_{s1}-casein. *Agric. Biol. Chem.* 51: 2557–2561.

Masuda O, Nakamura Y and Takano T. 1996. Antihypertensive peptides are present in aorta after oral administration of sour milk containing the peptides to spontaneously hypertensive rats. *J. Nutr.* 126: 3063–3068.

Mathew BC, Daniel RS and Augusti KC. 1996. Hypolipidemic effect of garlic protein substituted for casein in diet of rats compared to those of garlic oil. *Ind. J. Exp. Biol.* 34: 337–340.

Matsuoka H, Nakata M, Kohno K, Koga Y, Nomura G, Toshima H and Imaizumi T. 1996. Chronic L-arginine administration attenuates cardiac hypertrophy in spontaneously hypertensive rats. *Hypertension* 27: 14–18.

Matthews DM. 1972. Rates of peptides uptake by small intestine. In Elliott K and O'Connor M, Eds., *Peptide Transport in Bacteria and Mammalian Gut*, Ciba Foundation Symposium, Associated Scientific Publishers, Amsterdam, pp. 71–88.

Matthews DM, Lis MT, Cheng B and Crampton RF. 1969. Observations on the intestinal absorption of some oligopeptides of methionine and glycine in the rat. *Clin. Sci.* 37: 751–764.

Matthias D, Becker CH, Riezler R and Kindling PH. 1996. Homocysteine induced arteriosclerosis-like alterations of the aorta in normotensive and hypertensive rats following application of high doses of methionine. *Atherosclerosis* 122: 201–216.

Maubois JL and Leonil J. 1989. Peptides du lait à activité biologique. *Lait* 69: 245–269.

Maubois JL, Leonil J, Trouve R and Bouhallab S. 1991. Les peptides du lait à activité physiologique. III. Peptides du lait à effet cardiovasculaire: Activités antithrombotique et antihypertensive. *Lait* 71: 249–255.

Maxwell AJ and Cooke JP. 1998. Cardiovascular effects of L-arginine. *Curr. Opin. Nephrol. Hypertens.* 7: 63–70.

Mayer D and Voges A. 1972. The role of the pituitary in control of cholesterol 7α-hydroxylase activity in the rat liver. *Hoppe Seyler's Z. Physiol. Chem.* 353: 1187–1188.

Mayer J and Jones AK. 1953. Hypercholesterolemia in hereditary obese-hyperglycemic syndrome of mice. *Am. J. Physiol.* 175: 339–342.

Mazoyer E, Levy-Toledano S, Rendu F, Hermant L, Lu H, Fiat AM, Jollès P and Caen J. 1990. KRDS, a new peptide derived from lactotransferrin, inhibits platelet aggregation and release reaction. *Eur. J. Biochem.* 194: 43–49.

Mazoyer E, Bal dit Sollier C, Drouet L, Fiat AM, Jollès P and Caen J. 1992. Active peptides from human and cow's milk proteins: Effects on platelet function and vessel wall. In Paubert-Braquet M, Dupont C and Paoletti R, Eds., *Foods, Nutrition and Immunity: Effects of Dairy and Fermented Milk Products*, Vol. 1, S. Karger, Basel, pp. 88–95.

McCarron DA, Henry H and Morris C. 1982. Human nutrition and blood pressure regulation: An integrated approach. *Hypertension* 4 (Suppl. 3): 2–13.

McClelland JW and Shih JC. 1988. Prevention of hypercholesterolemia and atherosclerosis in Japanese quail by high intake of soy protein. *Atherosclerosis* 74: 127–138.

McCully KS. 1969. Vascular pathology of homocysteinemia: Implications for the pathogenesis of arteriosclerosis. *Am. J. Pathol.* 56: 111–128.

McCully KS. 1983. Vascular pathology of homocysteinemia. Homocysteine theory of arteriosclerosis. Development and current status. In Gotto AM and Paoletti R, Eds., *Atheroscler. Rev.* 11: 157–246.

McCully KS. 1996. Homocysteine and vascular disease. *Nat. Med.* 2: 386–389.

McCully KS. 1997. *The Homocysteine Revolution*, Keats, New Canaan, CT.

McCully KS. 1998. Homocysteine, folate, vitamin B6 and cardiovascular disease. *J.A.M.A.* 279: 392–393.

McCully KS and Wilson RB. 1975. Homocysteine theory of arteriosclerosis. *Atherosclerosis* 22: 215–227.

McDonald AM. 1987. Diet and blood pressure response: Effects of macronutrient intakes and alcohol. In Watson RR, Ed., *Nutrition and Heart Disease*, Vol. 2, CRC Press, Boca Raton, FL, 1–18.

McGregor D. 1971. The effects of some dietary changes upon the concentrations of serum lipid in rats. *Br. J. Nutr.* 25: 213–224.

McGregor GA. 1999. Nutrition and blood pressure. *Nutr. Metab. Cardiovasc. Dis.* 9 (Suppl.): 6–15.

McKinley MC. 2000. Nutritional aspects and possible pathological mechanisms of hyperhomocysteinaemia: An independent risk factor for vascular disease. *Proc. Nutr. Soc.* 59: 221–237.

McLachlan CNS. 2001. β-casein A₁, ischaemic heart disease mortality, and other illnesses. *Med. Hypotheses* 56: 262–272.

McNamara EA, Levitt MD and Slavin JL. 1986. Breath hydrogen and methane: Poor indicators of apparent digestion of soy fiber. *Am. J. Clin. Nutr.* 43: 898–902.

Meeker DR and Kesten HD. 1940. Experimental atherosclerosis and high protein diets. *Proc. Soc. Exp. Biol.* 45: 543–545.

Meeker DR and Kesten HD. 1941. Effect of high protein diets in experimental atherosclerosis of rabbits. *Arch. Pathol.* 31: 147–162.

Meer van der R. 1983. Is the hypercholesterolemic effect of dietary casein related to its phosphorylation state? *Atherosclerosis* 49: 339–341.

Meer van der R. 1988. Species dependent effects of dietary casein and calcium cholesterol metabolism. *Bull. Int. Dairy Fed.* 222: 24–27.

Meer van der R, de Vries HT. 1985. Differential binding of glycine- and taurine-conjugated bile acids to insoluble calcium phosphate. *Biochem. J.* 229: 265–268.

Meer van der R, Schöning R and de Vries H. 1985a. The phosphorylation state of casein and its differential hypercholesterolemic effect in rabbits and rats. In Beynen AC, Geelen LJH, Katan MB and Schouten JA, Eds., *Cholesterol Metabolism in Health and Disease: Studies in the Netherlands*, Ponsen and Looijen, Wageningen, pp. 151–157.

Meer van der R, de Vries H, West CE and de Waard H. 1985b. Casein-induced hypercholesterolemia in rabbits is calcium-dependent. *Atherosclerosis* 56: 139–147.

Meer van der R and Beynen AC. 1987. Species-dependent responsiveness of serum cholesterol to dietary proteins. *J. Am. Oil Chem. Soc.* 64: 1172–1177.

Meer van der R, de Vries HT and Van Tintelen G. 1988. The phosphorylation state of casein and the species-dependency of its hypercholesterolemic effect. *Br. J. Nutr.* 59: 467–473.

Meghelli-Bouchenak M, Boquillon M and Belleville J. 1987. Time course of changes in rat serum apolipoproteins during the consumption of different low protein diets followed by a balanced diet. *J. Nutr.* 117: 641–649.

Meghelli-Bouchenak M, Belleville J and Boquillon M. 1989a. Hepatic steatosis and serum very low-density lipoproteins during two types of low protein diets followed by a balanced diet. *Nutrition* 5: 321–329.

Meghelli-Bouchenak M, Boquillon M and Belleville J. 1989b. Serum lipoproteins composition and amount during the consumption of two different low protein diets followed by a balanced diet. *Nutr. Rep. Int.* 39: 323–343.

Meghelli-Bouchenak M, Belleville J, Boquillon M and Prost J. 1991a. Metabolism of serum VLDL-, LDL-, and HDL-apoproteins in rats on two different low protein diets. *Nutr. Res.* 11: 575–586.

Meghelli-Bouchenak M, Belleville J, Boquillon M, Scherrer B and Prost J. 1991b. Removal rates of rat serum (^{3}H) labeled very low-density lipoproteins after consumption of two different low-protein diets. *Nutr. Res.* 11: 587–597.

Mehta JL, Bryant JL and Mehta P. 1995. Reduction of nitric oxide synthase activity in human neutrophils by oxidized low-density-lipoproteins. Reversal of the effect of oxidized low-density-lipoproteins by high-density-lipoproteins and L-arginine. *Biochem. Pharmacol.* 50: 1181–1185.

Meinertz H, Nilausen H and Faergeman O. 1984. Effects of dietary soy protein and casein on plasma lipoproteins in normo-lipidemic subjects. *Circulation* 70 (Suppl. 2): 290, Abstract 1161.

Meinertz H, Faergeman O, Nilausen K, Chapman MJ, Goldstein S and Laplaud PM. 1988. Effects of soy protein and casein in low cholesterol diets on plasma lipoproteins in normolipidemic subjects. *Atherosclerosis* 72: 63–70.

Meinertz H, Nilausen K and Faergeman O. 1989. Soy protein and casein in cholesterol-enriched diets: Effects on plasma lipoproteins in normolipidemic subjects. *Am. J. Clin. Nutr.* 50: 786–793.

Meinertz H, Nilausen K and Faergeman O. 1990. Effects of dietary proteins on plasma lipoprotein levels in normal subjects: Interaction with dietary cholesterol. *J. Nutr. Sci. Vitaminol.* 36 (Suppl.): 157S–164S.

Meleady R and Graham I. 1999. Plasma homocysteine as a cardiovascular risk factor: Causal, consequential, or no consequence? *Nutr. Rev.* 57: 299–305.

Mendel CM, Cavlieri RR and Körhle J. 1992. Thyroxine (T4) transport and distribution in rats treated with EMD 21388, a synthetic flavonoid that displaces T4 from transthyretin. *Endocrinology* 130: 1525–1532.

Mendez J. 1964. Effect of dietary protein level and cholesterol supplementation prior to acute starvation on serum and liver lipids in the rat. *Metabolism* 13: 669–674.

Mendiola HG, Hubbard RW, Shavlik GW and Sanchez A. 1987. Fasting plasma amino acids in relation to serum lipids in human male subjects. *Nutr. Rep. Int.* 35: 1301–1312.

Meng QH, Höckerstedt A, Heinonen S, Wähälä K, Adlercreutz H and Tikkanen MJ. 1999. Antioxidant protection of lipoproteins containing estrogens: *In vivo* evidence for low and high-density lipoproteins as estrogen carriers. *Biochim. Biophys. Acta.* 1439: 331–340.

Mengheri E, Scarino ML, Vignolini F and Spadoni MA. 1982. Effect of a hot ethanol extracted faba bean protein concentrate on rat serum cholesterol distribution. *Nutr. Rep. Int.* 26: 751–758.

Mercer NJH. 1985. Cholesterol-enriched semipurified diets containing two levels of either casein or soy protein: Effect on plasma total cholesterol and lipoprotein-cholesterol in *Mongolian* gerbils. *Fed. Proc.* 44: 1497, Abstract 6356.

Mercer NJH, Carroll KK, Wolfe BM and Giovannetti PM. 1982. Plasma cholesterol, triglyceride and lipoprotein levels in healthy adult volunteers when dietary milk protein was replaced by soy protein. *Fed. Proc.* 41: 531.

Mercer NJH, Carroll KK, Giovanetti PM, Steinke FH and Wolfe BM. 1987. Effects on human plasma lipids of substituting soybean protein isolate for milk protein in the diet. *Nutr. Rep. Int.* 35: 279–287.

Meredith L, Liebman M and Graves K. 1989. Alterations in plasma lipid levels resulting from tofu and cheese consumption in adult women. *J. Am. Coll. Nutr.* 8: 573–579.

Merz-Demlow BE, Duncan AM, Xu X, Phipps WR and Kurzer MS. 1998. Effects of soy isoflavones on plasma lipoprotein concentrations over the menstrual cycle. *F.A.S.E.B. J.* 12: A237, Abstract 1385.

Merz-Demlow BE, Duncan AM, Wangen KE, Xu X, Carr TP, Phipps W and Kurzer MS. 2000. Soy isoflavones improve plasma lipids in normocholesterolemic premenopausal women. *Am. J. Clin. Nutr.* 71: 1462–1469.

Mhrova O, Hladover J and Urbanova D. 1988. Metabolic changes in the arterial wall and endothelial injury in experimental methioninemia. *Cor Vasa* 30: 73–79.

Middleton CC, Clarkson TB, Lofland HB and Prichard RW. 1967. Diet and atherosclerosis of *Squirrel* monkeys. *Arch. Pathol.* 83: 145–153.

Miettinen TA, Gylling H and Vanhanen H. 1988. Serum cholesterol response to dietary cholesterol and apoprotein E phenotype. *Lancet* 26: 1261 (Letter).

Miettinen TA, Gylling H and Vanhanen H and Hollus A. 1992. Cholesterol absorption, elimination and synthesis related to LDL kinetics during varying fat intake in men with different apo E phenotypes. *Arterioscler. Thromb. Vasc. Biol.* 12: 1044–1052.

Migliore-Samour D, Floc'h F, Jollès P. 1989. Biological active casein peptides implicated in immunomodulation. *J. Dairy Res.* 56: 357–362.

Miksicek RJ. 1995. Estrogenic flavonoids: Structural requirements for biological activities. *Proc. Soc. Exp. Biol. Med.* 208: 44–50.

Miller GJ and Miller NE. 1975. Plasma-high-density lipoprotein concentration and development of ischaemic heart-disease. *Lancet* 1: 16–19.

Miller M. 1999. The epidemiology of triglyceride as a coronary artery disease risk factor. *Clin. Cardiol.* 22 (Suppl. 2): II-1–II-6.

Milner JA. 1979. Mechanism for fatty liver induction in rats fed arginine-deficient diets. *J. Nutr.* 109: 663–670.

Milner JA and Perkins EG. 1978. Liver lipid alterations in rats fed arginine deficient diets. *Lipids* 13: 563–565.

Milner RDG. 1970. The stimulation of insulin release by essential amino acids from rabbit pancreas *in vitro. J. Endocrinol.* 47: 347–352.

Minami K. 1955. The effect of glycine and taurine to the calcium metabolism. *Biochem.* 27: 269–273.

Mitchell JH, Gardner PT and Duthie GG. 1997. Potential antioxidant activity of phytoestrogens. Symposium on Phytoestrogen Research Methods: Chemistry, Analysis, and Biological Properties, Tucson, AZ, Sept. 21–24, 1997, Abstract.

Miyata S, Matsushima O and Hatton GI. 1997. Taurine in rat posterior pituitary: Localization in astrocytes and selective release by hypoosmotic stimulation. *J. Comp. Neurol.* 381: 513–523.

Mizuno T, Abe H, Hirano R and Yamada K. 1988. Effect of supplementation of sulfur-containing amino acids to a low-soy protein diet containing cholesterol on plasma cholesterol level in rats. *J. Jap. Soc. Nutr. Food Sci.* 41: 441–448.

Mizushima S, Nara Y, Sawamura M and Yamori Y. 1996. Effects of oral taurine supplementation on lipids and sympathetic nerve tone. *Adv. Exp. Med. Biol.* 403: 615–622.

Mochizuki H, Oda H and Yokogoshi H. 1998a. Amplified effect of taurine on PCB-induced hypercholesterolemia in rats. International Taurine Symposium 1997, Tucson, AZ, Abstract, p. 28.

Mochizuki H, Oda H and Yokogoshi H. 1998b. Increasing effect of dietary taurine on the serum HDL-cholesterol concentration in rats. *Biosci. Biotechnol. Biochem.* 62: 758–579.

Mochizuki H, Takido J and Yokogoshi H. 1999a. Effect of dietary taurine on endogenous hypocholesterolemia in rats fed on phenobarbital-containing diets. *Biosci. Biotechnol. Biochem.* 63: 1298–1300.

Mochizuki H, Takido J, Oda H and Yokogoshi H. 1999b. Improving effect of dietary taurine on marked hypercholesterolemia induced by a high-cholesterol diet in streptozotocin-induced diabetic rats. *Biosci. Biotechnol. Biochem.* 63: 1984–1987.

Mochizuki H, Oda H and Yokogoshi H. 2001. Dietary taurine potentiates polychlorinated biphenyl-induced hypercholesterolemia in rats. *J. Nutr. Biochem.* 12: 109–115.

Mokady S and Einav. 1978. Effects of dietary wheat gluten on lipid metabolism in growing rats. *Ann. Nutr. Metab.* 22: 181–189.

Mokady S and Liener IE. 1982. Effect of plant proteins on cholesterol metabolism in growing rats fed atherogenic diets. *Ann. Nutr. Metab.* 26: 138–144.

Mokady S, Cogan U and Aviram M. 1990. Dietary tryptophan enhances platelet aggregation in rats. *J. Nutr. Sci. Vitaminol.* 36 (Suppl.): 177S–180S.

Mol MAE, de Smet R and Terpstra AHM. 1982. Effect of dietary protein and cholesterol on cholesterol concentration and lipoprotein pattern in the serum of chickens. *J. Nutr.* 112: 1029–1037.

Moncada S, Palmer RMJ and Higgs EA. 1991. Nitric oxide: Physiology, pathophysiology, and pharmacology. *Pharmacol. Res.* 43: 109–142.

Moore MC, Guzman MA, Schilling PE and Strong JP. 1981. Dietary atherosclerosis study on deceased persons. *J. Am. Diet. Assoc.* 79: 668–672.

Morand C, Rios L, Moundras C, Besson C, Remesy C and Demigne C. 1997. Influence of methionine availability on glutathione synthesis and delivery by the liver. *J. Nutr. Biochem.* 8: 246–255.

Morgan B, Heald M, Brooks SG, Tee JL and Green J. 1972. The interaction between dietary saponin, cholesterol and related sterols in the chick. *Poultry Sci.* 51: 677–682.

Mori A and Takeuchi Y. 1955. On the absorption of Ca to the intestinal tract. *Biochemistry* 26: 652–655.

Mori N and Hirayama K. 2000. Long-term consumption of a methionine-supplemented diet increases iron and lipid peroxide levels in rat liver. *J. Nutr.* 130: 2349–2355.

Moriguchi S, Toba M and Kishino Y. 1985. The effects of soybean protein on cell-mediated immunity in rats. *Nutr. Sci. Soy Protein Jpn.* 6: 38–44.

Morita I, Takahashi R, Ebisawa H, Fujita Y and Murota S. 1985. Effect of dietary protein level on platelet aggregation in rat. *Prostaglandins Leukot. Med.* 18: 143–149.

Morita T, Oh-hashi A, Takei K, Ikai M, Kasaoka S and Kiriyama S. 1997. Cholesterol-lowering effects of soybean, potato and rice proteins depend on their low methionine contents in rats fed a cholesterol-free purified diet. *J. Nutr.* 127: 470–477.

Morris ER. 1992. Physico-chemical properties of food polysaccharides. In Schweizer TF and Edwards CA, Eds., *Dietary Fibre — A Component of Food: Nutritional Function in Health and Disease*, Springer-Verlag, London, pp. 41–56.

Morris RJ and Hussey EW. 1965. A natural glycoside of medicagenic acid. An alfalfa blossom saponin. *J. Org. Chem.* 30: 166–170.

Morse EH, Merrow SB, Parker MA, Lewis EP and Newhall CA. 1966. Lipid metabolism and the sulfur-containing amino acids. *J. Am. Diet. Assoc.* 48: 496–500.

Mortensen PB. 1984. Dicarboxyllic acids and the lipid metabolism. *Danish Med. Bull.* 31: 121–145.

Morton MS, Wilcox G, Wahlquist ML and Griffiths K. 1994. Determination of lignans and isoflavonoids in female plasma following dietary supplementation. *J. Endocrinol.* 142: 251–259.

Moundras C, Rémésy C, Levrat MA and Demigné C. 1995. Methionine deficiency in rats fed soy protein induces hypercholesterolemia and potentiates lipoprotein susceptibility to peroxidation. *Metabolism* 44: 1146–1152.

Moundras C, Demigné C, Morand C, Levrat MA and Rémésy C. 1997. Lipid metabolism and lipoprotein susceptibility to peroxidation are affected by a protein-deficient diet in the rat. *Nutr. Res.* 17: 125–135.

Moundras C, Rémésy C, Levrat MA, Behr SR and Demigné C. 1998. Interaction between soy protein and soy fiber on lipid metabolism in the rat. *Am. J. Clin. Nutr.* 68 (Suppl.): 1521S.

Moyer AW, Kritchevsky D, Logan JB and Cox HR. 1956. Dietary protein and serum cholesterol in rats. *Proc. Soc. Exp. Biol. Med.* 92: 736–737.

Mozaffari MS, Azuma J, Patel C and Schaffer SW. 1997. Renal excretory response to saline load in the taurine-depleted and taurine-supplemented rat. *Biochim. Pharmacol.* 54: 619–624.

Mügge A and Harrison DG. 1991. L-arginine does not restore endothelial dysfunction in atherosclerotic rabbit aorta *in vitro*. *Blood Vessels* 28: 354–357.

Mullaly MM, Meisel H and Fitzgerald RJ. 1996. Synthetic peptides corresponding to α-lactalbumin and β-lactoglobulin sequences with angiotensin-I converting enzyme inhibitory activity. *Biol. Chem. Hoppe-Seyler* 377: 259–260.

Mullaly MM, Meisel H and Fitzgerald RJ. 1997. Identification of a novel angiotensin-I-converting enzyme inhibitory peptide corresponding to a tryptic fragment of bovine β-lactoglobulin. *F.E.B.S. Lett.* 402: 99–101.

Munro HN, Steele MH and Forbes W. 1965. Effect of dietary protein level on deposition of cholesterol in the tissues of the cholesterol-fed rabbit. *Br. J. Exp. Pathol.* 49: 489–496.

Murakami S, Yamagishi I, Asami Y, Ohta Y, Toda Y, Nara Y and Yamori Y. 1996a. Hypolipidemic effect of taurine in *Stroke-Prone Spontaneously Hypertensive* rats. *Pharmacology* 52: 303–313.

Murakami S, Nara Y and Yamori Y. 1996b. Taurine accelerates the regression of hypercholesterolemia in *Stroke-Prone Spontaneously Hypertensive* rats. *Life Sci.* 58: 1643–1651.

Murakami S, Kondo-Ohtay and Tomisawa K. 1999. Improvement in cholesterol metabolism in mice given chronic treatment of taurine and fed high-fat diet. *Life Sci.* 64: 83–91.

Muramatsu K, Sugiyama K and Ohishi A. 1987. Effect of plant and animal proteins supplemented with methionine on plasma cholesterol level in rats. *Nutr. Sci. Soy Protein Jpn.* 8: 98–103.

Muramatsu K and Sugiyama K. 1990. Relationship between amino acid composition of dietary protein and plasma cholesterol level in rats. In Beynen AC, Kritchevsky D and Pollak OJ, Eds., *Dietary Proteins, Cholesterol Metabolism and Atherosclerosis*, Monographs on Atherosclerosis, Vol. 16, S. Karger, Basel, pp. 97–109.

Murawski U and Egge H. 1978. Longevity study of age changes in serum lipid in rats. *Interdisciplinary Top. Gerontol.* 13: 75–80.

Murphy-Chutorian DR, Wexman MP, Grieco AJ, Heininger JA, Glassman E, Gaull GE, Steven KC, Feit F, Wexman K and Fox AC. 1985. Methionine intolerance: A possible risk factor for coronary heart disease. *J. Am. Coll. Cardiol.* 6: 725–730.

Murthy L, Finelli VN, Garside PS and Petering HG. 1982. Relationship of sufficient and abundant level of minerals to lipid and lipoprotein metabolism in male rats. *Nutr. Res.* 2: 699–714.

Muscari A, Bozzoli C, Gerratana C, Zaca' F, Rovinetti C, Zauli DA, La Placa M and Puddu P. 1988. Association of serum IgA and C4 with severe atherosclerosis. *Atherosclerosis* 74: 179–186.

Muscari A, Volta U, Bonazzi C, Puddu GM, Bozzoli C, Gerratana C, Bianchi FB and Puddu P. 1989. Association of serum IgA antibodies to milk antigens with severe atherosclerosis. *Atherosclerosis* 77: 251–256.

Muscari A, Puddu GM, Pozzoli C, Volta V, Sangiorgi Z, Bianchi FB, Descovich GC and Puddu P. 1992. Serum IgA antibodies to apoproteins and milk-proteins in severe atherosclerosis. *Ann. Ital. Med. Int.* 7: 7–12.

Mustafa A, Hamsten A, Holm G and Lefvert AK. 2001. Circulating immune complexes induced by food proteins implicated in precocious myocardial infarction. *Ann. Med.* 33: 103–112.

Myant NB. 1981. The plasma cholesterol: Composition and metabolism. In Myant NB, Ed., *The Biology of Cholesterol and Related Steroids*, Heinemann Medical Books, London, pp. 507–510.

Myant NB and Mitropoulos KA. 1977. Cholesterol 7 α-hydroxylase (review). *J. Lipid Res.* 18: 135–153.

Nagaoka S, Aoyama Y and Yoshida A. 1985. Effect of tyrosine and some other amino acids on serum level of cholesterol in rats. *Nutr. Rep. Int.* 31: 1137–1148.

Nagaoka S, Miyazaki H, Oda H, Aoyama Y and Yoshida A. 1990. Effect of excess dietary tyrosine on cholesterol, bile acid metabolism and mixed-function oxidase system in rats. *J. Nutr.* 1134–1190.

Nagaoka S, Kanamura Y and Kuzuya Y. 1991. Effects of whey protein and casein on the plasma and liver lipids in rats. *Agric. Biol. Chem.* 55: 813–818.

Nagaoka S, Kanamaru Y, Kuzuya Y, Kojima T and Kuwata T. 1992. Comparative studies on the serum cholesterol lowering action of whey protein and soybean protein in rats. *Biosci. Biotechnol. Biochem.* 56: 1484–1485.

Nagaoka S, Awano R, Nagata N, Masaoka M, Hori G and Hashimoto K. 1997. Serum cholesterol reduction and cholesterol absorption inhibition in Caco-2 cells by a soyprotein peptic hydrolysate. *Biosci. Biotechnol. Biochem.* 61: 354–356.

Nagata C, Takatsuka N, Kurisu Y and Shimizu H. 1998. Decreased serum cholesterol concentration is associated with high intake of soy products in Japanese man and women. *J. Nutr.* 128: 209–213.

Nagata Y, Imaizumi K and Sugano M. 1980. Effects of soya-bean protein and casein on serum cholesterol levels in rats. *Br. J. Nutr.* 44: 113–121.

Nagata Y, Tanaka K and Sugano M. 1981a. Further studies on the hypocholesterolaemic effect of soya-bean protein in rats. *Br. J. Nutr.* 45: 233–241.

Nagata Y, Tanaka K and Sugano M. 1981b. Serum and liver cholesterol levels of rats and mice fed soya-bean protein or casein. *J. Nutr. Sci. Vitaminol.* 27: 583–593.

Nagata Y, Ishiwaki N and Sugano M. 1982. Studies on the mechanism of antihypercholesterolemic action of soy protein and soy protein-type amino acid mixtures in relation to the casein counterparts in rats. *J. Nutr.* 112: 1614–1625.

Naim M, Gestetner B, Kirson I, Birk Y and Bandi A. 1973. A new isoflavone from soybeans. *Phytochemistry* 22: 237–239.

Nakaki T, Hishikawa K, Suzuki H, Saruta T and Kato R. 1990. L-arginine-induced hypotension. *Lancet* 336: 696 (Letter).

Nakaki T and Kato R. 1994. Beneficial circulatory effect of L-arginine. *Jpn. J. Pharmacol.* 66: 167–171.

Nakamura Y, Yamamoto N, Sakai K, Okubo A, Yamazaki S and Takano T. 1995a. Purification and characterization of angiotensine I-converting enzyme inhibitors from sour milk. *J. Dairy Sci.* 78: 777–783.

Nakamura Y, Yamamoto N, Sakai K, and Takano T. 1995b. Antihypertensive effect of sour milk and peptides isolated from it that are inhibitors to angiotensine I-converting enzyme. *J. Dairy Sci.* 78: 1253–1257.

Nakashima S, Koike T and Nozawa Y. 1991. Genistein, a protein tyrosine kinase inhibitor, inhibits thromboxane A_2-mediated human platelet responses. *Mol. Pharmacol.* 39: 475–480.

Nanami K, Oda H and Yokogoshi H. 1996. Antihypercholesterolemic action of taurine on streptozotocin-diabetic rats or on rats fed a high cholesterol diet. *Adv. Exp. Med. Biol.* 403: 561–568.

Nara Y, Yamori Y and Lowenberg W. 1978. Effect of dietary taurine on blood pressure in spontaneously hypertensive rats. *Biochem. Pharmacol.* 27: 2689–2692.

Narce M, Poisson JP, Belleville J and Chanussot B. 1992. Depletion of Δ9 desaturase (EC 1. 14. 99. 5) enzyme activity in growing rat during dietary protein restriction. *Br. J. Nutr.* 68: 627–637.

Nath NJ, Harper AE and Elvehjem CA. 1959. Diet and cholesterolemia. III. Effect of dietary proteins with particular reference to the lipids in wheat gluten. *Can. J. Biochem. Physiol.* 37: 1375–1384.

Nath NJ, Seidel JC and Harper AE. 1961. Diet and cholesterolemia. VI. Comparative effects of wheat gluten lipids and some other lipids in presence of adequate and inadequate dietary protein. *J. Nutr.* 74: 389–396.

Neprokoeff CM, Lakshmanan MR, Ness GC, Dugan RE, Porter JW. 1974. Regulation of the diurnal rhythm of rat liver beta-hydroxy-beta-methylglutaryl coenzyme A reductase activity by insulin, glucagon, cyclic AMP and hydrocortisone. *Arch. Biochem. Biophys.* 160: 387–396.

Nestel PJ. 1985. Dietary factors affecting lipoprotein metabolism. *Adv. Exp. Med. Biol.* 183: 253–263.

Nestel PJ, Yamashita T, Sasahara T, Pomeroy S, Dart A, Lomesaroff P, Owen A and Abbey M. 1997. Soy isoflavones improves systemic arterial compliance but not plasma lipids in menopausal and perimenopausal women. *Arterioscler. Thromb. Vasc. Biol.* 17: 3392–3398.

Nestel PJ, Pomeroy S, Kay S, Komesaroff P, Behrsing J, Cameron JD and West L. 1999. Isoflavones from red clover improve systemic arterial compliance but not plasma lipids in menopausal women. *J. Clin. Endocrinol. Metab.* 84: 895–898.

Nevala R, Vaskonen T, Vehniäinen J, Korpela R and Vapaatalo H. 2000. Soy based diet attenuates the development of hypertension when compared to casein based diet in spontaneously hypertensive rat. *Life Sci.* 66: 115–124.

Neves LB, Clifford CK, Kohler G, de Fremery D, Knuckles BE, Cheowtirakul C, Miller MW, Weir MC, and Clifford AJ. 1980. Effect of dietary protein from variety of sources on plasma lipids and lipoproteins of rats. *J. Nutr.* 110: 732–742.

Newburgh LH. 1919. The production of Bright's disease by feeding high protein diets. *Arch. Intern. Med.* 24: 359–377.

Newburgh LH and Squier TL. 1920. High protein diets and arteriosclerosis in rabbits by diets containing meat. *Arch. Intern. Med.* 26: 38–40.

Newburgh LH and Clarkson S. 1922. Production of arteriosclerosis in rabbits by diets rich in animal protein. *J.A.M.A.* 79: 1106–1108.

Newburgh LH and Clarkson S. 1923a. High protein diets and arteriosclerosis in rabbits. *Arch. Intern. Med.* 26: 38–40.

Newburgh LH and Clarkson S. 1923b. The production of arteriosclerosis in rabbits by feeding diets rich in meat. *Arch. Intern. Med.* 26: 653–676.

Newman HAI, Kummerow FA and Scott HM. 1958. Dietary saponins, a factor which may reduce liver and serum cholesterol levels. *Poultry Sci.* 37: 42–45.

Ni W, Tsuda Y, Sakono M and Imaizumi K. 1998. Dietary soy protein isolate, compared with casein, reduces atherosclerotic lesion area in apolipoprotein E-deficient mice. *J. Nutr.* 128: 1884–1889.

Nicolosi RJ. 1997. Dietary fat saturation effects of low-density-lipoprotein concentrations in various animal models. *Am. J. Clin. Nutr.* 65 (Suppl.): 1617S–1627S.

Nicolosi RJ and Wilson TA. 1997. The anti-atherogenic effect of dietary soybean protein concentrate in hamsters. *Nutr. Res.* 17: 1457–1467.

Nigro G, Comi LL, Coiudice A and Petretta V. 1971. La taurina mel trattamento della cardiopatic ischemiche e delle distrofie muscolari progressive. *Clin. Ther.* 56: 347–359.

Nikitin YP. 1962. Influence of vitamin E on lipids and blood coagulability in patients with atherosclerosis.

Nikkilä EA and Ollilla O. 1957. Effect of low protein diet on the serum lipids and atherosclerosis of cholesterol-fed chickens. *Acta Pathol. Microbiol. Scand.* 40: 177–180.

Nilausen K and Meinertz H. 1996. Variation in the plasma lipoprotein response to dietary soy protein in normolipemic men. Second International Symposium on the Role of Soy in Preventing and Treating Chronic Disease, Brussels, Sept. 15–18, 1996, Abstract, p. 23.

Nilausen K and Meinertz H. 1998. Variable lipemic response to dietary soy protein in healthy normolipemic men. *Am. J. Clin. Nutr.* 68, (Suppl.): 1380S–1384S.

Nilausen K and Meinertz H. 1999. Lipoprotein(a) and dietary proteins: Casein lowers lipoprotein(a) concentrations as compared with soy protein. *Am. J. Clin. Nutr.* 69: 419–425.

Nishida T, Takenaka F and Kummerow FA. 1958. Effect of dietary protein and heated fat on serum cholesterol and beta-lipoprotein levels, and on the incidence of experimental atherosclerosis in chicks. *Circ. Res.* 6: 194–202.

Nishida T, Ueno K and Kummerow FA. 1960. Effect of dietary protein on the metabolism of sodium acetate-1-C^{14} in chicks. *J. Nutr.* 71: 379–386.

Nishimoto K, Asako K, Iwahara M, Ino T and Ohtsuka C. 1983. The effects of taurine on hemodynamics in congenital heart disease, especially its effects on the left to right shunt. *Sulfur-Containing Amino Acids* 6: 213–219.

Nishizawa N, Oikawa M, Nakamura N and Hareyama S. 1989. Effect of lysine and threonine supplement on biological value of proso millet protein. *Nutr. Rep. Int.* 40: 239–245.

Nishizawa N and Fudamoto Y. 1995. The elevation of plasma concentration of high-density lipoprotein cholesterol in mice fed with protein from proso millet. *Biosci. Biotechnol. Biochem.* 59: 333–335.

Nishizawa N, Shimanuki S, Fujihashi H, Watanabe H, Fudamoto Y and Nagasawa T. 1996. Proso millet protein elevates plasma levels of high-density lipoprotein: A new food function of proso millet. *Biomed. Environ Sci.* 9: 209–212.

Noda K. 1970. Influence of insulin, hydrocortisone and thyroxine on fatty liver of rats fed a low-casein diet supplemented with methionine. *J. Nutr.* 101: 1390–1397.

Noda K. 1971. Effect of food intake on the liver lipid content of rats fed a low-casein diet with or without methionine supply. *Eiyo to Shokuryo* 24: 89–91.

Noda K. 1973. Effect of glutathione on lipogenesis in liver slices from rats fed a low-casein diet. *Agric. Biol. Chem.* 37: 843–848.

Noda K and Okita T. 1980. Fatty liver due to disproportionally added methionine to a low soybean diet and lipotropic action of phosphatides in rats. *J. Nutr.* 110: 505–512.

Nogowski L, Mackowiak P, Kandulska K, Szudelski T and Nowak KW. 1998. Genistein-induced changes in lipid metabolism of ovariectomized rat. *Ann. Nutr. Metab.* 42: 360–366.

Noguchi A, Takita T, Suzuki K, Nakamura K and Innami S. 1992. Effects of casein and soy-protein on α-linolenic acid metabolism in rats. *J. Nutr. Sci. Vitaminol.* 38: 579–591.

Norrell SE, Ahlbom A and Feychting M. 1986. Fish consumption and mortality from coronary heart disease. *B.M.J.* 293: 426.

Norton SA, Beames CG, Maxwell CV and Morgan GL. 1987. Effect of dietary whey upon the serum cholesterol of the pig. *Nutr. Rep. Int.* 36: 273–279.

Norum KR, Berg T, Helgerud P, and Drevon CA. 1983. Transport of cholesterol. *Physiol. Rev.* 63: 1343–1362.

Noseda G and Fragiacomo C. 1980. Effects of soybean protein diet on serum lipids, plasma glucagon, and insulin. In Noseda G, Lewis B and Paoletti R, Eds., *Diet and Drugs in Atherosclerosis*. Raven Press, New York, pp. 61–65.

Noseda G, Sirtori CR and Descovich GC. 1987. Cholesterol-lowering and high-density lipo-protein-raising properties of lecithinated soy proteins in type II hyperlipidemic patients In Schlierf G and Mörl H, Eds., *Expanding Horizons in Atherosclerosis Research*, Springer-Verlag, Berlin, pp. 317–320.

Novak M, Monkus EF, Buch M and Hahn P. 1979. Acetylcarnitine and free carnitine in body fluids before and after birth. *Pediatr. Res.* 13: 10–15.

Novak M, Monkus EF, Buch M, Lesme H and Silverio J. 1983. Effect of L-carnitine supple-mented soybean formula on plasma lipids of infants. *Acta Chir. Scand.* 517 (Suppl.): 149–155.

Novotny MJ, Hogan PM, Paley DM and Adams HR. 1991. Systolic and diastolic dysfunction of the left ventricle induced by dietary taurine deficiency in cats. *Am. J. Physiol.* 261: H121–H127.

Nuttall FQ, Gannon MC, Wald JL and Ahmed M. 1985. Plasma glucose and insulin profiles in normal subjects ingesting diets of varying carbohydrate, fat, and protein content. *J. Am. Coll. Nutr.* 4: 437–450.

Nuzum FR, Seegel B, Garland R and Osborne M. 1926. Arteriosclerosis and increased blood pressure. Experimental production. *Arch. Intern. Med.* 37: 733–744.

Nygärd O, Vollset SE, Refsum H, Stensvold I, Tverdal A, Nordrehaug JE, Ueland PM and Kvale G. 1995. Total plasma homocysteine and cardiovascular risk profile. The Hordaland Homocysteine Study. *J.A.M.A.* 274: 1526–1533.

Nygärd O, Nordrehaus JE, Refsum H, Farstad M, Ueland PM and Vollset PE. 1997. Plasma homocysteine levels and mortality in patients with coronary artery disease. *N. Engl. J. Med.* 337: 230–236.

Nygärd O, Vollset SE, Refsum H, Brattström L and Ueland PM. 1999. Total homocysteine and cardiovascular disease. *J. Intern. Med.* 246: 425–454.

Oakenfull DG. 1981. Saponins in food — a review. *Food Chem.* 7: 19–40.

Oakenfull DG, Fenwick DE, Hood RL, Topping DL, Illman RL and Storer GB. 1979. Effects of saponins on bile acids and plasma lipids in the rat. *Br. J. Nutr.* 42: 209–216.

Oakenfull DG and Topping DL. 1983. Saponins and plasma cholesterol. *Atherosclerosis* 48: 301–303.

Obarzaneck E, Velletri PA and Cutler JA. 1996. Dietary protein and blood pressure. *J.A.M.A.* 275: 1598–1603.

Obinata K, Maruyama T, Hayashi M, Watanabe T and Nittono H. 1996. Effect of taurine on the fatty liver of children with simple obesity. *Adv. Exp. Med. Biol.* 403: 607–613.

Oda H, Matsuoka S and Yoshida A. 1986. Effects of dietary methionine, cystine and potassium sulfate on serum cholesterol and urinary ascorbic acid in rats fed PCB. *J. Nutr.* 116: 1660–1666.

Oda H, Okumura Y, Hitomi Y, Ozaki K, Nagaoka S and Yoshida A. 1989. Effect of dietary methionine and polychlorinated biphenyls on cholesterol metabolism in rats fed a diet containing soy protein isolate. *J. Nutr. Sci. Vitaminol.* 35: 333–348.

Oda H, Fukui H, Hitomi Y and Yoshida A. 1991. Alteration of serum lipoprotein metabolism by polychlorinated biphenyls and methionine in rats fed a soybean protein diet. *J. Nutr.* 121: 925–933.

O'Dell BL. 1979. Effect of soy protein ion trace mineral availability. In Wilcke HL, Hopkins DT and Waggle DH, Eds., *Soy Protein and Human Nutrition*, Academic Press, New York, pp. 187–204.

Ogawa H. 1996. Effect of dietary taurine on lipid metabolism in normocholesterolemic and hypercholesterolemic *Stroke-Prone Spontaneously Hypertensive* rats. *Adv. Exp. Med. Biol.* 403: 107–115.

Ogawa H, Nishikawa T, Fukushima S and Sasagawa S. 1988. Studies on *Stroke-Prone Spontaneously Hypertensive rats (SHRSP.* fed a high-fat and high-cholesterol diet: Effects of taurine on serum lipoprotein metabolism in hypercholesterolemic rats. *Nippon Eiseigaku Zasshi Jpn.* 14: 648–658.

Ogawa H, Nishikawa T and Sasagawa S. 1991. Effect of cholesterol feeding on the compositions of plasma lipoproteins and plasma lipolytic activities in *SHRSP. Clin. Exp. Hypertens.* 13: 999–1008.

Ogawa T, Gatchalian-Yee M, Sugano M, Kimoto M, Matsuo T and Hashimoto Y. 1992. Hypocholesterolemic effect of undigested fraction of soybean protein in rats fed no cholesterol. *Biosci. Biotechnol. Biochem.* 56: 1845–1848.

Ohmura E, Aoyama Y and Yoshida A. 1986. Changes in lipids in liver and serum of rats fed a histidine-excess diet or cholesterol supplemented diets. *Lipids* 21: 748–753.

Okamoto E, Rassin DK, Zucker CL, Salen GS and Heird WC. 1984. Role of taurine in feeding the low-birth-weight infant. *J. Pediatr.* 104: 936–940.

Okamoto K. 1969. Spontaneous hypertension in rats. In Richter GW and Epstein MA, Eds., *International Review of Experimental Pathology*, Vol. 7, Academic Press, New York, pp. 227–270.

Okamoto K and Aoki K. 1963. Development of a strain of *Spontaneously Hypertensive* rats. *Jpn. Circ. J.* 27: 282–293.

Okamoto K, Yamori Y and Nagaoka K. 1974. Establishment of a strain of *Stroke-Prone SHR* rats. *Circ. Res.* 33:34 (Suppl. I): 143–153.

Okey R and Lyman MM. 1954. Dietary constituents which may influence the use of food cholesterol. II. protein, L-cystine and DL methionine intake in adolescent rats. *J. Nutr.* 53: 601–611.

Okey R and Lyman MM. 1956. Protein intake and liver cholesterol. Effects of age and growth of the test animals. *J. Nutr.* 58: 471–482.

Okey R and Lyman MM. 1957. Age differences in the effects of L-cystine and DL-methionine on liver cholesterol storage in the rats. *J. Nutr.* 61: 103–112.

Okita T and Sugano M. 1989. Effects of the type and level of dietary proteins on plasma lipids, fatty acids profile, and fecal steroid excretion in rats. *Agric. Biol. Chem.* 53: 659–666.

Okita T and Sugano M. 1990. Effects of dietary protein levels and cholesterol on tissue lipids of rats. *J. Nutr. Sci. Vitaminol.* 36 (Suppl. 2): 151S–156S.

Okuda T, Miyoshi H, Sasaki K, Satake R, Hiratuka Y and Koishi H. 1987. Effect of soya protein isolate on fecal sterol excretion and plasma cholesterol in young men. *Nutr. Sci. Soy Protein Jpn.* 9: 93–97.

Okuda T, Miyoshi H, Sasaki K, Satake R, Hiratuka Y and Koishi H. 1988. Effect of soya protein isolate on fecal sterol excretion and plasma cholesterol in young men (II). *Nutr. Sci. Soy Protein Jpn.* 9: 97–100.

Okuda T, Miyoshi H, Sasaki K, Satake R, Hiratuka Y and Koishi H. 1989. Effects of soybean on lipid digestibility and fecal excretion of neutral sterols in young men on high-cholesterol diet. *Nutr. Sci. Soy Protein Jpn.* 10: 67–70.

Okura A, Arakawa M, Oka H, Yoshinari T and Monden Y. 1990. Effect of genistein on topoisomerases activity and on the growth of [val12] HA-ras-transformed NI43T3 cells. *Biochem. Biophys. Res. Commn.* 157: 183–189.

Oleesky DA, Penney MDS and Firoozmand S. 1982. Serum L-arginine in hypercholesterolemia. *Lancet* 340: 487.

Olson AL, Rebouche CJ. 1987. Gamma-butyrobetaine hydroxylase activity is not rate limiting for carnitine biosynthesis in the human infant. *J. Nutr.* 117: 1024–1031.

Olson AL, Nelson SE and Rebouche CJ. 1989. Low carnitine intake and altered lipid metabolism in infants. *Am. J. Clin. Nutr.* 49: 624–628.

Olson RE, Vester JW, Gursey D, Davis N and Longman D. 1958a. The effect of low-protein diets upon serum cholesterol in man. *Am. J. Clin. Nutr.* 6: 310–324.

Olson RE, Jablonski JR and Taylor E. 1958b. The effect of dietary protein, fat and choline upon the serum lipids and lipoproteins of the rat. *Am. J. Clin. Nutr.* 6: 111–118.

Olson RE, Nichaman MZ, Nittka J and Dorman L. 1964. Effect of amino acid intake upon serum cholesterol in man. *J. Clin. Invest.* 43: 1233.

Olson RE, Nichaman MZ, Nittka J and Eagles JA. 1970a. Effect of amino acid diets upon serum lipids in man. *Am. J. Clin. Nutr.* 23: 1614–1625.

Olson RE, Bazzano G and d'Elia JA. 1970b. The effects of large amounts of glutamic acid upon serum lipids and sterol metabolism in man. *Trans. Am. Physicians* 83: 196–210.

Ooi TC and Ooi DS. 1998. The atherogenic significance of an elevated plasma triglyceride level. *Crit. Rev. Clin. Lab. Sci.* 35: 489–516.

Oomen CM, van Erk MJ, Feskens EJM, Kok FJ and Kromhout D. 2000a. Arginine intake and risk of coronary heart disease mortality in elderly men. *Arterioscler. Thromb. Vasc. Biol.* 20: 2134–2139.

Oomen CM, Feskens EJM, Räsänen L, Fidanza F, Nissinen AM, Menotti A, Kok FJ and Kromhout D. 2000b. Fish consumption and coronary heart disease mortality in Finland, Italy, and the Netherlands. *Am. J. Epidemiol.* 151: 999–1006.

Oosthuizen W, Vorster HH, Vermaak WJH, Smuts CM, Jerling JC, Veldman FJ and Burger HM. 1998. Lecithin has no effect on serum lipoprotein, plasma fibrinogen and macro molecular protein complex levels in hyperlipidaemic men in a double-blind controlled study. *Eur. J. Clin. Nutr.* 52: 419–424.

Ordovas JM. 1999. The genetics of serum lipid responsiveness to dietary interventions. *Proc. Nutr. Soc.* 58: 171–187.

Ortega MF. 1989. Effects of dietary lysine level and protein restriction on the lipids and carnitine levels in the liver of pregnant rats. *Ann. Nutr. Metab.* 33: 162–169.

Osada K, Kodama T, Minehira K, Yamada K, Sugano M. 1996. Dietary protein modifies oxidized cholesterol-induced alterations of linoleic acid and cholesterol metabolism. *J. Nutr.* 126: 1635–1643.

Oster KA. 1971. Plasmalogens diseases: A new concept of the etiology of the atherosclerotic process. *Am. J. Clin. Res.* 2: 30–35.

Otsuji S, Nakajima O, Waku S, Kojima S, Hosokawa H, Kinoshita I, Okubo T, Tamoto S, Takada K and Ishihara T. 1995. Attenuation of acetylcholine-induced vasoconstriction by L-arginine is related to the progression of atheroclerosis. *Am. Heart J.* 129: 1094–1100.

Ozaki Y, Yatomi Y, Jinnai Y and Kume S. 1993. Effects of genistein, a tyrosine kinase inhibitor, on platelet functions. Genistein attenuates thrombin-induced Ca^{2+} mobilization in human platelets by affecting polyphosphoinositide turnover. *Biochem. Pharmacol.* 46: 395–403.

Pacini N, Ferrari A, Zanchi R, Corti M and Greppi GF. 1989. The effects of protein dietary sources on serum cholesterol and bile acid microbiological transformation in rabbits. *Nutr. Rep. Int.* 39: 851–859.

Paigen B. 1995. Genetics of responsiveness to high-fat and high-cholesterol diets in the mouse. *Am. J. Clin. Nutr.* 62: 458S–462S.

Palmer JP, Walter RM and Ensink JW. 1975. Arginine-stimulated acute phase of insulin and glucagon secretion. I. In normal man. *Diabetes* 24: 735–740.

Palmer RMJ, Ferrige AG and Moncada S. 1987. Nitric oxide release accounts for the biological activity of endothelium-derived relaxing factor. *Nature* 327: 524–526.

Palmer RMJ, Ashton DS and Moncada S. 1988. Vascular endothelial cells synthetize nitric oxide from L-arginine. *Nature* 333: 664–666.

Pan W, Ikeda K, Takebe M and Yamori Y. 2001. Genistein, daidzein and glycitein inhibit growth and DNA synthesis of aortic smooth muscle cells from *Stroke-Prone Spontaneously Hypertensive* rats. *J. Nutr.* 131: 1154–1158.

Panza JA, Casino PR, Badar DM and Quyyumi AA. 1993. Effect of increased bioavailability of endothelium-derived nitric oxide precursor on endothelium-dependent vascular relaxation in normal subjects and in patients with essential hypertension. *Circulation* 87: 1475–1481.

Park CS. 1985. Influence of dietary protein on blood cholesterol and related metabolites of growing calves. *J. Anim. Sci.* 61: 924–930.

Park MSC and Liepa GU. 1982. Effects of dietary protein and amino acids on the metabolism of cholesterol-carrying lipoproteins in rats. *J. Nutr.* 112: 1892–1898.

Park MSC, Kudchodkar BJ and Liepa GU. 1987. Effects of dietary animal and plant proteins in the cholesterol metabolism in immature and mature rats. *J. Nutr.* 117: 30–35.

Park T, Lee K, and Um Y. 1998. Dietary taurine supplementation reduces plasma and liver cholesterol and triglyceride concentrations in rats fed a high-cholesterol diet. *Nutr. Res.* 18: 1559–1571.

Park T, Oh J and Lee K. 1999. Dietary taurine or glycine supplementation reduces plasma and liver cholesterol and triglyceride concentrations in rats fed a cholesterol-free diet. *Nutr. Res.* 19: 1777–1789.

Parker F, Migliore-Samour D, Floc'h F, Zerial A, Werner GH, Jollès J, Casaretto M, Zahn H and Jollès P. 1984. Immunomodulating hexapeptide from human casein: Amino acid sequence, synthesis and biological properties. *Eur. J. Biochem.* 145: 677–682.

Parker NT and Goodrun KJ. 1990. A comparison of casein, lactalbumin, and soy protein effect on the immune response to a T-dependent antigen. *Nutr. Res.* 10: 781–792.

Passananti GT, Guerrant NB and Thompson RQ. 1958. Effects of supplementary methionine and choline on tissue lipids and on the vascular structure of cholesterol-fed growing rats. *J. Nutr.* 66: 55–74.

Patel RP, Crawford JH, Barnes S and Darley-Usmar M. 1997. Dietary protection against heart disease: Does genistein have a role as an antioxidant? Symposium on Phytoestrogen Research Methods: Chemistry, Analysis, and Biological Properties, Tucson, AZ, Sept. 21–24, 1997, Abstract.

Pathirana C, Gibney MJ, Gallagher PJ and Taylor TG. 1979. The effects of antibodies to dietary protein on the development of atherosclerosis in cholesterol-fed rabbits. *Proc. Nutr. Soc.* 38: 26A, Abstract.

Pathirana C, Gibney MJ and Taylor TG. 1980. Effects of soy protein and saponins on serum and liver cholesterol in rats. *Atherosclerosis* 36: 595–596.

Pathirana C, Gibney MJ and Taylor TG. 1981. The effect of dietary protein source and saponins on serum lipids and the excretion of bile acids and neutral sterols in rabbits. *Br. J. Nutr.* 46: 421–430.

Pearson TA, LaCava J and Weil HFC. 1997. Epidemiology of thrombotic-hemostatic factors and their association with cardiovascular disease. *Am. J. Clin. Nutr.* 65 (Suppl.): 1764S–1782S.

Pedrinelli R, Ebel M, Catapano G, Dell'Omo G, Ducci H, Del Chicca M and Clerico A. 1995. Pressor, renal and endocrine effects of L-arginine in essential hypertensives. *Eur. J. Clin. Pharmacol.* 48: 195–201.

Pellum LK and Medeiros DM. 1983. Blood pressure in young adult normotensives: Effect of protein, fat, and cholesterol intakes. *Nutr. Rep. Int.* 27: 1277–1285.

Peluso MR, Winters TA, Shanahan MF and Banz WJ. 2000. Cooperative interaction between soy protein and its isoflavone-enriched fraction lowers hepatic lipids in male obese *Zucker* rats and reduces blood platelet sensitivity in male *Sprague-Dawley* rats. *J. Nutr.* 130: 2333–2342.

Penttinen J, Pennanen S and Liesivuori J. 2000. Indicators of L-arginine metabolism and cardiovascular risk factors. A cross-sectional study in healthy middle-aged men. *Amino Acids* 18: 199–206.

Peret U, Chanez M, Cota J and Macaire I. 1975. Effects of quantity and quality of dietary protein and variation in certain enzyme activities on glucose metabolism in the rat. *J. Nutr.* 105: 1525–1534.

Perry IJ. 1999. Homocysteine, hypertension and stroke. *J. Hum. Hypertens.* 13: 289–293.

Petering HG, Murthy L and O'Flaherty E. 1977. Influence of dietary copper and zinc on rat lipid metabolism. *J. Agric. Food Chem.* 25: 1105–1109.

Petry CJ, Ozanne SE, Wang CL and Hales CN. 1997. Early protein restriction and obesity independently induce hypertension in 1-year-old rats. *Clin. Sci. (Colch.)* 93: 147–152.

Pety MA, Kintz J and DiFracesco GF. 1990. The effects of taurine on atherosclerosis development in cholesterol-fed rabbits. *Eur. J. Pharmacol.* 180: 119–127.

Petzke KJ, Elsner A, Proll J, Thielecke F and Metges CC. 2000. Long-term high protein intake does not increase oxidative stress in rats. *J. Nutr.* 130: 2889–2896.

Pfeuffer M. 1989. Differences in the underlying mechanisms of cholesterol- and casein-induced hypercholesterolemia in rabbit and rat. *Atherosclerosis* 76: 89–91.

Pfeuffer M and Barth CA. 1986a. Modulation of very low-density lipoprotein secretion by dietary protein is age-dependent in rats. *Ann. Nutr. Metab.* 30: 281–288.

Pfeuffer M and Barth CA. 1986b. Rates of VLDL secretion and serum lipids. Interaction of dietary protein and carbohydrates. IX Symposium on Drugs Affecting Lipid Metabolism, Florence, October 22–25, Abstract, p. 164.

Pfeuffer M and Barth C. 1986c. Influence of different dietary proteins on VLDL secretion *in vivo. Kieler Milchwirtsschaftliche Forschungsberichte* 38: 199–204.

Pfeuffer M, Ahrens F, Hagemeister H and Barth CA. 1988a. Influence of casein versus soy protein isolate on lipid metabolism of minipigs. *Ann. Nutr. Metab.* 32: 83–89.

Pfeuffer M, Wuttke W and Barth CA. 1988b. Influence of dietary proteins on plasma growth hormone in rats. *Z. Ernährungswiss.* 27: 229–235.

Pfeuffer M and Barth CA. 1990. Lipid metabolism: Especially referring to the hypercholesterolemic effect of casein. *Bull. Int. Dairy Fed.* 253: 19–33.

Pfeuffer M and Barth CA. 1992. Dietary sucrose but not starch promotes protein-induced differences in rates of VLDL secretion and plasma lipid concentrations in rats. *J. Nutr.* 122: 1582–1586.

Philip B, Nampoothiri VK and Kuruo PA. 1978. Zinc and metabolism of lipids in normal atheromatous rats. *Ind. J. Exp. Biol.* 16: 46–50.

Philis-Tsimikas A and Witzum LJ. 1995. L-arginine may inhibit atherosclerosis through inhibition of LDL-oxidation. *Circulation* 92 (Suppl. 1): 422, Abstract.

Pick R, Stamler J and Katz LN. 1959. Effects of high-protein intakes on cholesterolemia and atherogenesis in growing and mature chickens fed high-fat high-cholesterol diets. *Circ. Res.* 7: 866–869.

Pick R, Savitri J, Katz LN and Johnson P. 1965. Effect of dietary protein level on regression of cholesterol induced hypercholesterolemia and atherosclerosis of cockerels. *J. Atheroscler. Res.* 5: 16–25.

Pilgeram LO and Greenberg DM. 1955. Cholesterol stimulation of phosphatidyl choline formation. *Circ. Res.* 3: 47–50.

Piliang WG, Djojosoebagio S and Suprayogy A. 1996. Soybean hull and its effect on atherosclerosis in non-human-primates (*Macaca fascicularis*). *Biomed. Environ. Sci.* 9: 137–143.

Pion PD, Kittleson MD, Rogers QR and Morris JG. 1987. Myocardial failure in cats associated with low plasma taurine: A reversible cardiomyopathy. *Science* 237: 766–768.

Polcak J, Melichar F, Sevelova D, Dvorak I and Slakova M. 1965. The effect of a meat enriched diet on the development of atherosclerosis in rabbits. *J. Atheroscler. Res.* 5: 174–180.

Polichetti E, Diaconescu N, Lechene de la Porte P, Mali L, Portugal H, Pauli AM, Lafont H, Tuchweber B, Yousef I and Chanussot F. 1996. Cholesterol-lowering effect of soyabean lecithin in normolipidaemic rats by stimulation of biliary lipid secretion. *Br. J. Nutr.* 75: 471–481.

Pond WG, Yen JT, Mersmann HJ and Haschek WM. 1986. Comparative effects of dietary protein and cholesterol-fat content on genetically lean and obese pigs. *J. Nutr.* 116: 1116–1124.

Ponzio de Azevedo AM, Azzolin IR and Perry MLS. 1994. Effect of methionine supplementation to a low-soybean protein diet on liver lipid metabolism. *Ann. Nutr. Metab.* 38: 301–306.

Portman OW. 1956. Effect of diets low in organic sulfur on metabolism of cholesterol-C^{14} in the rat. *Am. J. Physiol.* 186: 403–405.

Portman OW, Alexander M and Neuringer M. 1985. Dietary protein effects on lipoprotein and on sex and thyroid hormones in blood of *Rhesus* monkeys. *J. Nutr.* 115: 425–435.

Potter JD, Topping DL and Oakenful D. 1979. Soya products, saponins, and plasma cholesterol. *Lancet* 1: 233.

Potter JD, Illman RJ, Calvert GD, Oakenfull DG and Topping DL. 1980. Soya saponins, plasma lipids, lipoproteins and fecal bile acids: A double blind cross over study. *Nutr. Rep. Int.* 22: 521–528.

Potter SM. 1995. Overview of proposed mechanisms for the hypocholesterolemic effect of soy. *J. Nutr.* 125 (Suppl. 3): 606S–611S.

Potter SM. 1996. Soy protein and serum lipids. *Curr. Opin. Lipidol.* 7: 260–264.

Potter SM. 1998. Soy protein and cardiovascular disease: The impact of bioactive components in soy. *Nutr. Rev.* 56: 231–235.

Potter SM and Kies C. 1988. Methionine and cystine as factors associated with the hypercholesterolemic effect of soy protein. *F.A.S.E.B. J.* 2: A1213, Abstract 5331.

Potter SM and Kies C. 1989a. Self-selected dietary protein sources and serum lipid patterns of adolescent humans. *Nutr. Rep. Int.* 40: 863–870.

Potter SM and Kies C. 1989b. Serum lipid level as influenced by sulfur-containing amino acids and dietary protein source. *F.A.S.E.B. J.* 3: A955, Abstract 4232.

Potter SM and Kies C. 1990. Influence of sulfur-amino acid content variation in plant vs. animal protein on serum and tissue lipids in rats. *Plant Foods Hum. Nutr.* 40: 297–308.

Potter SM, Picciano MF and Tseng E. 1990. Influence of dietary proteins on plasma lipids of infants. *F.A.S.E.B. J.* 46: A367, Abstract 587.

Potter SM, Bakhit RM, Essex-Sorlie DL, Weingartner KE, Chapman KM, Nelson RA, Prabhudesai M, Savage WD, Nelson AI, Winter LW and Erdman JW Jr. 1993a. Depression of plasma cholesterol in men by consumption of baked products containing soy protein. *Am. J. Clin. Nutr.* 58: 501–506.

Potter SM, Jimenez-Flores R, Pollack J, Lone TA and Berber-Jimenez MD. 1993b. Protein-saponin interaction and its influence on blood lipids. *J. Agric. Food Chem.* 41:1287–1291.

Potter SM, Pertile J and Berber-Jimenez MD. 1996a. Soy protein concentrate and isolated protein similarly lower blood serum cholesterol but differently affect thyroid hormones in hamsters. *J. Nutr.* 126: 2007–2011.

Potter SM, Baum J, Surya P and Erdman JW Jr. 1996b. Effects of soy protein and isoflavones on plasma lipid profiles in postmenopausal women. Second International Symposium on the Role of Soy in Preventing and Treating Chronic Diseases, Brussels, Sept. 15–18, 1996, Abstract, p. 22.

Potter SM, Baum JA, Teng H, Stillman RJ, Shay NF and Erdman JW. 1998. Soy protein and isoflavones: Their effects on blood lipids and bone density in postmenopausal women. *Am. J. Clin. Nutr.* 68 (Suppl.): 1375S–1379S.

Prather ES. 1965. Effect of protein on plasma lipids of young women. *J. Am. Diet. Assoc.* 47: 181–185.

Pratt DE and Birac PM. 1979. Source of antioxidant activity of soybeans and soy products. *J. Food Sci.* 44: 1720–1722.

Prescott SL, Jenner DA, Beilin LJ, Margetts BM and Vandongen R. 1987. Controlled study of the effects of dietary protein on blood pressure in normotensive humans. *Clin. Exp. Pharmacol. Physiol.* 14: 159–162.

Prescott SL, Jenner DA, Beilin LJ, Margetts BM and Vandongen R. 1988. A randomized controlled trial of the effect on blood pressure of dietary non-meat protein versus meat protein in normotensive omnivores. *Clin. Sci.* 74: 665–672.

Price KB, Curl CL and Fenwick GR. 1986. The saponin content and sapogenol composition of the seed of 13 varieties of legumes. *J. Sci. Food Agric.* 37: 1185–1191.

Prost J and Belleville J. 1995. Animal or vegetable protein intakes (100, 200 or 300 g casein or soya-bean proteins/kg) differentially alter plasma distribution of cholesterol and triacylglycerols in rats. *Proc. Nutr. Soc.* 55: 105A, Abstract.

Prost J, Ait-Yahia D, Suarez-Rey ML, Arribi Z and Belleville J. 1995. Effect of animal or vegetable protein intakes (100, 200 or 300 g casein or soyabean proteins/kg) on membrane hepatocyte very-low-density-lipoprotein (VLDL) receptors. *Proc. Nutr. Soc.* 54: 7A, Abstract.

Prost J and Belleville J. 1996. Effect of animal or vegetable protein intakes (100, 200 or 300 g casein or soyabean proteins/kg) on VLDL, HDL and apolipoproteins in the rat. *Proc. Nutr. Soc.* 55: 106A, Abstract.

Prost J, Narce M, Peyron S and Belleville J. 1996. VLDL binding by isolated hepatocytes in rats fed on animal or vegetable protein diet (100, 200 or 300 g casein or soyabean proteins/kg). *Proc. Nutr. Soc.* 55: 70 A, Abstract.

Pucci E, Chiovato L and Pinchera A. 2000. Thyroid and lipid metabolism. *Int. J. Obesity* 24 (Suppl. 2): S109–S112.

Qian ZY, Jollès P, Migliore-Samour D and Fiat AM. 1995a. Isolation and characterization of sheep lactotransferrin, an inhibitor of platelet aggregation and comparison with human lactoferrin. *Biochem. Biophys. Acta* 1243: 25–32.

Qian ZY, Jollès P, Migliore-Samour D, Schoentgen F and Fiat AM. 1995b. Sheep κ-casein peptides inhibit platelet aggregation. *Biochim. Biophys. Acta* 1244: 411–417.

Qureshi AA, Solomon JA and Eichelman B. 1978. L-histidine induced facilitation of cholesterol biosynthesis in rats. *Proc. Soc. Exp. Biol. Med.* 159: 57–60.

Quyyumi AA, Dakak N, Mulcahy D, Andrews NP, Husain S and Panza JA. 1997. Nitric oxide activity in the atherosclerotic human coronary circulation. *J. Am. Coll. Cardiol.* 29: 308–317.

Raaij van JMA, Katan MB and Hautvast JGAJ. 1979. Casein, soya protein, serum cholesterol. *Lancet* 2: 958.

Raaij van JMA, Katan MB, Hautvast JGAJ and Hermus RJJ. 1981. Effect of casein versus soy protein diets on serum cholesterol and lipoprotein in young healthy volunteers. *Am. J. Clin. Nutr.* 34: 1261–1271.

Raaij van JMA, Katan MB, West CE and Hautvast JGAJ. 1982. Influence of diets containing casein, soy isolate and soy concentrate on serum cholesterol and lipoprotein in middle-aged volunteers. *Am. J. Clin. Nutr.* 35: 925–934.

Raaij van JMA, Katan MB and West CE. 1983. Influence of human diets containing casein and soy protein on serum cholesterol and lipoproteins in humans, rabbits and rats. In Gibney MJ and Kritchevsky D, Eds., *Animal and Vegetable Protein in Lipid Metabolism and Atherosclerosis*, Current Topics in Nutrition and Disease, Vol. 8, Alan R. Liss, New York, pp. 111–134.

Rabolli D and Martin RJ. 1977. Effects of diet composition on serum levels of insulin, thyroxine, triiodothyronine, growth hormone and corticosterone in rats. *J. Nutr.* 107: 1068–1078.

Radcliffe JD and Czajka-Narins DM. 1998. Partial replacement of dietary casein with soy protein isolate can reduce the severity of retinoid-induced hypertriglyceridemia. *Plant Foods Hum. Nutr.* 52: 97–108.

Rader DJ and Puré E. 2000. Genetic susceptibility to atherosclerosis. Insight from mice. *Circ. Res.* 86: 1013–1015.

Radomski W, Palmer RMJ and Moncada S. 1987. The role of nitric oxide and cGMP in platelet adhesion to vascular endothelium. *Biochem. Biophys. Res. Commn.* 148: 1482–1489.

Raheja KL and Linscheer WG. 1982. Comparative effects of soy and casein protein on plasma cholesterol concentrations. *Ann. Nutr. Metab.* 26: 44–49.

Raines EW and Ross R. 1995. Biology of atherosclerotic plaques: Possible role of growth factors in lesion development and the potential impact of soy. *J. Nutr.* 125: 624S–630S.

Rainwater DL, Kammerer CM and VandeBerg JL. 1999. Evidence that multiple genes influence baseline concentrations and diet response of Lp(a) in baboons. *Arterioscler. Thromb. Vasc. Biol.* 19: 2696–2700.

Raja PK and Jarowski CI. 1975. Utility of fasting essential amino acids plasma levels in formulation of nutritionnaly adequate diets. IV. Lowering of human plasma cholesterol and triglycerides by lysine and tryptophan supplementation. *J. Pharm. Sci.* 64: 691–692.

Ramalingswami V, Vickery AL, Stanbury JB and Hegsted DM. 1965. Some effects of protein deficiency on the rat thyroid. *Endocrinology* 77: 87–95.

Rango de F and Del Corso P. 1974. Modificazioni elettrocardiopatie ischemiche acute con taurina. *Clin. Terap.* 68: 261–270.

Rantala M, Savolainen MJ, Kervinen K and Kesäniemi YA. 1997. Apoprotein E phenotype and diet-induced alteration in blood pressure. *Am. J. Clin. Nutr.* 65: 543–550.

Rantala M, Rantala TT, Savolainen MJ, Friedlander Y and Kesäniemi YA. 2000. Apoprotein B gene polymorphisms and serum lipids: Meta-analysis of the role of genetic variation in responsiveness. *Am. J. Clin. Nutr.* 71: 713–724.

Rao PN and Rao GV. 1977. Alterations in serum lipids and blood glucose on high protein diet. *Ind. J. Exp. Biol.* 15: 380–381.

Ratnayake WM, Sarwar G and Laffey P. 1997. Influence of dietary protein and fat on serum lipids and metabolism of essential fatty acids in rats. *Br. J. Nutr.* 78: 459–467.

Ravel A, Roussel AM, Alary J and Laturaze J. 1988. Effects of varying dietary proteins on plasma lipids and rabbit platelet function. *Thromb. Res.* 49: 405–414.

Reaven G and Grecaberg RE. 1965. Experimental leucine-induced hypoglycemia in mice. *Metabolism* 14: 625–630.

Record IR, Dreosti IE, and McInerney JK. 1995. The antioxidant activity of genistein *in vitro. J. Nutr. Biochem.* 6: 481–485.

Redgrave TG. 1984. Dietary proteins and atherosclerosis. *Atherosclerosis* 52: 349–351 (Letter).

Reed D. 1984. Diet, blood pressure and multicollinearity. In Lovenberg W and Yamori Y, Eds., *Nutritional Prevention of Cardiovascular Disease*, Academic Press, Orlando, FL, pp. 155–166.

Reed D, McGee D, Yano K and Hankin J. 1985. Diet, blood pressure, and multicollinearity. *Hypertension* 7: 405–410.

Refsum H and Ueland PM. 1998. Recent data are not in conflict with homocysteine as a cardiovascular risk factor. *Curr. Opin. Lipidol.* 9: 533–539.

Reinli K and Block G. 1996. Phytoestrogens content of foods: A compendium of literature values. *Nutr. Cancer* 26: 123–148.

Reiser R, Henderson GR, O'Brien BC and Thomas J. 1977. Hepatic 3-hydroxy-3-methyl-glutaryl coenzyme-A reductase of rats fed semipurified and stock diets. *J. Nutr.* 107: 453–457.

Renner E, Schaafsma V and Scott KJ. 1989. Micronutrients in milk. In Renner E, Ed., *Micronutrients in milk and milk-based food products*. Elsevier, New York, pp. 1–70.

Reshef G, Gestetner B, Birk Y and Bondi A. 1978. Effect of alfalfa saponins on the growth and some aspects of lipid metabolism of mice and quails. *J. Sci. Food Agric.* 27: 63–72.

Rettura G, Padower J, Barbul A, Levenson SM and Seiffer E. 1979. Supplemental arginine increases thymic cellularity in normal and murine sarcoma virus inoculated mice and increases the resistance to murine sarcoma virus tumor. *J. Parenteral Enteral Nutr.* 3: 409–416.

Reusser ME and McCarron DA. 1994. Micronutrient effects on blood pressure regulation. *Nutr. Rev.* 52: 367–375.

Richard MJ, Julius AD and Wiggers KD. 1983. Effects of dietary protein and fat on cholesterol deposition and body composition of pigs. *Nutr. Rep. Int.* 28: 973–981.

Richardson M, Kurowska EM and Carroll KK. 1994. Early lesion development in the aortas of rabbits fed low-fat, cholesterol-free, semi-purified casein diet. *Atherosclerosis* 107: 165–178.

Ridout JH, Lucas CC, Patterson JM and Best CH. 1954. Preventive and curative studies on cholesterol "fatty liver" of rats. *Biochem. J.* 58: 301–306.

Rifkind BM. 1983. Nutrient-high-density lipoprotein relationships: An overview. *Prog. Biochem. Pharmacol.* 19: 89–109.

Rimm EB, Katan MB, Ascherio A, Stampfer MJ and Willett WC. 1996. Relation between intake of flavonoids and risk for coronary heart disease in male health professionals. *Ann. Intern. Med.* 125: 384–389.

Ritzel G. 1975. Evaluation von Ernährungserhebungen im Rahmen der Basler Studies III. Evaluation of nutrition surveys in the Basler Study III. In Brubacher G and Ritzel G, Eds., *Zur Ernährungssituation der Schweizerichen Bevölkerung*, Hans Huber, Bern, pp. 57–82.

Roberts DCK, West CE, Redgrave TG and Smith JB. 1974. Plasma cholesterol concentration in normal and cholesterol-fed rabbits: Its variation and hereditability. *Atherosclerosis* 19: 369–380.

Roberts DCK, Huff MW and Carroll KK. 1979. Plasma lipoproteins changes in suckling and weanling rabbits fed semipurified diets. *Lipids* 14: 566–571.

Roberts DCK, Stalmach ME, Khalil MW, Huntchinson JC and Carroll KK. 1981. Effects of dietary protein on composition and turnover of apoproteins in plasma lipoproteins of rabbits. *Can. J. Biochem.* 59: 642–647.

Roberts DCK and Samman S. 1990. Dietary protein and cholesterol metabolism — interactions of minerals. *J. Nutr. Sci. Vitaminol.* 36 (Suppl. 2): 119S–124S.

Roberts DF. 1985. Genetics and nutritional adaptations. In Blaxter K and Waterlow JC, Eds., *Nutritional Adaptation in Man*, J. Libbey, London, pp. 45–59.

Rodwell VW, Nordstrom JL and Mitchelen JJ. 1976. Regulation of HMG-CoA reductase. *Adv. Lipid Res.* 14: 1–74.

Rogers SR and Pesti GM. 1990. The influence of dietary tryptophan on broiler chick growth and lipid metabolism as mediated by dietary protein levels. *Poultry Sci.* 69: 746–756.

Rogers SR and Pesti GM. 1992. Effects of tryptophan supplementation of a maize-based diet on lipid metabolism in laying hens. *Br. Poultry Sci.* 33: 195–200.

Romano EL, Sotolongo-Pons M, Camejo G and Soyano A. 1984. Circulating immune complexes, immunoglobulins, complement, antibodies to dietary antigens, cholesterol and lipoprotein levels in patients with occlusive coronary lesions. *Atherosclerosis* 53: 119–128.

Rose RJ and Balloun SL. 1969. Effect of restricted energy and protein intake on atherosclerosis and associated physiological factors in cockerels. *J. Nutr.* 98: 335–343.

Rosenfeld ME. 1998. Inflammation, lipids, and free radicals: Lessons learned from the atherogene process. *Semin. Reprod. Endocrinol.* 16: 249–261.

Ross J and Oster KA. 1975. Milk-protein antibodies and myocardial infarction. *Lancet* 2: 1037.

Rossitch E Jr, Alexander E, Black PM and Cooke JP. 1991. L-arginine normalizes endothelial function in cerebral vessels from hypercholesterolemic rabbits. *J. Clin. Invest.* 87: 1295–1299.

Rossouw JE. 1998. Does estrogen have a role in the prevention of cardiovascular disease? *Nutr. Metab. Cardiovasc. Dis.* 8: 62–67.

Roth JS and Milstein SW. 1957. Some effects of excess methionine on lipid metabolism in the rat. *Arch. Biochem. Biophys.* 70: 392–400.

Rouse IL, Armstrong BK and Beilin LJ. 1983a. The relationship of blood presssure to diet and lifestyle in two religious populations. *J. Hypertens.* 1: 65–71.

Rouse IL, Beilin LJ, Armstrong BK and Vandongen R. 1983b. Blood pressure lowering effect of a vegetarian diet: Controlled trial in normotensive subjects. *Lancet* 1: 5–10.

Rouse IL and Beilin LJ. 1984. Vegetarian diet and blood pressure. *J. Hypertens.* 2: 231–240.

Rowland IR. 1991. Nutrition and gut microflora metabolism. In Rowland IR, Ed., *Nutrition, Toxicity and Cancer*, CRC Press, Boca Raton, FL, pp. 113–136.

Roy DM and Schneeman BO. 1981. Effect of soy protein, casein and trypsin inhibitor on cholesterol, bile acids and pancreatic enzymes in mice. *J. Nutr.* 111: 878–885.

Rudel LL and Pitts LL. 1978. Male-female variability in the dietary cholesterol-induced hyperlipoproteinemia of *Cynomolgus* monkeys (*Macaca fascicularis*). *J. Lipid Res.* 19: 992–1003.

Ruiz-Larrea MB, Mohan AR, Paganga G, Miller NJ, Bolwell GP and Rice-Evans J. 1997. Antioxidant activity of phytoestrogenic isoflavones. *Free Radical Res.* 26: 63–70.

Rukaj A and Sérougne C. 1983. Effect of excess dietary cystine ont the biodynamics of cholesterol in the rat. *Biochim. Biophys. Acta* 753: 1–5.

Russel R. 1990. The pathogenesis of atherosclerosis: A perspective for the 1990s. *Nature* 362: 800–809.

Rutherfurd KJ and Gill HS. 2000. Peptides affecting coagulation. *Br. J. Nutr.* 84 (Suppl.): S99–S102.

Ruys J and Hickie JB. 1976. Serum cholesterol and triglycerides levels in Australian adolescent vegetarians. *B.M.J.* 2: 87.

Ryzhenkov VE, Shanygina KI, Chistiakova AM, Miroshkina VN and Parfenova NS. 1984. Effect of arginine on the lipid and lipoprotein content of animal blood. *Vopr. Med. Khim.* 30: 76–79.

Sacks FM, Rosner B and Kass EH. 1974. Blood pressure in vegetarians. *Am. J. Epidemiol.* 100: 390–398.

Sacks FM, Castelli WP, Donner A and Kass EH. 1975. Plasma lipids and lipoprotein in vegetarians and controls. *N. Engl. J. Med.* 292: 1148–1151.

Sacks FM, Donner A, Castelli WP, Gronemeyer J, Pletka P, Margolius HS, Landsberg L and Kass EH. 1981. Effects of ingestion of meat on plasma cholesterol of vegetarians. *J.A.M.A.* 246: 640–644.

Sacks FM, Breslow JL, Wood PG and Kass EH. 1983. Lack of an effect of dairy protein (casein) and soy protein on plasma cholesterol in strict vegetarians. An experiment and a critical review. *J. Lipid Res.* 24: 1012–1020.

Sacks FM, Wood PG and Kass EH. 1984. Stability of blood pressure in vegetarians receiving dietary protein supplements. *Hypertension* 6: 199–201.

Sadoshima S, Busija D, Brody M and Heistad D. 1981. Sympathetic nerves protect against stroke in *Stroke-Prone Hypertensive* rats. A preliminary report. *Hypertension* 3 (Suppl. 1): 124.

Saeki S, Nishikawa H and Kiriyama S. 1987. Effects of casein or soybean protein on plasma cholesterol level in jejunectomized or ileectomized rats. *J. Nutr.* 117: 1527–1531.

Saeki S and Kiriyama S. 1988. Conservation of hyper- and hypo-cholesterolemic activities of dietary casein and soybean protein isolate after the administration of cholestyramine in the rat. *Nutr. Rep. Int.* 37: 565–573.

Saeki S and Kiriyama S. 1989. Effect of hypolipidemic drugs on plasma cholesterol levels characteristics of dietary casein and soybean. *Nutr. Rep. Int.* 39: 185–195.

Saeki S and Kiriyama S. 1990. Some evidence excluding the possibility that rat plasma cholesterol is regulated by the modification of enterohepatic circulation of steroids. In Beynen AC, Kritchevsky D and Pollak OJ, Eds., *Dietary Proteins Cholesterol Metabolism and Atherosclerosis*, Monographs on Atherosclerosis, Vol. 16, S. Karger, Basel, pp. 71–84.

Saeki S, Kanauchi O and Kiriyama S. 1990. Some metabolic aspects of the hypocholesterolemic effect of soybean protein in rats fed a cholesterol-free diet. *J. Nutr. Sci. Vitaminol.* 36 (Suppl.): 125S–131S.

Sakono M, Yoshida K and Yahiro M. 1993. Combined effects of dietary protein and fat on lipid metabolism in rats. *J. Nutr. Sci. Vitaminol.* 39: 335–343.

Sakono M, Fukuyama T, Ni WH, Nagao K, Ju HR, Sato M, Sakata N, Iwamoto H and Imaizumi K. 1997. Comparison between dietary soybean protein and casein of the inhibiting effect on atherogenesis in the thoracic aorta of hypercholesterolemic (ExHC) rats treated with experimental hypervitamin D. *Biosci. Biotechnol. Biochem.* 61: 514–519.

Sakuma I, Stuehr D, Gross SS, Nathan C and Levi R. 1988. Identification of arginine as a precursor of endothelium-derived relaxing factor. *Proc. Natl. Acad. Sci. U.S.A.* 85: 8664–8667.

Sakuma I, Togashi H, Yoshioka M, Saito H, Yamagida M, Tamura M, Kobayashi T, Yasuda H, Gross SS, and Levi R. 1992. NG-methyl-L-arginine, an inhibitor of L-arginine-derived nitric oxide synthesis, stimulates renal sympathetic nerve activity *in vivo*. *Circ. Res.* 70: 607–611.

Sambuichi EJ, Shizuka F and Kishi K. 1991. The influence of dietary protein on lipid peroxide formation in old, food restricted rats. *Nutr. Res.* 11: 1415–1426.

Samman S and Roberts DCK. 1984. The phosphorylation state of casein and its hyper-cholesterolemic effect: The role of divalent cations. *Atherosclerosis* 52: 347–348.

Samman S and Roberts DCK. 1987. The importance of the non-protein components of the diet in the plasma cholesterol response of rabbits to casein. Zinc and copper. *Br. J. Nutr.* 57: 27–33.

Samman S and Roberts DCK. 1988. The effect of zinc supplements on lipoproteins and copper status. *Atherosclerosis* 70: 247–252.

Samman S, Khosla P and Carroll KK. 1989. Effects of dietary casein and soybean protein on metabolism of radiolabelled low-density apolipoprotein B in rabbits. *Lipids* 24: 169–172.

Samman S, Khosla P and Carroll KK. 1990a. Influence of dietary minerals on apolipoprotein B metabolism in rabbits fed semipurified diets containing casein. *Atherosclerosis* 82: 69–74.

Samman S, Khosla P and Carroll KK. 1990b. Intermediate density lipoprotein-apolipoprotein B turnover in rabbits fed semipurified diets containing casein or soy protein. *Ann. Nutr. Metab.* 34: 98–103.

Samman S, Kurowska EM, Khosla P and Carroll KK. 1990c. Effects of dietary protein on composition and metabolism of plasma lipoprotein in rabbits. *J. Nutr. Sci. Vitaminol.* 36 (Suppl.): 95S–99S.

Samman S, Lyons Wall PM, Chan GS, Smith SJ, and Petoez P. 1999. The effects of supple-mentation with isoflavones on plasma lipids and oxidisability of low density lipo-protein in premenopausal women. *Atherosclerosis* 147: 277–283.

Samsonov MA, Pogozhaeva AV, Vasilev AV, Bogdanova SN, Pokrovskaia GR, Varsanovich EA and Orlova LA. 1993. Effect of anti-arteriosclerosis diet, containing soya protein isolate and omega–3–polyunsaturated fatty acids on the activity of mononuclear and platelet lysosomal hydrolases in patients with hypertension and ischemic heart dis-ease. *Vopr. Pitan.* (USSR) 1: 14–18.

Sanchez A, Register UD, Blankenship JW and Hunter CC. 1981. Effect of microwave heating of soyabeans on protein quality. *Arch. Latinoamer. Nutr.* 31: 44–51.

Sanchez A, Horning MC and Wingeleth DC. 1983. Plasma amino acids in human fed plant proteins. *Nutr. Rep. Int.* 28: 497–507.

Sanchez A, Horning MC, Shavlik GW, Wingeleth DC and Hubbard RW. 1985. Changes in levels of cholesterol associated with plasma amino acids in humans fed plant proteins. *Nutr. Rep. Int.* 32: 1047–1056.

Sanchez A, Rubano DA, Shavlik GW, Fagenstrom P, Register UD and Hubbard RW. 1988a. Separate effects of dietary protein and fat on serum cholesterol levels: Another view of amino acid content of proteins. *Arch. Latinoamer. Nutr.* 38: 239–250.

Sanchez A, Hubbard RW, Smit E and Hilton GF. 1988b. Testing a mechanism of control in human cholesterol metabolism: Relation of arginine and glycine to insulin and glu-cagon. *Atherosclerosis* 71: 87–92.

Sanchez A, Rubano, DA, Shavlik GW, Hubbard R and Horning MC. 1988c. Cholesterolemic effect of the lysine/arginine ratio in rabbits after initial early growth. *Arch. Latinoamer. Nutr.* 38: 229–238.

Sanchez A, Hubbard RW and Hilton GF. 1990. Hypocholesterolemic amino acids and the insulin glucagon ratio. In Beynen AC, Kritchevsky D and Pollak OJ, Eds., *Dietary Proteins, Cholesterol Metabolism and Atherosclerosis*, Monographs on Atherosclerosis, Vol. 16, S. Karger, Basel, pp. 126–138.

Sanchez A and Hubbard RW. 1991. Plasma amino acids and the insulin/glucagon ratio as an explanation for the dietary protein modulation of atherosclerosis. *Med. Hypotheses* 35: 324–329.

Sanno Y, Kimura T and Tanaka T. 1983. Effects of dietary proteins on serum levels of cholesterol and apolipoprotein in rats. *Nutr. Sci. Soy Protein Jpn.*, 4: 89–92.

Sargeant P, Farndale RW and Sage SO. 1993a. The tyrosine kinase inhibitors methyl 2,5-dihydroxycinnamate and genistein reduce thrombin-evoked tyrosine phosphorylation and Ca^{2+} entry in human platelets. *Fed. Eur. Biochem. Soc.* 315: 242–246.

Sargeant P, Farndale RW and Sage SO. 1993b. ADP- and thapsigargin-evoked Ca^{2+} entry and protein-tyrosine phosphorylation are inhibited by the tyrosine kinase inhibitors genistein and methyl-2,5-dihydroxycinnamate in fura-2-loaded human platelets. *J. Biol. Chem.* 268: 18151–18156.

Sarkkinen ES, Uusitupa MIJ, Pietinen P, Aro A, Ahola I, Penttilä I, Kervinen K and Kesäniemi YA. 1994. Long-term effects of three fat-modified diets in hypercholesterolemic subjects. *Atherosclerosis* 105: 9–23.

Sasaki J, Funakoshi M and Arakawa K. 1985. Effect of soybean crude fiber on the concentration of serum lipids and apolipoproteins in hyperlipemic subjects. *Ann. Nutr. Metab.* 29: 274–278.

Sato M, Nagao K, Sakono M, Ogawa H, Yamamoto K and Imaizumi K. 1996. Low protein diets posttranscriptionally repress apolipoprotein B expression in rat liver. *J. Nutr. Biochem.* 7: 381–385.

Satoh A, Hitomi M and Igarashi K. 1995. Effects of a spinach leaf protein concentrate on the serum cholesterol and amino acid concentration in rats fed a cholesterol-free diet. *J. Nutr. Sci. Vitaminol.* 41: 563–573.

Satoh T, Goto M and Igarashi K. 1993. Effects of protein isolates from radish and spinach leaves on serum lipid levels in rats. *J. Nutr. Sci. Vitaminol.* 39: 627–633.

Sautier C, Doucet C, Flament C and Lemonnier D. 1979. Effects of soy protein and saponin on serum, tissue and feces steroids in rats. *Atherosclerosis* 34: 233–241.

Sautier C, Dieng K, Flament C, Doucet C and Lemonnier D. 1982. Effects of dietary proteins and sodium phytate on the lipoproteins and the metabolism of sterols in rats. In Noseda G, Fragiacomo C, Fumagalli R and Paoletti R, Eds., *Lipoproteins and Coronary Atherosclerosis*, Elsevier, Amsterdam, pp. 271–279.

Sautier C, Dieng K, Flament C, Doucet C, Sequent LP, and Lemonnier D. 1983. Effects of whey protein, casein, soybean, and sunflower proteins on the serum, tissue, and fecal steroids in rats. *Br. J. Nutr.* 49: 313–319.

Sautier C, Flament C, Doucet C and Suquet JP. 1986. Effect of eight dietary proteins and their amino acid content on serum, hepatic and fecal steroids in the rat. *Nutr. Rep. Int.* 34: 1051–1061.

Sautier C, Flament C and Doucet C. 1990. Effects of animal and vegetable proteins on cholesterolemia and plasma lipoproteins in *Wistar* and *Brown-Norway* rats. In Beynen AC, Kritchevsky D, Pollak OJ, Eds., *Cholesterol Metabolism and Atherosclerosis*, Monographs on Atherosclerosis, Vol. 16, S. Karger, Basel, pp. 44–58.

Scarabottolo L, Trezzi E, Roma P and Catapano AL. 1986. Experimental hypothyroidism modulates the expression of the low density lipoprotein receptor by the liver. *Atherosclerosis* 59: 329–333.

Scarino L, Mengheri E, Vignolini F and Spadoni MA. 1979. Preliminary observations on the hypocholesterolaemic effect of faba beans. *Boll. Soc. Ital. Biol. Sper.* 55: 196.

Scebat L, Renais J and Groult N. 1980. Etude des lésions aortiques spontanées du lapin. Rôle possible de mécanismes humains. *Paroi artérielle* 6: 37–46.

Schaeffer EJ. 1997. Effects of dietary fatty acids on lipoproteins and cardiovascular disease risk: Summary. *Am. J. Clin. Nutr.* 65 (Suppl.): 1655S–1656S.

Schaffer SW and Azuma J. 1992. Review: myocardial physiological effects of taurine and their significance. *Adv. Exp. Med. Biol.* 315: 105–120.

Schaffer SW, Lombardini JB and Azuma J. 2000. Interaction between the actions of taurine and angiotensin II. *Amino Acids* 18: 305–318.

Schaffer WT. 1985. Effects of growth hormone on lipogenic enzyme activities in cultured rat hepatocytes. *Am. J. Physiol.* 248: E719–E725.

Schendel HE and Hansen JDL. 1958. Studies on fat metabolism in kwashiorkor. 1. Total serum cholesterol. *Metab. Clin. Exp.* 7: 731–741.

Schiff D, Chan G, Seccombe D and Hahn P. 1979. Plasma carnitine levels during intravenous feeding of the neonate. *J. Pediatr.* 95: 1043–1046.

Schmeisser DD, Kummerow FA and Baker DH. 1983. Effect of excess dietary lysine on plasma lipids of the chick. *J. Nutr.* 113: 1777–1783.

Schmeisser DD and Hrisco C. 1987. Soy protein is hypocholesterolemic but not hypoglycemic in the genetically obese mouse. *Fed. Proc.* 46: 1333, Abstract 5931.

Schmidt HHHW, Nau H, Wittfoht W, Gerlach J, Prescher KE, Klein MM, Niroomand F and Bohme E. 1988. Arginine is a physiological precursor of endothelium-derived nitric oxide. *Eur. J. Pharmacol.* 154: 213–216.

Schmidtmann M. 1926. Experimentelle Studien zur Pathogenese der Arteriosklerose. *Virchows Arch. Pathol. Anat. Physiol. Klin. Med.* 237: 1–21.

Schneeman BO and Gallaher D. 1980. Changes in small intestinal digestive enzyme activity and biles acids with dietary cellulose in rats. *J. Nutr.* 110: 584–590.

Schoene NW and Guidry CA. 1996. Genistein inhibits reactive oxygen species (ROS) formation during activation of rat platelets in whole blood. Second International Symposium on the Role of Soy in Preventing and Treating Chronic Diseases, Brussels, Sept. 15–18, 1996, Abstract, pp. 28–29.

Scholz KE, Beynen AC and West CE. 1982. Comparison between the hypercholesterolemia in rabbits induced by semipurified diets containing either cholesterol or casein. *Atherosclerosis* 44: 85–97.

Scholz KE, Beynen AC and West CE. 1983. Regression of casein and cholesterol induced hypercholesterolemia in rabbits. *Z. Ernährungwiss.* 22: 85–96.

Scholz-Ahrens KE, Hagemeister H, Unshelm J, Agergaard N and Barth CA. 1990. Response of hormones modulating plasma cholesterol to dietary casein or soy protein in minipigs. *J. Nutr.* 120: 1387–1392.

Schöne NW and Guidry CA. 1999. Dietary soy isoflavones inhibit activation of rat platelets. *J. Nutr. Biochem.* 10: 421–426.

Schouw van der YT, de Kleijn MJ, Peeters PH and Grobbee DE. 2000. Phytoestrogens and cardiovascular disease risk. *Nutr. Metab. Cardiovasc. Dis.* 10: 154–167.

Schriver de R. 1990. Cholesterol metabolism in mature and immature rats fed animal and plant protein. *J. Nutr.* 120: 1624–1632.

Schwandt P, Richter WO and Weisweiler P. 1981. Soybean protein and serum cholesterol. *Atherosclerosis* 40: 371–372.

Schwarzacher SP, Lim TT, Wang, Kernoff RS, Niebauer J, Cooke JP and Young AC. 1997. Local intramural delivery of L-arginine enhances nitric oxide generation and inhibits lesion formation after balloon angioplasty. *Circulation* 95: 1863–1869.

Schweizer TF, Bekhechi AR, Koellreuter B, Reimann S, Pometta D and Bron BA. 1983. Metabolic effects of dietary fiber from dehulled soybeans in humans. *Am. J. Clin. Nutr.* 38: 1–11.

Schweizer TF and Edwards CA. 1992. *Dietary Fibre — A Component of Food: Nutritional Function in Health and Disease*, Springer-Verlag, London.

Scott BB, McGuffin P, Swinburne ML and Losowski MS. 1976. Dietary antibodies and myocardial infarction. *Lancet* 2: 125–128.

Scott JM. 2000. Homocysteine and cardiovascular risk. *Am. J. Clin. Nutr.* 72: 333–334.

Seakins A and Waterlow JC. 1972. Effects of low protein diet on the incorporation of amino acids into rat serum lipoproteins. *Biochem. J.* 129: 793–795.

Seccombe DW, James L, Hahn P and Jones E. 1987. L-carnitine treatment in the hyperlipidemic rabbit. *Metabolism* 36: 1192–1196.

Seegraber FJ and Morril JL. 1982. Effect of soy protein on calves intestinal absorptive ability and morphology determined by scanning electron microscopy. *J. Dairy Sci.* 65: 1962–1970.

Sehlub J. 1999. Homocysteine metabolism. *Annu. Rev. Nutr.* 19: 217–246.

Seidel JC, Nath N and Harper AE. 1960. Diet and cholesterolemia. V. Effects of sulfur-containing amino acids and protein. *J. Lipid Res.* 1: 474–481.

Seidel JC and Harper AE. 1962. Effects of ethionine and methionine on serum lipids and lipoproteins. *Proc. Soc. Exp. Biol. Med.* 111: 579–582.

Seidel JC and Harper AE. 1963. Diet and cholesterolemia. VII. Effects of methionine, ethionine and *p*-fluorphenylalanine. *J. Lipid Res.* 4: 75–80.

Sekizaki H, Yokosawa R, Chinen C, Adachi H and Yamane Y. 1993. II. Synthesis of isoflavones and their attracting activity to *Aphanomyces euteiches zoospore*. *Biol. Pharm. Bull.* 16: 698–701.

Selhub J. 1999. Homocysteine metabolism. *Annu. Rev. Nutr.* 19: 217–246.

Selvam R and Ravichandran V. 1991. Effect of oral methionine and vitamin E on blood lipid peroxidation in vitamin B_6 deficient rats. *Biochem. Int.* 23: 1007–1017.

Sérougne C and Rukaj A. 1983. Plasma and lipoprotein cholesterol in rats fed L-amino acid-supplemented diets. *Ann. Nutr. Metab.* 27: 386–395.

Sérougne C, Férézou J and Rukaj A. 1984. Effect of excess dietary L-cystine on the rat plasma lipoproteins. *Ann. Nutr. Metab.* 28: 311–320.

Sérougne C, Férézou J and Rukaj A. 1987. A new relationship between cholesterolemia and cholesterol synthesis determined in rats fed an excess of cystine. *Biochim. Biophys. Acta* 921: 522–530.

Sérougne C, Mathé D and Lutton C. 1988. Induction of long-lasting hypercholesterolemia in the rat fed a cystine-enriched diet. *Lipids* 23: 930–936.

Sérougne C, Felgines C, Férézou J, Hajri T, Bertin C and Mazur A. 1995. Hypercholesterolemia induced by cholesterol- or cystine-enriched diets is characterized by different plasma lipoprotein and apolipoprotein concentrations in rats. *J. Nutr.* 125: 35–41.

Session VA, Martin A, Gomez-Muonz A, Brindley DN and Salter AM. 1993. Cholesterol feeding induces hypertriglyceridemia in hamsters and increases the activity of the Mg^{2+}-dependent phosphatidate phosphohydrolase in liver. *Biochim. Biophys. Acta* 1166: 238–243.

Setchell KDR. 1998. Phytoestrogens: The biochemistry, physiology, and implications for human health of soy isoflavones. *Am. J. Clin. Nutr.* 68 (Suppl.): 1333S–1346S.

Setchell KDR, Gosselin SJ and Welsh MB. 1987. Dietary estrogens — a probable cause of infertility and liver disease in captive cheetahs. *Gastroenterology* 93: 225–233.

Setchell KDR and Adlercreutz H. 1988. Mammalian lignans and phyto-oestrogens: Recent studies on their formation, metabolism and biological role in health and disease. In Rowland IR, Ed., *Role of the Gut Flora in Toxicity and Cancer*, Academic Press, London, pp. 315–345.

Shah NP. 2000. Effects of milk-derived bioactives: An overview. *Br. J. Nutr.* 84 (Suppl. 1): S3–S10.

Shapiro SL and Freedman L. 1955. Effect of essential unsaturated fatty acids and methionine on hypercholesterolemia. *Am. J. Physiol.* 181: 441–445.

Sharma RD. 1978. Isoflavones and hypercholesterolemia in rats. *Lipids* 14: 535–540.

Sharmanov TS, Maksimenko VB, Servetnik-Chalaia GK and Abdraimova SM. 1988. Effect of various dietary proteins on the processes of lipid transport in the blood serum. *Vopr. Pitan.* (USSR) 4: 45–48.

Shekelle RB, Missel LV, Paul O, Shryock AM and Stamler J. 1985. Fish consumption and mortality from coronary heart disease. *N. Engl. J. Med.* 313: 820 (Letter).

Shighe H, Ishikawa T, Higashi K, Yamashita T, Tomiyasu K, Yoshida H, Hosoai H, Ito T, Nakajima K, Ayaori M, Yonemura A, Suzukawa M and Nakamura H. 1996. Effect of soy protein isolate (SPI) and casein on the postprandial lipemia in normolipidemic men. *J. Nutr. Sci. Vitaminol.* 44: 113–127.

Shih DM, Welch C, and Lusis AJ. 1995. New insights into atherosclerosis from studies with mouse models. *Mol. Med. Today* 1: 364–372.

Shimokado K, Yokota T, Umezawa K, Sasaguri T and Ogata J. 1994. Protein kinase inhibitors inhibit chemotaxis of vascular smooth muscle cells. *Exp. Cell Res.* 220: 266–273.

Shimokado K, Umezawa K and Ogata J. 1995. Tyrosine kinase inhibitors inhibit multiple steps of the cell cycle of vascular smooth muscle cells. *Arterioscler. Thromb.* 14: 973–981.

Shore B and Shore V. 1974. An apolipoprotein preferentially enriched in cholesterol ester-rich very low density lipoproteins. *Biochem. Biophys. Res. Commn.* 58: 1–7.

Shore VG, Shore B and Hart RG. 1974. Changes in apolipoproteins and properties of rabbit very low density lipoproteins on induction of cholesterolemia. *Biochemistry* 13: 1579–1584.

Shorey RL and Davis JL. 1979. Effects of substituting soy for animal protein in the diets of young mildly hypercholesterolemic males. *Fed. Proc.* 38: 551, Abstract 1706.

Shorey RL, Bazan B, Lo GS and Steinke FH. 1981. Determinants of hypercholesterolemic response to soy and animal protein based diets. *Am. J. Clin. Nutr.* 34: 1769–1778.

Shorey RL, Day PJ, Willis RA, Lo GS and Steinke FH. 1985. Effects of soybean polysaccharide on plasma lipids. *J. Am. Diet. Assoc.* 85: 1461–1465.

Shull RL, Ershoff BH and Alfin-Slater RB. 1958. Effect of antioxidants on muscle and plasma lipids of vitamin E-deficient guinea pigs. *Proc. Soc. Exp. Biol. Med.* 98: 364–366.

Shutler SM, Walker AF and Low AG. 1987a. The choletesterol-lowering effect of legumes. I. Effects of the major nutrients. *Hum. Nutr. Food Sci. Nutr.* 41: 71–86.

Shutler SM, Walker AF and Low AG. 1987b. The cholesterol-lowering effect of legumes. II. Effects of fibre, sterols, saponins and isoflavones. *Hum. Nutr. Food Sci. Nutr.* 41: 87–102.

Sicuteri F, Fanciullacci M, Franci G, Giotti A and Guidotti A. 1970. Taurine as a therapeutic agent in vascular pain. *Clin. Med.* 77: 21–32.

Sidhu GS and Oakenfull DG. 1986. A mechanism for the hypocholesterolaemic activity of saponins. *Br. J. Nutr.* 55: 643–649.

Sidransky H. 1976. Nutritional disturbances of protein metabolism in the liver. *Am. J. Pathol.* 84: 649–667.

Sidransky H. 1990. Possible role of dietary proteins and amino acids in atherosclerosis. *Ann. N. Y. Acad. Sci.* 598: 464–481.

Sidransky H and Baba T. 1960. Chemical pathology of acute amino acid deficiencies. III. Morphological and biochemical changes in young rats fed valine- or lysine-devoid diets. *J. Nutr.* 70: 463–483.

Silagy C and Neil A. 1994. Garlic as a lipid-lowering agent — a meta-analysis. *J. R. Coll. Physicians* 28: 39–45.

Silk DBA, Marrs TC, Addison JM, Burston D, Clark ML and Matthews DM. 1973. Absorption of amino acids from a complex mixture simulating casein and a tryptic hydrolyzate of casein in man. *Clin. Sci. Mol. Med.* 45: 715–719.

Silk DBA, Clark ML, Marrs TC, Addison JM, Bursten D and Matthews DM. 1975. Jejunal absorption of an amino acid mixture simulating casein and an enzymatic hydrolyzate of casein prepared for oral administration to normal adults. *Br. J. Nutr.* 33: 95–100.

Simons LA, von Konigsmark M, Simons J and Celermajer DS. 2000. Phytoestrogen does not influence lipoprotein levels or endothelial function in healthy, postmenopausal women. *Am. J. Cardiol.* 85: 1297–1301.

Simopoulos AP. 1999. Genetic variation and nutrition. *Nutr. Rev.* 57: S10–S19.

Simopoulos AP and Nestel PJ. 1997. Genetic variation and dietary response. *World Rev. Nutr. Diet.* 80: 165 pp.

Simpson MV, Farber E and Tarver H. 1950. Studies on ethionine. I. Inhibition of protein synthesis in intact animals. *J. Biol. Chem.* 182: 81–89.

Singal SA, Hazon SJ, Snydertricker VP and Little-John JE. 1953. The production of fatty livers in rats on lysine and threonine deficient diets. *J. Biol. Chem.* 200: 867–871.

Singer AH, Tsao PS, Wang BY, Bloch DA and Cooke JP. 1995. Discordant effects of dietary L-arginine on vascular structure and reactivity in hypercholesterolemic rabbits. *J. Cardiovasc. Pharmacol.* 25: 710–716.

Sirtori CR, Agradi E, Conti F, Mantero O and Gatti E. 1977. Soybean protein diet in the treatment of type II hyperlipoproteinemia. *Lancet* 1: 275–278.

Sirtori CR, Gatti E, Mantero O, Conti F, Agradi E, Tremoli E, Sirtori M, Fraterrigo L, Tavazzi L and Kritchevsky D. 1979. Clinical experience with the soybean protein diet in the treatment of hypercholesterolemia. *Am. J. Clin. Nutr.* 32: 1645–1658.

Sirtori CR, Noseda G and Descovich GC. 1983. Studies on the use of a soybean protein diet for the management of human hyperlipoproteinemias. *Curr. Top. Nutr. Dis.* 8: 135–148.

Sirtori CR, Galli G, Lovati MR, Carrara P, Bosisio E and Galli-Kienle MG. 1984. Effects of dietary proteins on the regulation of liver lipoprotein receptors in rats. *J. Nutr.* 114: 1493–1500.

Sirtori CR, Even R and Lovati MR. 1993. Soybean protein diet and plasma cholesterol: From therapy to molecular mechanisms. *Ann. N. Y. Acad. Sci.* 676: 188–201.

Sirtori CR, Lovati MR, Manzoni C, Monetti M, Pazzucconi F and Gatti E. 1995. Soy and cholesterol reduction: Clinical experience. *J. Nutr.* 125: 598S–605S.

Sirtori CR, Manzoni C, Gianazza E, and Lovati MR. 1996. Soy and cholesterol reduction: Clinical experience and potential molecular mechanisms. Second International Symposium on the Role of Soy in Preventing and Treating Chronic Disease, Brussels, Sept. 15–19, 1996, Abstract, p. 24.

Sirtori CR, Gianazza E, Manzoni C, Lovati MR and Murphy PA. 1997. Role of isoflavones in the cholesterol reduction by soy protein in the clinic. Type II patients in the Italian studies with the soybean protein diet did not receive isoflavones. *Am. J. Clin. Nutr.* 65: 166–171.

Sirtori CR, Lovati MR, Manzoni C, Gianazza E, Bondioli A, Staels B and Auwerx J. 1998. Reduction of serum cholesterol by soy proteins: Clinical experience and potential molecular mechanisms. *Nutr. Metab. Cardiovasc. Dis.* 8: 334–340.

Sirtori CR, Pazzucconi F, Colombo L, Battistin P, Bondioli A, and Descheemaeker K. 1999. Double-blind study of the addition of high-protein soya milk vs. cow's milk to the diet of patients with severe hypercholesterolaemia and resistance to or intolerance of statins. *Br. J. Nutr.* 82: 91–96.

Sirtori CR. 2001. Reduction of LDL and total cholesterol with soy products. In Descheemaeker K and Debruyne I, Eds., *Soy and Health 2000: Clinical Evidence, Dietetic Applications*, Garant, Leuven, pp. 29–33.

Sjöblom L, Eklund A, Humble L, Ostlund-Lindqvist AM and Jönsson L. 1989. Effects of diet and metoprolol on lipid levels in the blood plasma and morphology of the heart and intramural branches of coronary arteries of spontaneously hypertensive male rats. A 9 month study. *Ann. Nutr. Metab.* 33: 284–296.

Sjöblom L and Eklund A. 1990. Dietary protein and fatty acid composition of liver lipids in the rat. *Biochim. Biophys. Acta* 1004: 187–192.

Sjöblom L, Eklund A, Humble L, Menschik-Lundin A and Ostlund-Lindqvist AM. 1991. Plasma very low density lipoprotein from male rats fed casein or soybean protein diets: A comparison of fatty acid composition and influence on prostanoid production. *J. Nutr.* 121: 1705–1713.

Sjövall J. 1959. Dietary glycine and taurine on bile acid conjugation in man. *Proc. Soc. Exp. Biol. Med.* 100: 676–678.

Sklan D. 1980. Digestion and absorption of casein at different dietary levels in the chick: Effect on fatty acid and bile absorption. *J. Nutr.* 10: 989–994.

Sklan D, Budowski P and Hurwitz S. 1979. Absorption of oleic and taurocholic acids from the intestine of the chick. Interactions and interference by proteins. *Biochim. Biophys. Acta* 573: 31–39.

Slag MF, Ahmed M, Gannon MC and Nuttal FQ. 1981. Meal stimulation of cortisol secretion: A protein induced effect. *Metabolism* 30: 1104–1108.

Slavin JL. 1991. Nutritional benefits of soy protein and soy fiber. *J. Am. Diet. Assoc.* 91: 816–819.

Slavin JL, Nelson NA, McNamara EA and Cashmere K. 1985. Bowel function of healthy men consuming liquid diet with and without dietary fiber. *J. Parent. Enter. Nutr.* 9: 317–321.

Slawinski M, Grodzinska L, Kostka-Trabka E, Bieron K, Goszcz A and Gryglewski RJ. 1996. L-arginine substrate for no synthesis: Its beneficial effects in therapy of patients with peripheral arterial disease: Comparison with placebo-preliminary results. *Acta Physiol. Hung.* 84: 457–458.

Smith DR. 1998. Animal models: Nutrition and lipoprotein metabolism. *Curr. Opin. Lipidol.* 9: 3–6.

Smith RL and Pickney ER. 1989. Diet, blood cholesterol and coronary heart disease: A critical review of the literature, Rev., Vector Enterprise, Santa Monica, CA.

Smith RS. 1989. Protein carbohydrate and fiber. In Smith RS, Ed., *Nutrition, Hypertension and Cardiovascular Disease*, 2nd ed., Lyncean Press, Portland, OR, pp. 130–144.

Snowdon DA, Philips RL and Fraser GE. 1984. Meat consumption and fatal ischemic heart disease. *Prev. Med.* 13: 490–500.

Solomon JK and Geison RI. 1978a. Effect of excess dietary L-histidine on plasma cholesterol levels in weanling rats. *J. Nutr.* 108: 936–943.

Solomon JK and Geison RI. 1978b. L-histidine-induced hypercholesterolemia: Characteristics of cholesterol biosynthesis in rat livers. *Proc. Soc. Exp. Biol. Med.* 159: 44–47.

Solomons NW and Cousins RJ. 1984. Zinc. In Solomons NW and Roenberg IH, Eds., *Absorption and Malabsorption of Mineral Nutrients*, Alan R. Liss, New York, pp. 125–197.

Sommariva D, Tirrito M, Bonfiglioli D, Pogliaghi I, Cabrini E, Bellintani L and Fasoli A. 1985. Changes in the serum lipoprotein pattern induced by two low-fat diets with a different vegetable content in hypercholesterolemic patients. *Atherosclerosis* 56: 119–124.

Spolarics Z, Lang CH, Baghy CJ and Spitzer JJ. 1991. Glutamine and fatty acid oxidation are the main sources of energy for Kupfer and endothelial cells. *Am. J. Physiol.* 261: G185–G190.

Sprecher DL. 1998. Triglycerides as a risk factor for coronary heart disease. *Am. J. Cardiol.* 82: 49U–56U.

Srebnik HH, Evans ES and Rosenberg LL. 1963. Thyroid function in female rats maintained on a protein-free diet. *Endocrinology* 73: 267–270.

Srinivasan SR, Radhakrishnamurthy B, Dalferes ER, Webber LS and Berenson GS. 1977. Serum lipoprotein responses to exogenous cholesterol in *Spider* monkeys: Effect of levels of dietary protein. *Proc. Soc. Exp. Biol. Med.* 154: 102–106.

Srinivasan SR, Radhakrishnamurthy B, Dalferes ER and Berenson GS. 1979. Serum α-lipoprotein responses to variation in dietary cholesterol, protein and carbohydrate in different nonhuman primate species. *Lipids* 44: 559–565.

Stähelin HB and Ritzel G. 1979. Effect of whey on plasma lipids. *Int. J. Vitam. Nutr. Res.* 49: 229–230.

Stähelin HB, Oberhänsli A, Vanner M, Jost M, Schneeberger H and Ritzel G. 1980. Effect of whey feeding on serum lipids in swine. In Noseda G, Lewis B and Paoletti R, Eds., *Diet and Drug in Atherosclerosis*, Raven Press, New York, pp. 41–46.

Stamler JE. 1979. Population studies. In: Levy RI, Rifkind BM, Dennis BM and Ernst ND, Eds., *Nutrition, Lipid and Coronary Heart Disease*, Raven Press, New York, pp. 25–88.

Stamler JS, Pick R and Katz LN. 1958a. Action of casein, egg albumin and corn germ on cholesterolemia and atherogenesis in cockerels. *Fed. Proc.* 17: 155.

Stamler JS, Pick R and Katz LN. 1958b. Effects of dietary proteins, methionine and vitamins on plasma lipids and atherogenesis in cholesterol fed cockerels. *Circ. Res.* 6: 442–446.

Stamler JS, Pick R and Katz LN. 1958c. Effects of dietary protein and carbohydrate level on cholesterolemia and atherogenesis in cockerel on a high-fat, high-cholesterol mash. *Circ. Res.* 6: 447–451.

Stamler JS, Caggiula A and Grandist GA. 1992. Relationship of dietary variables to blood pressure (BP) finding of the Multiple Risk factors Intervention Trial (MRFIT). *Circulation* 85: 867, Abstract 23.

Stamler JS, Osborne JA, Jaraki O, Rabini LE, Rabbani LE, Mullins M, Singel D and Loscalzo LE. 1993. Adverse vascular effects of homocysteine are modulated by endothelium-derived relaxing factor and related oxides of nitrogen. *J. Clin. Invest.* 91: 308–318.

Stamler JS and Slivka A. 1996. Biological chemistry of thiols in the vasculature and in vascular-related disease. *Nutr. Rev.* 54: 1–30.

Stange EF and Diestchy JM. 1984. Age-related decreases in tissue sterol acquisition are mediated by changes in cholesterol synthesis and not low density lipoprotein uptake in the rat. *J. Lipid Res.* 25: 703–713.

Starkebaum G and Harlan JM. 1986. Endothelial cell injury due to copper-catalyzed hydrogen peroxide generation from homocysteine. *J. Clin. Invest.* 77: 1370–1376.

Starokadomsky L and Ssobolew LW. 1909. Zur Frage der experimentellen Arteriosklerose. *Frankf. Z. Pathol.* 3: 912–925.

St Clair RW. 1997. Effects of estrogens on macrophage foam cells: A potential target for the protective effects of estrogens on atherosclerosis. *Curr. Opin. Lipidol.* 8: 281–286.

Stead IM, Brosnan ME and Brosnan JT. 2000. Characterization of homocysteine metabolism in the rat liver. *Biochem. J.* 350: 685–692.

Stein JH and McBride PE. 1998. Hyperhomocysteinemia and atherosclerotic vascular disease. *Arch. Intern. Med.* 158: 1301–1306.

Steinberg F and Villablanca A. 1998. Soy proteins decrease lipid and lipoprotein levels in pre- and post-menopausal women. *F.A.S.E.B. J.* 12: Part II, A817, Abstract 4738.

Steinbiss W. 1913. Uber experimentelle alimentare Atherosklerose. *Virschows Arch. Pathol. Anat. Physiol. Klin. Med.* 212: 152–187.

Steinke FH. 1992. Nutritional value of soybean protein foods. In Steinke FH, Waggle DH and Volgarev MN, Eds., *New Protein Foods in Human Health: Nutrition, Prevention and Therapy*, CRC Press, Boca Raton, FL, pp. 59–73.

Stemmer KL, Petering HG, Murthy L, Finelli VN and Menden EE. 1985. Copper deficiency effects on cardiovascular system and lipid metabolism in the rat; the role of dietary protein and excessive zinc. *Ann. Nutr. Metab.* 29: 332–347.

Stephan ZF, Lindsey S and Hayes KC. 1987. Taurine enhances low density lipoprotein binding. Internalization and degradation by cultured Hep G2 cells. *J. Biol. Chem.* 262: 6069–6073.

Stevenson RW, Stebbing N, Rudman CG, William PE and Cherrington AD. 1987. The synthetic 32–46 fragment of human growth hormone increases insulin and glucagon levels in the conscious dog. *Metabolism* 36: 400–404.

Stolzenberg-Solomon RZ, Miller ER 3rd, Maguire MG, Selhub J and Appel LJ. 1999. Association of dietary protein intake and coffee consumption with serum homocysteine concentration in an older population. *Am. J. Clin. Nutr.* 69: 467–475.

Story JA, Tepper SA and Kritchevsky D. 1976. Age-related changes in the lipid metabolism of the *Fisher 344* rats. *Lipids* 19: 544–552.

Story JA and Kritchevsky D. 1978. Bile acid metabolism and fiber. *Am. J. Clin. Nutr.* 31 (Suppl.): S199–S202.

Story JA, LePage SL, Petro MS, West LG, Cassidy MM, Lightfoot FG and Vahouny GV. 1984. Interactions of alfalfa plant and sprout saponins with cholesterol *in vitro* and in cholesterol-fed rats. *Am. J. Clin. Nutr.* 39: 917–929.

Stratum van P, Rudrun M, ten Hoor F, Wilson R and Pikaer NA. 1978. Effets physiologiques d'un régime alimentaire riche en protéines de soja chez l'homme. *Ann. Nutr. Metab.* 32: 377–389.

Strasberg SM, Ilson RG and Paloheimo JE. 1983. Bile salt-associated electrolyte secretion and the effect of sodium taurocholate on bile flow. *J. Lab. Clin. Med.* 101: 317–326.

Streilein JW and Hildreth EA. 1966. Tolerance to bovine γ-globulin in adult guinea pigs. *J. Immunol.* 96: 1027–1034.

Strong JP and McGill HC. 1967. Diet and experimental atherosclerosis in *Baboons. Am. J. Pathol.* 50: 669–690.

Stuckey NW. 1911. Uber die Veränderungen der Kaninchen Aorta unter der Wirkung reichlicher tierischer Nahrung. *Centralbl. Allg. Pathol. Pathol. Anat.* 22: 379–380.

Stuckey NW. 1912. Uber die Veränderungen der Kaninchen Aorta bei der Fütterung mit verschiedenen Fettsorten. *Centralbl. Allg. Pathol. Pathol. Anat.* 23: 910–911.

Subbiah MTR. 1977. Early dietary and medical intervention and the development of atherosclerosis. I. Effect of low-protein diet on the age-related accumulation of sterols and steryl-esters in aorta during spontaneous atherogenesis in the white *Carneau*-pigeon. *Nutr. Rep. Int.* 15: 223–229.

Subbiah MTR and Siekert RG Jr. 1977. Dietary restriction and the development of athero-sclerosis. *Br. J. Nutr.* 41: 1–6.

Suberville C. 1987. Relative contribution of cysteine and methionine to glutathione content and thyroid hormone levels in the rat. *Br. J. Nutr.* 58: 105–111.

Sugano M. 1983. Hypocholesterolemic effect of plant protein in relation to animal protein: Mechanism of action. In Gibney MJ and Kritchevsky D, Eds., *Animal and Vegetable Proteins in Lipid Metabolism and Atherosclerosis*, Current Topics in Nutrition and Disease, Vol. 8, Alan R. Liss, New York, pp. 51–84.

Sugano M, Tanaka K and Ide T. 1982a. Secretion of cholesterol, triglycerides and apolipo-protein A1 by isolated perfused liver from rat fed soy protein and casein or their amino acids mixtures. *J. Nutr.* 112: 855–862.

Sugano M, Ishiwaki N, Nagata Y and Imaizumi K. 1982b. Effects of arginine and lysine addition to casein and soya bean protein on serum lipids, apolipoprotein, insulin and glucagon in rats. *Br. J. Nutr.* 48: 211–221.

Sugano M, Ishiwaki N and Nakashima K. 1983. Hypocholesterolemic effect of soy protein isolate in rats. *Nutr. Sci. Soy Protein Jpn.* 4: 79–84.

Sugano M, Ishiwaki N and Nakashima K. 1984. Dietary protein-dependent modification of serum cholesterol level in rats. Significance of the arginine/lysine ratio. *Ann. Nutr. Metab.* 28: 192–199.

Sugano M, Ishida T and Koba K. 1988a. Protein-fat interaction on serum cholesterol level, fatty acids desaturation and eicosanoid production in rats. *J. Nutr.* 118: 548–554.

Sugano M, Yamada Y, Yodshida K, Hashimoto Y, Matsuo T and Kimoto M. 1988b. The hypocholesterolemic action of the undigested fraction of soybean protein in rats. *Atherosclerosis* 72: 115–122; erratum 1988; 74: 187.

Sugano M and Goto S. 1990. Steroid-binding peptides from dietary proteins. *J. Nutr. Sci. Vitaminol.* 36 (Suppl.): 147S–150S.

Sugano M, Goto S, Yamada Y, Yoshida K, Hashimoto Y, Matsuo T and Kimoto M. 1990a. Cholesterol-lowering activity of various undigested fractions of soybean protein in rats. *J. Nutr.* 120: 977–985.

Sugano M, Yamada Y, Goto S and Yoshida K. 1990b. Hypocholesterolemic effect of the undigested fraction of soy protein. In Beynen AC, Kritchevsky D and Pollak OJ, Eds., *Dietary Proteins Cholesterol Metabolism and Atherosclerosis*, Vol. 16, S. Karger, Basel, pp. 85–96.

Sugano M and Koba K. 1993. Dietary protein and lipid metabolism: A multifunctional effect. *Ann. N. Y. Acad. Sci.* 676: 215–222.

Sugiyama K. 1989. Importance of sulfur-containing amino acids in cholesterol metabolism. *Nippon Eiyö Shokuryö Gakkaishi*, 42: 353–363.

Sugiyama K, Kushima Y and Muramatsu K. 1984. Effect of methionine, cystine and taurine on plasma cholesterol level in rats fed a high cholesterol diet. *Agric. Biol. Chem.* 48: 2897–2899.

Sugiyama K, Ozawa M and Muramatsu K. 1985a. Dietary sulfur-containing amino acids and glycine as determinants factors in plasma cholesterol regulation in growing rats. *J. Nutr. Sci. Vitaminol.* 31: 121–125.

Sugiyama K, Kushima Y and Muramatsu K. 1985b. Effects of sulfur-containing amino acids and glycine on plasma cholesterol level in rats fed on a high cholesterol diet. *Agric. Biol. Chem.* 49: 3455–3461.

Sugiyama K, Ohkawa S, Muramatsu K and Keiichiro K. 1986a. Relationship between amino acid composition of diet and plasma cholesterol level in growing rats fed a high cholesterol diet. *J. Nutr. Sci. Vitaminol.* 32: 413–423.

Sugiyama K, Mizuno M and Muramatsu K. 1986b. Effects of individual amino acids on plasma cholesterol level in rats fed a high-cholesterol diet. *J. Nutr. Sci. Vitaminol.* 32: 623–633.

Sugiyama K, Akai H and Muramatsu K. 1986c. Effect of methionine and related compounds on plasma cholesterol level in rats fed a high cholesterol diet. *J. Nutr. Sci. Vitaminol.* 32: 537–549.

Sugiyama K and Muramatsu K. 1987. Effect of plant and animal proteins supplemented with methionine on plasma cholesterol level in rats. *Nutr. Sci. Soy Protein Jpn.* 8: 98–103.

Sugiyama K, Suzuki H and Muramatsu K. 1987. Effect of dietary choline on plasma and liver lipid levels in rats fed on a high cholesterol diet. *Agric. Biol. Chem.* 51: 2603–2605.

Sugiyama K, Ohishi A and Muramatsu K. 1988. Relationship between effect of methionine on plasma cholesterol level and dietary protein (casein and soy protein isolate) level in rats. *Nutr. Sci. Soy Protein Jpn.* 9: 86–92.

Sugiyama K, Ohishi A, Ohnuma T and Muramatsu K. 1989a. Comparison between the plasma cholesterol-lowering effect of glycine and taurine in rats fed on high cholesterol diets. *Agric. Biol. Chem.* 53: 1647–1652.

Sugiyama K, Ohishi A, Siyu H and Takeuchi H. 1989b. Effects of methyl-group acceptors on the regulation of plasma cholesterol level in rats fed high cholesterol diets. *J. Nutr. Sci. Vitaminol.* 35: 613–626.

Sugiyama K and Muramatsu K. 1990. Significance of the amino acid composition of dietary protein in the regulation of plasma cholesterol. *J. Nutr. Sci. Vitaminol.* 36 (Suppl.): 105S–110S.

Sugiyama K, Kanamori H and Tanaka S. 1993. Correlation of the plasma cholesterol-lowering effect of dietary glycine with the alteration of hepatic phospholipid composition in rats. *Biosci. Biotechnol. Biochem.* 57: 1461–1465.

Sugiyama K, Kanamori H, Akachi T and Yamakawa A. 1996. Amino acid composition of dietary proteins affects plasma cholesterol concentration through alteration of hepatic phospholipid metabolism in rats fed a cholesterol-free diet. *J. Nutr. Biochem.* 7: 40–48.

Sugiyama K, Yamakawa A, Kumazawa A and Saeki S. 1997. Methionine content of dietary protein affects the molecular species composition of plasma phosphatidylcholine in rats fed a cholesterol-free diet. *J. Nutr.* 127: 600–607.

Sulistiyani, Tumbelaka L, Sutanto J and Sajuthi D. 1998. The lack of effect of isoflavones on plasma lipid concentrations in ovariectomized *Cynomolgus* monkeys and LDL susceptibility to oxidation. *Am. J. Clin. Nutr.* 68 (Suppl.): 1521S–1522S.

Sullivan AC, Miller ON, Wittman JS and Hamilton J. 1971. Factors influencing the *in vivo* and *in vitro* rate of lipogenesis in rat liver. *J. Nutr.* 101: 265–272.

Sullivan MA, Duffy A, Dimarco N and Liepa G. 1985. Effects of various dietary animal and vegetable proteins on serum and biliary lipids and on gallstone formation in the hamster. *Lipids* 20: 1–6.

Sumino H, Sato K, Sakamaki T, Masuda H, Nakamura T, Kamla T and Nagai R. 1998. Decreased basal production of nitric oxidemic patients with heart disease. *Chest* 113: 317–322.

Sutton-Tyrell K, Bostom A, Selhub J and Zeigler-Johnson C. 1997. High homocysteine levels are independently related to isolated systolic hypertension in older adults. *Circulation* 96: 1745–1749.

Sved AF, Fernstrom JD and Wurtman RJ. 1979. Tyrosine administration reduces blood pressure and enhances brain norepinephrine release in *Spontaneously Hypertensive* rats. *Proc. Nat. Acad. Sci.* 76: 35110–35114.

Sved AF, van Italie CM and Fernstrom JD. 1982. Studies on the hypertensive action of L-tryptophan. *J. Pharm. Exp. Ther.* 221: 329–333.

Takeuchi H, Sugiura K, Imai Y, Goto N, Takeshima H and Yamamoto K. 2000. Effects of graded levels of dietary casein and corn oil on total cholesterol and triacylglycerol in plasma and liver of rats. *J. Nutr. Sci. Vitaminol.* 46: 280–284.

Takihara K, Azuma J, Awata N Ohta H, Hamaguchi T, Sawamura A, Tanaka Y, Kishimoto S and Sperelakis N. 1986. Beneficial effects of taurine in rabbits with chronic congestive heart failure. *Am. Heart J.* 112: 1278–1284.

Tall AR, Small DM, Atkinson D and Rudel LL. 1978. Studies on the structure of low density lipoprotein isolated from *Macaca fascicularis* fed an atherogenic diet. *J. Clin. Invest.* 62: 1354–1363.

Tanaka K and Nozaki Y. 1983. Effect of partial hydrolysates of casein and soy bean protein on serum lipoproteins and fecal neutral sterols. *J. Nutr. Sci. Vitaminol.* 29: 439–446.

Tanaka K, Imaizumi K and Sugano M. 1983a. Effects of dietary proteins on the intestinal synthesis and transport of cholesterol and apolipoprotein A-1 in rats. *J. Nutr.* 113: 1388–1394.

Tanaka C, Watanuki M and Nozaki Y. 1983b. Effect of soyabean protein on coprostanol production and cholesterol metabolism in cholesterol-fed rats. *J. Nutr. Sci. Vitaminol.* 29: 447–454.

Tanaka K and Sugano M. 1989a. Effect of addition of sulfur-containing amino acids and glycine to soybean protein and casein on serum cholesterol levels of rats. *J. Nutr. Sci. Vitaminol.* 35: 323–332.

Tanaka K and Sugano M. 1989b. Effects of modification of the arginine/lysine ratio of dietary proteins on absorption and turnover of cholesterol in rats. *Agric. Biol. Chem.* 53: 1351–1356.

Tanno N, Oikawa S, Koizumi M, Fujii Y, Hori S, Susuki N, Sakuma E, Kotake H, Namai K and Toyota T. 1989. Effect of taurine administration on serum lipid and biliary lipid composition in man. *Tokohu J. Exp. Med.* 159: 91–99.

Tao S, Tsou B, Wu S, Hsiao Z, Tsai R, Gao R, Lu C and Yu C. 1984. Blood pressure and dietary factors among farmers in Northern and Southern China. In Lovenberg W and Yamori Y, Eds., *Nutritional Prevention of Cardiovascular Disease*, Academic Press, Orlando, FL, pp. 101–113.

Tasker TE and Potter SM. 1993. Effect of dietary protein source on plasma lipids, HMGCoA reductase activity, and hepatic glutathione levels in gerbils. *J. Nutr. Biochem.* 4: 458–462.

Tatcher CD, Jacobson NL, Young JW and Richard MJ. 1984. Effects of sources of dietary fat and protein on tissue cholesterol. *Nutr. Res.* 4: 1013–1024.

Tateishi N. 1981. Relative contributions of sulfur-atoms of dietary cysteine and methionine to rat liver glutathione and proteins. *J. Biochem.* 90: 1603–1610.

Tawakol A, Omland T, Gerhard M, Wu JT and Creager MA. 1997. Hyperhomocyst(e)inemia is associated with impaired endothelium-dependent vasodilatation in humans. *Circulation* 95: 119–121.

Teisseidre PL, Frankel EN, Waterhouse AL, Peleg H and German JB. 1996. Inhibition of *in vitro* human LDL oxidation by phenolic antioxidants from grapes and wine. *J. Sci. Food Agric.* 70: 55–61.

Teixeira S, Potter SM, Weigel R, Hannum S, Erdman JW and Hassler CM. 1998. Dose-dependent effect of soy protein hypercholesterolemic men. *F.A.S.E.B. J.* 12: Part I, A237, Abstract.

Teixeira S, Potter SM, Weigel R, Hannum S, Erdman JW and Hassler CM. 2000. Effects of feeding 4 levels of soy protein for 3 and 6 weeks on blood lipids and apolipoproteins in moderately hypercholesterolemic men. *Am. J. Clin. Nutr.* 71: 1077–1084.

Temler RS, Dormond CA, Simon E and Peret J. 1983. Alteration in hepatic enzymes activities in rats fed increased levels of soya protein with or without methionine supplementation. *Nutr. Rep. Int.* 28: 253–265.

Teng H, Say NF and Potter SM. 1996. The influence of soy protein and isoflavones on LDL receptor mRNA in postmenopausal women. *F.A.S.E.B. J.* 10: A508, Abstract 2930.

Terasawa F, Hirano Y, Wada M, Takita T, Nakamura K and Innami S. 1994. Effects of dietary casein and soy-protein on metabolic conversion of docosahexaenoic acid in the liver of rat. *J. Nutr. Sci. Vitaminol.* 40: 353–362.

Terpstra AHM and Sanchez-Muniz FJ. 1981. Time course of the development of hypercholesterolemia in rabbits fed semipurified diets containing casein or soybean protein. *Atherosclerosis* 39: 217–227.

Terpstra AHM, Harkes L and van der Veen FH. 1981. The effect of different proportions of casein in semipurified diets on the concentration of serum cholesterol and lipoprotein composition in rabbits. *Lipids* 16: 114–119.

Terpstra AHM, van Tintelen G and West CE. 1982a. The effect of semipurified diets containing different proportions of either casein or soybean protein on the concentration of cholesterol in whole serum lipoproteins and liver in male and female rats. *Atherosclerosis* 42: 85–95.

Terpstra AHM, van Tintelen G and West CE. 1982b. The hypocholesterolemic effect of dietary soy protein in rats. *J. Nutr.* 112: 810–817.

Terpstra AHM, Woodward CJH, West CE and van Boven HGA. 1982c. A longitudinal cross over study of serum cholesterol and lipoproteins in rabbits fed on semipurified diets containing either casein or soybean protein. *Br. J. Nutr.* 47: 213–221.

Terpstra AHM, van Tintelen G and West CE. 1982d. Dietary protein and serum cholesterol in guinea pigs. *Nutr. Rep. Int.* 25: 726–731.

Terpstra AHM, Hermus RJJ and West CE. 1983a. The role of dietary protein in cholesterol metabolism. *World Rev. Nutr. Diet.* 42: 1–55.

Terpstra AHM, Hermus RJJ and West CE. 1983b. Dietary protein and cholesterol metabolism in rabbits and rats. In Gibney MJ and Kritchevsky D, Eds., *Animal and Vegetable Protein in Lipid Metabolism and Atherosclerosis*, Current Topics in Nutrition and Disease, Vol. 8, Alan R. Liss, New York, pp. 19–49.

Terpstra AHM, Beynen AC and West CE. 1983c. De invloed vande soort eiwit in de voeding op de serumcholesterolconcentratie bij mens en dier. *Voeding* 44: 308–313.

Terpstra AHM, Schutte JB and West CE. 1983d. Prevention of hypercholesterolemia in cholesterol-fed chickens by high-casein and high soya-bean protein diets. *Atherosclerosis* 46: 95–104.

Terpstra AHM, West CE, Fennis JTCM, Schouten JA and van der Veen A. 1984. Hypocholesterolemic effect of dietary protein versus casein in *Rhesus* monkeys (*Macaca mulatta*). *Am. J. Clin. Nutr.* 39: 1–7.

Terpstra AHM, Holmes JC and Nicolosi RJ. 1991. The hypocholesterolemic effect of dietary soybean protein versus casein in hamsters fed cholesterol-free or cholesterol-enriched semipurified diets. *J. Nutr.* 121: 944–947.

Terpstra AHM, Laitinen L, Stucchi AF and Nicolosi RJ. 1994. The effects of semipurified diets containing two levels (20% and 40%) of either casein or soybean protein isolate and concentrate on plasma lipids in hamsters. *Nutr. Res.* 14: 885–895.

Tew BY, Xu X, Wang HJ, Murphy PA and Hendrich S. 1996. A diet high in wheat fiber decreases the bioavailability of soybean isoflavones in a single meal fed to women. *J. Nutr.* 126: 871–877.

Thacker PA and Bowland JP. 1981. Effects of dietary propionic acid on serum lipids and lipoproteins of pigs fed diets supplemented with soybean meal or canola meal. *Can. J. Anim. Sci.* 61: 439–448.

Thacker PA, Salomons MO, Aherne FX, Milligan LP and Bowland JP. 1981. Influence of propionic acid on the cholesterol metabolism of pigs fed hypercholesterolemic diets. *Can. J. Anim. Sci.* 61: 969–975.

Thambyrajah J and Townend JN. 2000. Homocysteine and atherothrombosis — mechanisms for injury. *Eur. Heart J.* 21: 967–974.

Therond P, Abella A, Laurent D, Couturier M, Chalas J, Legrand A and Lindenbaum A. 2000. *In vitro* study of the cytotoxicity of isolated oxidized lipid low-density lipoprotein fractions in human endothelial cells: Relationship with the glutathione status and cell morphology. *Free Radical Biol. Med.* 28: 585–596.

Theuer RC and Sarett HP. 1970. Nutritive adequacy of soy infant formula in rats: Choline. *J. Agric. Food Chem.* 18: 913–916.

Thiagarajan D, Bennink MR and Mayle JE. 1997. Soy protein efficacy in reducing risk for cardiovascular diseases (CVD). *F.A.S.E.B. J.* 11: A170, Abstract 986.

Thomas FB, Mazzaferri EL, Crockett SE, Mekjian HS, Gruemer HD and Cataland S. 1976. Stimulation of secretion of gastric inhibitory polypeptide and insulin by intraduodenal amino acid perfusion. *Gastroenterology* 70: 523–527.

Thompson DB and Erdman JR. 1982. Phytic acid determination in soybean. *J. Food Sci.* 47: 513–517.

Thompson GR, Soutar AK, Spengel FA, Jadhav A, Gavigan SJ and Myant NB. 1981. Defects of receptor mediated low density lipoprotein catabolism in homozygous hypercholesterolemia and hypothyroidism *in vivo. Proc. Nat. Acad. Sci. U.S.A.* 78: 2591–2595.

Thorne S, Mullen MJ, Clarkson P, Donald AE and Deanfeld JE. 1988. Early endothelial dysfunction in adults at risk from atherosclerosis: Different response to L-arginine. *J. Am. Coll. Cardiol.* 32: 110–116.

Tikkanen MJ. 1997. Apolipoprotein E polymorphism and plasma cholesterol response to dietary change. *World Rev. Nutr. Diet.* 80: 15–21.

Tikkanen MJ, Huttunen JK, Enholm C and Pietinen P. 1990. Apolipoprotein E4 homozygoty predisposes to serum cholesterol elevation during high fat diet. *Arteriosclerosis* 10: 285–288.

Tikkanen MJ, Wähälä K, Ojala S, Vihma V and Adlercreutz H. 1998. Effect of soybean phytoestrogen intake on low density lipoprotein oxidation resistance. *Proc. Natl. Acad. Sci. U.S.A.* 95: 3106–3110.

Tikkanen MJ and Adlercreutz H. 2000. Dietary soy-derived isoflavone phytoestrogens. Could they have a role in coronary heart disease prevention? *Biochem. Pharmacol.* 60: 1–5.

Toborek M, Chmurzynska W, Manteuffel-Cymborowska M, Sikora E and Grzelakowska-Sztabert B. 1990. Enzymes of homocysteine remethylation and transsulfuration in methionine or cholesterol induced atherosclerosis in rabbits. In Curtis HC, Ghisla S and Blau N, Eds., *Chemistry and Biology of Pteridines 1989*, Walter deGruyter, Berlin, pp. 876–880.

Toborek M and Hennig B. 1994. Is methionine an atherogenic acid? *J. Opt. Nutr.* 3: 80–83.

Toborek M, Kopieczna-Grzebieniak E, Drozdz M and Wieczorek M. 1995. Increased lipid peroxidation as a mechanism of methionine-induced atherosclerosis in rabbits. *Atherosclerosis* 115: 217–224.

Toborek M and Hennig B. 1996. Dietary methionine imbalance endothelial cell dysfunction and atherosclerosis. *Nutr. Res.* 16: 1251–1266.

Toivanen A, Viljanen MK and Savilahti E. 1975. IgM and IgG anti-milk antibodies measured by radioimmunoassay in myocardial infarction. *Lancet* 2: 205–207.

Tomkins GM, Chaikoff IL and Bennett LL. 1952. Cholesterol synthesis by liver, effects of hypohysectomy. *J. Biol. Chem.* 189: 543–545.

Topping DL, Storer GB, Calvert GD, Illman RJ, Oakenfull DG and Welle RA. 1980a. Effect of dietary saponins on fecal bile acids and neutral sterols, plasma lipid and lipoprotein turnover in the pigs. *Am. J. Clin. Nutr.* 33: 783–786.

Topping DL, Trimble RP, Illman RJ, Potter JD and Oakenfull DG. 1980b. Prevention of dietary hypercholesterolemia in the rat by soy flour high and low in saponins. *Nutr. Rep. Int.* 22: 513–519.

Torre GM, Lynch VDP and Jarowski CI. 1980. Lowering of serum cholesterol and triglyceride levels by balancing amino acid intake in the rat. *J. Nutr.* 110: 1194–1196.

Torreilles J and Guerin MC. 1995. Des peptides isus de la caséine peuvent provoquer l'oxydation des LDL humaines par un processus dépendant des peroxydases et indépendant des métaux. *C. R. Soc. Biol.* 189: 933–942.

Tovar-Palacio C, Potter SM and Shay NF. 1997. Intake of soy protein and soy protein extracts alter blood cholesterol levels and hepatic apolipoprotein gene expression in the gerbil. *F.A.S.E.B. J.* 11: A170, Abstract 987.

Tovar-Palacio C, Hafermann JC, Paria BC, Kennedy KJ, Potter SM and Shay NF. 1998a. Interaction of dietary isoflavones and methionine supplementation: Their effect on cholesterol levels in gerbils. *F.A.S.E.B. J.* 12: A 207, Abstract 1205.

Tovar-Palacio C, Potter SM, Hafermann JC and Shay NF. 1998b. Intake of soy protein and soy protein extracts influences lipid metabolism and hepatic gene expression in gerbils. *J. Nutr.* 128: 839–842.

Tran L and Nicolosi RJ. 1997. Comparative effects of soy and rice protein concentrate on plasma lipoprotein levels and early atherosclerosis in hamsters. *F.A.S.E.B. J.* 11: A152, Abstract 884.

Tripathy K, Lotero H and Bolanos O. 1970. Role of dietary protein upon serum cholesterol level in malnourished subjects. *Am. J. Clin. Nutr.* 23: 1160–1168.

Truswell AS. 1964. Effect of surplus leucine intake on serum cholesterol in man. *Proc. Nutr. Soc.* 23: xlvi–xlvii.

Truswell AS, McVeigh S, Mitchell WD and Bronte-Stewart B. 1965. Effect in man of feeding taurine on bile acid conjugation and serum cholesterol levels. *J. Atheroscler. Res.* 5: 526–532.

Truswell AS and Hansen JDL. 1969. Fatty liver in protein-calorie malnutrition. *S. Afr. Med. J.* 43: 280–283.

Truswell AS and Beynen AC. 1992. Dietary fibre and plasma lipids: Potential for prevention and treatment of hyperlipidaemias. In Schweizer TS and Edwards CA, Eds., *Dietary Fibre — A Component of Food: Nutritional Function in Health and Disease*, Springer-Verlag, London, 295–332.

Tsai AC, Mott EL, Owen GM, Bennick MR, Lo GS and Steinke FH. 1983. Effects of soy polysaccharide on gastrointestinal functions, nutrient balance, steroids excretions, glucose tolerance, serum lipids and other parameters in humans. *Am. J. Clin. Nutr.* 38: 504–511.

Tsao PS, Theimeier G, Singer AH, Leung LL and Cooke JP. 1994a. L-arginine attenuates platelet reactivity in hypercholesterolemic rabbits. *Arterioscler. Thromb.* 14: 1529–1533.

Tsao PS, McEvoy LM, Drexler H, Butcher EC and Cooke JP. 1994b. Enhanced endothelial adhesiveness in hypercholesterolemia is attenuated by L-arginine. *Circulation* 89: 2176–2182.

Tseng E, Potter SM and Picciano MF. 1990. Dietary protein source and plasma lipid profiles of infants. *Pediatrics* 85: 548–552.

Tsuji K, Seki T and Iwao H. 1979. Cholesterol lowering effects of taurine and sulfur containing amino acids in serum and liver of rats. *Sulfur-Containing Amino Acids* 6:249–255.

Tsuji K, Ichikawa T, Nakagawa Y, Matsuura Y and Kawamura M. 1983. Hypocholesterolemic effect of taurine or taurocyamine feeding in cholesterol-fed rats. *Sulfur-Containing Amino Acids* 6: 239–248.

Tulp OL, Easton TA and Spencer VL. 1984. Effect of high protein-cafeteria feeding on serum cholesterol and atherogenesis in the corpulent rat. *Nutr. Res.* 4: 981–987.

Tumbelaka SL, Sutanto J and Sajuthi D. 1996. The lack of effect of isoflavones on plasma lipid concentrations in ovariectomized *Cynomolgus* monkeys and LDL susceptibility to oxidation. Second International Symposium on the Role of Soy in Preventing and Treating Chronic Diseases, Brussels, Sept. 15–18, 1996, Abstract, p. 26.

Tutel'ian VA, Vasil'ev AV and Ren LH. 1989. Antiatherogenic properties of the soy protein isolate 500EJ. *Patol. Fiziol. Eksp. Ter. USSR.* 4: 62–65.

Tyagi SC. 1999. Homocyst(e)ine and heart disease: pathophysiology of extracellular matrix. *Clin. Exp. Hypertens.* 21: 181–198.

Tyagi SC, Smiley LM and Mujumdar VS. 1999. Homocyst(e)ine impairs endocardial endothelial function. *Can. J. Physiol. Pharmacol.* 77: 950–957.

Tyroler HA. 2000. Coronary heart disease epidemiology in the 21st century. *Epidemiol. Rev.* 22: 7–13.

Tzonou A, Kalkadidi A, Trichopoulos A, Hsiah CC, Toupadaki N, Willett N and Trichopoulos D. 1993. Diet and coronary heart disease: A case-control study in Athens, Greece. *Epidemiology* 4: 511–516.

Uchida K, Nomura Y, Kadowaki M, Takeuchi N and Yamamura Y. 1977. Effect of dietary cholesterol on cholesterol and bile acid metabolism in rats. *Jpn. J. Pharmacol.* 27: 193–204.

Uchida K, Nomura Y, Kadowaki M, Takase H, Takano K and Tageuchi N. 1978. Age-related changes in cholesterol and bile acid metabolism in rats. *J. Lipid Res.* 19: 544–552.

Ueland PM, Refsum H, Beresford SAA and Vollset SE. 2000. The controversy over homocysteine and cardiovascular risk. *Am. J. Clin. Nutr.* 72: 324–332.

Ungerer T, Lelana RPA, Sajythi D, Soeparto I and Lelana ID. 1998. Tempe supplementation in high-cholesterol diets does not improve dyslipidemia in *Cynomolgus* monkeys. *Am. J. Clin. Nutr.* 68, (Suppl.): 1520.

Usami M, Seino Y, Seino S, Takemura J, Nakahara H, Ikeda M and Imura H. 1982. Effects of high protein diet on insulin and glucagon secretion in normal rats. *J. Nutr.* 112: 681–685.

Usui K, Kawaguchi A, Ozaki M, Niva M, Kimeno A, Kumisada K and Minakawi S. 1983. Taurine and hypertension, several clinical experiences. *Sulfur-Containing Amino Acids* 6: 221–228.

Utermann G, Kindermann I, Kaffarnik H and Steinmmetz A. 1984. Apolipoprotein E phenotypes and hyperlipidemia. *Hum. Genet.* 65: 232–236.

Vagenakis AG, Burger A, Portnay GI, Rudolph M, O'Brian JT, Aziki F, Arky RA, Nicod P, Ingbar SH and Braverman LE. 1975. Diversion of peripheral thyroxine metabolism from activating to inactivating pathways during complete fasting. *J. Clin. Endocrinol. Metab.* 41: 191–194.

Vahouny GV, Roy T, Gallo LL, Story JA, Kritchevsky D, Cassidy M, Grund BM and Trendwill CR. 1978. Dietary fiber and lymphatic absorption of cholesterol in the rat. *Am. J. Clin. Nutr.* 31 (Suppl.): S208–S212.

Vahouny GV, Chalcarz W, Satchithanandam S, Adamson I, Klurfeld DM and Kritchevsky D. 1984. Effects of soy protein and casein intake on intestinal absorption and lymphatic transport of cholesterol and oleic acid. *Am. J. Clin. Nutr.* 40: 1156–1164.

Vahouny GV, Adamson I, Chalcarz W, Satchithanandam S, Muesing R, Klurfeld DM, Tepper SA, Sanghvi A and Kritchevsky D. 1985. Effects of casein and soy protein on hepatic and serum lipids and lipoprotein lipid distributions in the rat. *Atherosclerosis* 56: 127–137.

Vallance P, Collier J and Moncada S. 1989. Effects of endothelium-derived nitric oxide on peripheral arteriolar tone in man. *Lancet* 2: 997–1000.

Vallance P, Leone A, Calver A, Collier J and Moncada S. 1992a. Accumulation of an endogenous inhibitor of nitric oxide synthesis in chronic renal failure. *Lancet* 339: 572–575.

Vallance P, Leone A, Calver A, Collier J and Moncada S. 1992b. Endogenous dimethylarginine as an inhibitor of nitric oxide synthesis. *J. Cardiovasc. Pharmacol.* 20 (Suppl. 12): 60S–62S.

Valsala P and Kurup A. 1987. Investigations on the mechanism of hypercholesterolemia observed in copper deficiency. *J. Biosci.* 12: 137–142.

Vance JE and Vance DE. 1985. The role of phosphatidylcholine biosynthesis in the secretion of lipoproteins from hepatocytes. *Can. J. Biochem. Cell Biol.* 63: 870–881.

Verbeva NP. 1965. The effect of vitamin E on the development of experimental atherosclerosis in rabbits. *Vopr. Pitan.* (USSR) 24: 42–49.

Verhoef P, Stampfer MJ, Buring JE, Gaziano JM, Allen RH, Stabler SP, Reynolds RD, Kok FJ, Kennekens CH and Willett WC. 1996. Homocysteine metabolism and risk of myocardial infarction relation with vitamin B6, B12 and folate. *Am. J. Epidemiol.* 143: 845–859.

Verrillo A, de Teresa A, Giarrusso PC and La Rocca S. 1985. Soybean protein diets in the management of type II hyperliproteinemia. *Atherosclerosis* 54: 321–331.

Vessby G, Karlstrom B, Lithell H, Gustaffson IB and Werner I. 1982. The effects of lipid and carbohydrate metabolism of replacing some animal protein by soy protein in a lipid-lowering diet for hypercholesterolaemic patients. *Hum. Nutr. Appl. Nutr.* 36A: 179–189.

Vesselinovitch D and Wissler RW. 1980. Reversal of atherosclerosis: Comparison of non-human primate models. In Gotto AM, Smith LC and Allen B, Eds., *Atherosclerosis*, Vol. 5, Springer-Verlag, Berlin, pp. 369–374.

Vigna GB, Pansini F, Bonaccorsi G, Albertazzi P, Donega P, Zanotti L, De Aloysio D, Mollica G and Fellin R. 2000. Plasma lipoproteins in soy-treated postmenopausal women: A double-blind, placebo-controlled trial. *Nutr. Metab. Cardiovasc. Dis.* 10: 315–322.

Villalon L, Tuchweber B and Yousef IM. 1987. Effect of a low protein diet on bile flow and composition in rats. *J. Nutr.* 117: 678–683.

Vinson JA, Dabbagh YA, Serry MM and Jang J. 1995. Plant flavonoids, especially tea flavonols, are powerful antioxidants using an *in vitro* oxidation model for heart disease. *J. Agric. Food Chem.* 43: 2800–2802.

Visser A and Thomas A. 1987. Review, soya protein products — their processing, functionality, and applications aspects. *Food Rev. Int.* 3: 1–32.

Viviani R, Seghi AM and Lenaz G. 1964. Fatty acid composition fatty livers in lysine- and threonine-deficient rats. *J. Lipid Res.* 5: 52–56.

Volgarev MN, Vysotsky VG, Meschery-Akova VA, Yatsyshina TA and Steinke FH. 1989. Evaluation of isolated soy protein foods in weight reduction with obese hypercholesterolemic and normocholesterolemic obese individuals. *Nutr. Rep. Int.* 39: 61–72.

Vollset SE, Heuch I and Bjelke E. 1985. Fish consumption and mortality from coronary heart disease. *N. Engl. J. Med.* 313: 820–821.

Voutilainen S, Lakka TA, Hämelahti P, Lehtimäki T and Poulsen HE. 2000. Plasma total homocysteine concentration and the risk of acute coronary events: The Kuopio Ischaemic Heart Disease Risk Factor Study. *J. Intern. Med.* 248: 217–222.

Vrecko K, Mlekusch W and Aloia RC. 1988. Effect of skim milk and whey diets on plasma lipid levels of rabbits in a cross-over study. *Atherosclerosis* 72: 11–17.

Wacker L and Hueck W. 1913. Über experimentelle Atherosklerose und Cholesterinämie. *Muench Med. Wochenschr.* 60: 2097–2100.

Waggle DH and Kolar CW. 1979. Types of soy products. In Wilcke HL, Hopkins DT and Waggle DH, Eds., *Soy Protein and Human Nutrition*, Academic Press, New York, pp. 19–51.

Wagner JD, Cefalu WT, Anthony MS, Litwak KN, Zhang L and Clarkson TB. 1997. Dietary soy protein and estrogen replacement therapy improve cardiovascular risk factors and decrease aortic cholesteryl ester content in ovariectomized *Cynomolgus* monkeys. *Metabolism* 46: 698–705.

Waki M, Tsushima M, Yamashita N, Ryohmoto K, Koh H, Komatsu R, Hara Y and Matsuyama T. 1996. Effect of soy protein on serum lipid, platelet aggregation and hemostatic markers and progression of atherosclerosis in hyperlipidemic patients. *Rep. Soy Protein Res. Commn. Jpn.* 17: 129–134.

Walker ARP and Arvidson VB. 1954. Fat intake, serum cholesterol concentrations and atherosclerosis in the South Africa Bantu. I. A low fat intake and age trend of serum cholesterol concentration in the South Africa Bantu. *J. Clin. Invest.* 33: 1358–1365.

Walker GR, Morse EH and Overley VA. 1960. The effect of animal protein and vegetable protein diets having the same fat content on the serum lipid levels of young women. *J. Nutr.* 72: 317–321.

Walter ED. 1941. Genistin (an isoflavone glucoside) and its aglucone, genistein, from soybeans. *J. Am. Chem. Soc.* 63: 3273–3276.

Walton KW, Scott PJ, Dykes PW and Dawies JWL. 1965. The significance of alterations in serum lipids in thyroid dysfunction. Part 2. Alteration in metabolism and turnover of ^{131}I low density lipoprotein in hypothyroidism and thyrotoxicosis. *Clin. Sci.* 29: 189–215.

Wang BY, Singer AH, Tsao PS, Drexler H, Kosek J and Cooke JP. 1994. Dietary arginine prevents atherogenesis in the coronary artery of the hypercholesterolemic rabbit. *J. Am. Coll. Cardiol.* 23: 452–458.

Wang HJ and Murphy PA. 1994a. Isoflavone content in commercial soybean foods. *J. Agric. Food Chem.* 42: 1666–1673.

Wang HJ and Murphy PA. 1994b. Isoflavone composition in American and Japanese soybeans in Iowa: Effects of varieties, year and location. *J. Agric. Food Chem.* 42: 1674–1679.

Wang MF, Yamamoto S, Chung HM, Chung SY, Miyatani S, Mori M, Okita T and Sugano M. 1995. Antihypercholesterolemic effect of undigested fraction of soybean protein in young females volunteers. *J. Nutr. Sci. Vitaminol.* 41: 187–195.

Wang W, Franke AA, Custer LJ and Le Marchand L. 1996. Antioxidant properties of dietary phenolic agents in a human LDL-oxidation *ex vivo* model. Second International Symposium on the Role of Soy in Preventing and Treating Chronic Diseases, Brussels, Sept. 15–18, 1996, Abstract, p. 28.

Wang W and Ballatori N. 1998. Endogenous glutathione conjugates occurence and biological functions. *Pharmacol. Rev.* 50: 335–356.

Wang X. 1999. A theory for the mechanism of homocysteine-induced vascular pathogenesis. *Med. Hypotheses* 53: 386–394.

Wangen KE, Duncan AM, Xu X and Kurzer MS. 2001. Soy isoflavones improve plasma lipids in normocholesterolemic and mildly hypercholesterolemic postmenopausal women. *Am. J. Clin. Nutr.* 73: 225–231.

Ward M, McNully H, Pentieva K, Partlin J, Strain JJ, Weir DG and Scott JM. 2000. Fluctuations in dietary methionine intake do not alter plasma homocysteine concentration in healthy men: A preliminary study. *J. Nutr.* 130: 2653–2657.

Ward M, McNully H, McPartlin J, Strain JJ, Weir DG and Scott JM. 2001. Effect of supplemental methionine on plasma homocysteine concentration in healthy men: A preliminary study. *Int. J. Vitam. Nutr. Res.* 71: 82–86.

Warden CH, Daluiski A and Lusis AJ. 1992. Identification of new genes contributing to atherosclerosis: The mapping of genes contributing to complex disorders in animal models. In Lusis AJ, Rotter JI and Sparkes RS, Eds., *Molecular Genetics of Coronary Artery Disease: Candidate Genes and Processes in Atherosclerosis*, Monographs in Human Genetics, Vol. 14, S. Karger, Basel, pp. 419–441.

Warshafsky S, Kamer RS and Sivak SL. 1993. Effect of garlic on total serum cholesterol: A meta-analysis. *Ann. Intern. Med.* 119: 599–605.

Warshaw AL, Walker WA and Isselbacher KJ. 1974. Protein uptake by the intestine: evidence for absorption of intact molecules. *Gastroenterology* 66: 987–992.

Wascher TC, Posch K, Wallner S, Hermetter A, Kostner GM and Graier WF. 1997. Vascular effects of L-arginine: Anything beyond a substrate for the NO-synthase? *Biochem. Biophys. Res. Commn.* 234: 35–38.

Washburn S, Burke GL, Morgan T and Anthony M. 1999. Effect of soy protein supplementation on serum lipoproteins, blood pressure, and menopausal symptoms in perimenopausal women. *Menopause* 6: 7–13.

Watanabe Y. 1980. Serial inbreeding of rabbits with heritable hyperlipidemia (*WHHL*-rabbit) incidence and the development of atherosclerosis and xanthoma. *Atherosclerosis* 36: 261–268.

Waterlow JC. 1975. Amount and rate of disappearance of liver fat in malnourished infants in Jamaica. *Am. J. Clin. Nutr.* 2: 1330–1336.

Watkins JB, Järvenpää AL, Sczepanik-van Leeuwen P, Klein PD, Rassin DK, Gaull GA and Räihä NC. 1983. Feeding the low-birth-weight infant. V. Effects of taurine, cholesterol and human milk on bile acid kinetics. *Gastroenterology* 85: 793–800.

Weck M, Hanefeld M, Lenothardt W, Haller K, Robowsky KD, Noack R and Schmandke H. 1983. Ackerbohnenproteindiät bei Hypercholesterolamie. *Die Nahrung* 27: 327–333.

Wei HC, Wei LH, Frenkel K, Bowen R and Barnes S. 1993. Inhibition of tumor promoter-induced hydrogen peroxide formation *in vitro* and *in vivo* by genistein. *Nutr. Cancer* 20: 1–12.

Weigand W, Hannapel E and Brand K. 1980. Effect of starvation and refeeding a high-protein or high-carbohydrate diet on lipid composition and glycogen content of rat livers in relation to age. *J. Nutr.* 110: 669–674.

Weigensberg Bin Stary HC and McMillan GC. 1964. Effect of lysine deficiency on cholesterol atherosclerosis in rabbits. *Exp. Mol. Pathol.* 3: 444–454.

Weinans GJB and Beynen AC. 1983. Plasma cholesterol concentrations in mice fed cholesterol-rich, semi purified diets containing casein or soybean protein. *Nutr. Rep. Int.* 28: 1017–1027.

Weiss HJ and Dietschy JM. 1974. Adaptive responses in hepatic and intestinal cholesterogenesis following ileal resection in the rat. *Eur. J. Clin. Invest.* 4: 33–41.

Weitzel GH, Schöen H, Gey F and Buddecke E. 1956. Fettlösliche Vitamine und Atherosklerose. *Hoppe-Seyler's Z. Physiol. Chem.* 304: 247–251.

Wennmalm A, Edlund A, Granström F and Wiklund O. 1995. Acute supplementation with the nitric oxide precursor L-arginine does not improve cardiovascular performance in patients with hypercholesterolemia. *Atherosclerosis* 118: 223–231.

Wesselkin NW. 1913. Über die Ablagerung von fettartigen Stoffen in den Organen. *Virchows Arch. Pathol. Anat. Physiol. Klin. Med.* 212: 225–235.

West CE, Deuring K, Ben Schutte J and Terpstra AHM. 1982. The effect of age on the development of hypercholesterolemia in rabbits fed semipurified diets containing casein. *J. Nutr.* 112: 1287–1295.

West CE, Beynen AC, Terpstra AHM, Scholz KE, Carroll KK and Woodward CJH. 1983a. The nature of dietary protein and serum cholesterol. *Atherosclerosis* 46: 253–256.

West CE, van Raaij JMA, Beynen AC, Hautvast JGAJ, Katan MB, Kuyvenhoven MW, Scholz KE and Terpstra AHM. 1983b. The influence of dietary protein on serum cholesterol in man and in experimental animals. *Kieler Milchwirshaftliche Forschungberichte* 35: 397–407.

West CE, Beynen AC, Scholz KE, Terpstra AHM, Schutte JB, Deuring K and van Gils LGM. 1984. Treatment of dietary casein with formaldehyde reduces its hypercholesterolemic effect in rabbits. *J. Nutr.* 114: 17–25.

West CE and Beynen AC. 1986. Are the atherogenic dietary proteins? *Verh. Dtsch. Ges. Inn. Med.* 92: 666–673.

West CE and Beynen AC. 1988. Are there atherogenic dietary proteins? In Barth CA and Fürst P, Eds., *Wahl der Nahrungsproteine, Dietary Protein in Clinical Nutrition*, JF Bergmann Verlag, München, pp. 27–34.

West CE, Spaaij CJ, Clous WM, Twisk HP, Goertz MP, Hubbard RW, Kuyvenhoven MW, Van der Meer R, Roszkowski WF, Sanchez A and Beynen AC. 1989. Comparison of the hypocholesterolemic effects of dietary soybean protein with those of formaldehyde-treated casein in rabbits. *J. Nutr.* 119: 843–856.

West CE, Beynen AC, Lapré JA, Lovati MR and Sirtori CR. 1990. Mechanism of the differential hypercholesterolemic effect of dietary casein and fish protein. *Bull. Int. Dairy Fed.* 253: 34–43.

West RO and Hayes OB. 1968. Diet and serum cholesterol levels: A comparison between vegetarians in a Seventh Day Adventist group. *Am. J. Clin. Nutr.* 21: 853–862.

Westerterp KR. 1999. Nutritional implications of gender differences in metabolism: Energy metabolism, human studies. In Tarnopolsky M, Ed., *Gender Differences in Metabolism: Practical and Nutritional Implications*, CRC Press, Boca Raton, FL, pp. 249–264.

Whalley de CV, Rankin SM, Hoult JR, Jessup W and Leakes DS. 1990. Flavonoids inhibit the oxidative modification of low density lipoproteins by macrophages. *Biochem. Pharmacol.* 39: 1743–1750.

White PL. 1981. Once more with feeding. *J.A.M.A.* 246: 677–678.

Whitehead RG and Dean RFA. 1964a. Serum amino acids in kwashiorkor. I. Relationship to clinical condition. *Am. J. Clin. Nutr.* 14: 313–320.

Whitehead RG and Dean RFA. 1964b. Serum amino acids in kwashiorkor. II. An abbreviated method of estimation and its application. *Am. J. Clin. Nutr.* 14: 320–330.

Whitehead RG and Dean RFA. 1964c. The metabolism of amino acids in kwashiorkor. *E. Afr. Med. J.* 41: 581–583.

Whiting SJ and McNally ME. 1989. Calciuric effect of diets high in soy, beef or lactalbumin protein in the rat. *Nutr. Rep. Int.* 40: 199–205.

Whitten PL and Naftolin F. 1992. Effects of a phytoestrogen diet on estrogen-dependent reproductive processes in immature female rats. *Steroids* 57: 56–61.

Widhalm K. 1986. Effect of diet on serum lipid and lipoprotein in hyperlipoproteinic children. In Beynen AC, Ed., *Nutritional Effects on Cholesterol Metabolism.* Transmondial, Voorthuizen, Netherlands, 133–140.

Widhalm K. 1996. Treatment of hypercholesterolemia in children by diet using soy protein. In Second International Symposium on the Role of Soy in Preventing and Treating Chronic Disease, Brussels, Sept. 15–18, 1996, Abstract, pp. 23–24.

Widhalm K. 1998. Treatment of hypercholesterolemia in children by diet using soy protein. *Am. J. Clin. Nutr.* 68, (Suppl.): 1519S–1520S.

Widhalm K, Brazda G, Schneider B and Kohl S. 1993. Effect of soy protein diet versus standard low fat, low cholesterol diet on lipid and lipoprotein levels in children with familial or polygenic hypercholesterolemia. *J. Pediatr.* 123: 30–33.

Wiebe SL, Bruce WM and McDonald BE. 1984. A comparison of the effect of diets containing beef protein and plant proteins on blood lipids of healthy young men. *Am. J. Clin. Nutr.* 40: 982–989.

Wiener RP, Yoshida M and Harper AE. 1963. Influence of various carbohydrates on the utilization of low protein rations by the white rat. *J. Nutr.* 80: 279–290.

Wigand G. 1959. Production of hypercholesterolemia and atherosclerosis in rabbits by feeding different fats without supplementary cholesterol. *Acta Med. Scand.* 166 (Suppl.) 351: 1–91.

Wilcox EB, Galloway LS and Taylor F. 1964. Effect of protein, milk intake, and exercise on athletes. *J. Am. Diet. Assoc.* 44: 95–99.

Wilcox JN and Blumenthal BF. 1995. Thrombotic mechanisms in atherosclerosis: Potential impact of soy proteins. *J. Nutr.* 125: 631S–638S.

Wilcox LJ, DeDreu LE, Borradaile NM and Huff MW. 1999. The soy phytoestrogens, genistein and daidzein, decrease apolipoprotein B secretion by HepG$_2$ cells. *Circulation* 100 (Suppl. 1): Abstract 565.

Wilcox MR and Galloway LS. 1961. Serum and liver cholesterol, total lipids and lipid phosphorus levels of rats under various dietary regimes. *Am. J. Clin. Nutr.* 9: 326–243.

Wilgram GF and Hartroft WS. 1955. Pathogenesis of fatty and sclerotic lesions in the cardiovascular system of choline-deficient rats. *Br. J. Exp. Pathol.* 36: 298–305.

Wilgram GF, Best CH and Blumenstein J. 1955a. Aggravating effect of cholesterol on cardiovascular changes in choline-deficient rats. *Proc. Soc. Exp. Biol. Med.* 89: 476–479.

Wilgram GF, Lewis LA and Blumenschein J. 1955b. Lipoproteins in choline deficiency. *Circ. Res.* 3: 549–552.

Wilgram GF and Blumenstein J. 1956. Aetiology of cardiovascular disease in choline deficiency. *Fed. Proc.* 15: 384–385.

Wilgram GF, Lewis LA and Best CH. 1957. The effect of choline and cholesterol on lipoprotein patterns of rats. *Circ. Res.* 5: 111–114.

Williams CL, Bollella M, Spark A and Puder D. 1995. Soluble fiber enhances the hypocholesterolemic effect of the Step I diet in childhood. *J. Am. Coll. Nutr.* 14: 251–257.

Williams J, Lang D, Smith JA and Lewis MJ. 1993. Plasma-L-arginine levels in a rabbit model of hypercholesterolemia. *Biochem. Pharmacol.* 46: 2097–2099.

Williams JE, Hedrick HB, Tumbleson ME, Grebing SE, Miller SJ and Ellersieck MA. 1985. Effect of feeding cooked ground beef on serum lipid and lipoprotein bound cholesterol concentrations in male swine. *Nutr. Rep. Int.* 31: 165–180.

Williams JK, Geary R, Clarkson TB and Tumbelaka L. 1997. Effects of soy isoflavones on arterial pathobiology of postmenopausal monkeys. Symposium on Phytoestrogen Research Methods: Chemistry, Analysis, and Biological Properties, Tucson, AZ, Sept. 21–24, 1997, Abstract.

Williams JK and Clarkson TB. 1998. Dietary soy isoflavones inhibit *in vivo* constrictor responses of coronary arteries to collagen-induced platelet activation. *Coron. Artery Dis.* 9: 759–764.

Williams JN Jr. 1964. Response of the liver to prolonged protein depletion. IV. Protection of succinic oxidase and succinic deshydrogenase by dietary methionine and cystine in a protein-free ration. *J. Nutr.* 82: 51–60.

Williams JN Jr and Jasik AD. 1963. A marked anti-lipotropic action of methionine. *Nature* 200: 472.

Williams JN Jr and Hurlebaus AJ. 1965a. Response of the liver to prolonged protein depletion. V. Neutral glycerides and cholesterol; production of fatty livers by certain amino acids in a protein-free ration. *J. Nutr.* 85: 73–81.

Williams JN Jr and Hurlebaus AJ. 1965b. Response of the liver to prolonged protein depletion. VI. Total phospholipids and plasmalogens, and protection of phospholipids by methionine and cystine. *J. Nutr.* 85: 82–88.

Williams PT, Krauss RM, Kindel-Joyce S, Dreon DM, Vranizan KM and Wood PD. 1986. Relationship of dietary fat, protein, cholesterol, and fiber intake to atherogenic lipoproteins in men. *Am. J. Clin. Nutr.* 44: 788–797.

Wilson C, Larson M, Hassan A and Potter S. 1992. Cholesterol metabolism in rabbits as influenced by dietary casein: Whey ratios. *F.A.S.E.B. J.* 6: A1107, Abstract 993.

Wilson TA and Nicolosi RJ. 1997. The hypocholesterolemia and antiatherogenic effect of soy lecithin in hypercholesterolemic hamsters: beyond linoleate. *F.A.S.E.B. J.* 11: A152, Abstract 883.

Wilson TA, Behr SR and Nicolosi RJ. 1998a. Addition of guar gum and soy protein increases the efficacy of the American Heart Association (AHA). Step 1 cholesterol-lowering diet without reducing high density lipoprotein cholesterol levels in non human primates. *J. Nutr.* 128: 1429–1433.

Wilson TA, Meservey CM and Nicolosi RJ. 1998b. Soy lecithin reduces plasma lipoprotein cholesterol and early atherogenesis in hypercholesterolemic monkeys and hamsters: beyond linoleate. *Atherosclerosis* 140: 147–153.

Wiseman H, O'Reilly JD, Adlercreutz H, Mallet AI, Bowey EA, Rowland IR and Sanders TAB. 2000. Isoflavones phytoestrogens consumed in soy decreased F_2-isoprostane concentrations and increase resistance of low-density lipoprotein to oxidation in humans. *Am. J. Clin. Nutr.* 72: 395–400.

Wissler RW, Eilert ML, Schroeder MA and Cohen L. 1954. Production of lipomatous and atheromatous lesions in the albino rat. *Arch. Path.* 57: 333–351.

Wolf A, Zalpour C, Theilmeier G, Wang BY, Ma A, Anderson B, Tsao PS and Cooke JP. 1997. Dietary L-arginine supplementation normalize platelet aggregation in hypercholesterolemic humans. *J. Am. Coll. Cardiol.* 29: 479–485.

Wolfe BM. 1995. Potential role of raising dietary protein intake for reducing risk of atherosclerosis. *Can. J. Cardiol.* 11 (Suppl.): 127G–131G.

Wolfe BM, Giovanetti PM, Cheng DCH, Roberts DCK and Carroll KK. 1981. Hypolipidemic effect of substituting soybean protein isolate for all meat and dairy protein in the diets of hypercholesterolemic men. *Nutr. Rep. Int.* 24: 1187–1198.

Wolfe BM and Grace DM. 1984. Mechanism of hypolipidemic effect of soy protein in conscious fed baboons. *Clin. Invest. Med.* 1 (Suppl.) 2: 71.

Wolfe BM and Giovanetti PM. 1985. Elevation on VLDL-cholesterol during substitution of soy protein for animal protein in diets of hypercholesterolemic Canadians. *Nutr. Rep. Int.* 32: 1057–1065.

Wolfe BM and Grace DM. 1987. Substitution of mixed amino acids resembling soy protein for mixed amino acids resembling casein in the diet reduces plasma cholesterol in slowly, but not rapidly fed or not fasted baboons. *Metabolism* 36: 223–229.

Wolfe BM and Giovanetti PM. 1992. High protein diet complements resin therapy of familial hypercholesterolemia. *Clin. Invest. Med.* 15: 349–359.

Wolmarans P, Benadé AJS, Kotze TJ, Daubitzer AK, Marais MP and Laubscher R. 1991. Plasma lipoprotein response to substituting fish for red meat in the diet. *Am. J. Clin. Nutr.* 53: 1171–1176.

Wong WW, Hachey DL, Clarke LL and Zhang S. 1995. Cholesterol synthesis and absorption by ^2H_2O and ^{18}O-cholesterol and hypocholesterolemic effect of soy protein. *J. Nutr.* 125 (Suppl.): 612S–618S.

Wong WW, Hachey DL, O'Brian Smith E, Stuff JE, Heird WC and Pownall HJ. 1996. Mechanisms for the hypocholesterolemic effect of soy protein in normocholesterolemic and hypercholesterolemic men. Second International Symposium on the Role of Soy in Preventing and Treating Chronic Disease, Brussels, Sept. 15–18, 1996, Abstract, p. 25.

Wong WW, O'Brian Smith E, Stuff JE, Hachey DL, Heird WC and Pownall HJ. 1998. Cholesterol-lowering effect of soy protein in normocholesterolemic and hypercholesterolemic men. *Am. J. Clin. Nutr.* 68, (Suppl.): 1385S–1389S.

Woodward CJH and Carroll KK. 1985. Digestibilities of casein and soya bean protein in relation to their effects on serum cholesterol in rabbits. *Br. J. Nutr.* 54: 355–366.

World Health Organization. 1983. Primary Prevention of Essential Hypertension, Report of a WHO Scientific Group, 686, World Health Organization, Geneva.

Wright SM and Salter AM. 1993. The effect of dietary casein and soyprotein on cholesterol metabolism in hamsters. *Biochem. Soc. Trans.* 21: 155S.

Wright SM and Salter AM. 1998. Effects of soy protein on plasma cholesterol and bile acid excretion in hamsters. Comp. *Biochem. Physiol. B, Biochem. Mol. Biol.* 119: 247–254.

Wu G, Ruan C, Drouet L and Caen J. 1992. Inhibition effects of KDRS, a peptide derived from lactotransferrin, on platelet function and arterial thrombus formation in dogs. *Haemostasis* 22: 1–6.

Wu G and Morris SM Jr. 1998. Arginine metabolism: Nitric oxide and beyond. *Biochem. J.* 336: 1–17.

Wu G, Flynn NE, Flynn SP, Jolly CA and Davis PK. 1999. Dietary protein or arginine deficiency impairs constitutive and inducible nitric oxide synthesis by young rats. *J. Nutr.* 129: 1347–1354.

Xu CF, Boerwinkle E, Tikkanen MJ, Huttunen JK, Humphries SE and Talmud PJ. 1990. Genetic variation at the apolipoprotein gene loci contribute to response of plasma lipids to dietary change. *Genet. Epidemiol.* 7: 261–275.

Xu X, Wang HJ, Murphy PA, Cook L and Hendrich S. 1994. Daidzein is a more bioavailable in soymilk isolate than in genistein in adult women. *J. Nutr.* 123: 825–832.

Xu X, Harris KS, Wang HJ, Murphy PA and Hendrich S. 1995. Bioavailability of soybean isoflavones depends upon gut microflora in women. *J. Nutr.* 125: 2307–2315.

Xu X, Wang HJ, Murphy PA and Hendrich S. 2000. Neither background diet nor type of soy foods affects short-term isoflavone bioavailability in women. *J. Nutr.* 130: 798–801.

Yadav NR and Liener IE. 1977. Reduction of serum cholesterol in rats fed vegetable protein or an equivalent amino acid mixture. *Nutr. Rep. Int.* 16: 383–389.

Yagasaki K and Kamakata M. 1984. Apolipoprotein synthesis by the fatty liver of rats fed a low whole egg protein diet. *Nutr. Rep. Int.* 29: 533–540.

Yagasaki K, Okada K, Takagi K and Irirkura T. 1984. Effect of 4-(4'-chlorobenzyloxy)benzyl nicotinate (KCD–232) on cholesterol metabolism in rats fed on amino acid imbalanced diet. *Agri. Biol. Chem.* 48: 1417–1423.

Yagasaki K, Ohsawa N and Funabiki R. 1986a. Effects of dietary amino acids, and role of thyroid hormone in methionine-induced endogenous hypercholesterolemia. *Nutr. Rep. Int.* 33: 321–328.

Yagasaki K, Machida M and Funabiki R. 1986b. Effects of dietary methionine, cystine, and glycine on endogenous hypercholesterolemia in hepatoma-bearing rats. *J. Nutr. Sci. Vitaminol.* 32: 643–651.

Yagasaki K, Aoki T and Funabiki R. 1986c. Serum and liver responses to methionine and cystine in rats fed diets with different casein levels. *Nutr. Rep. Int.* 34: 59–66.

Yagasaki K and Funabiki R. 1990. Effects of dietary supplemented amino acids on endogenous hypercholesterolemia in rats. *J. Nutr. Sci. Vitaminol.* 36 (Suppl.): 165S–168S.

Yagasaki K, Machida-Takehana M and Funabiki R. 1990. Effects of dietary methionine and glycine on serum lipoprotein profiles and fecal sterol excretion in normal and hepatoma-bearing rats. *J. Nutr. Sci. Vitaminol.* 36: 45–54.

Yagasaki K, Ebara K, Jujisawa K, Kawasaki M, Miura Y and Funabiki R. 1994. Reduction of hypercholesterolemia and proteinuria in nephritic rats by low-meat-protein diets. *J. Nutr. Sci. Vitaminol.* 40: 583–591.

Yamabe H and Lovenberg W. 1974. Increased incorporation of 14C-lysine into vascular proteins of the spontaneously hypertensive rats. *Eur. J. Pharmacol.* 29: 109–116.

Yamakoshi J, Piskula MK, Izumi T, Tobe K, Saito M, Kataoka S, Obata A and Kihuchi M. 2000. Isoflavone aglycone-rich extract without soy protein attenuates atherosclerosis development in cholesterol-fed rabbits. *J. Nutr.* 130: 1887–1893.

Yamamoto M and Yamamura Y. 1971. Changes in cholesterol metabolism in the ageing rat. *Atherosclerosis* 13: 365–374.

Yamamoto N, Akino A and Takano T. 1994. Antihypertensive effect of the peptides derived from casein by an extracellular proteinase from *Lactobacillus helveticus* CP790. *J. Dairy Sci.* 77: 917–922.

Yamamoto S, Kina T, Yamagata N, Kokubu T, Shinjo S and Asato L. 1993. Favorable effects of egg white protein on lipid metabolism in rats and mice. *Nutr. Res.* 13: 1453–1457.

Yamamoto S, Yamamoto T, Chung HM, Wang MF, Shinjo S, Komatsu T. 1996. Anticholesterolemic effect of the undigested fraction of soybean protein. Second International Symposium on the Role of Soy in Preventing and Treating Chronic Disease, Brussels, Sept. 15–18, 1996, Abstract, p. 25.

Yamanaka Y, Tsuji K, Ichikawa T, Nakagawa Y and Kawamura M. 1985. Effect of dietary taurine on cholesterol gallstone formation and tissue cholesterol contents in mice. *J. Nutr. Sci. Vitaminol.* 31: 225–232.

Yamanaka Y, Tsuji K and Ichikawa T. 1986. Stimulation of chenodesoxycholic acid excretion in hypercholesterolemic mice by dietary taurine. *J. Nutr. Sci. Vitaminol.* 32: 287–296.

Yamashita J and Hayashi S. 1990. The effect of dietary protein source on plasma cholesterol level and fecal steroid excretion in obese mice. *J. Nutr. Sci. Vitaminol.* 36: 545–558.

Yamashita J, Yoshiko F, Kamimura M and Hayashi SI. 1990. Different effects of soy protein on cholesterol metabolism in rats and mice. In Beynen AC, Kritchevsky D and Pollack OJ, Eds., *Dietary Proteins, Cholesterol Metabolism and Atherosclerosis*, Monographs on Atherosclerosis, Vol. 16, S. Karger, Basel, pp. 36–43.

Yamashita T, Sasahara T, Pomeroy SE, Coollier G and Nestel PJ. 1998. Arterial compliance, blood pressure, plasma leptin and plasma lipids in women are improved with weight reduction equally with a meat-based diet and a plant-based diet. *Metabolism* 47: 1308–1314.

Yamauchi F and Suetsuna K. 1993. Immunological effects of dietary peptide derived from soya-bean protein. *J. Nutr. Biochem.* 4: 450–457.

Yamauchi-Takihara K, Azuma J and Kishimoto S. 1986. Taurine protection against experimental arterial calcinosis in mice. *Biochem. Biophys. Res. Commn.* 140: 679–683.

Yamori Y. 1981. Environmental influences on the development of hypertensive vascular diseases in *SHR* and related models, and their relation to human disease. In Worcel M, Bonvalet JP, Langer SZ, Menard J and Sassard J, Eds., *New Trends in Arterial Hypertension*, INSERM Symposium 17, Elsevier/North Holland, Amsterdam, pp. 305–320.

Yamori Y. 1989. Hypertension and biological dietary markers in urine and blood. A progress report from the CARDIAC Study Group. In Yamori Y and Strasser T, Eds., *New Horizons in Preventing Cardiovascular Diseases*, Elsevier, Amsterdam, pp. 111–126.

Yamori Y, Horie R, Akiguchi I, Ohtaka M, Nara Y and Fukase M. 1976a. New models of *Spontaneously Hypertensive* rats (SHR) for studies on stroke and atherogenesis. *Clin. Exp. Pharmacol. Physiol.* 3: 199–203.

Yamori Y, Nakada T and Lovenberg W. 1976b. Effect of antihypertensive therapy on lysine incorporation into vascular protein of the *Spontaneously Hypertensive* rats. *Eur. J. Pharmacol.* 38: 349–358.

Yamori Y, Horie R, Ikeda K, Nara Y and Lovenberg W. 1979a. Prophylactic effect of dietary protein on stroke and its mechanisms. In Yamori Y, Lovenberg W and Freis ED, Eds., *Perspectives in Cardiovascular Research*, Vol. 4: *Prophylactic Approach to Hypertensive Diseases*, Raven Press, New York, pp. 497–504.

Yamori Y, Tsunematsu T, Note S, Ishikawa S and Fukase M. 1979b. Nutritional improvement for stroke prevention. In Yamori Y, Lovenberg W and Fries S, Eds., *Perspectives in Cardiovascular Research*, Vol. 4: *Prophylactic Approach to Hypertensive Diseases*, Raven Press, New York, pp. 587–593.

Yamori Y, Nara Y, Kihara M, Horie R, Ooshima A, Iritani N and Fukuda E. 1980. Possible involvement of taurine in pathological cholesterol metabolism of arteriolipidosis prone rats. *Sulfur-Containing Amino Acids* 3: 107–113.

Yamori Y, Horie R, Nara Y, Ikeda M, Ooshima A and Fukase M. 1981a. Genetics of hypertensive diseases: Experimental studies on pathogenesis, detection of predisposition and prevention. *Adv. Nephrol.* 10: 51–74.

Yamori Y, Kihara M, Nara Y, Ohtaka H, Horie R, Tsunematsu T and Notes S. 1981b. Hypertension and diet: Multiple regression analysis in a Japanese farming community. *Lancet* 1: 1204–1205.

Yamori Y, Nara Y, Horie R, Ooshima A and Lovenberg W. 1981c. Pathophysiological role of taurine in blood pressure regulation in *Stroke-Prone Spontaneously Hypertensive* rats (SHR). In Shaffer S and Baskins S, Eds., *The Action of Taurine on Excitable Tissue*, Spectrum Press, New York, pp. 391–403.

Yamori Y, Horie R, Akiguchi I, Kihara M, Nara Y and Lovenberg W. 1982. Symptomological classification in the development of stroke in *Stroke-Prone Spontaneously Hypertensive* rats. *Jpn. Circ. J.* 46: 274–283.

Yamori Y, Horie R, Nara Y, Kihara M, Jujiwara K, Nabika T, Mano M and Ikeda K. 1984a. Nutritional causation and prevention of cardiovascular diseases. Experimental evidence in animal models and man. In Lovenberg W and Yamori Y, Eds., *Nutritional Prevention of Cardiovascular Disease*. Academic Press, Orlando, FL, pp. 37–51.

Yamori Y, Horie R, Tanase H, Fujiwara K, Nara Y and Lovenberg W. 1984b. Possible role of nutritional factors in the incidence of cerebral lesions in *Stroke-Prone Spontaneously Hypertensive* rats. *Hypertension* 6: 49–53.

Yamori Y, Horie R, Nara Y, Tagami M, Kihara M, Mano M and Ishino H. 1987. Pathogenesis and dietary prevention of cerebrovascular diseases in animal models and epidemiological evidence for the applicability in man. In Yamori Y and Lenfant C, Eds., *Prevention of Cardiovascular Diseases*, Elsevier, Amsterdam, pp. 163–177.

Yamori Y, Nara Y, Mizushima S, Mano M, Sawamura M, Kihara M and Horie R. 1992a. International cooperative study on the relationship between dietary factors and blood pressure: A preliminary report fron the cardiovascular diseases and alimentary comparison (CARDIAC) study. *Nutr. Health* 8: 77–90.

Yamori Y, Nara Y, Mizushima S, Murakami S, Ikeda K, Sawamura M, Nabika T and Horie R. 1992b. Gene environment interaction in hypertension, stroke and atherosclerosis in experimental models and supportive findings from a world-wide cross-sectional epidemiological survey: A WHO-CARDIAC study. *Clin. Exp. Pharmacol. Physiol.* 19: 43–52.

Yamori Y, Mizushima S, Ueda M, Sawamura M and Nara Y. 1994. Nutritional factors for hypertension and major cardiovascular diseases: International cooperative studies for dietary prevention. *Deutsche Med. Woch.* 15: 1825–1841.

Yamori Y, Nara Y, Ikeda K and Mizushima S. 1996. Is taurine a preventive nutritional factor of cardiovascular diseases or just a biological marker of nutrition? *Adv. Exp. Biol.* 403: 623–629.

Yan CC, Bravo E and Cantafora A. 1993. Effect of taurine levels on liver lipid metabolism: An *in vivo* study in the rat. *Proc. Soc. Exp. Biol. Med.* 202: 88–96.

Yanaura S and Sakamoto M. 1975. Influence of alfalfa meal on experimental hyperlipidemia. *Folia Pharmacol. Jpn.* 71: 387–383.

Yao Z and Vance DE. 1988. The active synthesis of phosphatidylcholine is required for very low density lipoprotein secretion from rat hepatocytes. *J. Biol. Chem.* 263: 2998–3004.

Yashiro A, Shinobu O and Sugano M. 1985. Hypocholesterolemic effect of soybean protein in rats and mice after peptic digestion. *J. Nutr.* 115: 1325–1336.

Yeh SJC and Léveillé GA. 1969. Effect of dietary protein on hepatic lipogenesis in the growing chick. *J. Nutr.* 98: 356–366.

Yeh SJC and Léveillé GA. 1972. Cholesterol and fatty acids synthesis in chick fed different levels of protein. *J. Nutr.* 102: 349–357.

Yeh SJC and Léveillé GA. 1973. Influence of dietary protein level on plasma cholesterol turnover and fecal steroid excretion in the chick. *J. Nutr.* 103: 407–411.

Yerushalmy J and Hilleboe HE. 1957. Fat in the diet and mortality from heart disease. A methodologic note. *N. Y. State J. Med.* 57: 2343–2354.

Yokogoshi H, Yasuda A, Quazi S and Yoshida A. 1985. Effect of the supplementation of sulfur amino acids to a diet containing soy protein isolate on lipid metabolism in rats. *Agric. Biol. Chem.* 49: 2865–2873.

Yokogoshi H, Mochizuki H, Nanami K, Hida Y, Miyachi F and Oda H. 1999. Dietary taurine enhances cholesterol degradation and reduces serum and liver cholesterol concentrations in rats fed a high-cholesterol diet. *J. Nutr.* 129: 1705–1712.

Yoshida A, Moritoki K and Noda K. 1966. Plasma lipids of rats with fatty liver owing to amino acid imbalances. *Eiyo to Shokuryo* 19: 291–296.

Yoshida K, Yashiro M and Ahiko K. 1988. Effects of addition of arginine, cystine, and glycine to the bovine milk-simulated amino acid mixture on the level of plasma and liver cholesterol in rats. *J. Nutr. Sci. Vitaminol.* 34: 567–576.

Yoshida A, Fukui H, Aoyama Y and Oda H. 1990a. Comparative studies on soy protein and rice protein for cholesterol metabolism in rats. *J. Nutr. Sci. Vitaminol.* 36 (Suppl.): 137S–139S.

Yoshida A, Aoyama Y, Oda H and Okumura Y. 1990b. Characteristic effect of soy and rice protein on cholesterol metabolism in rats. In Beynen AC, Kritchevsky D and Pollack OJ, Eds., *Dietary Proteins, Cholesterol Metabolism and Atherosclerosis*, Monographs on Atherosclerosis, Vol. 16, S. Karger, Basel, pp. 1–10.

Young VR. 1991. Soy protein in relation to human protein and amino acid nutrition. *J. Am. Diet. Assoc.* 91: 828–835.

Young VR, Wayler A, Garza C, Steinke FH, Murray E, Rand WM and Scrimshaw NS. 1984a. A long-metabolic balance study in young men to assess the nutritional quality of an isolated soy protein and beef proteins. *Am. J. Clin. Nutr.* 39: 8–15.

Young VR, Puig M, Queiroz E, Scrimshaw NS and Rand WM. 1984b. Evaluation of the protein quality of an isolated soy protein in young men: Relative nitrogen requirements and effect of methionine supplementation. *Am. J. Clin. Nutr.* 39: 16–24.

Yount NY, McNamara DJ, Al-Othman AA and Ley KY. 1990. The effect of copper deficiency on rat hepatic-hydroxy-methylglutaryl coenzyme A reductase activity. *J. Nutr. Biochem.* 1: 21–27.

Yu X, Li Y and Xiong Y. 1994. Increase of an endogenous inhibitor of nitric oxide synthesis in serum of high cholesterol fed rabbits. *Life Sci.* 54: 753–758.

Yuan YV and Kitts DD. 1993. Milk product and constituent protein effects on plasma and hepatic lipids and systolic blood pressure of normotensive rats. *Food Res. Int.* 26: 173–179.

Yudkin J. 1957. Diet and coronary thrombosis: Hypothesis and fact. *Lancet* 2: 155–162.

Zaki M, Niwa M, Wei LJ, Yamashiro K, Tsuchiyama H and Nawatari I. 1980. Effect of taurine on blood pressure and fat metabolism in experimental hypertension. *Sulfur-Containing Amino Acids* 3: 115–121.

Zambón D, Ros E, Casals E, Sanllehy C, Bertomeu A and Campero A. 1995. Effect of apolipoprotein E polymorphism on the serum lipid response to a hypolipidemic diet rich in monounsaturated fatty acids in patients with hypercholesterolemia and combined hyperlipidemia. *Am. J. Clin. Nutr.* 61: 141–148.

Zeiher AM, Drexler H, Wollschlaeger H and Just H. 1991. Modulation of coronary vasomotor tone in humans: Progressive endothelial dysfunction with different early stages of coronary atherosclerosis. *Circulation* 83: 391–401.

Zeisel SH. 1981. Dietary choline: biochemistry, physiology, and pharmacology. *Annu. Rev. Nutr.* 1: 95–121.

Zhang SH, Reddick RL, Piedrahita JA and Maeda N. 1992. Spontaneous hypercholesterolemia and arterial lesions in mice lacking apolipoprotein E. *Science* 258: 468–471.

Zhang X. 1992. Influence of Dietary Proteins on Cholesterol Metabolism and Nephrocalcinosis. Thesis, Utrecht University.

Zhang X and Beynen AC. 1990. Dietary fish proteins and cholesterol metabolism. In Beynen AC, Kritchevsky D and Pollack OJ, Eds., *Dietary Proteins, Cholesterol Metabolism and Atherosclerosis*, Monographs on Atherosclerosis, Vol. 16, S. Karger, Basel, pp. 148–152.

Zhang X and Beynen AC. 1993a. Influence of dietary fish proteins on plasma and liver cholesterol concentrations in rats. *Br. J. Nutr.* 69: 767–777.

Zhang X and Beynen AC. 1993b. Lowering effect of dietary milk-whey protein v. casein on plasma and liver cholesterol concentrations in rats. *Br. J. Nutr.* 70: 139–146.

Zhou B, Wu X, Tao SQ, Yang J, Cao TX, Zheng RP, Tian XZ, Lu CQ, Miao HY, Ye FH, Zhu LG, Zhu C, Jiang JP, He HQ, Ma F, Du FC and Bin W. 1989. Dietary patterns in 10 groups and the relationship with blood pressure. Collaborative Study Group for Cardiovascular Diseases and their Risk Factors. *Chin. Med. J.* 102: 257–261.

Zhou B, Zhang X, Zhu A, Zhao L, Zhu S, Ruan L, Zhu L and Liang S. 1994. The relationship of dietary animal protein and electrolytes to blood pressure: A study on three Chinese populations. *Int. J. Epidemiol.* 23: 716–722.

Zhu B, Sun Y, Sievers RE, Shuman JL, Glantz SA, Chatterjee K, Parmley WW and Wolfe CL. 1996. L-arginine decreases infarct size in rats exposed to environmental tobacco smoke. *Am. Heart J.* 132: 91–100.

Zicha J and Kunes J. 1999. Ontogenic aspects of hypertension development: Analysis in the rat. *Physiol. Rev.* 79: 1227–1282.

Zilversmith DB. 1973. A proposal linking atherogenesis to the interaction of endothelial lipoprotein lipase with triglyceride-rich lipoproteins. *Circulation* 33: 633–638.

Zommara M, Tachibana N, Sakono M, Suzuki Y, Oda T, Hashiba H and Imaizumi K. 1996. Whey from cultured skim milk decreases serum cholesterol and increases antioxidant enzymes in liver and red blood cells in rats. *Nutr. Res.* 16: 293–302.

Zuphten van LFM and Den Bieman MGCW. 1981. Cholesterol response in inbred strain of rats, *Rattus norvegicus. J. Nutr.* 111: 1833–1838.

Zuphten van LFM, Den Bieman MGCW, Hülsmann WC and Fox RR. 1981. Genetic and physiological aspects of cholesterol accumulation in hyperresponding and hyporesponding rabbits. *Lab. Anim.* 15: 61–67.

Amino Acid Index

ALANINE

Katan et al. 1982; Sautier et al. 1983; Sugiyama et al. 1989b, 1996; Atwal et al. 1997.

ARGININE

Jones 1964; Williams and Hurlebaus 1965a, 1965b; Jones et al. 1966; Harper et al. 1970; Palmer et al. 1975; Milner and Perkins 1978; Hermus and Dallingha-Thie 1979; Rettura et al. 1979; Milner 1979; Aoyama and Ashida 1979; Kritchevsky 1979; Czarnecky and Kritchevsky 1979; Kritchevsky 1980b; Huff and Carroll 1980a, 1980b; Barbul et al. 1980a, 1980b; Aoyama et al. 1981; Terpstra et al. 1981; Kovanen et al. 1981; Nagata 1981b; Kritchevsky et al. 1982a; Balogun et al. 1982; Katan et al. 1982; Sugano et al. 1982b; Oleeski et al. 1982; Gibney 1983; Chao et al. 1983; Schmeisser et al. 1983; West et al. 1983a; Sugano et al. 1984; Ryzhenkov et al. 1984; Sanchez et al. 1985; Kohls et al. 1985; Vahouny et al. 1985; Forsythe 1986; Jacques et al. 1986; Kohls et al. 1987; Radomski et al. 1987; Palmer et al. 1987, 1988; Thorne et al. 1988; Yoshida et al. 1988; Mizuno et al. 1988; Sanchez et al. 1988a, 1988b, 1988c; Schmidt et al. 1988; Sakuma et al. 1988; Vallance et al 1989; Tanaka and Sugano 1989b; Ignarro 1989a, 1989b; Sugiyama et al. 1989b; Jacques et al. 1990; Girerd et al. 1990; Kugiyama et al. 1990; De Schriver et al. 1990; Sanchez et al. 1990; Creager et al. 1990; Russel 1990; Nakaki et al. 1990; Mügge and Harrison 1991; Moncada et al. 1991; Rossitch et al. 1991; Lentz and Sadler 1991; Calver et al. 1991; Drexler et al. 1991b; Cooke et al. 1991, 1992; Cooke and Tsao 1992; Chin et al. 1992; Vallance et al. 1992b; Creager et al. 1992; Kuo et al. 1992; Hishikawa et al. 1992; Kuo et al. 1992; Kanno et al. 1992; Imaizumi et al. 1992; Jeserich et al. 1992; Sakuma et al. 1992; Horigome and Cho 1992; Williams et al. 1993; Ebel et al. 1993; Barbul 1993; Panza et al. 1993; Hishikawa et al. 1993; Baudoin et al. 1993; Bode-Böger et al. 1994; Nakaki and Kato 1994; Yu et al. 1994; Li et al. 1994; Jun and Wennmalm 1994; Casino et al. 1994; Wang et al. 1994; Tsao et al. 1994a; Singer et al. 1995; Engelman et al. 1995; Philis-Tsimikas and Witzum 1995; Kharitonov et al. 1995; MacAllister et al. 1995; Higashi et al. 1995; Carroll and Kurowska 1995; Adams et al. 1995; Otsuji et al. 1995; de Caterina et al. 1995; Pedrinelli et al. 1995; Böger et al. 1995, 1996a, 1996b; Bode-Böger et al. 1996b; Jeremy et al. 1996; Gryglewski et al. 1996; Slawinski et al. 1996; Chauhan et al. 1996; Matsuoka et al. 1996; Davies et al. 1996; Zhu et al. 1996; Chen et al. 1996; Garini et al. 1996; Kurowska and Carroll 1996; Clarkson et al. 1996; Adams et al. 1997a, 1997b; Böger et al. 1997; Campese et al. 1997; Wascher et al. 1997; Chowienczyk and Ritter 1997; Quyyumi et al. 1997, Adams et al. 1997a, 1997b, 1997c;

Lubec et al. 1997; Hutchinson et al. 1997; Atwal et al. 1997; Aji et al. 1997; Kayashita et al. 1997; Schwarzacher et al. 1997; Wolf et al. 1997; Giroux et al. 1998; Cooke 1998; de Lorgeril 1998; Maxwell and Cooke 1998; Wu and Morris 1998; Sumino et al. 1998; Wu et al. 1999; Campisi et al. 1999; Giroux et al. 1999a, 1999b; Ignarro et al. 1999; Mantha 1999; Penttinen et al. 2000; Oomen et al. 2000a; Kurowska 2001.

CYSTEINE AND CYSTINE

Mann et al. 1953; Fillios and Mann 1954; Okey and Lyman 1954, 1956, 1957; Mann 1960; Mann et al. 1960; Seidel et al. 1960; Léveillé and Sauberlich 1964; Williams 1964; Williams and Hurlebaus 1965a, 1965b; Morse et al. 1966; Guidotti et al. 1967; Burns and Self 1969; Harper et al. 1970; Feland et al. 1973; Itokawa et al. 1973; Jackson and Burns 1974; Aoyama et al. 1977; Myant and Mitropoulos 1977; Tateishi 1981; Nagata et al. 1981a; Rukaj and Sérougne 1983; Sautier et al. 1983; Sérougne and Rukaj 1983; Sérougne et al. 1984; Cho et al. 1984; Sugiyama et al. 1984, 1985b, 1986b; Oda et al. 1986; Yagasaki et al. 1986b, 1986c; Suberville 1987; Sérougne et al. 1987, 1988; Aoyama et al. 1988; Potter and Kies 1988; Mizuno et al. 1988; Yoshida et al. 1988; Tanaka and Sugano 1989a; Potter and Kies 1989b, 1990; Hagemeister et al. 1990; Yagasaki and Funabiki 1990; Sugiyama and Muramatsu 1990; Muramatsu and Sugiyama 1990; Aljawad et al. 1991; Aoyama et al. 1992a, 1992b; Tasker and Potter 1993; Fujisawa et al. 1994, 1995; Sérougne et al. 1995; Atwal et al. 1997; Aoyama et al. 1998.

ETHIONINE

Simpson et al. 1950; Farber et al. 1950; Feinberg et al. 1954; Furman et al. 1957; Seidel and Harper 1962, 1963.

GLUTAMIC ACID

Williams and Hurlebaus 1965a, 1965b; Bazzano 1969; Bazzano et al. 1970; Olson et al. 1970a, 1970b; Garlich et al. 1970; Bazzano et al. 1972; Sautier et al. 1983; Hinshaw et al. 1990; Spolarics et al. 1991.

GLYCINE

Bremer 1955, 1956; Herrmann 1959; Sjövall 1959; Harper et al. 1970; Benevenga and Harper 1970; Kerr 1972; Feland et al. 1973; Hermus and Dallinga-Thie 1979; Aust et al. 1980; Katan et al. 1982; Ryzhenkov et al. 1984; Sugiyama et al. 1985a, 1985b, 1986a, 1986b; Yagasaki et al. 1986b; Beynen and Lemmens 1987; Yoshida et al. 1988; Sanchez et al. 1988b; Tanaka and Sugano 1989a; Sugiyama et al. 1989a; Sanchez et al. 1990; Muramatsu and Sugiyama 1990; Yagasaki et al. 1990; Yagasaki and Funabiki 1990; Horigome and Cho 1992; Kurowska and Carroll 1993; Sugiyama et al. 1993, 1997; Morita et al. 1997; Atwal et al. 1997; Giroux et al. 1998, 1999a; Park et al. 1999.

L-HISTIDINE

Kerr et al. 1965; Williams and Hurlebaus 1965a, 1965b; Kerr et al. 1966; Harper et al. 1970; Geison and Waisman 1970; Gerber et al. 1971; Aoyama and Ashida 1972; Solomon and Geison 1978a, 1978b; Qurehsi et al. 1978; Harvey et al. 1981; Aoyama et al. 1983a; Nagaoka et al. 1985; Ohmura et al. 1986; Aoyama et al. 1991; Kurowska and Carroll 1993.

ISOLEUCINE

Williams and Hurlebaus 1965a, 1965b; Harper et al. 1970; Mahgoub and Abu-Jayyab 1984, 1987; Kurowska and Carroll 1993.

LEUCINE

Truswell 1964; Williams and Hurlebaus 1965a, 1965b; Harper et al. 1970; Kurowska and Carroll 1993; Maghoub and Abu-Jayyab 1984, 1987; Kurowska and Carroll 1994; Carroll and Kurowska 1995.

LYSINE

Singal et al. 1953; Sidransky and Baba 1960; Viviani et al. 1964; Weigensberg et al. 1964; Williams and Hurlebaus 1965a, 1965b; Kerr et al. 1965, 1966; Harper et al. 1970; McGregor 1971; Aoyama and Ashida 1972; Banerjee and Chakrabarti 1973; Yamabe and Lovenberg 1974; Jarowski and Pytelewski 1975; Yamori et al. 1976b; Kritchevsky 1979; Czarnecki and Kritchevsky 1979; Hevia et al. 1980a, 1980b; Hevia and Visek 1980; Park and Liepa 1982; Mokady and Liener 1982; Sugano et al. 1982b; Aoyama et al. 1983b; Kurup et al. 1983; Schmeisser et al. 1983; Mahgoub and Abu-Jayyab 1984; Kihara et al. 1984; Yamori et al. 1984b; Kohls et al. 1985; Vahouny et al. 1985; Nagaoka et al. 1985; Bassat and Mokady 1985; Sanchez et al. 1985; Mahgoub and Abu-Jayyab 1987; Kohls et al. 1987; Sanchez et al. 1988a, 1988c; Sugiyama et al. 1989b; Fernandez Ortega 1989; Ortega 1989; Lovenberg and Yamori 1990; Kurowska and Carroll 1992, 1993, 1994; Zhou et al. 1994; Carroll and Kurowska 1995; Kurowska and Carroll 1996; Aoyama et al. 1998; Giroux et al. 1998, 1999a, 1999b; Kurowska 2001.

LYSINE/ARGININE RATIO

Jones 1964; Weigensberg et al. 1964; Jones et al. 1966; Mokady and Einav 1978; Hermus and Dallingha-Thie 1979; Kritchevsky 1979; Czarnecki and Kritchevsky 1979; Jarrousse et al. 1980; Kritchevsky 1980b; Huff and Carroll 1980a, 1980b; Terpstra et al. 1981; Nagata et al. 1981b; Kritchevsky et al. 1982a; b; c; Sugano et al. 1982b; Katan et al. 1982; Mokady and Liener 1982; West et al. 1983a; Gibney 1983; Kritchevsky et al. 1984; Sugano et al. 1984; Vahouny et al. 1985; Jacques et al. 1986; Sanchez et al. 1988a, 1988b, 1988c; Tanaka and Sugano 1989b; Bergeron and Jacques 1989; Jacques et al. 1990; Sanchez et al. 1990; Hagemeister et al. 1990; de Schriver 1990; Horigome and Cho 1992; Chinellato et al. 1992; de Abreu and Millan 1994.

METHIONINE

Mann et al. 1953; Okey and Lyman 1954; Fillios and Mann 1954; Shapiro and Freedman 1955; Portman 1956; Jones et al. 1957; Okey and Lyman 1957; Roth and Milstein 1957; Harper 1958; Passananti et al. 1958; Seidel et al. 1960; de Groot 1960; Nath et al. 1961; Léveillé et al. 1962a; Seidel and Harper 1962, 1963; Klavins 1963; Williams and Jasik 1963; Bagchi et al. 1963; Williams 1964; Williams and Hurlebaus 1965a, 1965b; Morse et al. 1966; Yoshida et al. 1966; Hill 1966; Yoshida et al. 1966; McCully 1969; Harper et al. 1970; Benevenga and Harper 1970; Theuer and Sarrett 1970; Noda 1970, 1973; Aoyama et al. 1973; Carroll and Hamilton 1975; McCully and Wilson 1975; Hamilton and Carroll 1976; Krishnawamy and Rao 1977; Kim et al. 1978; Hermus and Dallinga-Thie 1979; Noda and Okita 1980; Neves et al. 1980; Tateishi 1981; Yamori et al. 1981c; Kato et al. 1982; Schaffer and Azuma 1982; Aoyama et al. 1983a, 1983b; Kurup et al. 1983; McKully 1983; Terpstra et al. 1983b; Mahgoub and Abu-Jayyab 1984; Yagasaki et al. 1984; Sugiyama et al. 1984, 1985a, 1985b; Murphy-Chutorian et al. 1985; Yokogoshi et al. 1985; Nagaoka et al. 1985; Oda et al. 1986; Yagasaki et al. 1986a, 1986b, 1986c; Sugiyama et al. 1986b, 1986c; Finkelstein and Martin 1986; Sugiyama and Muramatsu 1987; Muramatsu et al. 1987; Horie et al. 1987; Mahgoub and Abu-Jayyab 1987; Sugiyama et al. 1987, 1988; Fau et al. 1988; Mizuno et al. 1988; Potter and Kies 1988; Hennig and Chow 1988; Oda et al. 1989; Tanaka and Sugano 1989a; Hitomi and Yoshida 1989; Lynch and Strain 1989; Sugiyama et al. 1989b; Leclerc et al. 1989; Potter and Kies 1989b, 1990; Chiji et al. 1990; Toborek et al. 1990; Yagasaki and Funabiki 1990; Anderson et al. 1990; Yagasaki et al. 1990; Saeki et al. 1990; Muramatsu and Sugiyama 1990; Selvam and Ravichandran 1991; Chandrasiri 1991; Lentz and Sadler 1991; Aljawad et al. 1991; Oda et al. 1991; Horigome and Cho 1992; Kang et al. 1992; Kurowska and Carroll 1992, 1993; Satoh et al. 1993; Stamler et al. 1993; Tasker and Potter 1993; Kurowska and Carroll 1994; Ponzio de Azevedo et al. 1994; Hennig et al. 1994a; Guttormsen et al. 1994; Toborek and Hennig 1994; Wang et al. 1994; Yagasaki et al. 1994; Carroll and Kurowska 1995; Bostom et al. 1995; Moundras et al. 1995; Koyama 1995; Fujisawa et al. 1995; Auboiron et al. 1995; Toborek et al. 1995; Kurowska and Carroll 1996; Toborek and Hennig 1996; Matthias et al. 1996; Loscalzo 1996; Lentz et al. 1996; den Heijer et al. 1996; Verhoef et al. 1996; Sugiyama et al. 1996, 1997; Freyburger et al. 1997; Morita et al. 1997; Harpel 1997; Tawakol et al. 1997; Divine et al. 1998; Bellamy et al. 1998; Aoyama et al. 1998; de Jong et al. 1998; Giroux et al. 1998, 1999a, 1999b; Mann et al. 1999; Selhub 1999; Lambert et al. 1999; Constans et al. 1999; Stolzenberg-Solomon et al. 1999; Guthikonda and Haynes 1999; Gregory et al. 2000; Fukagawa et al. 2000; Mhrova et al. 2000; Mori and Hirayama 2000; Ward et al. 2000, 2001; Mochizuki et al. 2001.

PHENYLALANINE

Williams and Hurlebaus 1965a, 1965b; Harper et al. 1970; Aoyama and Ashida 1972; Mahgoub and Abu-Jayyab 1984; Nagaoka et al. 1985; Mahgoub and Abu-Jayyab 1987; Kurowska and Carroll 1993.

SERINE

Harper et al. 1970; Sugiyama et al. 1993; Stead et al. 2000.

TAURINE

Kato 1951; Mori and Takeuchi 1955; Minami 1955; Bremer 1955, 1956; Sjövall 1959; Herrmann 1959; Mann 1960; Mann et al. 1960; Seidel et al. 1960; Truswell et al. 1965; Gottfries et al. 1966; Guidotti et al. 1967; Becattini 1967; Jacobsen and Smith 1968; Burns and Self 1969; Harper et al. 1970; Nigro et al. 1971; Feland et al. 1973; Hamaguchi and Aoyagi 1974; de Rango and Del Corso 1974; Cagliarducci 1974; Jackson and Burns 1974; Lombardini 1975; Nara et al. 1978; Baskin and Finney 1979; Yamori et al. 1979a; Zaki et al. 1980; Kibe et al. 1980; Yamori et al. 1981c; Batta et al. 1982; Chao et al. 1983; Hardison and Grundy 1983; Strasberg et al. 1983; Tsuji et al. 1983; Nishimoto et al. 1983; Kohashi et al. 1983; Watkins et al. 1983; Usui et al. 1983; Sugiyama et al. 1984; Okamoto et al. 1984; Himeno et al. 1984; Azuma et al. 1984, 1985; Gaul et al. 1985; Yamanaka et al. 1985, 1986; Sugiyama et al. 1986c; Cantafora et al. 1986; Oda et al. 1986; Dlouha and McBroom 1986; Yamagauchi-Takihara et al. 1986; Horie et al. 1987; Pion 1987; Stephan et al. 1987; Awata et al. 1987; Bellentani et al. 1987a; b; Mizuno et al. 1988; Ogawa et al. 1988; Oda et al. 1989; Tanno et al. 1989; Ikeda et al. 1989; Sugiyama et al. 1989a; Pety et al. 1990; Muramatsu and Sugiyama 1990; Pety et al. 1990; Goodman and Shihabi 1990; Muramatsu and Sugiyama 1990; Cantafora et al. 1991; Novotny et al. 1991; Gandhi et al. 1992; Fox and Sturman 1992; Schaffer and Azuma 1992; Elizarowa et al. 1993; Yan et al. 1993; Cantafora et al. 1994; Kim et al. 1995; Huang and Rao 1995; Ogawa 1996; Nanami et al. 1996; Obinata et al. 1996; Mizushima et al. 1996; review in Yamori et al. 1996; Murakami et al. 1996a, 1996b; Mozaffari et al. 1997; Miyata et al. 1997; Mochizuki 1998a, 1998b, 1999a, 1999b; Park et al. 1998, 1999; Murakami et al. 1999; Yokogoshi et al. 1999; Schaffer et al. 2000; Mochizuki et al. 2001.

THREONINE

Singal et al. 1953; Viviani et al. 1964; Williams and Hurlebaus 1965a, 1965b; Harper et al. 1970; Aoyama and Ashida 1972; Bassat and Mokady 1985; Sugiyama et al. 1986b, 1989b; Hitomi and Yoshida 1989; Fukuda et al. 1990; Sidranski 1990; Yagasaki et al. 1994; Fujisawa et al. 1994; Aoyama et al. 1998.

TRYPTOPHAN

Williams and Hurlebaus 1965a, 1965b; Harper et al. 1970; Aoyama and Ashida 1972; Raja and Jarowski 1975; Sidranski 1976; Sved et al. 1979; Heron et al. 1980; Sved et al. 1982; Mahgoub and Abu-Jayyab 1984; Lovenberg 1984; Kohls et al. 1985; Fregly and Fater 1986; Mahgoub and Abu-Jayyab 1987; Fregly et al. 1987, 1988; Sidranski 1990; Lark et al. 1990; Mokady et al. 1990; Rogers and Pesti 1990; Nakaki et al. 1990; Aviram et al. 1991; Rogers and Pesti 1992; Engelberg 1992; Kurowska and Carroll 1993; Nakaki and Kato 1994; Baldo-Enzi et al. 1996.

TYROSINE

Williams and Hurlebaus 1965a, 1965b; Harper et al. 1970; Aoyama and Ashida 1972; Sved et al. 1979; Yamori et al. 1980; Sved et al. 1982; Sautier et al. 1983; Nagaoka et al. 1985; Jacques et al. 1988a, 1990; Nagaoka et al. 1990; Muramatsu and Sugiyama 1990; Kuchel 1998.

VALINE

Williams and Hurlebaus 1965a, 1965b; Harper et al. 1970; Kurowska and Carroll 1993; Sugiyama et al. 1996; Yagasaki et al. 1994.

Index